T0231250

ANNUAL PROGRESS IN CHILD PSYCHIATRY AND CHILD DEVELOPMENT 1986

ANNUAL PROGRESS IN CHILD PSYCHIATRY AND CHILD DEVELOPMENT 1986

Edited by

STELLA CHESS, M.D.

Professor of Child Psychiatry
New York University Medical Center

and

ALEXANDER THOMAS, M.D.

Professor of Psychiatry
New York University Medical Center

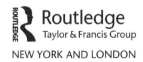

Routledge
Taylor & Francis Group

NEW YORK AND LONDON

Copyright © 1987 by BRUNNER/MAZEL, INC.

Published by Routledge

711 Third Avenue,

New York, NY 10017

All rights reserved. No part of this book may be reproduced by any process whatsoever without the written permission of the publisher.

Library of Congress Card No. 68-23452

ISBN 0-87630-437-4

ISSN 0066-4030

MANUFACTURED IN THE UNITED STATES OF AMERICA

Publisher's Note

The publisher has gone to great lengths to ensure the quality of this reprint but points out that some imperfections in the original may be apparent.

CONTENTS

ANNUAL PROGRESS IN
CHILD PSYCHIATRY AND
CHILD DEVELOPMENT
1986

Part I
INFANCY STUDIES

Research studies of the psychological capacities of the infant continue to produce fruitful findings that have both theoretical and practical significance.

The paper by Meltzoff represents a carefully designed and executed study of imitation by infants of their parents. The ability to imitate is one important modality of learning and also comprises a highly important element in the child's progressive ability to utilize parents and others as role models.

Meltzoff's finding that as early as 14 months of age infants are capable of imitating a specific act of the parent, not only immediately, but even 24 hours later, suggests that the capacity for memory is greater and appears earlier than previously thought. As the author indicates, this ability may play a significant role in learning and socialization in infancy. One cautionary note, with which we are sure the author will agree, is necessary: Meltzoff's findings of the infant's capacity for imitation should not be used as evidence that the influence of the parent as a role model in infancy remains basic and fixed throughout the child's subsequent development. Other influential figures in the child's life, as well as sociocultural factors, may serve to attenuate, modify, or intensify the influence of the parent as a role model as the child grows older.

The paper by Dunn, Plomin, and Nettles takes up a different issue of the parent-child relationship in infancy, but one that also bears significantly on the question of whether mothers behave consistently or differently toward their infant siblings. As the authors point out, previous reports by others have been contaminated by maternal observations and ratings when the siblings were of different ages. Many factors may influence the mother's behavior toward her children who are of different ages. Dunn and her coworkers avoided the problem by making their maternal observations and ratings when each of the two siblings was 12 months old. Their detailed ratings (by factor analysis) of the mother's behavior yielded three factors—affection, verbal attention, and control and restriction—three highly important elements in a mother's behavior toward her infant child. Their finding that the mothers varied widely in these behaviors, but that, whatever their pattern, they behaved very similarly toward their two siblings at the same age in infancy, is of interest for several reasons. We know that one-year-old siblings can vary significantly in temperament and other behavioral features, and yet here is evidence that this is not due to differential treatment by their mothers in the first year of life. It is, of course, possible that the mothers may vary in their treatment of their infants in some other important dimension, but this remains to be adequately demonstrated. It may be possible, on the other hand, as the authors suggest, that different treatment of the children by the parents becomes more evident and developmentally significant as the children grow older. The authors cite several references that suggest this possibility. We have also found evidence to this effect in our interviews in the New York Longitudinal Study with the mothers of temperamentally difficult children. In the first year interviews these mothers tended to give positive, affectionate descriptions of their children. In the second year their positive attitudes were expressed less enthusiastically. By the third year a number were ambivalent, with their positive statements admixed with negative and even hostile expressions of the stresses and problems their difficult children were imposing on them.

It is clear that the findings of Dunn and her coworkers provide important evidence in the debate in developmental psychology and child psychiatry over the extent of the mother's influence in the child's first year of life on his or her future developmental course. The mother-child relationship is of course a significant force in shaping the child's development. But if the mother treats her children the same in the first year, and yet the children are different from each other, then we have to ask how much of these differences in the infants is due to the mother's functioning.

PART I: INFANCY STUDIES

1

Immediate and Deferred Imitation in Fourteen- and Twenty-Four-Month-Old Infants

Andrew N. Meltzoff

University of Washington, Seattle

A laboratory procedure is developed that can be used to assess imitation in the second year of life. The procedure uses a blind scoring technique and incorporates control conditions to distinguish infant imitation from spontaneous production of the target behavior. The procedure is used in 2 experiments evaluating the imitation of a simple action with a novel toy. The experiments assess both immediate and deferred imitation in each of 2 age groups, 14-month-olds and 2-year-olds. The deferred imitation task involved a 24-hour delay between the modeling and response periods. There was strong evidence that 2-year-old infants could perform both the immediate and deferred imitation tasks, which was expected. The results also showed that 14-month-olds could succeed in both tasks. The discussion considers the implications of the deferred imitation results in light of current data and theorizing concerning representational capacities and long-term memory in infancy.

Reprinted with permission from *Child Development*, 1985, Vol. 56, 62-72. Copyright 1985 by the Society for Research in Child Development.

This research was supported by grants from NSF (BNS 8309224) and the MacArthur Foundation. I am greatly indebted to Craig R. Harris for assistance and insightful suggestions on all phases of this project. I also thank Laralee Jasper and Calle Fisher for their help. Patricia K. Kuhl and Alison Gopnik provided helpful comments on an earlier draft of this paper.

There is near-universal acceptance of the view that imitative processes play an important role in the early cognitive and social development of the child. There is also an increasing consensus that the developmental course of imitation in infancy needs further empirical investigation.

Recent laboratory studies have shown that young infants are more proficient imitators than had previously been thought. Meltzoff and Moore (1977, 1983a), Jacobson (1979), and Field, Woodson, Greenberg, and Cohen (1982) have reported that infants in the first month of life are capable of imitating facial gestures displayed by an adult experimenter. Discussion continues about what mechanism underlies this early behavior (Meltzoff, 1985; Meltzoff & Moore, 1983b, 1985; Uzgiris, 1979), but such findings suggest that revisions may be needed in the standard accounts of imitative development, which place the onset of such behavior at about 1 year of age. They also suggest that it may be profitable to reexamine the imitative abilities of older infants, particularly in the 1–2-year-old age range itself, where there have been relatively few controlled laboratory experiments.

The study of imitation in this older age range raises several interesting methodological issues. First, there is the problem of distinguishing imitation from spontaneous behaviors that may happen to match the target behavior. Most of the early studies of imitation in the second year did not include the controls necessary to make this distinction (Mehrabian & Williams, 1971; Paraskevopoulos & Hunt, 1971; Rodgon & Kurdek, 1977; Uzgiris, 1972; Uzgiris & Hunt, 1975).[1] In these studies, various models were presented and infants were scored according to whether or not they performed similar behaviors during a given response period. Imitation was inferred if the infant produced a behavior that matched the adult's. Imitation development was inferred if older infants produced more behavior matching the target than did younger infants.

Such designs do not provide unambiguous evidence from which to draw inferences about the existence of imitation and its development. First, they do not provide conclusive evidence for imitation, because control conditions were not used to assess the spontaneous production of the target behaviors in absence of exposure to the model. The demonstration of imitation requires more than showing that infants produce behaviors that match the adult target behaviors. It also requires that the

---

[1]These studies of imitation explored a broad range of infant skills and did not attempt to use strict, experimentally controlled procedures, perhaps out of necessity given their breadth.

infants' productions are above the spontaneous rate when the infants have not been exposed to the target behavior at all. Second, inferences about imitative development cannot unambiguously be drawn from data showing that older infants produce more of the target behavior than do younger infants. For some of the behaviors under study, it is possible that older infants have a higher spontaneous rate of the target behavior than do younger infants. Imitative development is not assessed simply by testing whether the rate of the target behavior increases as a function of age, but by testing whether there is a differential increase in the rate of the target behavior in modeling versus the control conditions as a function of age.

There are only a few studies of imitation in older infants that attempted to distinguish the spontaneous production of the target behavior from imitation by including control conditions to assess baseline rates (e.g., Abravanel, Levan-Goldschmidt, & Stevenson, 1976; Killen & Uzgiris, 1981; McCall, Parke, & Kavanaugh, 1977). The results from these laboratory experiments suggest that older infants are rather poor imitators, certainly poorer than the earlier, less well-controlled studies had suggested.

For example, Abravanel et al. tested for imitation of 22 items in infants up to 15 months old. The items were simple acts such as patting an object, shaking a bell, and squeezing a toy. The results showed imitation (i.e., significant differences between the modeling and nonmodeling conditions) for only eight of the 22 items. These results are much weaker than the classic views of infant imitation would have predicted (Piaget, 1962), given the simple tasks used and the age range tested. Likewise, when spontaneous rates were taken into account, the Killen and Uzgiris study was unable to find significant imitation of simple acts such as shaking or banging in infants less than 16 months of age (see their Table 2), although there was some suggestion of mimicking conventional actions such as drinking from a cup at younger ages. Similarly, McCall et al. reported rather poor imitative performance below 18 months.

There are, however, two reasons for caution in interpreting these laboratory experiments. First, the type of tasks and their sheer number (up to 22 items in a repeated-measures design) may have dampened infants' performance. Abravanel et al. and McCall et al. both noted that their experimental procedures may well have "perplexed" or "puzzled" the infants. Second, despite adding needed controls, these newer experimental studies retained some of the methodological shortcomings of the earlier work. Neither the stimulus presentations nor the response periods were of fixed duration. This opens the possibility that the experimenter could wait longer for an imitative response at the older ages, or on certain tasks, and thus obtain biased developmental or task efforts. Moreover, these experiments did not ensure that the scorer was kept uninformed about the experimental condition. The studies were video-taped (a potential improvement upon the earlier work using "live" scoring); however, the experimenter's behavior was visible on the videotape, and thus scorers were still informed about the behavior shown to the infants. A rigorous test of infant imitation requires that the infant's behavior be scored by an observer who is uninformed about the experimental condition.

Most recent studies of infant imitation have focused on tasks in which the infant is allowed to copy what he sees with no temporal delay. From the point of view of both social and cognitive development, it is also interesting to investigate the development of infants' ability to imitate after a delay. Imitative processes can play only a limited role in early socialization and learning as long as the infant is limited to copying the adult actions immediately after witnessing them and cannot yet duplicate actions that have been absent from the perceptual field for some time. A common age estimate for the onset of deferred imitation is about 18–24 months (McCall et al., 1977), and it has been suggested that infants below this age may lack the perceptual-cognitive sophistication, in terms of long-term recall memory and representational capacities, to succeed on such tasks (Flavell, 1977; McCall et al., 1977).

Despite its relevance for social- and cognitive-developmental theory, deferred imitation has not been the focus of much experimental work. The only laboratory experiment focused on deferred imitation was the McCall et al. study, which contained the methodological shortcomings noted earlier. The study demonstrated deferred imitation, but was conducted with 2-year-olds, an age at which most theorists and observers would expect such behavior. What was left untested was whether the ability to perform deferred imitation first emerged at about 18–24 months, as McCall et al. and others have argued, or whether even younger infants can also succeed on such tasks.

There were three goals of the present studies: *(a)* to develop a methodologically sound test of imitation in the second year of life by using blind scoring techniques and incorporating control conditions to distinguish true imitation from spontaneous behavior emitted without exposure to the model; *(b)* to test for the existence of immediate and deferred imitation in 2-year-old infants, an age at which most theorists would predict both to occur; *(c)* to assess immediate and deferred imitation in 14-month-old infants. A demonstration of deferred imitation under strict laboratory-controlled conditions in infants younger than the 18–24 month age range would provide new data bearing on imitative development, memory, and representation in infancy.

STUDY 1

Method

Subjects. The subjects were 60 normal 2-year-old infants. The mean age at the time of first test was 104.8 weeks (SD = .56, range = 103.6–105.4). The mean birth weight was 8.0 pounds (SD = .98, range = 5.8–9.8). All the subjects were full-term (over 37 weeks gestation and 5.5 pounds at birth) according to maternal report. There were equal numbers of males and females. An additional five subjects were eliminated from the study: four for not returning for the second visit and one for refusing to touch the test object. These eliminations were distributed approximately equally across test conditions.

Test environment and apparatus. The test room (3.2 × 2.1 m) was unfurnished except for the test equipment. The parent and experimenter faced each other across a small (1.2 × .60 m) black table, with the infants on their parents' laps. A camera to the left (10m) of the experimenter was focused to include the infant's torso, head, and most of the tabletop. The experiment was electronically timed by a character generator that mixed the elapsed time in .10-sec increments onto the videotapes. Friends and family observed the test session through a one-way mirror in an adjacent room.

Stimulus. The object used during the experiment was a specially constructed, unfamiliar toy that could be pulled apart and put back together again. It consisted of two plain wooden squares (2.5 × 2.5 cm), each with a 7.5-cm length of rigid tubing extending from it. The plastic tubing attached to one square was 1.3 cm in diameter; the tubing attached to the other was slightly smaller, .95 cm in diameter. It was thus possible for one piece to fit inside the other. When the test object was placed on the table it gave the appearance of a solid, one-piece, dumbbell-shaped toy consisting of two wooden squares with a gray plastic tube attaching them. The object could be pulled apart by grasping the two wooden cubes and exerting an outward force of 4.91 kg·m/s². The object was constructed to meet these specifications because pilot studies indicated that infants under 2 years old could pull it apart, but that it fit together snugly enough to prevent it from falling apart accidentally if banged.

Procedure. Each subject and parent was escorted to a reception room.

For approximately 10 min the infant was allowed to explore the room, while the male experimenter described the test procedure to the parent. Next, the infant and parent were brought to the test room and the infant given approximately 2 more minutes to acclimate to that environment, while the experimenter handed the infant a series of small rubber warm-up toys to explore. Once the infant seemed comfortable, the experiment began.

Each infant was randomly assigned to one of the two groups according to whether he or she was to partake in the "immediate" ($N = 30$) or "deferred" ($N = 30$) test. Within each group, infants were randomly assigned to one of three test conditions such that there were 10 infants in each, including equal numbers of males and females. The three conditions were the baseline control, the activity control, and the imitation test.

In the imitation condition the experimenter brought the toy up from below the table to about the center of his chest. Once the infant fixated the toy, the experimenter pulled it apart with a very definite movement. He then reassembled it and repeated the act, pulling it apart in the same way two more times. This stimulus presentation period lasted for 20 sec. The toy was then lowered below the table edge and immediately brought back into view and placed on a spot 17 cm away and directly in front of the infant. A 20-sec response period was then timed, starting from when the infant touched the object. During this response period, the experimenter fixated the spot where he had placed the toy, assumed a relaxed facial pose, and said nothing, regardless of the infant's response.

In the baseline condition, the toy was simply brought up from below the table and placed on the same spot in front of the infant. As before, a 20-sec response period was timed from when the infant first touched the object, and the experimenter again fixated a spot on the table.

It can be argued that the baseline condition alone is not a sufficient control for assessing imitation. Infants who see the experimenter pick up and play with the toy may be especially interested in the object and promoted to engage in nonspecific manipulations of it. Such nonspecific manipulations might lead infants to discover by chance that the toy can be pulled apart, thus yielding significantly more of the target behavior (toy pulling) in the modeling condition versus the baseline condition. A more rigorous test of imitation would be to include a control condition in which the experimenter performs a second behavior with the same toy at approximately the same rate of movement. If the infant pulls the object apart significantly more often after seeing the pull-apart demonstration than after seeing the experimenter perform this control action, then one can be more secure in inferring imitation.

This was the procedure followed in the activity-control condition. The experimenter brought the toy up from below the table to about chest height in the identical way as before. When the infant fixated the object, it was moved in a circle and returned to the starting point. The experimenter then paused before repeating the action two more times. The diameter of the circle traced by the object was the same as the linear movement used in pulling apart the toy in the imitation condition (42 cm). The timing of the three demonstrations was kept the same as the imitation condition, and the entire stimulus-presentation period again lasted 20 sec. After this, the toy was briefly lowered beneath the table and then placed on a spot 17 cm away and directly in front of the infant. The 20-sec response period was then timed.

The same three test conditions were used to assess imitation in the "deferred" group. The only difference in procedure was that a 24-hour delay was interposed between the modeling and the response periods (delay range = 24.0–24.5 hours). In the imitation condition, the infants were given the warm-up procedure, shown the pulling movement, and then sent home until the next day. In the activity-control condition, the infants were given the warm-up, shown the circle movement, and sent home. In the baseline condition, the infants simply came into the experimental room, went through the warm-up, and then were sent home. The test on day 2 was identical for all three conditions. The experimenter brought the toy up from below the table, placed it on the spot in front of the child, and timed the 20-sec response period identically as before.

Scoring. The videotapes shown to the scorer did not contain any record of the experimental condition. The scorer was shown 60 20-sec response periods in a random order, all of which started when the infant first touched the toy. The scorer used paper and pencil to record whether or not the infant pulled apart the object, and if so, the latency to pull. The toy was scored as having been pulled apart the moment that the two halves of it were visibly separated. Intra- and interobserver agreement was assessed by having all 60 periods scored twice by one scorer and once by a second, independent scorer. For the dichotomous judgment of whether or not the infant pulled apart the toy in a given response period, there was 100% agreement for both the intra- and the interobserver assessments. The intra- and the interobserver agreements for the latency measures were both .99, as measured by Pearson correlations. The largest disagreement in the latency-to-pull measure was .10 sec.

Results and Discussion

Preliminary analyses revealed that there were no sex differences in the number of subjects who pulled apart the object ($p > .50$). Nor were there any significant differences between the proportion of infants pulling apart the toy in the baseline versus activity control conditions ($p > .50$). The data were therefore collapsed across these factors for subsequent analyses.

The results clearly support the hypothesis that the subjects were imitating. The number of subjects who produced the target behavior as a function of experimental condition is displayed in Table 1. Collapsing across delay and considering all 60 subjects together, infants were over three times as likely to produce the target behavior after it was modeled (75%) than in the control condition (23%), $\chi^2(1) = 13.20$, $p < .001$. As expected, the results from the immediate group alone provide the strongest evidence for imitation. For that group, 80% of the infants exposed to the model produced the target behavior, as compared to 20% in the control condition, $\chi^2(1) = 7.66$, $p < .01$. However, there was also evidence for deferred imitation. After the 24-hour delay, 70% of the subjects matched the target, as compared to only 25% in the control condition, $\chi^2(1) = 3.91$, $p < .05$. There was no significant reduction in imitation for the deferred versus immediate test groups. This can be seen by inspection and is shown statistically by a chi-square test for homogeneity (Fleiss, 1981), which reveals no significant difference ($p > .50$) between the two chi-square tables just reported.

The latency scores for all those infants who produced the target behavior were also analyzed using a two-way ANOVA, examining the ef-

TABLE 1

PERCENTAGE OF 24-MONTH-OLDS PRODUCING THE TARGET BEHAVIOR IN THE
IMMEDIATE- AND DEFERRED-IMITATION TESTS

| | CONDITION | | | | |
| | Imitation | | Controls | | |
TEST TYPE	%	N	%	N	χ^2
Immediate	80	10	20	20	7.66**
Deferred	70	10	25	20	3.91*

*$p < .05$.
**$p < .01$.

fects of test condition (control vs. imitation) and delay (immediate vs. deferred). There was a significant main effect for test condition, $F(1,20)$ = 24.70, $p < .001$, indicating that the infants in the imitation condition were faster to produce the target behavior than those in the control condition. The mean latency in the imitation condition was 2.00 sec (SD = 2.32), as compared to 9.53 (SD = 4.92) in the control condition. There was no main effect of delay ($p > .50$) and no delay × test condition interaction ($p > .50$).[2]

This experiment shows that 2-year-olds can imitate a simple action with an unfamiliar toy. The data provide evidence not only for immediate imitation but also for deferred imitation, when infants are forced to delay their imitation of a display for 24 hours after it was perceived. The long delay did little to dampen the imitation effect. Infants were as likely to imitate after a 24-hour delay as they were immediately. A second study was therefore undertaken to determine whether younger infants, 14-month-olds, could also succeed on these imitation tasks. According to some theorists (McCall et al., 1977), the 14-month-old group should succeed on the immediate imitation task but fail on the deferred task.

---

[2]The results demonstrate imitation of toy pulling. It might also be noted that a second act was shown to infants as part of the "activity control" condition, namely, holding the toy with both hands and moving it in a circle. Infants were not observed to perform full and precise circling movements in response. However, some infants seemed to mimic aspects of the modeled behavior by making small twirling or twisting motions with the toy after observing this movement. The morphology of these reactions varied across infants, which made behavioral scoring difficult. However, we sought to substantiate our impressions by using a forced-choice "perceptual judgment" scoring procedure (Meltzoff & Moore, 1983b). On the basis of watching the videotape of the 20-sec response period, a scorer who was blind to the test conditions made a forced-choice judgment as to which of the two control conditions an infant was in (baseline or circle-movement). The scorer also wrote down the basis of the judgment. The results supported our initial observations: There was evidence that the scorer could distinguish the infants' reactions in the two control conditions (65% correct; $p < .05$, binomial test, one-tailed), and inspection of the scorer's written record showed that there were more observations of twisting, twirling, rolling, and other directed manipulatory activity in the activity-control than the baseline condition. This underscores our basic idea that the activity control was useful to incorporate when testing for the imitation of the toy-pulling act, because in that condition the infants were prompted to manipulate the toy. It also lends support to the notion that infants will sometimes mimic certain features of a display even without duplicating it precisely. The manner in which motor constraints and other factors interact to influence whether infants try to imitate at all, and when they do what features of the display they choose to duplicate, is an interesting topic that must be left for future studies.

STUDY 2

Method

The test environment, stimulus, and procedure were identical to those already described. The subjects were 120 14-month-olds. Half were randomly assigned to the immediate and half to the deferred group (delay range = 24.0–25.5 hours). The mean age at the time of the first test was 60.8 weeks (SD = .62, range = 59.7–61.9). The mean birth weight was 7.8 pounds (SD = 1.0, range = 5.9–9.8). All subjects were full-term according to maternal report.

Within both the immediate and deferred groups, there were three test conditions, as previously described, with equal numbers of males and females in each test condition. Fourteen additional subjects were eliminated from the study, three for excessive fussing, eight for refusal to pick up the toy, and three for not returning for the second visit. These eliminations were distributed approximately equally across test conditions. The scoring was done exactly as described in Study 1. There was 100% intra- and interobserver agreement for the dichotomous judgment of whether or not the target behavior was produced in a given response period. Intra- and interobserver Pearson r's for the latency were, respectively, .98 and .99.

Results and Discussion

Preliminary analyses revealed no differences in the production of the target behavior as a function of sex of the subjects ($p > .20$) or for the baseline versus activity-control conditions ($p > .50$). Therefore, in subsequent analyses the data were collapsed across these factors.

The results provide strong evidence for imitation. Considering all 120 subjects, infants were over four times as likely to produce the target behavior after seeing it modeled (60%) than they were in the control condition (14%), $\chi^2(1) = 25.42$, $p < .001$. As predicted, there were significant results in the immediate imitation group alone, $\chi^2(1) = 14.81$, $p < .001$. Table 2 shows that about 75% of the infants produced the target behavior after seeing it modeled, as compared to 20% of the controls. There were also significant results in the deferred imitation group, $\chi^2(1) = 9.49$, $p < .01$. After the 24-hour delay, 45% of the infants in the imitation condition produced the target behavior, as compared to 7.5% of the controls. There was no significant difference in the strength of the imitation effect in the immediate versus deferred groups,

TABLE 2

PERCENTAGE OF 14-MONTH-OLDS PRODUCING THE TARGET BEHAVIOR IN THE
IMMEDIATE- AND DEFERRED-IMITATION TESTS

	CONDITION				
	Imitation		Controls		
TEST TYPE	%	N	%	N	χ^2
Immediate	75	20	20	40	14.81***
Deferred	45	20	7.5	40	9.49**

**$p < .01$.
***$p < .001$.

as revealed by a chi-square test for homogeneity comparing the two chi-square tables just reported ($p > .50$).

The latency scores for subjects producing the target behavior were analyzed using a two-way ANOVA examining test condition (control vs. imitation) and delay (immediate vs. deferred). There was a significant main effect of test condition, $F(1,31) = 19.17$, $p < .001$. The infants in the imitation condition were faster to produce the target behavior. The mean latency in the imitation condition was 4.02 sec (SD = 3.58), as compared to 9.83 sec (SD = 5.06) in the control. There was no main effect of delay ($p > .30$). The test condition × delay interaction could not be validly assessed due to the small number of subjects producing the target behavior in one of the cells. (In the control condition in the deferred test, only three infants pulled the toy apart.)

The power of the modeling on the infants' subsequent behavior is best illustrated by combining the results from the two studies. Figure 1 shows that over both studies ($N = 180$), 65% of the infants in the imitation condition produced the target behavior, in contrast to only 17% in the control condition. Moreover, it depicts the remarkable speed with which this imitative behavior was produced. As shown, the probability of infants spontaneously producing the target behavior within the first 5 sec of the response period in the control condition was near zero; it simply was not a high probability event if infants were not shown the behavior. Yet 52% of the infants in the imitation condition produced it. Indeed, in the imitation condition, most (79%) of the infants who produced the target behavior did so within 5 sec of first touching the toy.

This captures what one sees in testing the infants. The infants go directly to reproducing the behavior themselves without much fumbling with the novel object. Even the younger infants do this, and they do so

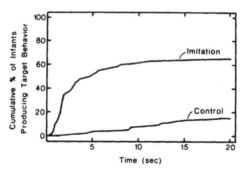

FIG. 1.—Cumulative percentage of infants in the imitation ($N = 60$) and control ($N = 120$) conditions producing the target behavior as a function of time.

even in the deferred imitation task. (The mean latency to pull for the young infants after the 24-hour delay was only 5.02 sec.) The infants reached out to the toy and pulled it apart without engaging in exploratory manipulations before imitating. Evidently a short demonstration with an unfamiliar toy has profound influence on the subsequent actions of infants for as long as 24 hours later. Moreover, even the 14-month-old infants need not reconstruct what they saw through trial and error, but can remember it well enough to duplicate the act immediately.

GENERAL DISCUSSION

These experiments demonstrate that 14- and 24-month-olds can imitate a simple action with an unfamiliar object, both immediately and after a 24-hour delay. They provide the first experimental demonstration that infants as young as 14 months old are capable of performing deferred imitation. The results have implications both for the design of imitation experiments and for theories of infant memory and representational development.

Design Implications

The present studies developed a rigorous test procedure for assessing imitation in the second year. The design improved upon previous research by using blind scoring techniques and incorporating controls to distinguish between imitation and spontaneous production of the target response. Two types of controls were used. The first was a baseline control in which infants were simply given the test object to manipulate without any prior exposure to it. In the second control condition, the experimenter used the test object to demonstrate a different movement from the target behavior but at approximately the same rate. These controls were introduced to help distinguish true imitation from the spontaneous production of the target behavior that would occur even in the absence of seeing the model.

The pattern of results illustrates the importance of including these controls when assessing imitation. For the 14-month-olds in the deferred imitation condition, 45% produced the target behavior after the 24-hour delay. Is this sufficient evidence for deferred imitation? In order to answer this question, we need to know how many infants would be expected to produce this behavior spontaneously, without seeing the adult demonstration. The control conditions show that infants are very unlikely to produce the target behavior on their own, without previous exposure to the demonstration. Only 7.5% of them did so. The comparison of the controls versus the imitation conditions is significant and thus permits the inference of deferred imitation within the 14-month-old group. The results allow us to conclude that the infants were basing their behavior on the perception of the modeled action—that it was not a chance event or one occurring simply because infants had previously seen the experimenter handling the test object.[3]

While 45% of the younger group produced the target behavior after the delay, 70% of the older group did so. If we had not included the control groups, these data might be taken for a developmental change in imitative capacities per se. However, the experiment shows that this inference cannot legitimately be drawn, because the controls showed comparable increases in the production of the target behavior as a function of age. In the control condition after the delay, only 7.5% of the younger infants produced the target behavior, whereas fully 25% of the older infants did so. Evidently, the younger infants simply had a lower probability of producing the target behavior after a delay than did the older infants, and this held true regardless of whether or not the infant saw the target behavior demonstrated.

From the point of view of *imitation*, the critical point is not that more

---

[3]The findings show that 14-month-olds are capable of performing deferred imitation, at least of this particular action under the conditions of this test. It is a matter for further research to determine whether or not there are interesting restrictions on the type of actions that can be so imitated or on the length of delay that young infants can tolerate before this behavior is disrupted. Such tests would, of course, need to be conducted using the controls outlined in the text.

of the older infants produced the target behavior in the imitation condition than did the younger infants, but that the older infants were about three times more likely to produce the target behavior in the imitation than in the control condition (70% vs. 25%), and the younger infants were six times more likely to do so (45% vs. 7.5%). Each age group thus demonstrated significant deferred imitation (more of the target behavior in the imitation than in the age-matched control condition, as shown in the bottom rows of Tables 1 and 2). Moreover, a chi-square test for homogeneity (Fleiss, 1981) reveals no significant difference between the deferred imitation results at 24 months (70% vs. 25%) and 14 months (45% vs. 7.5%).

The foregoing discussion shows that development may sometimes result in changes in infants' tendencies to produce the target behavior (in both the imitative or control conditions), but not necessarily in imitative capabilities per se. This point was confounded in many previous studies, which did not include controls to assess the rate of spontaneous production. The present results do not, of course, permit the inference that there is *no* developmental change in infants' imitative abilities. Rather, they underscore the need to separate changes in imitation per se from changes in the proclivity to perform the target action in the absence of exposure to the model.[4]

Given the current findings of both immediate and deferred imitation in both age groups, one might also ask why some previous laboratory studies reported weaker statistical effects at these and older ages than did the present study. In previous studies, infants have been given a long list of imitative tasks to perform in a repeated-measures design. For example, Abravanel et al. presented infants with up to 22 items in a single test session, including bell ringing, hand clapping, and spoon stirring. On some trials the natural sounds associated with these actions (e.g., the ringing of the bell) were eliminated. Our pilot studies indicated that such procedures were poor elicitors of imitation. The infants often became engaged in other problems, such as why a noise-making bell was now being shaken without any resulting noise. They also tended to persist in imitating what they had just done. For these reasons, the present

---

[4]There may be many reasons, aside from ones having to do with imitation per se, why the younger infants in the delay condition had an overall lower tendency to produce the target behavior (in both the imitation and control conditions). For example, these infants seemed particularly apt to reach out and offer the toy to the experimenter on day 2. This attempt at reestablishing social contact with the experimenter they had briefly seen the day before may have dampened their tendency to produce the target behavior. Again this underscores the need for the control conditions outlined in the text.

experiments required infants to imitate one action with an unfamiliar toy that they could have no preconceptions about. When the theoretical debate revolves around infants' underlying imitative capacities, such as whether infants of a certain age have the ability to delay their imitation until a later point in time, it may be judicious to design studies with a small number of carefully chosen test items.

Implications for Infant Memory

Developmental theorists have found it useful to retain some distinction between recognition and recall memory (Flavell, 1977). Much recent work in the infant cognition literature has focused on recognition memory. The present studies complement this literature by providing a useful technique for assessing infant recall memory.

Using habituation and paired-comparison test procedures, developmentalists have evaluated the impact of several factors on subsequent recognition memory: familiarization period (Fagan, 1974), delay interval (Cornell, 1979; Fagan, 1973; Pancratz & Cohen, 1970), interference (Cohen, DeLoache, & Pearl, 1977), stimulus characteristics (Caron & Caron, 1969; Fagan, 1972), and age (Fantz, 1964; Wetherford & Cohen, 1973). The picture that has emerged from these studies is that infant visual *recognition* memory is extremely robust, with the absence of recognition being more of the exception than the rule, even after significant delays (Cohen & Gelber, 1975; Fagan, 1977; Olson, 1976). The work on *recall* memory, however, has been much more meager. Interesting hypotheses about the late development of this capacity remain largely untested. Although recognition memory has been postulated to be a primitive capacity, the ability to recall objects or events in their absence has been postulated to be a sensitive index of developmental level (Flavell, 1977; Kagan, Kearsley, & Zelazo, 1978; Piaget, 1952, 1954; Sophian, 1980).

One way to demonstrate that infants recall something that is now absent is through object-permanence tasks. Some investigators have systematically varied the interval between the occlusion of the object and the beginning of search in an attempt to assess recall memory. Most of the results to date are compatible with the theoretically based notion that recall memory is a fragile and late-developing capacity in infants. For example, Gratch, Appel, Evans, LeCompte, and Wright (1974) reported that 9-month-olds successfully recovered a hidden object when allowed to search after no delay, but that search fell to chance when delays as short as 1–7 sec were introduced. Using a related object-hiding procedure, Webb, Massar, and Nadolny (1972) reported that 14-month-olds could not tolerate a delay of more than 10 sec. DeLoache (1980) recently suggested that more favorable estimates might be obtained from more naturalistic research with familiar objects being hidden in a home environment, and her observations suggest that by 18–30 months old, at least, infants can demonstrate some recall after an overnight delay.

The present studies provide a different and complementary test procedure that can be used to investigate aspects of infant recall memory. In the deferred imitation task, infants are shown a certain action and then a delay is interposed before the response is allowed. In order to reproduce the now-absent action, the infant must access an internal representation to guide his or her present behavior. If infants accurately reproduce the action, it indicates that they can do more than simply recognize that the current scene is related to the old one. It illustrates that they can recall or "reconstruct" what they have seen. Thus deferred imitation can be used to tap some form of recall memory in preverbal infants (Kagan, 1981; Meltzoff, 1981, 1985; Piaget, 1962; Watson, in press; Werner & Perlmutter, 1979).

The present studies demonstrated deferred imitation in 14-month-old infants after delays as long as 24 hours. The test object was not familiar to the infant, nor was the test environment designed to be naturalistic. Nonetheless, the retention interval, 24 hours, was the same as shown by DeLoache with far older children (18–30-month-olds), and like that work, provides a more favorable estimate of long-term recall capacities than was originally suggested by Gratch et al. (1974) and Webb et al. (1972) using their particular object-search procedures.

Object-search tasks and deferred imitation are similar in that infants must govern their motor actions on the basis of a stored representation of a now-absent object or event, and not simply recognize two scenes as similar. The two tasks also have clear and obvious differences. For example, in the object permanence case, infants must represent a particular object in a spatial location, whereas in the deferred imitation task, it is not a particular object in space but an absent action that must be stored. As such, this new work on deferred imitation provides a converging technique for investigating non-recognition forms of memory in infants.

Future experiments using deferred imitation designs of the type developed here could investigate parameters such as delay, interference, stimulus characteristics, and perhaps, most interestingly, their interaction with age or developmental level as measured by other tasks. Converging tests of infant memory using paired-comparison, habituation, object permanence, and deferred imitation procedures would not only increase our knowledge about memory development, but may also help to clarify the differences between the types of representational processes involved in these different cases.

Regardless of this future research, the present studies show that infants as young as 14 months can profit from observation, and can use this visual experience to direct their behavior at a significantly later point in time. This suggests that imitation could, in principle, play a useful role in learning and socialization during infancy (Meltzoff, 1985).

REFERENCES

Abravanel, E., Levan-Goldschmidt, E., & Stevenson, M. B. (1976). Action imitation: The early phase of infancy. *Child Development, 47,* 1032-1044.

Caron, R. F., & Caron, A. J. (1969). Degree of stimulus complexity and habituation of visual fixation in infants. *Psychonomic Science, 14,* 78-79.

Cohen, L. B., DeLoache, J. S., & Pearl, R. A. (1977). An examination of interference effects in infants' memory for faces. *Child Development, 48,* 88-96.

Cohen, L. B., & Gelber, E. R. (1975). Infant visual memory. In L. B. Cohen & P. Salapatek (Eds.), *Infant perception: From sensation to cognition* (Vol. 1, pp. 347-403). New York: Academic Press.

Cornell, E. H. (1979). Infants' recognition memory, forgetting and savings. *Journal of Experimental Child Psychology, 28,* 359-374.

DeLoache, J. S. (1980). Naturalistic studies of memory for object location in very young children. In M. Perlmutter (Ed.), *New directions for child development: No. 10. Children's memory* (pp. 17-32). San Francisco: Jossey-Bass.

Fagan, J. F. III (1972). Infants' recognition memory for faces. *Journal of Experimental Child Psychology, 14,* 453-476.

Fagan, J. F. III (1973). Infants' delayed recognition memory and forgetting. *Journal of Experimental Child Psychology, 16,* 424-450.

Fagan, J. F. III (1974). Infant recognition memory: The effects of length of familiarization and type of discrimination task. *Child Development, 45,* 351-356.

Fagan, J. F. III (1977). Infant recognition memory: Studies in forgetting. *Child Development, 48,* 68-78.

Fantz, R. L. (1964). Visual experience in infants: Decreased attention to familiar patterns relative to novel ones. *Science, 146,* 668-670.

Field, T. M., Woodson, R., Greenberg, R., & Cohen, D. (1982). Discrimination and imitation of facial expressions by neonates. *Science, 218,* 179-181.

Flavell, J. (1977). *Cognitive development.* Englewood-Cliffs, NJ: Prentice-Hall.

Fleiss, J. L. (1981). *Statistical methods for rates and proportions* (2d ed.). New York: Wiley.

Gratch, G., Appel, K. J., Evans, W. F., LeCompte, G. K., & Wright, N. A. (1974). Piaget's stage IV object concept error: Evidence of forgetting or object conception? *Child Development, 45,* 71-77.

Jacobson, S. W. (1979). Matching behavior in the young infant. *Child Development, 50,* 425-430.

Kagan, J. (1981). *The second year.* Cambridge, MA: Harvard University Press.

Kagan, J., Kearsley, R. B., & Zelazo, P. R. (1978). *Infancy: Its place in human development.* Cambridge, MA: Harvard University Press.

Killen, M., & Uzgiris, I. C. (1981). Imitation of actions with objects: The role of social meaning. *Journal of Genetic Psychology*, **138**, 219-229.

McCall, R. B., Parke, R. D., & Kavanaugh, R. D. (1977). Imitation of live and televised models by children one to three years of age. *Monographs of the Society for Research in Child Development*, **42**(5, Serial No. 173).

Mehrabian, A., & Williams, M. (1971). Piagetian measures of cognitive development for children up to age two. *Journal of Psycholinguistic Research*, **1**, 113-126.

Meltzoff, A. N. (1981). Imitation, intermodal coordination, and representation in early infancy. In G. Butterworth (Ed.), *Infancy and epistemology* (pp. 85-114). Brighton: Harvester.

Meltzoff, A. N. (1985). The roots of social and cognitive development: Models of man's original nature. In T. M. Field & N. Fox (Eds.), *Social perception in infants* (pp. 1-30). Norwood, NJ: Ablex.

Meltzoff, A. N., & Moore, M. K. (1977). Imitation of facial and manual gestures by human neonates. *Science*, **198**, 75-78.

Meltzoff, A. N., & Moore, M. K. (1983a). Newborn infants imitate adult facial gestures. *Child Development*, **54**, 702-709.

Meltzoff, A. N., & Moore, M. K. (1983b). The origins of imitation in infancy: Paradigm, phenomena, and theories. In L. P. Lipsitt (Ed.), *Advances in infancy research* (Vol. **2**, pp. 265-301). Norwood, NJ: Ablex.

Meltzoff, A. N., & Moore, M. K. (1985). Cognitive foundations and social functions of imitation and intermodal representation in infancy. In J. Mehler & R. Fox (Eds.), *Neonate cognition: Beyond the blooming, buzzing confusion* (pp. 139-156). Hillsdale, NJ: Erlbaum.

Olson, G. M. (1976). An information-processing analysis of visual memory and habituation in infants. In T. J. Tighe & R. N. Leaton (Eds.), *Habituation: Perspectives from child development, animal behavior, and neurophysiology* (pp. 239-277). Hillsdale, NJ: Erlbaum.

Pancratz, C. N., & Cohen, L. B. (1970). Recovery of habituation in infants. *Journal of Experimental Child Psychology*, **9**, 208-216.

Paraskevopoulos, J., & Hunt, J. McV. (1971). Object construction and imitation under differing conditions of rearing. *Journal of Genetic Psychology*, **119**, 301-321.

Piaget, J. (1952). *The origins of intelligence in children*. New York: International Universities Press.

Piaget, J. (1954). *The construction of reality in the child*. New York: Basic.

Piaget, J. (1962). *Play, dreams and imitation in childhood*. New York: Norton.

Rodgon, M. M., & Kurdek, L. A. (1977). Vocal and gestural imitation in 8-, 14-, and 20-month-old children. *Journal of Genetic Psychology*, **131**, 115-123.

Sophian, C. (1980). Habituation is not enough: Novelty preferences, search, and memory in infancy. *Merrill-Palmer Quarterly*, **26**(3), 239-257.

Uzgiris, I. C. (1972). Patterns of vocal and gestural imitation in infants. In F. J. Mönks, W. W. Hartup, & J. deWit (Eds.), *Determinants of behavioral development* (pp. 467-471). New York: Academic Press.

Uzgiris, I. C. (1979). Die Mannigfaltigkeit der Imitation in der frühen Kindheit. In L. Montada (Ed.), *Brennpunkte der Entwicklungspsychologie* (pp. 173-193). Stuttgart: Kohlhammer.

Uzgiris, I. C., & Hunt, J. McV. (1975). *Assessment in infancy*. Urbana: University of Illinois Press.

Watson, J. S. (in press). Memory in infancy. In J. Piaget, J. P. Bronkart, & P. Mounoud (Eds.), *Encylcopedie de la pleidade: La psychologie*. Paris: Gallimard.

Webb. R. A., Massar, B., & Nadolny, T. (1972). Information and strategy in the young child's search for hidden objects. *Child Development, 43,* 91-104.

Werner, J. S., & Perlmutter, M. (1979). Development of visual memory in infants. In H. W. Reese & L. P. Lipsitt (Eds.), *Advances in child development and behavior* (Vol. 14, pp. 1-56). New York: Academic Press.

Wetherford, M. J., & Cohen, L. B. (1973). Developmental changes in infant visual preferences for novelty and familiarity. *Child Development, 44,* 416-424.

2

Consistency of Mothers' Behavior Toward Infant Siblings

Judith F. Dunn

*Cambridge University, Madingley,
Cambridge, England*

Robert Plomin and Margaret Nettles

University of Colorado, Boulder

How similarly do mothers behave toward infant siblings? We explored this question in 50 families in which mothers were videotaped while interacting with each of two siblings when each child was 12 months old. The average age difference between the siblings was 35 months. Maternal behavior was reliably assessed, and factor analysis of the data yielded three factors: affection, verbal attention, and control. The results indicate that the mothers behaved very similarly towards their two siblings at the same age in infancy: The consistency of maternal behavior toward the siblings approached the reliability of the measures. Although results might differ for older children, and for siblings of different ages, these data suggest that differential maternal treatment of children of the same age in infancy is unlikely to

Reprinted with permission from *Developmental Psychology*, 1985, Vol. 21, 1188–1195. Copyright 1985 by the American Psychological Association, Inc.

Data from the Colorado Adoption Project were obtained with the support of grants from the National Science Foundation (BNS-7826204 and BNS 8200310) and the National Institute of Child Health and Human Development (HD-10333). The ratings and analyses of the sibling data presented in this article were supported by a grant from the Colorado Node of the MacArthur Research Network on the Transition from Infancy to Early Childhood and were conducted while the first author was supported by the MacArthur Transition Network. We thank Rebecca G. Miles for her editorial advice in the preparation of this article.

be a major source of the marked individual differences that have been observed within pairs of siblings.

Measures of personality and psychopathology reveal differences between siblings growing up in the same family that are almost as great as those between unrelated children growing up in separate families (Rowe & Plomin, 1981; Scarr & Grajek, 1982). This notable finding suggests, as pointed out by Maccoby and Martin (1984), that many of the family environment and parental child-rearing variables that we have presumed to be important in influencing children's development in fact account for little of the variance among children. What factors do contribute to the differences between siblings? One possibility is that parents behave differently toward different children and that growing up in the "same" family environment involves different experiences with the parents for each child. Until now there has been relatively little direct systematic evidence from which to judge the contribution that differential parental treatment may make to the development of individual differences within pairs of siblings.

Studies of average group differences in parents' behavior toward their children suggest that parental treatment may differ within families from one sibling to another. For instance, mothers of first-born children have been reported to be more directive and intrusive (Hilton, 1967; Rothbart, 1971), more attentive (Koch, 1954), more inconsistent (Sears, Maccoby, & Levin, 1957), less indulgent (Newson & Newson, 1976), and more persistent and less effective at feeding (Thoman, Turner, Leiderman, & Barnett, 1970) than are mothers of later-born children. A few studies have examined differential treatment of children within the same family (e.g., Abramvitch, Pepler, & Corter, 1982; Bryant & Crockenberg, 1980; Jacobs & Moss, 1976). However, these studies also focus primarily on average differences in treatment within families for first-born and later-born siblings, rather than considering the general issue of consistency of mothers' behavior toward siblings. For example, mothers were reported by Jacobs and Moss to show less social, affectionate, and caretaking behavior with their second-born than with their first-born children at 3 months of age; in Bryant and Crockenberg's study of 7- to 10-year-olds, mothers were reported to be more responsive and more intrusive with their later-born than with their first-born children. No significant parity differences were reported by Abramovitch and her colleagues. Only three studies have included analyses of the consistency of maternal behavior to successive siblings. Jacobs and Moss report significant stability in social, affectionate, and caretaking behavior toward two siblings; Dunn and Kendrick (1982) found stability in maternal play with siblings; and Abramovitch and her colleagues report significant correlations for both positive and negative maternal behavior toward older and younger siblings.

However, the siblings in all but one of these studies of differential parental treatment were of different ages when the mother's behavior was studied. Differences in maternal behavior toward the two children may well have reflected differences in the mother's response to the ages and needs of the two children. In other words, studies of different-aged siblings might assess differential responding of mothers to younger and older children rather than differential responding to two children per se. To examine the issue of differential treatment, we require information on mothers' behavior toward their children at equivalent age points and in similar situations. Although Jacobs and Moss's (1976) data on maternal behavior toward two siblings when each child was 3 months old suggest that mothers may be quite consistent in their behavior, their study focused on average differences in mothers' treatment of siblings as a function of birth order and sex.

How much and in what ways parents do behave differently toward their different children remains an open question, even though extant data suggest that parents may be quite consistent in their behavior toward siblings. In this article, we present observational data on 50 mothers and 100 children: The mothers were studied with their two children in similar situations when each child was 12 months old. These families are part of a larger sample of families taking part in the Colorado Adoption Project (Plomin & DeFries, 1983) and are the first families who are participating in the study with both their first and their second child. We focus here on the question of whether there are systematic differences in the behavior of the mothers toward their two children during playful interactions and in a feeding situation.

METHOD

Sample

The study is based on 50 two-child families who are taking part in the Colorado Adoption Project, a longitudinal, prospective study of behavioral development (Plomin & DeFries, 1983, 1985). Although 65 of the 100 siblings are biological siblings in nonadoptive families, 35 adopted infants were included in order to explore the possibility of genetic influences on maternal treatment (Plomin, Loehlin, & DeFries, 1985) by comparing differences in maternal treatment for genetically unrelated adoptee pairs and biological sibling pairs. Both adoptive and nonadoptive families are representative of middle-class families in terms of paternal occupational status (Plomin & DeFries, 1985). Occupational status was assessed with the "new" National Opinion Research Center rating (based on the 1970 census as revised by Hauser and Featherman, 1977); the mean rating for paternal occupation is 51.5. Mean values for educational level are 15.8 and 15.2 years for fathers and mothers, respectively. The interval between the siblings ranges from 14 months to 74 months, with a mean of 35 months. The sample includes 59 boys and 41 girls, 21 same-sex sibling pairs, and 29 opposite-sex sibling pairs.

Procedure

Each of the 100 siblings was visited at home when he or she was 12 months old. During the 3-hr visit, measures of mental and motor development, temperament assessments, and assessments of the home environment (described by Plomin & DeFries, 1985) were obtained, and two 5-min sequences of the mother and infant interacting were videotaped. The videotaped observations were made in a feeding situation (lunch or snack) and in a free-play situation in which the mother was asked to play with the infant in whatever manner they would mutually enjoy. Thus the mother was observed interacting separately with each of the two siblings when they were 12 months of age.

Despite their brevity, the videotaped situations have proved to be "behaviorally intense" and to yield reliable information about mothers' behavior toward their infants. Concerning the possible intrusiveness of videotape equipment, mothers reported in interviews that the hand-held camera had little effect on their own or their infant's behavior because the situations (feeding and free play) were engrossing and because the rapport between the mothers and infants and the tester was good. The tester was in the home for at least 1 hr before videotaping began.

Maternal Behavior Measures

The mothers' behavior toward their two children—each child observed separately with the mother at 12 months of age—during the feeding situation and the free-play situation was coded from the videotapes. The 10 min of observation time were divided into 10-s time units, and each occurrence of any 14 categories of maternal behavior listed in Table 1

Table 1
Categories of Maternal Behavior

1. Mother holds, or touches affectionately	M kisses, cuddles, caresses, holds, or makes other affectionate gesture.
2. Mother laughs	
3. Mother accepts[a]	Verbal indication by M that she accepts or approves of some behavior (verbal or nonverbal) by C (e.g., "Good." "That's the way."): May be a question (e.g., C shows M a toy. M says "Yes, is it a dog?"): May be approving suggestion about C's actions toward others (e.g., C turns toward camera with a toy. M says, "You going to show it to Judy?")
4. Mother directs[a]	M's verbal directions, instructions, commands, and requests: May be positive or negative (the vast majority are positive), i.e., directive or intrusive statements.
5. Mother rejects[a]	M's verbal rejections of either words or actions, e.g., "No, it's not a dog, it's a kitty."
6. Mother prohibits	Verbal prohibition by M
7. Mother questions	
8. Mother vocalizes	M talks to C, but vocalization is not included in any other category.
9. Mother refers to feelings	Explicit verbal reference by M to C's wants, needs, feeling state, likes, dislikes
10. Mother shows	M demonstrates toy or object to C or points to focus C's attention.
11. Mother gives	
12. Mother imitates	
13. Mother positive affect	Positive affect is recorded if M speaks to C in a positive warm tone of voice or smiles.
14. Mother negative affect	Negative affect is recorded if M speaks to C in negative tone of voice.

Note. M = mother. C = child.
[a]From Nelson (1973).

during each 10-s time unit was recorded. Categories of behavior were selected to include aspects of warm and affectionate behavior toward the child (Categories 1, 2, 13); responsiveness to the child (Category 3); controlling, restrictive, or punitive behavior (Categories 4, 5, 6, 14); other aspects of verbal behavior toward the child (Categories 7, 8, 9); and interest in showing and giving the baby objects and imitating the baby (Categories 10, 11, 12). Negative physical contact (mother pushes, hits, or shakes infants) and games (reciprocal play that involves two or more "turns") were also rated but omitted from analysis because they were infrequently observed during the videotape sessions. Categories 3–5 were originally used by Nelson (1973) in a study of language acquisition, but in a longitudinal study of mother–child relationships proved to index differences in maternal behavior toward 1-year-olds of considerably broader significance than their importance in language acquisition (Dunn, 1977). Differences between mothers in Category 9 (reference to child's feelings) have also been shown to be related to differences in a wide range of child-centered behaviors, which in turn are related differences in children's behavior over time (Dunn & Kendrick, 1982).

RESULTS

Descriptive Statistics

Complete data were obtained for 46 mother–sibling–sibling triads for each measure; these data were the focus of our analyses. Table 2 lists the means and standard deviations for the 14 measures of maternal behavior summed over the feeding and free-play situations for the 92 children in the study. The means indicate that the videotaped observations capture a considerable amount of maternal behavior. For example, on the average, mothers touched their children affectionately 3 times, vocalized more than 61 times, and gave their children objects 6 times. The standard deviations show that the mothers differed substantially in their behavior toward 12-month-olds.

The focus of the study is individual variability in a mother's behavior toward her two children at the same age in the same situations. To examine this issue, individual differences analyses—specifically, analyses of the correlations between mothers' behavior toward each of two siblings—are more illuminating than are comparisons of groups differing in sex or birth order, because such analyses encompass the variance explained by all such group differences. Differences in maternal consistency are not necessarily revealed by group comparisons: It is quite possible, for example, for there to be no average difference in maternal responsiveness toward siblings differing in sex, birth order, or other sibling status variables, and yet for mothers to treat their two siblings differentially. Nonetheless, given the interest in the literature in such group differences, we conducted t tests for maternal behavior comparing mothers of first-born versus second-born siblings, same-sex versus opposite-sex siblings, boys versus girls, and biological versus adoptive siblings. The analyses yielded few significant mean differences, and those that emerged explained little variance.

Out of 56 comparisons, only 2 yield a difference significant at $p < .05$, which is the number expected on the basis of chance alone. Mothers affectionately touched their first-born more than their second-born child (the respective means are 4.7 vs. 2.1, a difference that is significant at $p < .05$, but explains less than 6% of the variance). Mothers prohibited opposite-sex siblings more than same-sex siblings ($Ms = 1.6$ vs. 0.5). There was a tendency for mothers to question girls more than boys and

Table 2
Means, Standard Deviations, and Reliabilities of Measures

Category	M	SD	Intercoder reliability	Test-retest reliability
1. Touches affectionately	3.42	5.38	.80*	.67*
2. Laughs	13.00	8.13	.92*	.73*
3. Accepts	14.73	11.12	.75*	.86*
4. Directs	24.52	18.01	.91*	.58*
5. Rejects	2.94	3.74	.78*	.63*
6. Prohibits	1.05	1.84	.74*	.26
7. Questions	29.50	16.49	.97*	.78*
8. Vocalizes	61.52	27.38	.76*	.77*
9. Refers	8.48	6.39	.92*	.58*
10. Shows	10.20	6.02	.67*	.19
11. Gives	6.33	4.64	.87*	.20
12. Imitates	2.13	3.58	.88*	.12
13. Positive affect	23.98	11.25	.90*	.90*
14. Negative affect	0.17	0.49	.82*	.61*

Note. N for means and standard deviations is 92; for intercoder reliability and test-retest reliability, the sample sizes were 28 and 18, respectively.
*$p < .05$.

to vocalize more to girls than to boys (Ms = 33.14 vs. 26.90 and 67.2 vs. 57.5, respectively). However, these differences are only marginally significant ($p < .10$).

Rater Reliability and Test–Retest Reliability

The next question addressed the extent to which the variability in the mothers' behavior is reliable. Table 2 also lists intercoder reliabilities for the first 28 videotapes. The average rater reliability is .87 for the 14 categories of maternal behavior. Reliability was rechecked halfway through the coding of 10 videotapes. The agreement at this halfway stage ranged from .72 to 1.0, with a mean of .89.

Test–retest reliabilities were calculated for 18 mothers observed with their infants on two occasions, 2 weeks apart. Maternal behaviors in the feeding and free-play situations were summed within each of the 14 categories. The test–retest correlations, listed in Table 2, indicate that the 10-min observations did provide moderately reliable indexes of the mothers' behavior. The average test–retest reliability is .53.

Factor Analysis

The measures of maternal behavior were submitted to factor analysis. Initially, factor analyses were conducted separately for observations of the feeding situation and of free play and for observations of the first and of the second child. For both the feeding situation and free play, and for both the first and second child, the analyses revealed highly similar factor structures. For purposes of data reduction and clarity of presentation, therefore, the factor structure is reported for the combined data on the feeding and play situations and the first and second children.

Three factors, which together accounted for 61.1% of the total variance, were rotated. The first rotated factor was defined primarily by measures of positive affection and acceptance by the mother; it accounted for 63.3% of the rotated variance. The variables loading above .50 on this first factor were positive affect (.94), laughs (.82), and accepts (.71). The second factor was defined by measures of verbal behavior and accounted for 24.6% of the rotated variance. The measures loading most highly on this factor were questions (.85), vocalizes (.76), and refers to feelings (.56). The third factor, which accounted for 12.2% of the variance, was defined by measures of maternal control and restrictive behavior. The variables loading most highly were rejects (.88), negative affect (.62), prohibits (.57), and directs (.50). The three factors thus apparently reflect three dimensions of maternal behavior: positive affection, verbal behavior, and control.

Scales were constructed to represent these factors. For each factor, measures loading more than .50 on the factor were standardized as z scores, and then the z scores were summed. Thus scales for maternal affection, maternal verbal behavior, and maternal control were created. The test–retest reliabilities for the three scales are .83, .62, and .55, respectively, which again suggest that mothers are consistent over 2 weeks' time in their behavior toward their infants.

Consistency of Mothers' Behavior Toward Two Siblings

The major purpose of the present study was to explore the consistency of mothers' behavior toward two siblings, when each siblings was 12 months of age and was observed in the same situations. Consistency was assessed by examining correlations between mothers' behaviors toward the two siblings for the three scale scores and for the 14 categories of maternal behavior. The correlations in these measures were computed initially for the feeding and the free-play situations separately and were next computed between the two situations. The correlations were very similar in the two situations and were high between the two situations, with 12 of the 14 correlations between the two situations being significant at $p < .01$. For brevity and clarity of presentation, the correlations are reported, therefore, for the combined data for the two situations. The results, presented in Table 3, show that mothers were strikingly consistent in their behavior toward their two children. Maternal consistency involves not just consistency in behavior toward two different children but also consistency over 3 years' time—the average age difference between the two siblings is 35 months. For this reason, maternal consistency needs to be evaluated in relation to the test–retest reliabilities, which are therefore shown for the three scale scores and listed again in Table 3 for the 14 categories of maternal behavior. It can be seen that for the scale scores, maternal consistency approaches the test-retest reliabilities.[1]

---

[1]When the scores are corrected for unreliability, the correlations for the three scales of maternal behavior average .70, suggesting the 70% of the variance in maternal behavior is consistent for the two siblings. In this case, the correlation is not squared because the issue is the extent to which variance in mothers' behavior is consistent (i.e., covaries or is shared in common) for the two children in a family. Correlations are squared when the issue is the extent to which variance in one variable can be explained by variance in the

Similar results on the whole were obtained for the 14 categories of behavior, although the results are more variable, as would be expected from the use of single ratings rather than scales. The maternal consistency correlations vary as a function of the test–retest reliabilities of the categories and, again, most of the reliable variance in maternal behavior for the 14 categories is consistent for the two siblings.

Age Gap Between Siblings

Maternal consistency toward the two siblings for each of the three factor scales was correlated with the age gap between the children in

Table 3
Correlations Between Mothers' Behavior Toward Two Children, Each
Observed at 12 Months of Age

Scales and categories of maternal behavior	Correlation	Test-retest reliability
Affection Scale	.58*	.83*
Verbal Scale	.45*	.62*
Control Scale	.37*	.55*
1. Touches affectionately	.15	.67*
2. Laughs	.41*	.73*
3. Accepts	.26*	.86*
4. Directs	.49*	.58*
5. Rejects	.44*	.63*
6. Prohibits	.03	.26
7. Questions	.57*	.78*
8. Vocalizes	.38*	.77*
9. Refers	.26*	.58*
10. Shows	.03	.19
11. Gives	.31*	.20
12. Imitates	.30*	.12
13. Positive affect	.60*	.90*
14. Negative affect	.09	.61*

*$p < .05$.

other variable. The situation is analogous to test theory—test–retest reliability is true variance, which is calculated simply as the correlation—not the correlation squared—between measurements at two times. This issue is explained in the context of covariance among relatives in an article entitled "A Note on Why Genetic Correlations Are Not Squared" (Jensen, 1971). Regardless of the corrections for reliability, the correlations in Table 3 suggest substantial consistency in the behavior of mothers toward two siblings.

months. For the scales of the factors of maternal affection and maternal control, the correlations were not significant. For the maternal verbal behavior scale there was a low, but positive, correlation (.28) between the age gap between the children and the inconsistency of the mother's verbal behavior. That is, mothers with closely spaced children tended to be more consistent in their verbal behavior toward the siblings than mothers with a large age gap between the children.

Same-Sex Different-Sex Siblings

Comparisons of the maternal consistency correlations in families with same-sex and with different-sex siblings showed no significant differences in the two groups.

Biological and Adoptive Siblings

Given the substantial similarity in mothers' responding to their two children, it is unlikely that their behavior is influenced by genetic differences between the siblings. Nonetheless, as a preliminary check on the possibility, we compared correlations for mothers' behavior toward biological siblings (32 pairs) with correlations for mothers' behavior toward adoptive siblings (14 pairs). If mothers treat siblings differently because of genetic differences between them, then mothers of adoptive siblings—who are genetically unrelated to each other—will treat their two children more differently than will mothers of biological siblings. In other words, if mothers are influenced by genetic differences between their two children, then correlations for mothers' behavior toward adoptive siblings should be lower than the correlations for behavior toward biological siblings. We examined correlations separately for adoptive and biological siblings for the three scale scores. For two scales, mothers' verbal behavior and mothers' control, correlations for adoptive siblings and biological siblings were nearly identical. However, mothers' affection yielded a correlation of .37 for adoptive siblings and .70 for biological siblings. Although the difference in correlations is not significant, it is in the direction expected if mothers' behavior is influenced by genetic differences between their children. This pattern of results is particularly interesting because Rowe (1983) has found in two separate twin studies that measures of parental affection show genetic influence, whereas measures of parental control do not. Correlations for the 14 specific measures gave similar results. Given the small sample sizes of adoptive and biological siblings, the finding clearly needs replication before it can be regarded with confidence, but it does indicate that further research in this area would be useful.

DISCUSSION

The mothers in this study showed very similar behavior toward their two children when both were 12 months old, during observations that were made on average 35 months apart. Mothers' affectionate behavior and their verbal attention to their children, as well as their more controlling and directive behaviors, all were remarkably consistent toward their two children. This striking degree of consistency was not, in fact, what we had expected to find. The range of differences among mothers was considerable. Mean group differences explained little of the variability in mothers' behavior, however. Mothers tended to be more consistent in their verbal behavior toward closely spaced siblings than toward widely spaced siblings, but few significant mean group differences emerged for birth order, sex, or comparisons between same-sex and opposite-sex pairs. The lack of birth order differences might be considered surprising in view of the differences reported by Jacobs and Moss (1976) and by Thoman and her colleagues (Thoman et al., 1970). However, these studies were focused on infants at 3 months or under. It is quite plausible that the uncertainty and lack of experience with which primiparous mothers handle their new babies, which undoubtedly contribute to these differences, have decreased by 1 year. Indeed there is systematic evidence to show that during feeding interactions the primiparous/multiparous differences apparent during the first few days of a life decrease markedly (Dunn & Richards, 1977).

If a significant difference in birth order had been found and accounted for substantial variance, this would have led to *inconsistency* in that particular variable. The high consistency in the maternal variables in a sample containing equal numbers of children of different birth order, sex, and same-sex, different-sex pairs in itself indicates that these do not contribute in an important way to the variation.

The rationale for the study was not only to establish how mothers behaved toward siblings but also to assess the extent to which mothers' differential treatment of siblings could be a factor in explaining the marked sibling differences that are known to exist. The results imply that mothers' differential treatment of siblings as infants of the same age is not likely to be of major importance in contributing to individual differences between the siblings.

The findings also have implications for understanding the causes of differences in maternal behavior. Even though they indicate that mothers treat their children similarly, siblings within a family *are* different. For example, the average correlation for parental ratings of temperament for the siblings in the present sample is .22; sibling (fraternal twin) correlations for temperament measures in other studies are about .30 (Goldsmith, 1983). For the Bayley Mental Developmental Index, the average weighted sibling correlation in three studies of 1-year-olds is .22 (McCall, 1972; Nichols & Broman, 1974; Wilson, 1983). If infant siblings within a family are so different, and yet mothers show such similar affection, verbal behavior, and directive control toward them, it appears that differences in these aspects of maternal behavior primarily reflect characteristics of the mother, not the infant. What this implies is that we may need to reconsider current theories of the direction of influence in the mother–infant relationship. Over the past 15 years there has been a welcome recognition of the importance of the role of the infant as an influence on the interaction between mother and child. Yet the findings reported here suggest that the affection, verbal behavior, and directive control that mothers show toward their 12-month-old babies during feeding and playful interactions reflect maternal rather than infant characteristics.

The findings of the present study are limited in two important respects. The first concerns the nature of the observations. The observation period was very brief, and the presence of a videocamera and observer meant that negative, hostile, or punitive behavior by the mother was very rarely shown. What was captured on the videotapes was more typical of the "best" exchanges between mother and child. We cannot then assume that there would be no differences in the more hostile behaviors toward first-born and later-born children. However, the high test–retest reliabilities of the affection and verbal behavior scales indicate that we can have confidence in the findings that there is marked consistency in these aspects of maternal behavior toward successive children within the same family.

The second caution concerns the age of the children. It is, of course, possible that differential treatment of the children within a family becomes more evident and more developmentally important as children grow from infancy to childhood. Given the dramatic changes during the second year in children's social, cognitive, and emotional behavior, and the parallel changes in parental views of problem behavior and their own capacity to control their children (Carey, 1985), it seems quite possible that by 2 or 3 years of age, differences in parental behavior toward their various children, especially in the areas of *control,* might well be apparent. A theory predicting that children increasingly evoke such differences in their parents has been proposed by Scarr and McCartney (1983). Information on parental behavior toward different children within a family as the children grow up will make it possible to test one essential feature of such a model.

REFERENCES

Abramovitch, R., Pepler, D., & Corter, C. (1982). Patterns of sibling interaction among preschool-age children. In M. Lamb & B. Sutton-Smith (Eds.), *Sibling relationships: Their nature and significance across the lifespan* (pp. 61–86). Hillsdale, NJ: Erlbaum.

Bryant, B., & Crockenberg, S. (1980). Correlates and dimensions of prosocial behavior: A study of female siblings with their mothers. *Child Development, 51*, 529-544.

Carey, W. B. (1985). Clinical interactions of temperament: Transitions from infancy to childhood. In R. Plomin & J. Dunn (Eds.). *The study of temperament: Changes, continuities, and challenges.* (11, 151–162). Hillsdale, NJ: Erlbaum.

Dunn, J. B., (1977). Patterns of early interaction: Continuities and consequences. In H. R. Schaffer (Ed.), *Studies in mother-infant interaction* (pp. 457–474). New York: Academic Press.

Dunn, J. B., & Richards, M. P. M. (1977). Observations on the developing relationship between mother and baby in the newborn period. In H. R. Schaffer (Ed.), *Studies in mother-infant interaction* (pp. 438–456). New York: Academic Press.

Dunn, J., & Kendrick, C. (1982). *Siblings: Love, envy and understanding.* Cambridge, MA: Harvard University Press.

Goldsmith, H. H. (1983). Genetic influences on personality from infancy to adulthood. *Child Development, 54*, 331-355.

Hauser, R. M., & Featherman, D. L. (1977). *The process of stratification: Trends and analysis.* New York: Academic Press.

Hilton, I. (1967). Differences in the behavior of mothers toward first- and later-born children. *Journal of Personality and Social Psychology, 7*, 282-290.

Jacobs, B. S., & Moss, H. A. (1976). Birth order and sex of sibling as determinants of mother-infant interaction. *Child Development, 47*, 315-322.

Jensen, A. R. (1971). A note on why genetic correlations are not squared. *Psychological Bulletin, 75*, 223-224.

Koch, H. L. (1954). The relation of "primary mental abilities" in five- and six-year-olds to sex of child and characteristics of his sibling. *Child Development, 25*, 207-223.

Maccoby, E. E., & Martin, J. A. (1984). Socialization in the context of the family: Parent-child interaction. In P. H. Mussen (Ed.), *Handbook of child psychology (4th ed.): Vol. IV. Socialization, personality, and social development* (pp. 1–101). New York: Wiley.

McCall, R. B. (1972). Similarity in developmental profile among related pairs of human infants. *Science, 178*, 1004-1005.

Nelson, K. (1973). Structure and strategy in learning how to talk. *Monographs of the Society for Research in Child Development, 38* (1, Serial No. 149).

Newson, J., & Newson, E. (1976). *Four years old in an urban community.* Harmondsworth, U.K.: Pelican.

Nichols, P. L., & Broman, S. H. (1974). Familial resemblance in infant mental development. *Developmental Psychology, 10*, 442-446.

Plomin, R., & DeFries, J. C. (1983). The Colorado Adoption Project. *Child Development, 54,* 276-289.

Plomin, R., & DeFries, J. C. (1985). *Origins of individual differences in infancy: The Colorado Adoption Project.* New York: Academic Press.

Plomin, R., Loehlin, J. C., & DeFries, J. C. (1985). Genetic and environmental components of "environmental" influences. *Developmental Psychology, 21,* 391-402.

Rothbart, M. K. (1971). Birth order and mother-child interaction in an achievement situation. *Journal of Personality and Social Psychology, 17,* 113-120.

Rowe, D. C. (1983). A biometrical analysis of perceptions of family environment: A study of twin and singleton kinships. *Child Development, 54,* 416-423.

Rowe, D. C., & Plomin, R. (1981). The importance of nonshared (E_1) environmental influences in behavioral development. *Developmental Psychology, 17,* 517-531.

Scarr, S., & Grajek, S. (1982). Similarities and differences among siblings. In M. E. Lamb & B. Sutton-Smith (Eds.), *Sibling relationships: Their nature and significance across the lifespan* (pp. 357-381). Hillsdale, NJ: Erlbaum.

Scarr, S., & McCartney, K. (1983). How people make their own environment: A theory of genotype-environment correlations. *Child Development, 54,* 424-435.

Sears, R. R., Maccoby, E., & Levin, H. (1957). *Patterns of child rearing.* Evanston, IL: Rowe & Peterson.

Thoman, E. B., Turner, A. M., Leiderman, P. H., & Barnett, C. R. (1970). Neonate-mother interaction: Effects of parity on feeding behavior. *Child Development, 41,* 1103-1111.

Wilson, R. S. (1983). The Louisville Twin Study: Developmental synchronies in behavior. *Child Development, 54,* 298-316.

Part II

DEVELOPMENTAL ISSUES

This year's selection covers a number of issues, all of which are of value both theoretically and practically.

The paper by Scarr points up an issue that requires strong and continuous emphasis. The meaning we give to research data, the variables we choose to investigate, the data we select as important and those we ignore or minimize, the theories we generate—all these are shaped by the biases of the particular historical period. As Scarr puts it, "At different times and places, facts invented in one theory become different facts in another. In each generation, psychologists have pet variables that serve loyally within the theoretical boundaries of the scientific wisdom of that time." (We might add that this generalization applies to psychiatrists as much as to psychologists.) Scarr illustrates this thesis by a number of pertinent and vivid examples. Her view of the validity of our theories and research data is, however, in no way nihilistic or pessimistic. Rather, she points up the positive implications of the constant reminder to ourselves and others of the limits imposed by the particular historical period in which we live and work. Scientific knowledge is always imperfect, and any of our pet theories may not be infallible. To believe otherwise always has the danger of distorting science into its opposite-ideological dogmatism.

The paper by Wilson takes up the issue of the vulnerability of children born small in weight for gestational age (SGA). Such children are now considered to be at higher risk for impaired mental development. Wilson's data indicate that this generalization does not hold for SGA twins, as contrasted to singleton infants. Even for the very small twin infants (below 1,750 grams birth weight), slowness in development was evident at 3 years, but had been overcome by 6 years. SES status and the mother's educational level were important variables in influencing this process of resiliency. Wilson's data remind us that there may be subgroups that are exceptions to generalizations regarding high risk factors, and that short-range effects may not have long-range consequences. The need for long-term followup is clear before we generalize. Wilson concludes with the optimistic note that "Under supportive conditions, most at-risk infants will recoup from early trauma and progress toward a level commensurate with their targeted capabilities." This principle of resiliency in a child's development is an important conclusion, with the *caveat* that the author points out—namely the need for "supportive conditions." The risk comes not from the early trauma as such, but from trauma plus an impoverished environment.

The paper by MacDonald also considers the issue of risk and resiliency from an examination of the concept of sensitive periods and the influence of early experience on the child's social development. It is worth pointing up that the term "sensitive period" has supplanted the previously favored term "critical period." The latter term implied that if the child missed an important experience at a certain age period, he or she could not make up this loss at a later period. By contrast the term "sensitive period" implies that specific experiences can exert a greater influence at one particular age period than another, but this does not mean that the child who misses this experience at that age is doomed to a permanent deficit. MacDonald points up this issue from his review of the literature: "We have come a long way from supposing that behavior is absolutely fixed at an early age by genetic factors or that after a sensitive period it is impossible to change behavior." He does suggest, however, that the plasticity of behavior declines with age, but that even this can be overcome, at least partially, by sufficient intensity of appropriate remedial measures at later ages. Like Wilson, MacDonald emphasizes "the power of environmental events and the buffering ability of the organism."

The paper by Horner gives us a scholarly and critical analysis of the popular classical psychoanalytic concepts of symbiosis and infantile omnipotence. He traces these ideas as they evolved in psychoanalytic writings until their full formulation by Margaret Mahler. From this review he questions the validity of the evidence for these concepts and their usefulness for contemporary developmental theory and research. Horner cites a statement by Mahler and her coworkers that touches on a basic issue in science. "Whereas there is no conceivable method by which the validity of the hypothesis of a symbiotic phase of the mother-infant dual unity can be proven, it is just as impossible, we think, to empathically or otherwise provide or militate for acceptance of the contrary hypothesis." We ourselves have heard a number of prominent psychoanalysts present this same "defense" of one or another basic psychoanalytic concept—that by their very nature their validity cannot be demonstrated or disproven by the established methods of scientific research. But if this is the case, then such theories are outside the realm of science, and represent, as Horner suggests, "poetic" constructions. It is certainly true that a creative scientist may make a giant "poetic" leap in developing a new theory that is only barely suggested by the evidence at hand. But when this happens, it is then necessary to undertake a research effort that can produce data from which the theory can either be validated or falsified.

The last paper in this section, by Murphy and Vogel, tells the poignant story of the short life of a boy, David, who was born with a severe combined immune deficiency and lived his 12½ years of life in a sterile isolator. He was of superior IQ and his school achievement test scores were above grade level. Motor coordination and dexterity skills were excellent. But he lived in a drastically limited environment, which the authors describe vividly. Our professional interest in this extraordinary case history is the drastically distorted view of the world David had, in spite of his cognitive assets. The authors spell out these distortions and link them clearly and specifically to the boy's physical environment which severely limited his life experiences. Perception and cognition are shaped by many factors, but actual life experience is vital for their development.

3

Constructing Psychology: Making Facts and Fables for Our Times

Sandra Scarr

University of Virginia, Charlottesville

Like other scientists, psychologists construct knowledge. To sensory data we attribute meaning in theoretically guided inventions of "facts." At different times and places, facts invented in one theory become different facts in another. In each generation, psychologists have pet variables that serve loyally within the theoretical boundaries of the scientific wisdom of that time. I argue that pet variables can blind us to other theories and other variables that could compete for our affections. I examine what makes theories and facts plausible and propose a continuum of persuasion, determined by the contexts of the theorists. Contemporary research on lead exposure and on parent–child interaction are examined as examples of "facts" that can become different "facts" in other theories.

All the world's a stage, but the script is not *As You Like It*, it is *Rashomon*. Each of us has our own reality of which we try to persuade others. Facts

Reprinted with permission from *American Psychologist*, 1985, Vol. 40, 499–512. Copyright 1985 by the American Psychological Association, Inc.

This article is based on the Presidential Address to Division 7 at the annual meeting of the American Psychological Association in Anaheim, California on August 27, 1983.

I wish to express my appreciation to Carol Fleisher Feldman for many stimulating discussions on these and many other issues. Research presented in this article was conducted under the sponsorship of the Bermuda Government, the W. T. Grant Foundation, and the U.S. Environmental Protection Agency.

do not have an independent existence. Rather, facts are created within theoretical systems that guide the selection of observations and the invention of reality. In this article I hope to explain how this should change our claims about research, not discredit them.

If one adopts, as I do, a constructionist position on epistemology, then knowledge of all kinds, including scientific knowledge, is a construction of the human mind. Sensory data are filtered through the knowing apparatus of the human senses and made into perceptions and cognitions. The human mind is also constructed in a social context, and its knowledge is in part created by the social and cultural context in which it comes to know the world. Knowledge of the world is therefore always constructed by the human mind in the working models of reality in the sciences. If this is not evident, consider for a moment the vast differences in our concepts of the world before Galileo, Darwin, Einstein, and Freud.

We do not discover scientific facts; we invent them. Their usefulness to us depends both on shared perceptions of the "facts" (consensual validation) and on whether they work for various purposes, some practical and some theoretical.

THE IMPORTANCE OF BELIEFS IN SCIENTIFIC KNOWLEDGE

It is also true that we cannot perceive or process knowledge without the constraints of belief. One example of the personal constraint on knowledge is found in eyewitness accounts of crimes (Loftus, 1979). Fleeting impressions of criminal behavior are elaborated by individuals into complete accounts that they believe to be "true." The wrong people are identified as the criminals, and events are construed in ways that are consistent with the observer's emotions and prejudices. When such events are videotaped and reviewed repeatedly by observers, a different consensus of the event emerges, one that is not consistent with the eyewitness account of the observer at the scene. The problem is that the eyewitness to a crime or other emotional event gleans only partial knowledge from the immediate experience. The eyewitness fills in the gaps in his or her knowledge by plausible constructions of what "must have" or "should have" happened to make sense of the scene. Unfortunately, the eyewitness account is often at variance with that of observers who can review the event more than once in the calm of a videotape viewing room. Emotional responses and personal prejudices color knowledge of such events.

Should we accept the eyewitness as an analogue to scientific knowledge? I argue that there are only quantitative differences between scientific inquiry and the eyewitness account. Each scientist approaches scientific problems with a theoretical viewpoint, whether explicit or implicit. Theory guides inquiry through the questions raised, the framework of inquiry, and the interpretation of the results. Each scientist seeks to find "facts" to assimilate into his or her world view. Thus, each of us is biased by the human tendency to seek "facts" that are congruent with our prior beliefs.

In everyday life, the biases of information seeking and interpretation are personal. In science, these biases are shared preferences for one theoretical perspective or another—social and cultural biases in the "facts" gathered and believed. But they can be seen as very much the same kind of biases as those of everyday life, except that they are shared beliefs among members of the scientific community. Their common acceptance in science may seem to give them a status in reality that they do not have.

SOCIOCULTURAL BIASES IN KNOWLEDGE

Although I am in sympathy with most of the current cultural ethos, let us be clear that we change our scientific lenses as the culture changes. Information gained from research is likely to be assimilated into current views. It is unlikely that current views will be challenged by any need to accommodate to discrepant information, because the "facts" gathered will not be construed as challenging to our current perspective.

One example from developmental psychology will illustrate this point. Since World War II the divorce rate has risen to proportions that some consider intolerable. Currently in the United States, half of the children born will live some of their developing years in a single-parent family. The rate of illegitimacy is now such that about one fourth of all births are to unmarried mothers. Scientists are not immune to cultural views. Thus, in the 1950s and 1960s, many social scientists looked for evidence of damage to children from "broken" homes. Families without fathers at home were studied extensively for their bad effects on the son's masculinity and were thought to result in poor mathematical skills and poor personal adjustment. Daughters were considered at risk for poor psychosocial development. The implicit, or sometimes explicit, assumption of the investigators of the period was that families without a masculine presence were doomed to inadequacy as rearing environments for children.

Like the eyewitness to a crime, the investigators of father-absent families filled in the gaps in their constructed knowledge by construing outcomes as unfortunate, whatever they were. Thus, sons who were less stereotypically masculine were lamented, as were daughters who were less stereotypically feminine.

Along came the women's movement, and the scientific assumptions about father-absent families changed. Suddenly, we have alternative family forms or nontraditional families (Lamb, 1982). Now, the scientific assumptions are that women are capable both of working outside the home and of being adequate parents for their children. It is no longer a virtue for sons to be supermasculine; they should be "caring males," able to tend children, cook, and clean, as well as work outside of the house, because their adult roles will include shared responsibilities for the home. Daughters who are competent at occupational skills as well as at homemaking are approved as the women of the future. Even the single-parent family may have strengths that were overlooked by a previous generation of investigators. Such virtues as androgyny (having the good characteristics of both sexes) are applauded by social scientists, not because they have been discovered but because they have been invented. Androgyny is the summative virtue of the 1970s, wrought by the women's movement and the Vietnam War.

This example is not intended to parody developmental psychology, which is no more or less susceptible to the foibles of the human perceiver than any other field. Inquiries into the nonhuman subject matter of physics and chemistry may seem less biased by the human observer, because the subject matter seems less directly related to the human condition. But the leaders of research in the physical sciences have been the most vocal commentators on the powerful effects of the human observer on "discovered fact" (see Rorty, 1979). No, we all share the problems of the human knower.

We should not be disturbed that science is constructed knowledge. Rather, the recognition of our own role in scientific knowledge should make more modest our claim to truth as the discovery of everlasting natural laws. Science construed as procedures of knowing and persuading others is only one form of knowing by the rules of one game. There are other games in town, some like art more intuitive, some like religion more determined by revelation and faith. In science there is a more democratic competition of ideas at any one time with a rule of fairness in the procedures that govern the scientists. Unlike religion, there are no revealed truths with claims of unchanging verity.

SCIENCE AS RULES OF KNOWING

In my definition, science is an agreed-upon set of procedures, not constructs or theories. At any one time there are prevailing views with favored constructs to explain and make consistent the facts as we construe them. But it is the procedures for gathering observations (sensory data) that are the rules of the scientific enterprise.

Psychology has developed good techniques to avoid the personal biases of knowers through requirements for reliability and validity. The "facts" must be reproducible across some units of time and across similar populations and situations. Thus, the single eyewitness problem of personal bias and limited perception can be reduced. Observations that are shared among observers and that prove useful can be separated from those that are not useful, are idiosyncratic, and are based on limited experience.

The admission that reality is a construction of the human mind does not deny the heuristic value of the construction. Indeed, we get around in the world and invent knowledge that is admirably useful. But the claim that science and reality are human constructions denies that there is any one set of facts that is absolute and real. Instead, it asserts that there are many sets of "facts" that arise from different theory-guided perceptions.

Proximal and Distal Variables: Is One Set More Real?

Psychologists have a distinct preference for proximal variables to explain behavior. From the 1920s until the last decade, most of our theoretical lenses had a very short focus that blurred or ignored distal events, at both biological and sociological levels of analysis. Even though our horizons have expanded, most psychologists retain a preference for nearby causal explanations. We should question the wisdom of this near-sightedness.

In the 1970s Bronfenbrenner rediscovered the other social sciences and urged psychologists to incorporate expanded views of the context in which development occurs. Children have not only an immediate family but contexts of neighborhood, community, and society in which they do or do not get medical care, day care, and school lunches. Parents have work lives and friendship groups that affect how much time of what quality they spend with the children, and so forth. It seems to me that a sociocultural level of analysis is essential to understanding behavior.

The lifespan developmentalists have expanded the sociocultural view to include cohort and historical facts about behavior. It is not the same to be 20 in 1985 as it was in 1935 or 1965. The Great Depression and the Vietnam War presented their generations with realities different from the Reaganomics we now face, for better or for worse.

Behavior geneticists, ethologists, and neurobiologists have reminded psychologists of biological effects on behavior and the importance of evolutionary theory for psychology. After all, how can we understand attachment, intelligence, or sexual attraction without a consideration of the evolved nature of the human being and his or her genetic individuality? How can we understand mind without brain?

It seems to me that we should use whatever we know to illuminate the questions at hand, as long as we keep our levels of analysis straight. Some psychologists' variables are neurological; others are sociological. As long as they know that the systems with which they deal are organized at levels other than a behavioral one, I consider their facts theoretically related to psychological facts. At least, I must account for their facts when I build theories at a behavioral level.

Problems arise, however, when levels of analysis are confused. Different levels of analysis do not compete. Each lower level is a constituent of the next higher, and in no sense can one account for the other. Yet they are all interrelated with implications for the others. In my view, they are nested "truths." Each level has its stipulated facts that arise from the theoretical framework in which the facts are invented, and each is useful to address questions formulated within that theoretical frame. But the levels cannot compete with or supplant one another.

Rather, hierarchical models of nested theories can account more fully for the behavioral phenomena we cherish. As I will argue later, pitting proximal and distal variables against each other in competing models can enrich our theoretical lives and save us fruitless attempts at intervention.

PERSUASIVE MODELS

Scientific theories are judged by their persuasive power in the community of scientists (Rorty, 1979). They advance and decline through discussions among scientists. Scientists conduct theory-ridden searches for new kinds of observations that become facts more easily within their theories than in the perspectives of competing theories. By this process of fact-building, scientific ideas evolve. By *evolve*, I mean change, not necessarily progress. Rather than accumulate, scientific knowledge may undergo metamorphoses of interpretation (Kuhn, 1970), as when the sun replaces the earth as the center of our universe and the motivation of young children is reinterpreted as basically benign rather than evil and willful. The sociocultural and historical context of the investigator is clearly a major determinant of what is likely to be believed by the investigator and by colleagues. The most persuasive views of the era form the working assumptions of most scientists of that time.

How do models persuade? What distinguishes plausible from implausible models? Most of us would agree on two criteria of plausibility: temporal priority and directional effects. Some models incorporate variables that have clear temporal priority over others, as in longitudinal studies and in studies of the possible effects on children of certain parental characteristics that were established before their children were born. It is implausible to think that a person's motor skills at age 2 were influenced by his or her motor skills at age 14, and it is implausible to think that an individual's friendships in high school were affected by the birth of a child five years later. In Western thought, we accept the idea that the past can affect future events but not the reverse; thus, we are persuaded by temporally ordered rather than disordered models.

Occasionally, models include variables with clearly directional effects that are not subsumed by temporal priority. Some contextual effects, such as those of unemployment rates on adolescents' recreational pursuits and school size on participation in many high school activities, have clear directional effects. It is highly unlikely, under our current assumptions, that unemployment rates are influenced by how adolescents spend their time or that the numbers of students who join teams and clubs determines the size of a high school.

In most theories, fundamental causes do not lie right next to the events they are to explain. Distal variables are better candidates for the status of causes that underlie events in even the most behavioral theories. Distal variables seem to have directional priority over more proximal ones for reasons of temporal priority and "underlyingness." In Western thought, temporal priority is a sine qua non of directional priority and cannot be violated. Although we may refer to backward conditioning, we mean that the organism imparts meaning to its present representation of previous events and alters its response accordingly, not that the causal order of events is truly reversed. The reconstruction of memories is a contemporary reprocessing of present memories, not evidence for present events affecting past events.

In theories of social interaction, distal variables nearly always have causal priority over proximal ones for both temporal and underlying causes. For example, parents' educational levels are more likely to be thought to affect how often they read to their children, rather than that reading to children causes parents to be better educated. More educated parents are more likely to enjoy reading, believe it to be important for children, and carry out a systematic program of reading to their offspring. Although the reverse is not totally implausible (reading to children might increase the parents' reading skills and motivation to obtain more education), this explanatory direction seems less plausible in the absence of other evidence, because we know that most adults complete their education before their children are preschoolers. Thus, there is a continuum of plausibility from completely implausible to probably plausible to really persuasive. The latter end of the continuum of plausibility represents what most psychologists currently believe.

In social and developmental psychology, most of the models we specify about human interactions have variables with neither temporal nor directional priorities that can escape challenge. Rather, parents and children, teachers and students, and siblings and peers are observed to interact and appear to influence each other's behaviors. Currently, psychologists seem to favor proximal over distal variables as more "real" explanations of the effects of people on each other. I want to question our devotion to theories about immediate, proximal events (potentially efficient causes in Aristotle's sense) and propose that underlying causes (final causes in Aristotle's usage) occur at greater distances from behavioral phenomena and often have more profound implications for science and intervention.

Correlated Events

The psychological world in which we conduct research is, in my view, a cloud of correlated events to which we as human observers give meaning. In the swirling cloud of interacting organisms and environments, most events merely co-occur. As investigators, we construct a story (often called a theory) about relations among events. We select a few elements and put them into a study. By so doing we necessarily eliminate other variables a priori from possible analysis, and we preconstrue causal relations among the events. One cannot avoid either the theoretical preconceptions or the selection of variables to study, but one can avoid exaggerated claims for the causal status of one's favorite model.

Take, for example, a problem on which I worked with six distinguished colleagues over the past year—lead (Pb) poisoning in children. Everyone agrees that lead in large doses is not good for children. Lead poisoning damages developing brains. But how much lead is enough to cause noticeable biological and behavioral effects? In other words, how low do lead emissions in gasoline and other industrial products have to be to inflict no lasting damage on the biological and psychological development of children? The economic consequences of this decision involve millions of dollars of industrial products, so that an easy position of "no lead is good lead" will not help in the decisions.

As might be imagined, exposure to lead is not random in the population. As usual, the poor and minorities live closest to lead smelters, live more often in old buildings painted with lead paint, and live closest to heavy motorized traffic. Their exposure to lead is many times that of middle-class suburban children. Figure 1 shows a simplified confound of Pb (X_1) with socioeconomic status (SES; X_2) in the prediction of IQ scores of exposed and unexposed children (Y).

The most notable effects claimed for moderate to low lead exposure are lower IQ and poorer perceptual motor skills. Of course, the very same lower SES children are also reputed to have lower IQ and perceptual motor skills for other reasons, such as poorly educated parents, poor nutrition, child abuse, genes for lower IQ, father absence, poverty,

Figure 1
Illustration of the Confounding of Two Variables,
X_1 and X_2 in the Prediction of Y

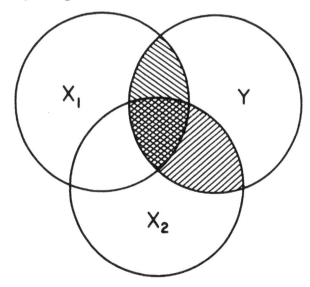

large families. and other afflictions. In other words, lead exposure is *confounded* with a host of other bad conditions, each of which may be independently correlated with lower test scores. How then shall we assess the effects of lead exposure?

Necessarily, some of the variance between lower SES and Pb exposure is truly confounded (the cross-hatched area in the figure) and cannot be disentangled. Psychology has developed various fancy statistical techniques, called covariance and regression models, to deal with correlated predictors such as SES and lead exposure. These techniques can allocate confounded variance among the correlated predictors, but they cannot provide a reliable estimate of the effects of any one variable as it would behave if it were isolated from the others.

In recent studies, investigators have entered a few or several confounding variables into the regression equation before the entry of Pb exposure. Unfortunately, the prior entry of confounded SES variables can underestimate the effects of Pb by attributing to SES the truly confounded variance. In the real world, if poverty means exposure to lead, among other disadvantages, then such an analysis will mask the effects of lead per se.

On the other hand, inadequate controls for the SES and other variables through fallible measures can overestimate the effects of Pb. If parental SES is poorly assessed, its imperfect reliability will leave some of the confounded variance to Pb. Exaggerated claims for lead effects can result.

Studies of naturally exposed and unexposed children, who differ on a host of other variables that can independently affect outcomes such as IQ, *cannot* provide perfect estimates of the effects of low to moderate lead exposure per se.

Direct and Indirect Inferences

An excellent article on the problems of causal inference from field studies by Feldman and Hass (1970) highlighted the differences between experimental and correlational research. Each design has virtues and deficiencies in the direct and indirect inferences that can be made. Correlational studies sample existing groups and describe their differences on one or more dependent variables. From correlational studies we can make direct inferences about naturally occurring differences between groups but only indirect inferences about the causes of those differences. Thus, from the studies of children with low to moderate lead exposures we can make direct inferences about existing differences but only indirect inferences about the underlying causes of those differences. Experimental studies can make direct inferences about the situations in which differences *can* occur but only indirect inferences about how they *do* occur in existing populations.

In field studies of lead exposure, we can describe the correlated cloud of events that differentiate lead-exposed from nonexposed children, but we can make only indirect inferences about why those differences occur and what role lead exposure plays. An experimental approach would permit direct inferences about the possible effects of Pb. Of course, we cannot experimentally expose random samples of the population to lead, so the isolated effects of lead exposure per se cannot be ethically studied in human populations. Even if we could experimentally vary lead exposure in human populations, we could make only indirect inferences about lead effects in existing populations. Such experimental studies would be open to competing hypotheses, such as the differential susceptibilities of some groups to the ill effects of Pb exposure, possible interactions of lead and nutrition, lead as a cause, rather than a result, of existing SES differences, and so forth. Both correlational and experimental studies would seem to be required to permit direct inferences about existing group differences and about the causes of those differences. I will show, however, that problems of causal inference will not be solved by even so grand a strategy.

PLAUSIBLE AND IMPLAUSIBLE MODELS

Suppose that an investigator decided to study the effects (beware already!) of parental management techniques on children's intellectual and emotional development. The investigator has read Bell (1979) and Baumrind (1971) and is prepared to think that children may have some reciprocal effects on their parents as well. To avoid the more obvious problems of correlational studies, in which the direction of effects is hopelessly muddled, the investigator chooses temporal priority to order the variables. The study will be longitudinal and will show the relative impact of parental behaviors at Time 1 on children's behaviors at Time 2 and the effects of children's behaviors at Time 1 on parental behaviors at Time 2—the familiar cross-lag analysis.

Now suppose that the investigator decided to take both proximal measures of the interactions of parents and their children and more distal measures of parent and child characteristics that are not bound by the interactional situations. Having been influenced by trait theories of intelligence and personality, the investigator tests cross-situational traits and situational variables in explanatory models of parent–child reciprocal influence.

Parental Predictors

In an actual study, based on the above model, my colleagues and I looked at two proximal parental variables: maternal control of children rated from 15-minute observations of teaching situations, and scores from interviews with mothers about their methods of disciplining their children in the face of typical misbehaviors.[1] Both measures have suitably high reliabilities and have been scored to yield a positive to negative dimension of parental management techniques. At the positive end are reasoning, explaining, and other verbal ways of dealing with young children. At the negative end is physical punishment. In the middle are various moderate to severe forms of admonishment.

The prediction of children's Stanford-Binet IQ scores over an 18-month period (Time 1 to Time 2) is quite good. Both positive control techniques observed and positive discipline scored from the discipline interview significantly predict children's IQ concurrently ($rs = .42–.49$) and 18 months later, with an R^2 of .23 (see Figure 2).

Psychologists with a proximal model might stop there, write their papers, and "prove" that positive parental management has a beneficial effect on intellectual development. The inference usually drawn from this sort of result is that parents who do not manage their children in positive ways could have more intelligent children if they did. The implications for intervention with parents are implicit, if not explicit. If only psychologists could help all parents to behave positively toward their children, their children would turn out to be brighter. As the editor of a developmental journal, I receive many papers of this sort.

As an investigator, however, I could not resist examining the following result, shown in Figure 3. When two more distal variables, the mother's education and her vocabulary score on the Wechsler Adult Intelligence

[1]Research on mother–child interaction is part of a larger project in collaboration with Kathleen McCartney, J. Conrad Schwarz, Elizabeth Hrncir, Barbara Caparulo, David Furrow, Conchita Ming, the staff of the Child Development Project of Bermuda, and Michael Radford, consultant to the project.

The 125 families from whom the data were collected are 94% of all eligible families with young children in the parish of Devonshire, a representative sample of Bermudian families. Additional information about the project can be obtained by writing to Sandra Scarr, Department of Psychology, Gilmer Hall, University of Virginia, Charlottesville, Virginia 22901.

Figure 2
Proximal Maternal Behaviors as Predictors of Child's IQ

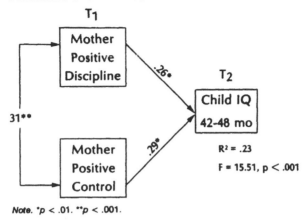

T₁

Mother Positive Discipline

.26*

T₂

Child IQ 42-48 mo

R² = .23
F = 15.51, p < .001

31**

Mother Positive Control

.29*

Note. *p < .01. **p < .001.

Figure 3
Proximal and Distal Maternal Predictors of Child's IQ

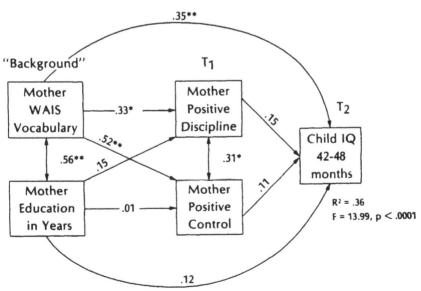

.35**

"Background"

T₁

T₂

Mother WAIS Vocabulary

.33*

Mother Positive Discipline

.15

Child IQ 42-48 months

.56**

.52**

.31*

R² = .36
F = 13.99, p < .0001

.15

Mother Education in Years

.01

Mother Positive Control

.11

.12

Note. *p < .01. **p < .001.

Scale (WAIS), are put into the equation, the mother's IQ dominates the prediction of her child's IQ. The mother's IQ determines in large part how she behaves toward her child in the teaching situation and contributes to her discipline techniques. Her educational level is of little importance to her behavior or to her child's IQ, once her own IQ is estimated from her vocabulary score. The only significant predictor of the child's IQ at 3½ to 4 years of age is the mother's WAIS vocabulary score.

The implications of this result for improving children's intellectual functioning by intervention in mothers' control and discipline techniques are dismal. Even if we could dramatically improve a mother's positive behaviors toward her child, her improved behavior would have little payoff in the child's IQ score. Although the proximal results promised some payoff for children's intellectual outcomes, a more distal variable undercut that model.

Perhaps this result is peculiar to IQ. Let us look at the children's communication skills, determined by scores from the Cain-Levine Social Competence Scale (Cain, Levine, & Elzey, 1963) that was answered by the mothers. Again, the mother's positive control and discipline techniques at Time 1 predict the child's communication skills at Time 2, as shown in Figure 4. If only all mothers would manage their children in more positive ways, their children would be better able to carry messages, remember instructions, answer the telephone, and tell stories.

Figure 4
Proximal Maternal Predictors of Child's Communication Skills

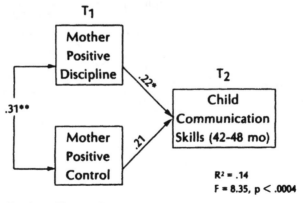

$R^2 = .14$
$F = 8.35, p < .0004$

Note. $^*p < .02.$ $^{**}p < .01.$

Figure 5
Proximal and Distal Maternal Predictors of Child's Communication Skills

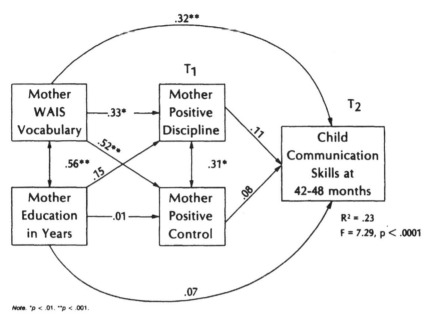

Note. *p < .01. **p < .001.

But again, the importance of these proximal predictors pales in comparison to the mother's vocabulary score, as shown in Figures 4 and 5. Children with good communication scores have mothers with high WAIS vocabulary scores. Any importance of maternal management techniques is mediated by maternal IQ. Mothers who are smarter behave in more benign ways toward their children, and their children have better verbal skills. Improving mothers' discipline and control techniques will not dramatically improve children's language skills, even though the proximal results seemed to offer this hope.

Perhaps these results apply only to cognitive outcomes for children. Let us look at social adjustment. The Childhood Personality Scale (Cohen & Dibble, 1974) was rated by both mothers and observers. The average of their scores was entered into a principal components analysis, which resulted in one large dimension of social adjustment—high expressiveness and attention and low apathy and introversion—as shown in Table 1.

Figure 6 shows that positive maternal discipline predicts a well-adjusted child. Mothers who handle their children in benign ways have

Table 1
Social Adjustment Factor: Combined Ratings of
the Childhood Personality Scale by
Mothers and Raters

Component	Rating
Attention	.61
Expressiveness	.76
Introversion	−.81
Apathy	−.80

Note. The eigenvalue is 2.26.

Figure 6
Proximal Maternal Predictors of
Child's Social Adjustment

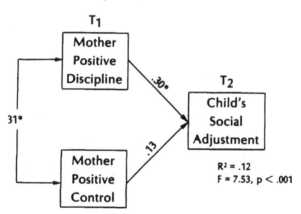

Note. *$p < .01$.

children who are more expressive and attentive and less withdrawn. The relationship between positive maternal discipline and child adjustment is sustained after the two maternal IQ and education variables are entered into the equation. This model is shown in Figure 7. Maternal vocabulary does not make a statistically reliable contribution to the child's social adjustment, apart from its contribution to the mother's discipline techniques. Changing mothers' discipline and control techniques could have some payoff for children's social adjustment.

Thus, we can see that the proximal variables of maternal control and

Figure 7
Proximal and Distal Maternal Predictors of Child's Social Adjustment

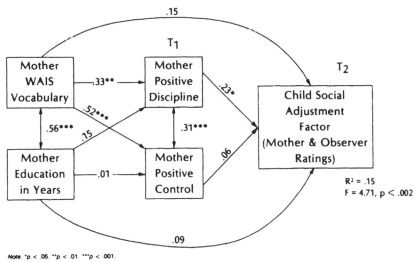

Note. *p < .05. **p < .01. ***p < .001.

discipline techniques can mask the relationships between maternal IQ and the child's intellectual skills but contribute directly to the child's social adjustment. With a theoretical model that included only proximal variables, we could not have perceived a difference in the prediction of children's social and intellectual outcomes. Without testing proximal versus distal variables, we would not have invented differential models for social and intellectual development and potential forms of intervention.

Child Predictors

Now let us examine children's effects on parents, again longitudinally. What effects do what characteristics of children have on their parents' behaviors toward them? I present only the full models to save space. We can see in Figure 8 that cooperative children are also those who score higher on the Stanford-Binet and have better communication and adaptive and self-help skills. In the model with only proximal variables, we would have "found" that children's cooperation in the teaching task was very important in "determining" how their mothers control them while teaching the toy sort (r = .37 over 18 months from test to retest). In the full model, however, we can see that intelligent children "cause" their mothers to behave in positive ways toward them.

Figure 8
Proximal and Distal Characteristics of Children as Predictors of Maternal Control Techniques

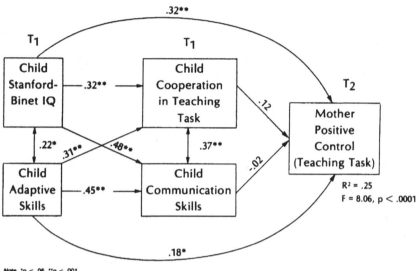

Note. *p < .05. **p < .001.

Children who are intelligent also have mothers who discipline them in positive ways (see Figure 9), according to their mothers' replies to 15 vignettes of typical child misbehaviors. The correlation of the child's IQ with the mother's discipline techniques is .40, both when the child is 24 and 48 months of age. Nothing the child is observed to do proximally controls this much variance in the mother's behavior toward him or her. Although there are positive and statistically reliable relationships between children's proximal behaviors and maternal handling, they are better explained, one might say mediated, by the child's IQ. Little variance is explained by the proximal effects of children's behaviors on their mother's behaviors.

Actually, I do not believe that intelligent children directly cause their mothers to behave more positively toward them, because the model does not take into account the mother–child IQ connection or the connection between maternal intelligence and maternal behaviors. Mothers who are intelligent have children who are intelligent; intelligent mothers behave in more benign and positive ways toward their children, who may also evoke more positive handling from their mothers. The world of parent–child interaction is fraught with inferential pitfalls.

Figure 9

Proximal and Distal Characteristics of Children as Predictors of Maternal Discipline Techniques

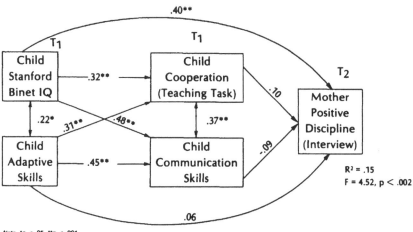

Note. *p < .05. **p < .001.

I can "demonstrate" with the same data that bright children cause their mothers to be better educated. As Figure 10 shows, high-IQ two-year-olds with good communication skills produce mothers with higher educational levels, regardless of whether the children cooperate in a teaching task. Implausible, you say! I agree that this model is implausible, because we have independent information about the educational histories of adults that make it very unlikely for a mother to obtain more education or to drop out of school according to her preschooler's IQ score. To imagine that preschoolers' intelligence determines their mothers' educational levels violates both criteria of plausibility: temporal and underlying.

Confounded Truths

What would our inferences be if we could randomly assign discipline techniques to mothers and cooperation levels to children? Perhaps an experimental design would permit direct inferences about the effects of discipline per se on children and the effects of cooperative and un-cooperative children on mothers' behaviors, without the confoundings of background variables and the co-occurrence of maternal and child characteristics. Unfortunately, as with Pb exposure, such an experiment

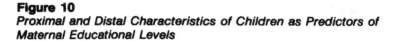

Figure 10
Proximal and Distal Characteristics of Children as Predictors of Maternal Educational Levels

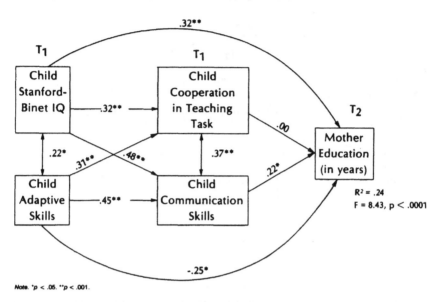

Note. *$p < .05$. **$p < .001$.

would not be feasible, ethical, or desirable. An experiment that divorces behavior from context would not generalize to the population of parents and children in the real world, where all of these variables co-occur. The system in which parental and child behaviors occur *is*, in my view, intrinsically confounded. The truth about this world cannot be simulated by the isolation of single variables, because parent and child characteristics have nonadditive effects on each other (see Scarr & McCartney, 1983; Scarr & Weinberg, 1978). Bright parents have intellectually responsive children and provide a more stimulating rearing environment for them, and the children evoke and generate for themselves more intellectual stimulation than less bright children. One plus one about parents and children does not equal two.

As Feldman and Hass (1970) indicated, experimental and correlational studies provide different kinds of direct inferences. There are causal statements about socially important issues, such as lead exposure and maternal–child behaviors, about which we can make only indirect inferences. I believe that in studies of such events we are limited in the causal inferences we can draw from the cloud of correlated events that appear to us as sensory data. We *must* make inferences about their meaning, but we should be mindful that our "facts" are products of our own theories, and they must compete with others' "facts." Our problems with inference will not be solved by reliance on the complementarity of experimental and correlational studies. Our problems reside in the theoretical lenses of our theories that focus on some pet variables and invent some facts and not others. We are blind to others' theories and facts, even those based on the same observations.

Making Models Plausible

Why do we find the models that claim that parents' and children's *behaviors* affect each other more plausible than the idea that children's intellectual traits affect their mothers' educational levels? Do we have independent information about the effects of parental and child behaviors on one another? I think not. We judge as plausible those models that specify parent–child, proximal behavioral influences because alternative formulations have not been considered, or have been thought illegitimate in recent years. It is unpopular to consider the possibility that most of what we observe about parent–child effects may be determined more by the parents' and child's distal characteristics, especially by genetic variation in their behaviors, than by mutual behavioral influences.

Although mute on the subject of genetic variation in behavior, both Lerner (Lerner & Busch-Rossnagel, 1981) and Wachs (Wachs, 1983; Wachs & Gruen, 1982) propose theories of organism–environment interaction, in which people evoke and experience different environments, based on their own physical and behavioral characteristics. Lerner's and Wachs's views are discrepant from the prevailing psychology of main effects, in which everyone is affected in the same way by the same, observable events. I predict that their views, forecast by Bem (Bem & Allen, 1974; Bem & Funder, 1978) will become the dominant psychological lens of the 1980s. Psychological studies will focus on person-situation interactions and invent new facts about the differential effects of environments on individuals.

A more radical challenge to current theory focuses on genetic variation in behavior. Consider the possibility that the behavior of most parents has little influence on their children's intellectual development. In the absence of neglect and abuse, perhaps children merely develop according to their own genetic blueprints in a supportive environment. Wilson's (1978, 1983) description of a genetic blueprint for intelligence, following Waddington's idea of a growth path, accommodates such "facts" quite well. According to Wilson, the ebbs and flows of intellectual development from infancy to adolescence can be far better explained as features of individual patterns of growth than as the result of any pattern of environmental influence.

Perhaps parents respond to the characteristics of their children in the only ways they know, and bright parents have more benign strategies than others. If one entertains this model, then parental behaviors are more or less correlated with those of their children as an epiphenomenon. If the parents' own characteristics are expressed in their parenting techniques and transmitted to their children genetically, then a correlation of parent and child behaviors can arise without any proximal influence of parents on their children or vice versa. This is an extreme view of the nature of parent–child effects, but is it any more one-sided than the currently popular theories based on pet proximal views? I do not think so.

The theory of genotype → environment effects that McCartney and I presented (Scarr & McCartney, 1983) predicts that children's intellectual and social experiences are largely of their own making. Different people at different ages evoke and actively seek different experiences. In this view, what people experience cannot be indexed by observations of environments to which they are exposed. What people experience in any given environment depends on what they attend to, how much they learn, how much reinforcement they feel they get for what behaviors. And what they experience in any given environment is a function of genetic individuality and developmental status. The additional lenses in this theory are genetic individuality and a developmental program that changes the active genotype across the lifespan, which in turn changes the experiences that people glean from their environments.

The plausibility of theories such as those put forth by Lerner, Wachs, Wilson, and Scarr and McCartney will be judged by the community of psychologists. We will discuss and judge their plausibility, not on any grounds of logical priority but on how consonant such theories are with our historical times and cultural places. To be plausible, they must correspond to other theories of reality and be coherent by the criteria of plausibility.

The remarkable feature of this process of making plausible models is that the same observations that were facts under the previous theories easily become different facts under the new. Facts about people's robust individuality in the face of different environments are invented by naturists from the *same* observations that have been used by nurturists to create facts about people's exquisitive sensitivity to variations in their environments. According to one theory, a child is made of china and can be broken by any environmental blow. In another theory's view, a child is made of magic plastic and can bend under unusual environmental pressures but will not break. Rather than suffer permanent damage from bad experiences, this child resumes his or her shape when released and continues to function without too many dents. Each set of facts is theoretically determined—necessarily so. The nature of the scientific enterprise is to persuade one's colleagues of the plausibility of one's theoretically derived facts.

Is the scientific enterprise, then, a cockpit of competing claims? That is one way to look at it. A more positive view is that science has a distribution of ideas that evolve through competition (Toulmin, 1973). The idea of evolution applied to ideas does not imply that a single view will dominate, however. On the contrary, well-adapted populations of animals and ideas are individually variable. There is no need to choose a single lens for psychology when we can enjoy a kaleidoscope of perspectives. In our own intellectual population we should construct the richest account we can of human behavior, which will include variables from several levels of analysis and alternative theoretical accounts. Because we *do* construct science and reality, we might as well give it breadth, depth, and some excitement.

IMPLICATIONS FOR SCIENCE AND INTERVENTION

Some may fear that the constructivist view of science leads to nihilism and withdrawal from efforts to improve human lives. Are we immobilized by the realization that what we perceive are "facts" of our own making? Can we no longer be agents of change because we recognize the boundaries of our own constructions? I do not think that such pessimism is required by this view. Rather, I think we are obligated as citizen–scientists to make the best theories we can and to act on their implications for intervention.

A constructivist view does imply that diagnoses of problems and intervention strategies are products of their own times and spaces in the same way as any other construction of reality. But that does not make them bad or useless. On the contrary, interventions, like other forms of reality, must be theory driven and must have contexts—social, cultural, and historical. Without a theory of the importance of early experience, we would not have had Head Start. If we had a theory about the importance of adolescence, we might have had Teen Start—which might not have been a bad idea, if it had occurred during the baby boom years when there was a glut of adolescents on the school and job scene. With a theory about the fixity of genetic traits, we had the eugenics movement. With a theory about genetic variability of a probabilistic sort, we could have more respect for individual differences in behavior. With this theoretical lens, we would blame parents less for their problem children and praise them less for their wonderful ones.

If we had recognized the temporal nature of the father-absence problem, we might have acted differently toward black families and teenage mothers. Intervention programs with mother–child families were driven by deficit theories. What if we had viewed father-absent families as blessed by mother–child integration, without the distractions of a sexual partner for mother? (Could this be another kind of sainthood?) Could one conceive of the mother–child household as beneficial for children?

Suppose we had considered alternative theories about early experience and the permanence of everyday traumas. We might have spent less time looking for far-flung sequelae of temporary maternal separations and more time looking at people's current lives. Suppose we thought, like the ancients, that children's sensibilities began at the age of 7. We might have worried less about mother–infant bonding and more about the emotional effects of peer group rejection. If we had considered more distal variables, we might have put more money into effective public transportation than into job training for the unemployed, who could not reach potential jobs even if trained. If we had conceptualized the school problems of blacks in the 1970s as ignorance of the norms of the majority culture, rather than as racial discrimination, we might have launched second-culture programs rather than Affirmative Action.

The effectiveness of the theory-spawned interventions will be judged in the same cultural context that generated the theories in the first place. Therefore, arguments about the efficacy of interventions will take place within a discussable range of beliefs. How can we go wrong? Or right?

Let us examine the disadvantages and the advantages of a constructivist science and intervention. The disadvantage of this view over the current realism is that we may feel less certain of what we are doing. How can we know what is right, if there is no right? The feeling can resemble the loss of faith in a familiar and comforting religion. Theories make conflicting claims that cause us to think and choose—uncomfortable processes for many people. We are thrown onto our own resources to invent a plausible story in the face of certain ambiguity.

The advantage of this view is that we can make more modest claims about the ultimate Truth, which leaves us less embarrassed when other theories replace our favorite view. A second and more important advantage is that we can modify our ineffective attempts to change others' behaviors more easily, because we recognize that we may have constructed the problem inappropriately for the time and space. It makes easier the invention of other questions and other approaches to a perceived problem.

The implication of this appraisal of science and policy is that arguments about intervention strategies are constrained within discussable limits. Conversations about what to do to improve people's lives can take place within a framework of shared images of human nature and proper human relations. This is not to say that important variations are not present in the current cultural ethos. Indeed, vigorous advocates of mental health programs compete for funds with others who advocate medical interventions, better education, and other means by which they optimistically intend to improve people's lives. But no one of any influence calls for public whippings, isolation of babies from their mothers, the reinstatement of slave labor, or a return to the orphanages of yesteryear. No, our current views of human society preclude such popular ideas from the past.

Any given theory and the intervention it launches are of limited usefulness—limited by the sociocultural time and space in which they occur. Why should we expect more? Why should we want more? The major disadvantage of realism in science is that it deludes believers into searching to discover facts that exist apart from theories about them. It seems to me much harder to be flexible in theory construction and intervention strategies if one believes there is a reality out there to be mirrored (Rorty, 1979). A constructivist view frees us to think the unthinkable, because our view of "reality" is constrained only by imagination and a few precious rules of the scientific game. The problem is to persuade our scientific peers and policymakers that our variation on the cultural theme is the wave of the future.

REFERENCES

Baumrind, D. (1971). Current patterns of parental authority. *Developmental Psychology Monographs, 4,* 99–103.

Bell, R. Q. (1979). Parent, child, and reciprocal influences. *American Psychologist, 34,* 821–826.

Bem, D. J., & Allen, A. (1974). On predicting some of the people some of the time: The search for cross-situational consistencies in behavior. *Psychological Review, 81,* 506–520.

Bem, D. J., & Funder, D. (1978). Predicting more of the people more of the time: Assessing the personality of situations. *Psychological Review, 85,* 485–501.

Cain, L. F., Levine, S., & Elzey, F. F. (1963). *Cain-Levine Social Competency Scale.* Palo Alto, CA: Consulting Psychologists Press.

Cohen, D. J., & Dibble, E. (1974). Companion instruments for measuring children's competence and parental style. *Archives of General Psychiatry, 30,* 805–815.

Feldman, C. F., & Hass, W. A. (1970). Controls, conceptualization, and the interrelation between experimental and correlational research. *American Psychologist, 25,* 633–635.

Kuhn, T. (1970). *The structure of scientific revolutions* (2nd ed.). Chicago: University of Chicago Press.

Lamb, M. (1982). *Non-traditional families.* Hillsdale, NJ: Erlbaum.

Lerner, R. M., & Busch-Rossnagel, N. A. (1981). Individuals as producers of their own development: Conceptual and empirical bases. In R. M. Lerner & N. A. Busch-Rossnagel (Eds.), *Individuals as producers of their own development: A lifespan perspective.* New York: Academic Press.

Loftus, E. F. (1979). *Eyewitness testimony.* Cambridge, MA: Harvard University Press.

Rorty, R. (1979). *Philosophy and the mirror of nature.* Princeton: Princeton University Press.

Scarr, S., & McCartney, K. (1983). How people make their own environments: A theory of genotype → environment effects. *Child Development, 54,* 424–435.

Scarr, S., & Weinberg, R. A. (1978). The influence of family background on intellectual attainment. *American Sociological Review, 43,* 674–692.

Toulmin, S. (1973). *Human understanding.* Chicago: University of Chicago Press.

Wachs, T. D. (1983). The use and abuse of environment in behavior-genetic research. *Child Development, 54,* 396–407.

Wachs, T. D., & Gruen, G. E. (1982). *Early experience and human development.* New York: Plenum.

Wilson, R. S. (1978). Synchronies in mental development: An epigenetic perspective. *Science, 202,* 939–948.

Wilson, R. S. (1983). The Louisville twin study: Developmental synchronies in behavior. *Child Development, 54,* 298–316.

4

Risk and Resilience in Early Mental Development

Ronald S. Wilson

University of Louisville
School of Medicine

Mental development scores were examined for two groups of at-risk twins throughout their childhood—those classified as small for gestational age (SGA), and those twins falling below 1,750 g birth weight. The SGA twins showed only a modest deficit in IQ scores as compared to the full twin sample, and thus these small-for-date infants did not appear to be at special risk. The twins below 1,750 g, however, did show a very significant deficit in IQ scores ($p < .001$) throughout childhood. When the recovery patterns were examined for this group, upper socioeconomic status (SES) twins appeared to recover completely, whereas lower SES twins remained significantly depressed. Mother's education was significantly related to recovery from 24 months onward, which suggests that maternal intelligence plays a prominent role in determining the level of recovery. When monozygotic twins of markedly unequal birth weight were compared, the twins who weighed less than 1,750 g attained the same level of IQ scores at 6 years as did their heavier co-twins. Among these genetic replicates, the initially powerful effects of low birth weight did not exert a long-term handicapping effect on mental development. The data argue for

Reprinted with permission from *Developmental Psychology*, Vol. 21, 795-805. Copyright 1985 by the American Psychological Association, Inc.

Preparation of this article was supported, in part, by a grant from the John D. and Catherine T. MacArthur Foundation. I am indebted to Marilyn Riese for a critical reading of the manuscript.

a high degree of resilience in mental development in the face of prenatal stress and for a powerful effect of heritage and home environment in guiding the recovery from early deficit.

Few topics have received as much attention in recent years as that of the infant who is delivered at risk, and the potential handicaps that risk condition may impose (e.g., Lipsett & Field, 1982). Improvements in neonatal care are now sustaining many infants who would have previously died, and many high-risk pregnancies now produce infants who seem to prosper and thrive.

Given the high incidence of prematurity among at-risk infants, it is not surprising to find deficits in early mental functioning. Often such infants are placed in intervention or enrichment programs to help overcome the early deficits. It is also true that many studies of risk infants draw from indigent or low socioeconomic status (SES) populations, where there may be a confounding of pregnancy-related risks with the influence of heritage and home environment.

From the perspective of mental development, there are two basic questions concerning risk and recovery. First, do pregnancy-related risks such as low birth weight and premature delivery impose a long-term deficit on mental development? Second, if not all cases are equally susceptible to risk, what factors determine which cases will recover and which ones will not?

Twins offer a powerful resource to study the relationship between risk and recovery. Twin pregnancies are typically treated as risk pregnancies because of intrauterine crowding and limitations in nourishment for the fetuses. Furthermore, even with improved prenatal care, the incidence of mortality and morbidity for twin births is somewhat higher than for singletons (MacGillivray, 1979).

However, twin pregnancies are spread across the entire spectrum of families, from the disadvantaged to the affluent, and in this sense they avoid the bias of dealing only with indigent families. Furthermore, twin gestation is regarded as something of a clinical test case for many perinatal risk factors that may have both immediate and long-term consequences (Medical Research Council of Canada, 1981). Therefore, a longitudinal study of mental development in infant twins offers a sharply focused opportunity to explore the relationship between risk and intellectual development in a broadly representative sample.

In addition, monozygotic (MZ) twins offer a rare natural experiment with genetic replicates to examine certain risk factors. Specifically, if one twin falls into a clear risk category (say below 1,750 g birth weight), how does this twin's mental development compare with the MZ co-twin who was not in the risk category?

The great advantage of an MZ co-twin control is that it furnishes a direct measure of what the expected level should be for that zygote and thus allows a precise estimate of deficit. In the absence of such matched controls, the assessment of recovery is based on whether the infant reaches the average level for its peer group, and this may overestimate the infant's likely attainments, whether at risk or not.

METHOD AND PROCEDURE

The results reported in this article are drawn from an ongoing longitudinal twin study described in more detail elsewhere (Wilson, 1983). The twins were recruited from the entire socioeconomic range in the metropolitan Louisville, Kentucky area, with a special effort made to retain low-SES families in the sample. Each twin family was assigned an SES score based on the occupational rating scale for the head of household (Reiss, 1961).

The twins were recruited as newborns, and they made periodic visits for testing throughout their childhood. About 30 new pairs were added each year, and the total sample size now exceeds 450 pairs of twins. Zygosity for same-sex twin pairs was determined by blood-typing on 22 or more red-cell antigens (Wilson, 1980). For the full sample, 50.5% of the twins were MZ, and 49.5% were dizygotic (DZ). Measures of birth size and gestational age were drawn from the medical records of the participating hospitals.

Tests and Ages

The twins were administered the Bayley Scales of Infant Development to age 24 months (Bayley 1969), the revised Stanford–Binet at age 3 years (Terman & Merrill, 1973), and the Wechsler Preschool and Primary Scale of Intelligence (WPPSI) to age 6 years (Wechsler, 1967). The twins in each pair were tested by separate examiners and within 2 weeks of their birthday.

The scores on all tests (Mental Development Index [MDI] for the Bayley; IQ for the Binet and WPPSI) were expressed in standard score form, with $M = 100$ and $SD = 16$ (15 for the WPPSI). Due to progressive recruiting, many pairs have not completed six full years of testing, but nearly two thirds of the twins have been tested over at least 4 consecutive years. The patterns of deficit and recovery were thus drawn from cases that had been assessed on a regular basis during childhood.

RESULTS

As a background for interpreting the results from twins at risk, the data for the complete twin sample may be briefly reviewed (Wilson, 1983). The mean mental development scores remained consistently in the range of 89 to 92 between 6 months and 3 years of age, then moved steadily upward to 100.1 at 6 years. Apparently there was a modest but long-sustained decrement in early mental functioning that arose from prematurity of the entire twin sample—on average, the twins were born 2.5 weeks before their due date and were nearly 1,000 g below the average singleton's birth weight.

But from 3 years onward, there was a steady incremental gain in IQ scores that brought the twins up to singleton norms by school age. On a samplewide basis, the effects of prematurity waned in successive years, and individual differences in intelligence were more consistently displayed. By 6 years, the stability of IQ scores for individual twins over a 1-year period was $r = .86$, whereas at 12 months the corresponding measure of 1-year stability was only $r = .48$.

The mental development scores also showed a changing pattern of relationships with certain key variables relating to birth size and family status. Among the latter, birth weight and gestational age were moderately correlated ($r = .52$), but neither showed any significant relationship to parental education or socioeconomic status ($rs < .08$). The degree of prematurity for individual twins was thus spread equally across all social strata represented in the sample. Education and family status was strongly related ($r = .71$), however, and there was a high degree of assortative mating for education among the parents ($r = .68$).

The changing pattern of relationships between these core variables and the twins' mental development scores was of particular interest, because it had a direct bearing on which twins were low scorers initially and which ones later recovered. The correlations were computed at six marker ages, and the results are displayed in Figure 1.

Birth weight and gestational age showed a strong initial correlation with mental test scores—the smaller, more premature infants scored lower during the first year. But these correlations steadily declined until leveling off at .15 by 6 years of age. The individual differences in prematurity that exerted such a strong effect in infancy were ultimately

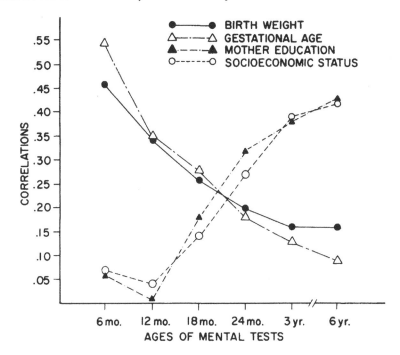

Figure 1. Correlations of demographic variables with twins' mental development scores during childhood.

overcome by school age, and the ordering of IQ scores at 6 years bore only a distant relationship to these measures of birth status.

By contrast, parental education and family status became increasingly correlated with childhood IQ scores, after showing no initial relationship during the first year.[1] As prematurity waned, and as individual differences in intelligence became more securely established, the contributions of heritage and home environment steadily increased as predictors of offspring IQ scores. Thus although prematurity exerted a potent but short-lived suppressor effect, the influences of heritage and home en-

---

[1] Father's education was omitted from Figure 1 because it was a virtual duplicate of mother's education and SES.

vironment seemed to furnish more of a latent resource that was progressively mobilized during childhood.[2]

Risk and Mental Development

With this as a perspective for the entire sample, we turn to those infants who would clearly be designated as at-risk infants. The definition of risk has been subject to some drift in recent years, and as mentioned earlier, working with indigent samples poses a special confounding problem when examining the effects of birth status on long-term mental development.

In the present analysis, two separate but frequently employed criteria of risk were used. The first criterion took into account the link between birth weight and gestational age, and identified those infants who were small for gestational age (SGA). This criterion was intended to detect those infants who had experienced unusual growth restriction as adjusted for length of pregnancy. Any infant whose weight fell below the 10th percentile for its gestational age was designated as SGA.

The singleton norms of Battaglia and Lubchenco (1967) have frequently been used for identifying SGA infants, and consequently these norms were applied to the twins in each category of gestational age.[3] Once identified, these SGA twins were then examined for potential decrements in mental development during childhood. The results are presented in Table 1.

---

[2] It is worth noting that infant mental development as measured in the first year is only distantly related to the elements of intelligence measured at school age. As described earlier (Wilson, 1977), primitive sensorimotor functions are the major component of infant mental development; but as the child matures, the mental functions increasingly resemble the analytic and integrative capabilities of the school-age child. The transition begins to occur after 18 months, and thus a precocious infant will not necessarily hold that advantage to a later age. Similarly, prematurity has its major suppressive effect on early sensorimotor functions but only a negligible effect on later intelligence. Plotting the mental test scores on a common axis does not imply that exactly the same functions are measured at each age. It does, however, signify whether a child is advanced or delayed for the basic capabilities measured at each age and whether an early deficit will automatically pull down the test scores at a later age.

[3] Because the average birth weight of twins fell progressively below the singleton norms as gestational age increased (Wilson, 1985), using the 10th-percentile cutting score produced an unusual distribution of SGA twins. Only two twins qualified as SGA through 34 weeks, but 69 twins qualified as SGA at 39-40 weeks. The majority of SGA twins were thus close to term for date of delivery, but they were considerably undersized by virtue of growth suppression. If intrauterine growth retardation due to crowding and marginal nutrition had a detrimental effect on mental development, it should be evident in this sample.

Table 1

Mental Development Scores For Small for Gestational Age (SGA) Twins

Variable	Ages					
	6 mo.	12 mo.	18 mo.	24 mo.	3 yr.	6 yr.
MDI/IQ scores	91.4	87.3	87.6	89.0	85.4	97.0
Deficit	−0.4	−2.2	−3.3*	−2.2	−5.0**	−4.0**

Note. For the SGA sample, birth weight *M* = 2,120 g; *mdn* gestational age = 39 weeks, *mdn n* for MDI/IQ scores = 110, mo. = month, yr. = year, MDI = 'Mental Development Index.
* *p* < .05. ** *p* < .01, for SGA deficit (*mdn df* = 658).

The SGA twins showed a significant but modest deficit from 3 years onward when compared with all non-SGA twins. In view of the large degrees of freedom, even this difference was of limited importance as a source of variance for individual test scores. When growth suppression was imposed by the special conditions of a twin pregnancy, it had little bearing on long-term mental development. A caveat should be added, however, that some SGA singletons may display long-term deficits, because growth retardation in singletons may be symptomatic of more pervasive developmental problems.

Infants Below 1,750 g

The second main criterion of risk involved all those infants who fell below 1,750 g in birth weight, regardless of gestational age. Many of these infants were very early deliveries (28–34 weeks), but they did not qualify as SGA because their weights exceeded the 10th-percentile weights of Battaglia and Lubchenco (1967).

In 14 pairs, both twins were below 1,750 g. Other cases came from pairs in which the co-twin was considerably heavier than the twin below 1,750 g, and these pairs furnished ideal matched controls for evaluating deficit and recovery in growth-suppressed infants.

Initially, the mental development scores were computed at each age for all infants below 1,750 g. These scores are shown in Table 2, and related demographic variables are shown in Table 3.

There was a very pronounced lag in early mental development for these low-birth weight (LBW) infants; and although the initial deficit of 19 points was eventually reduced to 9 points, there was no evidence of further recovery for this group until these children reached school age. In contrast to the SGA twins, these infants did seem to be at some long-term disadvantage for mental development.

The demographic measures showed that these infants were 975 g

Table 2

Mental Development Scores for All Twins Below 1,750 g Birth Weight

Variable	Ages					
	6 mo.	12 mo.	18 mo.	24 mo.	3 yr.	6 yr.
MDI/IQ scores	74.3	73.6	78.6	82.3	81.2	91.4
Deficit	−19.0*	−17.0*	−12.8*	−9.3*	−9.0*	−9.5*

Note. N = 63; *mdn N* for MDI/IQ scores = 48. MDI = Mental Development Index, mo. = month, yr. = year.
* *p* < .001.

Table 3

Demographic Variables for All Twins Below 1,750 g Birth Weight

Measure	Demographic variables				
	Birth weight	Gestational age	Mother's education	Father's education	SES
Mean values	1,545 g	33.6 wk.	12.4 yr.	12.5 yr.	36.7
Deficit	−975 g	−3.9 wk.	−0.1 yr.	−0.6 yr.	−6.3

Note. N = 63. SES = socioeconomic status, wk. = week, yr. = year.

smaller and nearly 4 weeks more premature than was the full twin sample. In addition, the family measures of parental education and socioeconomic status was somewhat depressed for this sample.

What effect did this stringent selection of at-risk infants have on the relationship between mental development and the demographic variables, as previously displayed for the full sample in Figure 1? If very low birth weight had a pervasive detrimental effect on mental development, it might markedly alter the pattern of relationships.

The correlations were computed at each age, and the results are plotted in Figure 2. Birth weight was omitted because all cases were below 1,750 g, but the other variables were retained intact.

Gestational age showed a strong initial association with early mental development, but after a marked decline over 18 months, the correlations stabilized in the low .20s. The LBW infants born closer to term had higher mental development scores at 6 months, but they maintained only a modest advantage in later years. As in the case of the full sample, this long-term advantage was not substantial enough to reach significance, so the variation in gestational age among LBW twins was ineffective as a predictor of 6-year IQ scores.

By contrast, the variables of mother education and socioeconomic status had a zero-order relationship with mental development in the first

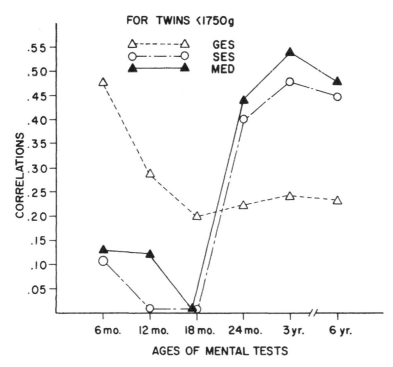

Figure 2. Correlations of demographic variables with mental development scores for twins whose birth weight was less than 1,750 g. (GES = gestational age, SES = socioeconomic status, MED = mother's education).

18 months but then made a precipitous gain at 24 months. Thereafter, the correlations remained in the high .40s, signifying that LBW infants from advantaged homes and parents tended to have higher IQ scores in the pre-school years.

The stringent selection of LBW twins appeared to accentuate and sharpen the original relationship—the curve inflection was much more pronounced and the correlations were higher than for the full sample. It would suggest that the LBW infants making the greatest recovery in mental development were those from advantaged families.

Recovery and Socioeconomic Status

To examine this more closely, the LBW sample was arrayed by SES, and the distribution was divided into three blocks. The upper and lower blocks were designated as high SES and low SES, respectively. The mental development scores were then computed for each group,[4] and the results are presented in Table 4. The accompanying demographic variables for both groups are shown in Table 5.

The mental development scores were substantially depressed in both groups through 18 months of age, and there was no significant difference between groups. From 24 months on, however, the high-SES group gained markedly and their scores significantly exceeded the low-SES group. By 6 years, the mean IQ score for high-SES twins was a full standard deviation above the low-SES mean; and even with a small sample $(n = 17)$, the difference was highly significant.

How did these groups compare with the entire twin sample? The mean mental development scores for each group are plotted in Figure 3.

The curves showed that the upper and lower SES groups moved in parallel through 18 months, then diverged sharply at 24 months. Subsequently, the high-SES group recovered fully to the overall twin mean at 3 years and remained equivalent through age 6.

By contrast, low-SES twins never offset the deficit after 18 months, although they did show the relative upshift between 3 and 6 years that was evident for all twins. Therefore, LBW twins from high-SES families

Table 4

Differences in Recovery for Low-SES and High-SES Infants, All Below 1,750 g Birth Weight

| Group | Mental development scores | | | | | |
	6 mo.	12 mo.	18 mo.	24 mo.	3 yr.	6 yr.
Low SES	73.0	74.1	77.9	75.6	73.6	86.5
High SES	76.8	77.7	80.7	88.2	88.5	101.1
Difference	−3.8	−3.6	−2.8	−12.6*	−14.9*	−14.6**

Note. SES = socioeconomic status, mo. = month, yr. = year.
* $p < .05$. ** $p < .005$.

Table 5

Demographic Variables for Low-SES and High-SES Infants, All Below 1,750 g Birth Weight

| Group | Demographic variables | | | | |
	SES range	GES	MED	FED	N
Low SES	1–25	32.6 wk.	11.4 yr.	10.8 yr.	17
High SES	46–87	35.1 wk.	14.2 yr.	14.5 yr.	17

Note. SES = socioeconomic status, wk. = week, yr. = year, GES = gestational age, MED = mother's education, FED = father's education.

---

[4] For this comparison between SES groups, the scores were averaged in those pairs with both twins below 1,750 g, so that each entry represented an independent case.

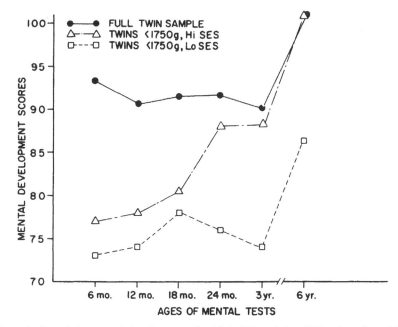

Figure 3. Trends in mental development for high-SES and low-SES twins whose birth weight was less than 1,750 g. (SES = socioeconomic status).

showed complete recovery by 6 years, whereas LBW twins from low-SES families were still significantly depressed below the 6-year norms.

What factors associated with SES might be implicated for these clear-cut differences in mental development? On first glance, the high-SES families would likely have provided a more supportive and stimulating environment during childhood, and this would have promoted a fuller recovery.

This factor was certainly important, but as Table 5 showed, the two SES groups were also substantially different in measures of parental education. The latter was intriguing because education was already in place as a variable when the twins were born, and it furnished an approximate measure of intelligence for the parents.

Multiple Regression Analysis

Accordingly, the three SES groups were recomposed into a single group of LBW infants, and a multiple regression analysis was performed, with four demographic variables as predictors. The analysis identified the single strongest predictor of the mental test scores at each age, then added any subsequent predictor making an independent contribution after the first predictor had been partialed out. The joint predictive value for all variables was expressed as a multiple correlation.

The analysis was performed at three criterion ages, and the results are presented in Table 6.

At 12 months, no predictor variable yielded a significant correlation with the mental test scores, and consequently there was no multiple correlation. At 3 and 6 years, however, all variables except gestational age yielded significant initial correlations with the criterion measures.[5]

The strongest predictor was mother's education, and once it was removed, no other predictor added significantly to the correlation. The partial *r*s ranged from .21 to .26, which for this size sample were too small to be significant. All of the systematic variance was captured by mother's education, and it exhausted the variance otherwise associated with socioeconomic status and father's education. For this risk sample of LBW twins, the strongest linkage between preschool IQ scores and family characteristics was via mother's education, as a presumptive marker of maternal intelligence.

These results generally corresponded to the more extensive results found for the complete sample of twins, as reported elsewhere (Wilson, 1983). In the complete sample, father's education was the strongest pre-

Table 6

Regression Analysis of Four Predictors With Mental Development Scores For Infants Below 1,750 g Birth Weight

| Predictors | Criterion Ages | | | | |
| | 12 months | 3 years | | 6 years | |
	Original *r*	Original *r*	Partial *r*	Original *r*	Partial *r*
Gestational age	.31	.16	.13	.28	.24
Mother's education	.19	.61[a]	—	.60[a]	—
Father's education	.10	.54	.26	.54	.25
Socioeconomic status	.10	.51	.21	.54	.23
Multiple correlation	—	.61[a]		.60[a]	

[a] Mother's education was the only significant contributor to multiple correlation; when extracted, none of the partial *r*s for remaining variables was significant.

[a] $p < .001$.

---

[5] These correlations are slightly higher than shown in Figure 2 due to averaging scores for those pairs with both twins below 1,750 g. See Footnote 4 for explanation.

dictor of 6-year IQ, but both mother's education and SES entered as significant supplementary predictors. With an increased sample size for the LBW twins, it might be expected that all three predictors would contribute significantly to the multiple correlation as well.

Perhaps the crucial conclusion is that measures of parental education and SES related in a powerful way to 6-year IQ scores for high-risk infants, and thereby identified the infants most likely to recover from the effects of very low birth weight. The risk factor did not abolish the basic relationship between family status and offspring IQ; if anything, the stress of very low birth weight may have enhanced the correlation between parental capability and offspring IQ.

Within-Pair Comparisons for LBW Twins

If recovery was significantly related to family-status variables, then how complete was the recovery in pairs that were discordant for risk but matched for heritage and home environment? As mentioned earlier, the unique contribution of MZ twins in assessing risk is that they furnish ideal matched controls on these variables. In pairs with a marked difference in birth weight, as may occur with the placental transfusion syndrome, the deficit imposed by low birth weight and the extent of recovery may be precisely calibrated by comparison of the LBW twin with his or her heavier co-twin.

For this analysis, 12 MZ pairs were selected in which the smaller twin was below 1,750 g, and the heavier co-twin averaged 815 g more than the LBW twin. Because the primary concern was any longstanding decrement in intelligence, the 6-year IQ scores were taken as the criterion measure, and a paired comparison test was performed on the IQ scores of the heavier and lighter twins.

The average deficit for the lighter twins was -2.0 points, which was nonsignificant ($p > .20$), and the within-pair correlation for these discordant MZ pairs was $R_{MZ} = .89$. The latter value was virtually identical to the MZ correlation for the full sample ($R_{MZ} = .88$), so the major birth weight differences for these 12 pairs did not amplify the differences in IQ scores.

Thus these data showed no evidence of a long-term deficit in mental development assignable to low birth weight by itself. Under the most stringent selection of at-risk infants matched with their much heavier genetic replicates, there was no significant deficit in mental functioning. It appeared that the common genotype was able to reach through the inequalities of prenatal growth and bring both twins to a common level.

If there was a residual effect, it was subtle indeed and was not detected by a standard intelligence test.

As a final analysis of risk, the 6-year IQ scores were plotted for all 40 pairs in which one or both twins were below 1,750 g. The smaller twin in each pair was designated as the index twin, and was always below 1,750 g. The heavier co-twin ranged from being very close in weight (and also below 1,750 g), to being nearly twice as large.

For ease of display, the pairs were plotted in blocks according to the magnitude of difference in birth weight. The first block contained those pairs with both twins below 1,750 g; the final block contained those pairs with the heavier co-twin averaging 1,235 g more than the index twin. As shown in Figure 4, MZ pairs and DZ pairs were separately identified, as were the heavier and lighter members within each pair. Collectively, this figure represented all twin pairs in which one or both twins were subject to risk as defined by low birth weight.

Looking first at the score differences within pairs, the MZ twins were generally close and the differences were small—the median IQ difference was 5 points, and the within-pair correlation was $R_{MZ} = .88$. It may be noted that the 12 MZ pairs plotted in the final two blocks furnished the cases for the preceding analysis of large birth weight differences, so there was no change in MZ concordance when all 23 LBW pairs were analyzed. If anything, the score differences were slightly smaller among MZ pairs with large birth weight differences than for MZ pairs closer in birth weight, as plotted in the first two blocks.

Turning to the DZ pairs, the score differences were somewhat larger and the within-pair correlation was $R_{DZ} = .66$, comparable to the full sample DZ correlation of .60. No significant deficit was found in the heavier-lighter comparison—in fact, the lighter twin was slightly higher ($p = .25$). In both zygosity groups of LBW twins, the birth weight differential had no significant effect on measured intelligence at 6 years of age.

If there was any distinctive trend in Figure 4, it was the somewhat lower scores for those pairs plotted in the first two blocks, in which both twins were very lightweight. The mean IQ score was about 11 points below the 6-year norm, and the median gestational age for these twins was 33 weeks, about 4.5 weeks less than the average. For these pairs, the extremes of very low birth weight and early delivery did seem to be linked to some long-terem deficit in IQ.

When these pairs were analyzed more closely, however, a large proportion of the twins (46%) came from the lowest SES families, and the measures of parental education were somewhat lower. Thus the family-status variables linked with incomplete recovery in the prior analyses (Figure 3 and Table 4) were also disproportionately represented among these pairs of very low birth weight twins. The apparent deficit in IQ scores appeared to issue more from family-status variables rather than from low birth weight itself.

From this perspective, it is time to set aside low birth weight as a ready explanation for decrements in IQ. It showed no significant relationship when tested with matched controls, as in the discordant MZ pairs; and on a sample-wide basis, its association with school-age IQ was limited to those pairs in which both twins were very small, the duration of pregnancy was short, and the family-status variables were below average. The question may then be raised whether low birth weight stands in a causal relationship to intellectual deficit via the mechanism of poor prenatal nutrition, or whether it was one symptom in a broader constellation of deficiencies.

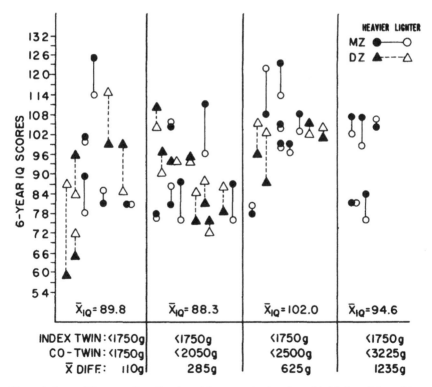

Figure 4. 6-year IQ scores for all pairs with one or both twins with birth weights of less than 1,750 g. (MZ = monozygotic, DZ = dizygotic).

The effects of prenatal malnutrition have been widely studied in recent years, and many of the results are surveyed in a volume edited by Lloyd-Still (1976). It appears that malnutrition interacts with other variables such as socioeconomic status and postnatal care, and it is difficult to weigh its contribution independently of these other factors. Its role is perhaps less ominous than was previously feared.

An auxiliary hypothesis that might be considered is a link between early initiation of labor (and thus premature delivery), and a higher risk potential in the fetus affecting many developmental processes. Premature delivery represents an intermediate step back toward spontaneous abortion, and it might be speculated that such premature infants make up a selective sample prejudiced in one of two possible ways: (2) a poor intrauterine environment that is inadequate to sustain full-term fetal growth, or (b) a fetus that is genetically at greater risk for inadequate development. In the latter case, if the elaborate mechanisms regulating prenatal growth are compromised by marginal instructions in the genetic programming, then the cases most at risk for premature birth may be susceptible to deficiencies in other areas of development. Thus the association between extreme prematurity and below-average intelligence may have a common root at the genotypic level, where the manifold coding of growth processes may have been biased toward higher risk potential (Wilson, 1977).

Risk and Resilence

Although the prior analyses have dwelt on the predictions of which infants will recover fully and which ones will not, perhaps the most heartening feature of these data is the pronounced gain shown by all risk infants up to school age. The effects of risk are not immediately overcome in the first 2 years, but even the low-SES infants showed a substantial upward gain between 3 years and 6 years of age.

There are recuperative capabilities and qualities of resilience even among risk infants that steadily compensate for the burden of prematurity. Such qualities bring into focus the fact that developmental processes are continuous and ongoing, and they possess intrinsic self-correcting tendencies. In fact, Waddington (1971) identified this as one of the cardinal properties of developmental processes.

> The characteristic of the pathways of development . . . is that the course they pursue is resistant to modification. If we act . . . to divert it from its normal course, we find that it

tends, after the initial fluctuation, to get back to the trajectory along which it had begun to travel. (pp. 19–20)

The course of mental development certainly appears to follow this principle—prematurity is a powerful suppressor, but the recovery processes steadily offset the initial deficit and restore the zygote to its targeted pathway. There may be differences in the timing of recovery, perhaps even differences in buffering against the impact of risk conditions; but the main message is that resilience is a prime characteristic of mental functioning. Under supportive conditions, most at-risk infants will recoup from early trauma and progress toward a level commensurate with their targeted capabilities.

REFERENCES

Battaglia, F. C., & Lubchenco, L. O. (1967). A practical classification of newborn infants by weight and gestational age. *Journal of Pediatrics, 71*, 159-163.

Bayley, N. (1969). *Bayley scales of infant development.* New York: Psychological Corporation.

Lipsett, L., & Field, T. M. (Eds.). (1982). *Infant behavior and development: Perinatal risk and newborn behavior.* Norwood, NJ: Ablex.

Lloyd-Still, J. D. (Ed.). (1976). *Malnutrition and intellectual development.* Littleton, MS: MTP Press.

MacGillivray, I. (Ed.). (1979). Proceedings of workshop of International Society of Twin Studies on twin pregnancy. *Acta Geneticae Medicae et Gemellologiae, 4,* 249-382.

Medical Research Council of Canada. (1981). *Report of the MRC committee on clinical trials.* Hamilton, Ontario: Author.

Reiss, A. J. (1961). *Occupations and social status.* New York: Free Press of Glencoe.

Terman, L. M., & Merrill, M. A. (1973). *Stanford-Binet Intelligence Scale: 1972 norms edition.* Boston: Houghton-Mifflin.

Waddington, C. H. (1971). Concepts of development. In E. Tobach, L. R. Aronson, & E. Shaw (Eds.), *The biopsychology of development,* (pp. 17-23). New York: Academic Press.

Wechsler, D. A. (1967). *Wechsler Preschool and Primary Scale of Intelligence.* New York: Psychological Corporation.

Wilson, R. S. (1977). Mental development in twins. In A. Oliverio (Ed.), *Genetics, environment, and intelligence* (pp. 305-334). Amsterdam, The Netherlands: Elsevier.

Wilson, R. S. (1980). Bloodtyping and twin zygosity: Reassessment and extension. *Acta Geneticae Medicae et Gemellologiae, 29,* 103-129.

Wilson, R. S. (1983). The Louisville twin study: Developmental synchronies in behavior. *Child Development, 54,* 298-316.

Wilson, R. S. (1985). Growth and development of human twins. In F. Falkner & J. M. Tanner (Eds.), *Human growth* (2nd ed., pp. 204-208). New York: Plenum Press.

PART II: DEVELOPMENTAL ISSUES

5

Early Experience, Relative Plasticity, and Social Development

Kevin MacDonald

University of Illinois at Urbana, Champaign

This paper examines the roles of early experience and relative plasticity in the development of social behavior in animals and humans. It is concluded that (1) long-term effects of early experience variables can be found in the animal and human literature; (2) there are age differences in the relative susceptibility to environmental influences during development; and (3) the power of environmental events and the buffering ability of the organism are crucial variables affecting the outcome of organism–environment interactions.

The theory of sensitive periods during behavioral development postulates that age-based periods are optimal or most vulnerable to environmental stimulation (Bateson, 1979; Immelmann & Suomi, 1981; Scott, 1979). This theory has guided much research but has come under fire recently from a variety of directions, especially regarding human development (Cairns, 1979; Clarke & Clarke, 1976; Kagan, Kearsley, & Zelazo, 1978; Sameroff, 1975; Scarr & McCartney, 1983). This paper is a review of data and theory relevant to the proper status of this concept in our views of human and animal social development.

Reprinted with permission from *Developmental Review*, 1985, Vol. 5, 99-121. Copyright 1985 by Academic Press, Inc.

I thank Patrick Bateson, Benson Ginsburg, Gilbert Gottlieb, Richard Lerner, Eugene Gollin, Ross Parke, J. P. Scott, and Steven Suomi for their encouragement and advice on previous versions of the manuscript. Send reprint requests to Kevin MacDonald, Department of Psychology, Trinity College, Hartford, CT 06106.

SENSITIVE PERIODS

The concept of a sensitive period hypothesizes age-based periods during which the organism is most vulnerable to environmental stimulation. Bateson (1979) points out that a large variety of terms have been used to describe basically the same phenomenon and that no term has received general adoption. The basic phenomenon is nicely summed up by Bateson (1979) as "the conviction that experience can exert a greater influence at some times of life than others" (p. 470). I will use the term "sensitive period," or speak of relative plasticity, i.e., relative susceptibility to environmental influences. The latter terminology seems appropriate in cases where there is no sharply delimited period of susceptibility to environmental influences, but rather a gradual decline in sensitivity. This model appears best suited to most of the data on early experience covered in this paper.

Although this general description applies to instances of sensitive periods, the term usually refers to behavioral systems in which there is at least some internal control, in the sense of Bateson (1976), over the relative sensitivity to the environment of different ages. For example, Bateson (1976) shows that both internal and external factors are implicated in influencing the onset of the sensitive period for filial imprinting in birds. There is presumably wide variation in the degree of internal and external control of sensitive period phenomena, and different mechanisms in different species for achieving this control (Bateson, 1976; Gollin, 1981). This suggests that there is no rigid distinction between sensitive periods resulting from differences in developmental level and those due to internal maturational change, but rather a continuum from greater to lesser environmental control. For example, an infant's cognitive level may mediate its reaction to verbal stimulation (Uzgiris, 1980) and in turn affect whether stimulation at a particular age has any effect on development. The infant's cognitive level may in turn be influenced by a variety of internal and external events, just as in the case of imprinting in birds.

However, if differential sensitivity to environmental stimuli is controlled completely externally, there would be age specificity (Wachs & Gruen, 1982) but not a true sensitive period. As a possible example of age specificity, Wachs and Gruen (1982) summarize data showing that parental restriction of exploration between 12 and 48 months of age is negatively related to cognitive performance, but there are no effects prior to age 1 or after age 4. The authors note that the lack of effect after age 4 may simply indicate that home restrictiveness becomes less critical as the child gets older and can leave home. Thus finding an effect of an environmental variable between ages 1 and 4 may be due simply to the cultural practice of allowing older children outside the home more often.

Despite the fact that the mechanisms and degree of internal control underlying sensitive periods may differ, there may be some general aspects of sensitive periods which are capable of providing some insights into these phenomena. In particular, I will be concerned with what may loosely be termed the intensity of the environmental stimulus and how this dimension interacts with differential plasticity. Schnierla (1957) was the first to emphasize the importance of the intensity of the stimulus as a general dimension in producing approach–withdrawal reactions. A paradigmatic example relating intensity of stimulus to the notion of sensitive periods comes from work on early handling of rodents. Denenberg (1968) reported data showing that handling or shocking rats with 0.2 mA at 2 days of age was ineffective in raising avoidance learning scores of adult rats, while such stimulation at 4 days was effective. However, if the level of shock is increased to 0.5 mA, an effect is found at 2 days of age. Moreover, handling, a less intense stimulus, is more effective on days 1–10 than on days 11–20. This leads naturally to an "intensity hypothesis" according to which the effect depends on the intensity of the stimulus and the age of the animal, results highly congruent with the notion of a sensitive period as described above. Henderson (1980) points out that the relation between intensity of stimulus and the effect on the organism is curvilinear in the case of early handling, with very high levels of stimulation being associated with deleterious effects on the animal. (See also Hutchings, 1962.)

Another example comes from the imprinting literature. Immelmann (1972) found a sensitive period for sexual imprinting lasting from 13 to 40 days of age for the zebra finch. Birds housed with the foster species during the sensitive period and subsequently housed with conspecifics still preferred the foster species when mating. Immelmann and Suomi (1981) point out that sexual imprinting is reversible but that the degree of reversibility depends on the age at social contact with the bird's own species as well as the duration of the contact. If only 3 or 7 days of contact are provided, the effects of cross fostering are irreversible up to the 40th day of life, but 30 or 60 days are effective as late as 57 or 71 days of age. These results indicate that the intensity of appropriate stimulation, in this case the duration of exposure to conspecifics, is a crucial parameter in reversing the effects of early experience.

As an example of the generality of this phenomenon, intensity of stimulus appears to be a basic feature of social behavior in humans. Early parent–child social interactions involve the regulation of affective arousal. Stern (1977) and Brazelton, Koslowski, and Main (1974) document the fluctuating, cyclic nature of early mother–infant interaction. Interactions typically build to a peak of excitement followed by a period of gaze aversion or withdrawal on the part of the infant when the interaction becomes too intense. Stern states that there is an optimal range for the intensity of social stimulation:

> [T]he stimulus events cannot be too weak, or too powerful, or too simple or too complex, or too familiar or too novel. Successive events cannot be too repetitive or attention is lost and excitement falls below the optimal range, and affect becomes neutral. On the other hand, successive stimuli cannot be too drastically dissimilar or the infant will not be able to engage them cognitively. (p. 72)

This passage emphasizes the fact that in addition to intensity, social stimuli may have other properties which affect their ability to result in affective arousal and thus also quite possibly their impact upon the recipient. Berlyne (1960, 1966), in developing a general theory of arousal, noted that, besides the intensity of the stimulus, such attributes of the stimulus as novelty, surprisingness, incongruity, complexity, and uncertainty affect ability to arouse the recipient. There appears to be a general trend in development for the child to be able to control and modulate higher levels of arousal, i.e., he/she develops an increasing capacity for more intense levels of affectively arousing social stimulation (Sroufe, 1979). Thus, father–child physical play with 3- to 4-year-old children often involves stimulation that would be far too intense for infants (MacDonald & Parke, 1984). Arousal-modulating ability appears to be a fundamental aspect of social behavior. Recently Zentall and Zentall (1983) have proposed that childhood behavior disorders involve deficiencies in arousal-regulating mechanisms and Zuckerman, Buchsbaum, and Murphy (1980) have argued for a general biological trait corresponding to individual differences in arousal due to novel stimuli.

Bateson (1983) gives several examples in which stimuli that are particularly effective in altering behavior can be interpreted as involving the manipulation of the intensity of a stimulus, quite possibly mediated by the emotional effect of the stimulus. Wild horses can be made submissive in as little as 15 min by means of drastic strangulation of the horse with a rope around its neck, and he describes anecdotal cases where similarly severe methods have been used successfully to socialize dogs. Bateson also discusses evidence that brainwashing, religious conversion, and psychotherapy appear to be facilitated by states of arousal brought about by the manipulation of emotionally charged stimuli, and evidence is presented that these effects could be mediated by noradrenergic systems in the brain.

It should be stressed that it is the intensity or duration of an ecologically relevant stimulus that is important. The findings that high levels of noise in the home are negatively related to IQ (Wachs, 1979) does not mean that higher levels of stimulation must be comprehensible to the child and attended to by the child.

Finally, the concept of a sensitive period can be considered to imply differences in the buffering ability of the organism at different ages. As will be seen below, however, some behaviors appear to develop in a wide variety of normal environments, and it is necessary to develop a notion of buffering. A behavioral system is well buffered if and only if there are no environmental events which attune or induce the behavior in the language of Gottlieb (1976) and Aslin (1981). (See also Gollin, 1981.) Following Scarr (1976) the application of the well-buffered model is restricted to normal environmental variation. However, if it can be shown that rearing in even highly abnormal environments results in essentially normal behavior, then the well-buffered model also applies. An example fitting this model comes from Scarr (1976) who argues that sensorimotor intelligence is well buffered since it occurs in a very wide range of human cultures and rearing environments. In addition, some cognitive abilities in monkeys occur even after social isolation (Gluck, Harlow, & Schlitz, 1973).

In this essay I am concerned with evidence for or against the existence of long-range effects of particular early environmental variables and evidence for or against age-based changes in susceptibility to environmental effects. In addition, I discuss aspects of the stimulus that appear important in reversing the effects of early experience and present data showing that some aspects of social behavior are well buffered in the above-defined sense.

SOCIAL BEHAVIOR IN NONHUMAN PRIMATES AND CANIDS

Harlow's group pioneered the investigation of long-term effects of various rearing paradigms in rhesus monkeys. Monkeys reared with peers (together–together) and subsequently housed singly showed several differences in behavior at 7 years of age from monkeys raised with mother and peer contact (Chamove, Rosenblum, & Harlow, 1973). The differences included highly abnormal infant-directed aggression as well as "suicidal" aggression toward adults and juveniles. Monkeys raised with the mother alone for 8 months are described as fairly normal, but with more extreme scores on bodily contact, affection, and aggression than mother–peer raised monkeys (Harlow & Harlow, 1969). The well-known isolation paradigm produces a host of highly abnormal effects in rhesus monkeys, including social indifference with vacant staring, stereotypical movements, self-clutching, aggression, and inadequate mothering (Harlow & Harlow, 1969). The effects of isolation vary between different species of monkeys, indicating variation in the degree of buffering of social behavior. Sackett, Ruppenthal, Fahrenbruch, Hold, and Greenough (1981) found that isolated crab-eating macaques showed a degree of social behavior comparable to nonisolated controls even though in isolation they exhibited behavior typical of the isolation syndrome. Pigtailed macaques were intermediate to the rhesus and crab-eating macaques in showing normal social behavior after isolation.

Long-term effects of separation have been found by Spencer-Booth & Hinde (1971) and Stevenson-Hinde, Zunz, and Stillwell-Barnes (1980) in rhesus monkeys. These effects are species specific, with bonnet macaques showing no signs of behavioral disturbance during or after separation (Kaufman & Rosenblum, 1969). As with the isolation paradigm with monkeys, there are clear indications of species differences in the buffering abilities of the organism.

These data indicate long-term effects of some differences in rearing environments. Other major alterations are consistent with quite normal social behavior, and are examples of well-buffered behavioral systems. For example, Suomi and Harlow (1975) have found normal social behavior in monkeys raised with surrogate mothers but given 2-h periods of interaction with peers 5 days per week (surrogate–peer rearing condition). As another example, Ruppenthal, Arling, Harlow, Sackett, and Suomi (1976) found that although many aspects of maternal behavior were adversely affected by isolation during development, some aspects of maternal behavior occurred even without the motherless mothers being reared by conspecifics or ever seeing the birth of an infant, indicating that these aspects of maternal behavior are buffered against even very extreme environmental disruptions. (Further examples of well-buffered behaviors are given below.)

The canid data using the isolation paradigm of rearing without adults suggest considerably more buffering than is the case with rhesus monkeys. Wolf cubs reared without parents show all the normal behavior of the species (Rabb, Woolpy, & Ginsburg, 1967). Fuller (1967) and Fuller and Clark (1966a, 1966b) isolated beagles and wirehaired terriers from 3 to 16 weeks and then subjected them to four 7-min arena tests each week until week 19. Comparison to controls showed a diminution of treatment effects over the testing period for beagles, with wirehaired terriers completely unaffected by isolation. Handling the animals gently before the arena tests resulted in almost completely normal behavior for the beagles, suggesting that behavioral deficits were the result of stress consequent to emerging into a strange environment rather than due to any basic behavioral deficit. Fox (1971) found that dogs reared with cats from 3½ to 16 weeks of age showed deficits in reacting to their own species, but showed recovery within 2 weeks, at which time socialization was complete. Cairns and Werboff (1967) also found normal mating behavior in 4 of 6 female dogs paired with a rabbit from 4 to 9 weeks of age. In a second experiment, Fox (1971) reported that dogs hand reared from birth and isolated from 3½ to 12 weeks of age tended to be deficient in play behavior with other dogs, but recovery was rapid, and deficits are described as occurring only early in the period of socialization. In addition, MacDonald and Ginsburg (1981) found that wolves with restricted rearing from 4 weeks of age to 24 weeks of age showed immediate cessation of stereotyped behaviors common during isolation as well as rapid occurrence of normal play behavior when paired with conspecifics. The buffering of behavioral development is not complete, however, since isolation of dogs from 4 weeks to between 8 and 24 months of age has been shown to result in persistent behavioral disturbances (Melzack & Thompson, 1956; Thompson & Heron, 1954), an effect possibly due to the length of the isolation treatment or breed differences in susceptibility to the effects of isolation. In addition, several studies have shown that isolated dogs are subordinate to normals and less aggressive (Fisher, 1955; Fuller, 1967), and MacDonald and Ginsburg (1981) found that isolated wolves tended to have exaggerated personalities compared to controls. Long-term effects on the socialization of dogs to humans have also been found (Freedman, King, & Elliot, 1961), and Pfaffenberger and Scott (1959) found long-term effects of early confinement in a kennel on later reaction to unfamiliar situations and ability to accept training.

There is considerable evidence that the age of the animal is a crucial interactant in whether long-range effects occur, although in several cases it cannot be concluded that there is differential sensitivity to the environment as a function of age. The effects of isolation in rhesus monkeys are more profound if isolation lasts until 12 months of age rather than only 6 months, and isolating the animals only for the first 3 months of life has no important long-range consequences (Harlow & Harlow, 1969). Although these results are consistent with a cumulative effect of isolation as proposed by Bloom (1964) for the effects of deprivation on cognitive development, isolation early in life presumably is far more devastating in its effects on social development than isolation of juveniles or adults. The age of peer separation is also crucial, with juvenile rhesus monkeys showing very little reaction to repeated peer separations (McKinney, Suomi, & Harlow, 1972), although if the animal shows strong attachments to the group from which it is separated, much more depressive behavior is observed (Suomi, Eisele, Grady, & Harlow, 1975). Ruppenthal et al. (1976) found that the effects of isolation rearing on maternal behavior showed an inverse relationship between age of initial introduction to conspecifics and the probability of adequate maternal behavior. Finally, a sensitive period for the effects of separation from the mother has been indicated but not rigorously delineated (McKinney, Kleise, Suomi, & Moran, 1973).

Freedman et al. (1961) demonstrated a sensitive period for the socialization of puppies to humans by showing that exposure to humans for 2-week periods was most effective between weeks 5 and 7 and relatively ineffective before or after this age. If animals were not exposed to humans prior to the 14th week, socialization did not occur despite continued handling. Fourteen weeks of age was also the cutoff point for producing the effects of the kennel dog syndrome (Pfaffenberger & Scott, 1959), and age is an important variable in socializing wolves (Woolpy & Ginsburg, 1967).

The evidence for long-term effects of early experience and age-dependent differential sensitivity to environmental effects does not, of course, preclude important interactions with later experience. In the case of well-buffered behavioral systems, as described above, simple restoration of the normal environment is sufficient to result in normal behavior. However, the normal environment is not sufficient to alter the behavior of isolate-reared monkeys. Here intensive therapy over a 26-week period involving younger therapist monkeys resulted in essentially normal behavior in these animals (Novak, 1979; Suomi & Harlow, 1972). A follow-up study (Cummins & Suomi, 1976) found no differences between the rehabilitated isolates and mother–peer raised animals at 2½ years, except that the isolates still engaged in more self-clasping. Novak (1979) found that rehabilitated male monkeys failed to perform the double foot clasp mount essential to reproduction, but could interact normally in other ways with age-matched monkeys. Suomi, Delizio, and

Harlow (1976) successfully rehabilitated separation-induced depressive disorders in rhesus monkeys by providing them with opportunities to interact with same-age monkeys. Finally, Woolpy and Ginsburg (1967) successfully socialized adult wolves long after the optimal age for socialization by a method of gradual habituation.

Two aspects of the stimulus situation appear to be relevant to producing interactions with later experience. First, the stimulus must be ecologically appropriate. Suomi and Harlow (1972) state that the success of the therapy of isolate-reared monkeys was because therapists at 3 months of age emitted appropriate behaviors—social clinging, primitive play, and lack of aggression—which the isolates need. In the peer-separation experiments, same age monkeys were appropriate therapists because the subjects already had a normal repertoire of social behavior.

Second, there is evidence that what one might broadly refer to as an intensity dimension, as described above, is relevant. Suomi et al. (1976) found that increasing the number of interaction sessions and the number of social partners was necessary to reverse separation-induced depressive disorders in rhesus monkeys. The method of Woolpy and Ginsburg (1967) involved the regulation of the affective state of the animal by ensuring that the animal was not overwhelmed by emotionally arousing stimuli. The goal of the therapist was to overcome the fear of the animal by gradually increasing the levels of social stimulation. The duration of the stimulus is also clearly important in producing the effects of isolation, since 12 months of isolation is far more devastating than 6 months (Harlow & Harlow, 1969) and is presumably a factor in successful therapy as well.

The animal data clearly do not result in any general principles regarding the importance of early experience in development. There are wide variations between species in the importance of early experience, later experience, and the degree of genetic buffering of the behavioral phenotype. Plotkin and Oldling-Smee (1981) point out that all aspects of the developing phenotype, including the capacity to respond to particular stimuli at particular ages and the relative buffering from environmental effects, are nested within the genetic level of analysis. This means that although the information gained by the organism via interactions with the environment is not passed on genetically, the capacity to do so must be. Plasticity itself must therefore be viewed as a biological adaptation with a genetic basis that has been subject to natural selection. Intraspecific and interspecific differences in plasticity resulting from genetic variation are to be expected. Behavioral plasticity is a two-edged sword: An organism with a high degree of plasticity is able to respond to environmental contingencies but is also susceptible to environmental variations that may be maladaptive. The adaptiveness of plasticity must ultimately depend on a general tendency for environmental programming of phenotypes to be a reliable route to adaptiveness. For example, the ethological theory of attachment proposes an "environment of evolutionary adaptedness" which resulted in the reliable production of adaptive phenotypes in children. However, since the system relies heavily on environmental contingencies, maladaptive environmental programming of phenotypes is an important possibility, especially in view of the massive changes in the social and economic environment that have occurred during the course of human evolution (MacDonald, 1984). Natural selection has apparently resulted in quite different degrees to which even the advanced social mammals require stimulation during development in order to develop normative phenotypes. Moreover, within a species some social behaviors, such as some aspects of maternal behavior in rhesus monkeys, may develop even in extremely abnormal circumstances while other aspects seem to be much more susceptible to environmental disruptions (Ruppenthal et al., 1976). Finally, behavior genetic analysis has shown the potential importance of individual genetic differences in response to environmental input. Thus Ginsberg (1969) reported results showing that early handling during a sensitive period has major effects on some inbred mouse strains but not others. Individual genetic differences may well be one important reason for the wide range of outcomes reported in the human literature on early experience (see below).

In summary, the data for monkeys and canids suggest considerable buffering of normal social behavior from the effects of some types of behavior even in highly abnormal environments, but that for some species environmental influences can have long-range effects during sensitive periods, after which complete remediation is difficult and depends on the ecological appropriateness of the stimulus situation as well as on what has been described as an intensity dimension. The data show that natural selection has resulted in species differences in the importance of early experience, the extent of behavioral buffering, and the susceptibility of the organism to environmental influences during development.

SOCIAL BEHAVIOR IN HUMANS

Much research on humans on the effects of early rearing experiences has focused on a proposed necessity for appropriate attachment behavior during the early years. This view was originally proposed by Bowlby

(1951) and was based on data showing profound effects of rearing in certain orphanages. These early studies have been widely criticized on methodological grounds and as confounding a great many variables, particularly the conditions within the institution, repeated separations, and age at institutionalization (Bronfenbrenner, 1968; Casler, 1968; Clarke & Clarke, 1976; O'Conner, 1968). Casler (1968) suggests that long-term effects of institutionalization are due to stimulus deprivation. This would also indicate a pervasive effect of early experience. Nevertheless, recent data from studies of children in more adequate institutions suggest that long-range effects due to abnormal attachment may indeed occur.

These data derive primarily from studies of children who have been adopted or institutionalized and are in some ways far from ideal. Dependent measures are often of questionable reliablity and validity, unlike the case with the attachment construct used in developmental research where major efforts have been undertaken to address these problems. (See for example Waters, Wippman, & Sroufe, 1979). At present, research using the strange situation paradigm has not experimentally manipulated variables such as age and attachment experience in order to determine the relative plasticity of attachment classification at various ages, and long-term continuity of behavior may well be due to current rearing conditions rather than an early sensitive period (Lamb, Thompson, Gardner, Charnov, & Estes, 1984). The available data from studies of institutionalization and adoption have not been derived from the strange situation procedure, but the data are reasonably consistent and have been used to minimize the importance of early experience. (See, for example, Cairns, 1979; Clarke & Clarke, 1976; Kagan et al., 1978.) In the following section these studies are reviewed in order to show that the data are consistent with long-term effects of some early experience variables and differences in relative plasticity in development.

Wolkind (1974) found that admission to an institution prior to 2 years of age was significantly associated with disinhibition, "a mixture of superficial overfriendliness and inappropriate reaction" in an interview. Of 43 children admitted prior to 2 years of age, 17 showed disinhibition, while of 49 admitted after age 2, only 2 showed disinhibition. Antisocial behavior did not show this relationship, although rates of antisocial behavior were quite high for the sample as a whole. The author interprets the data as showing a long-range effect of lack of normal attachment prior to age 2.

Tizard (1978) studied children from an institution that discouraged close relationships with the adults, but was otherwise considered stimulating. At follow-up at age 8, about half of the sample of adopted children showed behavioral abnormalities, including a higher prevalence of indiscriminate affection and poorer ratings by teachers for socialization with other children, irritability, and restlessness. Many of the children had normal attachments with their adoptive parents and the parents were generally satisfied with the adoptions. These results are congruent with animal data, summarized by Cairns (1979), showing that attachments can develop quite late in life. The difficulties appeared to come more in relationships with other adults and with peers. The author concludes that the first 2 years of life may be critical in shaping normal attachment behavior, but it is not known to what extent the results are irreversible. A previous study based on the same data and sometimes cited to support the lack of long-range effects of abnormal attachment behavior (Clarke & Clarke, 1976) and performed by the same author (Tizard & Rees, 1975) in fact strongly suggested pathological effects of early institutionalization. The earlier data were interpreted as showing no differences in a total problem score between institutionalized children and working class controls. In fact, however, these two groups showed quite different types of problems, with the institutionalized children scoring higher on poor concentration, problems with peers, temper tantrums, and clinging. Attachment behavior was more immature in the institutionalized group, and the institutionalized children were described by nurses as having shallow affections. The authors also describe these children as showing the disinhibited behavior noted by Wolkind (1974): shallow, indiscriminate overfriendliness.

Recently these conclusions have been replicated by Dixon (unpublished; discussed in Rutter, 1982). This study is notable because it used many of the same measures as Tizard, used direct observations rather than ratings, and contrasted children raised by foster parents with children raised in residential nurseries. Both groups differed from normals, but children raised in the residential nurseries without the opportunity to form attachments were much more deviant.

Two studies suggest that early institutional rearing does not preclude good adjustment if the child has an adult figure with whom he/she can form a lasting and deep relationship. Wolins (1970) found that good adjustment in two orphanages was not generally associated with early versus late admission but was associated with a "warm, close relationship" with adults or older children inside the institution. Similarly Pringle and Bossio (1960) found that good results were associated with "a friend outside." All five children with an adult relationship were described as well adjusted. The authors concluded that the child who is rejected early in life and remains unwanted is likely to become insecure, maladjusted, and educationally backward. Some such children were described as having "affectionless character" as noted in the studies of Tizard and Wolkind described above. These studies suggest that institution rearing is compatible with a good outcome if the emotional needs of the child are met in the institution but clearly cannot be used to argue that early attachment relationships are unimportant.

Moreover, if intervention is particularly intensive and ecologically appropriate, minimal maladjustment can be expected, results quite consistent with a theory of differential plasticity. Flint (1978) substantially reversed the decline in social behavior in a group of institutionalized children with a program emphasizing a very high child–staff ratio, a particular adult to whom the child was special, as well as a large number of professionals. Particularly noteworthy was the inclusion of relatively intense, affectively arousing physical styles of play into the intervention program. Recent research has shown physical play to be common between parents, particularly fathers, and children, and may well represent an important biological adaptation between parents and children (MacDonald, 1983, 1984). (See Parke & Suomi, 1981, for a review). Such play is extremely arousing and affectively salient to the child and has been found to be associated with social competence in children (MacDonald & Parke, 1984). This may well be a case in which increasing the intensity of social stimuli had therapeutic effects. Yet despite up to 2½ years of intensive intervention and subsequent adoption and follow-up support, the children showed lower Vineland Social Maturity scores at all ages up to age 15. Although this may have been the result of staff encouragement of dependency, case study data show continuing, long-term inadequate peer relations and maladjustment for some.

Adoption studies are often interpreted as involving separations from an established relationship or as involving multiple caretaking and hence as possibly involving abnormal attachment. Several studies often cited as showing the lack of effect of early experience in fact suggest lingering pathology in many cases. Rathbun, DiVirglio, and Waldfogel (1958) presented data showing considerable resiliency in foreign adoptees after being adopted in the United States: "With a few exceptions" they were described as not suffering from frozen affect or indiscriminate friendliness. Nevertheless, nothing was known of their previous history and the authors caution that the sample was nonrandom and that the children may have been selected on the basis of ability to cope with stressful conditions and the presence of good relations with people before adoption. A follow-up study (Rathbun, McLaughlin, Bennet, & Garland,

1965) reported the adjustment of 12 of 33 individuals was problematic or disturbed. Some children who were disturbed soon after adoption became well adjusted, but the authors depict a second pattern in which older children with poor adjustment originally were rated as problematic on follow-up, suggesting less malleability in the older children.

A study by Kadushin (1970) is often cited as showing the resiliency of older adoptees. However, the criterion of success used was the satisfaction of the parents. The data do suggest the feasibility of later adoption but also indicate long-term effects of early adversity. For example, 60% of the parents believed their adopted children were set in their ways. Abnormal separation anxiety was often observed and several showed the shallow, indiscriminate affection noted in several studies discussed above. Moreover, the older the child at the time of placement, the greater the prospects of unfavorable outcome, data highly consistent with declining plasticity regarding the molding of social behavior. A recent study by Cadoret and Cain (1980) points out how very early breaks in caretaking can have long-range effects. These investigators found that multiple mothering during the first 3–6 months of life was associated with antisocial behavior at age 10–17. These infants were separated at birth from their mothers and reared at a university-run orphanage until adopted. During this period they were cared for by 17–30 students in 5-day rotation. This relationship between multiple mothering and later antisocial behavior remained when effects due to antisocial personality, alcoholism, and other psychiatric disorders in the biological and adoptive parents and adoptive siblings, as well as divorce or separation in the adoptive parents, were partialed out.

Earlier literature, summarized by Pringle (1966), gives overwhelming evidence that age of adoption is an important variable: Later adoptions have less favorable outcomes and children adopted late have increased risk of behavior disorders. A recent review (Hersov, 1977) also concludes that adopted children are more often represented in psychiatric populations and that the diagnosis of antisocial behavior or conduct disorder is often made. While experience prior to placement is merely one of several factors implicated in these results, the adoption data do support the conclusion that major breaks in caretaking may have long-range effects.

Long-term effects for separation due to long or repeated hospitalization during childhood have also been found. Douglas (1975) and Quinton and Rutter (1976) both studied large independent samples of children retrospectively. Douglas found an association between long or repeated hospitalization and troublesome behavior, poor reading, delinquency, and unstable job pattern during adolescence. Furthermore, a sensitive period for these effects between 6 months and 3 years of age was indicated. This time span fits well with data showing that strong attachments do not begin until the latter part of the first year (Bowlby, 1973). Quinton and Rutter found similar long-term effects, even after correcting for family discord, a factor not included by Douglas. Both studies included several other variables, such as socioeconomic class, later hospitalization, and size of family, and both conclude that there is strong evidence for a causal relation between the outcome measures and early hospitalization.

The above case studies indicate long-term effects of particular environments in many cases, but it is important to note that the effects are by no means universal. Less than half of the subjects in the Wolkind (1974) study were adversely affected, and in the Tizard (1978) study between 39 and 69% of the sample exhibited problem behaviors. In the studies of Douglas (1975) and Quinton and Rutter (1976) only about 40% of the subjects were adversely affected. These results suggest that other factors are involved in the outcome, and recent research on vulnerability (Werner & Smith, 1982) suggests that many factors affect resiliency. From the present perspective it is important to note that better outcomes were generally achieved depending on the early experience or early adjustment prior to adoption. Thus Kadushin (1970) points out that the natural mother's relationship to the adopted child, if warm and accepting, was positively related to outcome and he reviews other adoption studies showing that better outcome was invariably associated with less exposure to pathological early environments, suggesting a graded outcome depending on the severity of environmental disruptions, as predicted by the theory of sensitive periods described above. Tizard (1978) found that children who were well adjusted within the institution tended to be well adjusted later as well. Later experience is also important, as seen for example by the fact that in the Tizard study adoption generally resulted in improvement in problem behavior while restoring children to poor environments with their natural parents was associated with generally worse outcomes. The results of Wolins (1970), Pringle and Bossio (1960), and Flint (1978) all show that adequate relations with adults or older children can ameliorate or eliminate the effects of institutional rearing.

Further evidence for graded effects depending on the severity of the early stress comes from work on prenatal and perinatal stressors in humans. Werner and Smith (1982) found a variety of relationships between the severity of prenatal and perinatal risk factors and long-term outcome in the Kauai longitudinal study. Developmental examinations at 20 months revealed a direct relationship between the severity of perinatal stress and the proportion of children rated as below normal on physical, social, or intellectual development, a trend especially pronounced among the moderate and severely stressed children. At age 10 the differences between stressed and unstressed groups were attenuated but were still quite strong for the group of severely stressed infants. At age 18 four of the five surviving severely stressed infants had persistent physical, learning, or mental health problems. The group rated as moderately stressed had three times the rate of serious mental problems, twice the rate of mental retardation, and, for girls, over twice the rate of teenage pregnancy. Sixty percent of the children in need of long-term mental health care at age 10 had moderate perinatal stress, low birthweight, congenital defects, or CNS dysfunctions. Seventy-five percent of these individuals contacted mental health agencies during adolescence, often for severe and persistent mental health problems. Only one third of them had improved by age 18. Graded effects on cognitive development depending on the severity of prenatal and perinatal stress have also been found by Sigman, Cohen, and Forsythe (1981), Broman (1979), and Winick, Meyer, and Harris (1975).

In summary, the human data on the consequences of failure to form early attachment relationships or the formation of defective early attachments support the existence of long-range effects and differential plasticity, although interaction with later environments undoubtedly can ameliorate the effects of those conditions. It is noteworthy that two studies (Tizard, 1978; Wolkind, 1974) found that age 2 was the cutoff point. Children who had not developed normal attachments by this age tended to be abnormal later, and in the case of Tizard (1978), this occurred despite removal to a normal environment. These results suggest that there is greater plasticity before age 2 than after, although there is no reason to suppose that there is no plasticity at all after this age, especially since Flint (1978) showed that considerable progress was possible with children after age 2, given an intensive therapeutic regimen. Nor does this imply that major breaks in attachments at very early ages cannot have long-range effects if later environments before or after age 2 do not alter the situation. A decrease in plasticity after age 2 is also consistent with the data reviewed by Lamb et al. (1984), indicating considerable instability of attachment classification associated with changing life circumstances in the second year of life. It is also noteworthy that Dennis (1973) found that age 2 marked a point after which removal of severely deprived children to better environments had less effect on cognitive development than removal before this age.

Early Experience and Normal Social Development

The above data indicate that (1) there are age-based differences in plasticity for human social behavior; (2) long-range effects of early experience variables can occur; (3) whether the long-range effects occur depends crucially on the appropriateness and intensity of the subsequent environments. It does not follow that these considerations are relevant for the understanding of behavior under normal circumstances. It could be argued that major breaks in caretaking, lack of attachment figures, and repeated hospitalizations represent extreme environments that are not encountered by the great majority of humans and, although they are of considerable theoretical importance, they are of little importance in explaining normal variation in social behavior. Scarr and McCartney (1983) distinguish between inhumane, abusive environments and normal environments. The latter environments contribute importantly to development, but essentially everyone benefits from them, so that individual differences are the result of factors other than the caretaking environment. Early experience and differential plasticity depending on age may be important, but only for the relatively small number of individuals affected by these extreme environments.

Such a position is attractive from the point of view presented above, since the power of the environment is crucial in determining both the effects of early experience as well as the effects of subsequent environments. The extreme environments typical of the studies reviewed above are far more likely, therefore, to have long-range effects. Nevertheless, given that the data from these severe environmental stressors indicate declining plasticity at later ages, this declining plasticity may well have important effects on the stability of behavior within the normal range and therefore on the long-range effects of attachment classifications. Unfortunately, longitudinal studies of the effects of environmental stressors on attachment classification have not compared the effects of similar levels of stress on attachment classification, or on the variables associated with attachment classification, at different ages in order to rigorously test this hypothesis. There is general agreement that attachment classification in the first 2 years of life tends to reflect current parent–child relationships and can be influenced by changes in these relationships

(Lamb et al., 1984; Thompson, Lamb, & Estes, 1983; Waters, 1983). These relationships apparently show considerable plasticity in the first 2 years of life, but such data are consistent with the possibility of decreasing plasticity after age 2. Such a theory would imply that attachment or its correlates assessed at later ages would be more likely to represent persistent traits of the individual, relatively immune from environmental disruptions. Decreasing plasticity would also predict an increasing stability of individual differences in longitudinal studies, and this has in fact been found (Moss & Susman, 1980). Attachment classification in the first 2 years of life would then be seen as providing a foundation for later development (Sroufe, 1984), subject to the proviso that relatively extreme environmental stressors occurring later in life could alter the child's behavior.

As was the case with the animal data, however, some aspects of human social behavior are most reasonably viewed as well buffered from environmental effects and thus do not vary in response to the normal range of environmental variation. For example, children reared in a very inadequate orphanage (Dennis, 1973) were nevertheless able to work well at menial jobs, although marriage, especially for the women, was a rarity, and there was a high rate of psychiatric problems for these individuals. Unlike the study of cognition where stage conceptions are well accepted, there is no conceptualization of social behavior which would allow for the description of cross-cultural universals of social behavior which occur in a very wide range of human cultures and normal rearing environments. The study of social behavior has been far more concerned with dimensions which reflect individual differences than with emphasizing commonalities of social behavior. Central notions such as that of attachment are tools for assessing individual differences but even insecurely attached individuals possess a wide range of social skills. Just as everyone achieves sensorimotor intelligence in all normal human environments, the basic social tasks of infancy are mastered by all. A step in this direction has been taken by Kagan (1982), who notes that the development of self-concept occurs with pretty much the same timetable in all human cultures. The social environment may be necessary for its development, but there is no reason to suppose that important individual differences are the result of specific experiences, much as is the case with the visual system in which the eye requires patterned stimulation but any patterns are inadequate. As McCall (1979) has pointed out with respect to cognitive development, by emphasizing individual differences we may ignore developmental functions. These latter may not be dependent on specific environmental stimulation.

CONCLUSION

There is good evidence for differential plasticity depending on age in the animal and human data. The evidence indicates that, after the time of maximum plasticity, considerable time, intensity of appropriate stimulus, or both must be expended to reverse the effects of early experience. The organism is viewed as increasingly refractory to change from environmental sources. In some extreme cases reversal may be impossible. The importance of the intensity of appropriate stimulus should be emphasized since it is generally missing from discussions of reversibility. Instances where the intensity of appropriate stimulus is an important factor in predicting the effects of early experience and whether reversal occurs have been discussed above, and the intensity of the stimulus in conjunction with the age of the organism are clearly the most important variables affecting the outcome of organism–environment interactions. Since humans appear to retain significant plasticity throughout development, the intensity of appropriate stimulus becomes of immense practical importance, since it is far easier to manipulate than is the biological basis for declining plasticity. The appropriate model is one in which the anatomical and physiological structures underlying behavior are present regardless of age, but these structures become increasingly refractory to stimulation so that in some cases reversal is not possible with the present technology. There is no support for the thesis that experience is necessary for producing the structures themselves so that after the sensitive period behavior would be irreversible. Such a theory would predict a complete lack of sensitivity to stimuli at later ages, not the gradually declining sensitivity actually found. The fact that social stimulation does vary in affective intensity suggests that this dimension may be important in reversing the effects of early experience. This conclusion is suggested by the work of Woolpy and Ginsburg (1967), Suomi et al. (1976), Flint (1978), as well as the cases discussed by Bateson (1983) and is consistent with a large body of literature indicating the importance of arousal regulation in social development (Zentall & Zentall, 1983; Zuckerman et al., 1980). Such findings suggest that affectively arousing styles of parent–child interaction such as those discussed by Stern (1977) and MacDonald and Parke (1984) may be central to social development. If indeed the affective systems are biological systems which provide graded responses depending on the intensity of social stimulation it would be expected that manipulating the affective environment of the organism could have important consequences on the social behavior of the organism. (See MacDonald, 1984, for a biological theory of affective development that emphasizes the effects of affective regulation during development.)

In conclusion, we have come a long way from supposing that behavior is absolutely fixed at an early age by genetic factors or that after a sensitive period it is impossible to change behavior. Nevertheless, there are too many data showing otherwise to reject the idea that there are important constraints on plasticity for human and animal behavior. This fact does not, of course, prevent us from finding ways to intervene with individuals who have suffered early environmental insults. Indeed, the theory of sensitive periods suggests that the intensity of an ecologically appropriate stimulus can, at least up to a point, overcome the organism's declining plasticity, and Lerner (1984) has emphasized the ultimate plasticity of all of life, including the genes themselves. The fact of declining plasticity merely indicates what we already know, that successful interventions are not at present easily come by.

REFERENCES

Aslin, R. N. (1981). Experiential influences and sensitive periods in perceptual development: A unified model. In R. N. Aslin, J. R. Alberts, & M. R. Petersen (Eds.), *Development of perception*. New York: Academic Press.

Bateson, P. P. G. (1976). Rules and reciprocity in behavioral development. In P. P. G. Bateson & R. A. Hinde (Eds.). *Growing points in ethology*. Cambridge, U.K.: Cambridge Univ. Press.

Bateson, P. P. G. (1979). How do sensitive periods arise and what are they for? *Animal Behavior*, **27**, 470-486.

Bateson, P. P. G. (1983). The interpretation of sensitive periods. In A. Oliverio & M. Zapella (Eds.), *The behavior of human infants*. New York: Plenum.

Berlyne, D. E. (1960). *Conflict, arousal, and curiosity*. New York: McGraw–Hill.

Berlyne, D. E. (1966). Curiosity and exploration *Science (Washington, D.C.);* **153**, 25-33.

Bloom, B. (1964). *Stability and change in human characteristics*. Chicago: Univ. of Chicago Press.

Bowlby, J. (1951). *Maternal care and mental health*. Geneva: World Health Organization.

Bowlby, J. (1973). *Separation, anxiety and anger*. New York: Basic Books.

Brazelton, T. B., Koslowski, B., & Main, M. (1974). The origins of reciprocity: The early mother–infant interaction. In M. Lewis & L. A. Rosenblum (Eds.), *The effect of the infant on its caretaker*. New York: Wiley.

Broman, S. H. (1979). Prenatal anoxia and cognitive development in early childhood. In T. M. Field (Ed.), *Infants born at risk*. New York: SP Medical & Scientific Books.

Bronfenbrenner, U. (1968). Early deprivatin in mammals: A cross-species analysis. In G. Newton & S. Levine (Eds.), *Early experience and behavior*. Springfield, IL: Thomas.

Bronfenbrenner, U. (1977). Toward an experimental ecology of human development. *American Psychologist*, **32**, 513-531.

Cadoret, R. J., & Cain, C. (1980). Sex differences in predictors of antisocial behavior in adoptees. *Archives of General Psychiatry*, **37**, 1171-1175.

Cairns, R. B. (1979). *Social development.* San Francisco: Freeman.

Cairns, R. B., & Werboff, J. (1967). Behavioral development in the dog: An interspecific analysis. *Science (Washington, D.C.),* **158,** 1070-1072.

Casler, L. (1968). Perceptual deprivation in institutional settings. In G. Newton & S. Levine (Eds.), *Early experience and behavior.* Springfield, IL: Thomas.

Chamove, A. S., Rosenblum, L. A., & Harlow, H. F. (1973). Monkeys raised with only peers: A pilot study. *Animal Behavior,* **21,** 316-325.

Clarke, A. D. B., & Clarke, A. M. (1976). *Early experience: Myth and evidence.* New York: Free Press.

Cummins, M. S., & Suomi, S. J. (1976). Long term effects of social rehabilitation in rhesus monkeys. *Primates,* **17,** 43-52.

Denenberg, V. H. (1968). A consideration of the usefulness of the critical period hypothesis as applied to the stimulation of rodents in infancy. In G. Newton & S. Levine (Eds.), *Early experience and behavior.* Springfield, IL: Thomas.

Dennis, W. (1973). *Children of the creche.* New York: Appleton.

Douglas, J. W. B. (1975). Early hospitalization and later disturbances of behavior. *Developmental Medicine and Child Neurology,* **17,** 456-480.

Fisher, A. E. (1955). *The effects of differential early treatment on the social and exploratory behavior of puppies.* PhD dissertation, Pennsylvania State University.

Flint, B. M. (1978). *New hope for deprived children.* Toronto: Toronto Univ. Press.

Fox, M. L. (1971). *Integrative development of brain and behavior in the dog.* Chicago: Univ. of Chicago Press.

Freedman, D. G., King, J. A., & Elliot, O. (1961). Critical period in the social development of the dog. *Science (Washington, D.C.),* **133,** 1016-1017.

Fuller, J. L. (1967). Experiential stress and later behavior: Emergence stress is postulated as the basis for behavioral deficits seen in dogs following isolation. *Science (Washington, D.C.),* **158,** 1645-1652.

Fuller, J. L., & Clark, L. D. (1966a). Effects of rearing with specific stimuli on the post-isolation behavior of dogs. *Journal of Comparative and Physiological Psychology,* **61,** 258-263.

Fuller, J. L., & Clark, L. D. (1966b). Genetic and treatment factors underlying the post-isolation syndrome in dogs. *Journal of Comparative and Physiological Psychology,* **61,** 251-257.

Ginsburg, B. E. (1969). Genotypic variables affecting response to postnatal stimulation. In J. A. Ambrose (Ed.), *Stimulation in early infancy.* New York/London: Academic Press.

Gluck, J. P., Harlow, H. F., & Schlitz, K. A. (1973). Differential effect of early enrichment and deprivation in the rhesus monkey *(Maccaca mulatta). Journal of Comparative and Physiological Psychology,* **84,** 598-604.

Gollin, E. S. (1981). Development and plasticity. In E. S. Gollin (Ed.), *Developmental plasticity: Behavioral and biological aspects of variations in development.* New York: Academic Press.

Gottlieb, G. (1976). The roles of early experience in the development of behavior and the nervous system. In G. Gottlieb (Ed.), *Studies in the development of behavior and the nervous system* (Vol. 3). New York: Academic Press.

Harlow, H. F., & Harlow, M. K. (1969). Effects of various mother–infant relationships on rhesus monkey behavior. In B. M. Foss (Ed.), *Determinants of infant behavior.* London: Methuen.

Henderson, N. O. (1980). Effects of early experience on the behavior of animals: The second 25 years of research. In E. C. Simmel (Ed.), *Early experience and early behavior.*

New York: Academic Press.

Hersov, L. (1977). Adoption studies. In M. Rutter & L. Hersov (Eds.), *Child psychiatry.* London: Blackwell.

Immelmann, K. (1972). Sexual and other long term effects of imprinting in birds and other species. In D. Lehrman, R. Hinde, & E. Shaw (Eds.), *Advances in the study of behavior* (Vol. 4). New York: Academic Press.

Immelmann, K., & Suomi, S. (1981). Sensitive phases in development. In K. Immelmann, G. Barlow, L. Petrinovich, & M. Main (Eds.), *Behavioral development.* New York: Cambridge Univ. Press.

Kadushin, A. (1970). *Adopting older children.* New York: Columbia Univ. Press.

Kagan, J. (1982). The emergence of self. *Journal of Child Psychology and Psychiatry,* **23,** 363-381.

Kagan, J., Kearsley, R., & Zelazo, P. (1978). *Infancy.* Cambridge, MA: Harvard Univ. Press.

Kaufman, I., & Rosenblum, L. (1969). The waning of the mother–infant bond in two species of macaques. In B. M. Foss (Ed.), *The determinants of infant behavior* (Vol. 4). London: Methuen.

Lamb, M. E., Thompson, R. A., Gardner, W., Charnov, E. L., & Estes, D. (1984). Security of infantile attachment as assessed in the "strange situation": Its study and biological interpretation. *Behavioral and Brain Sciences.*

Lerner, R. M. (1984). On the nature of human plasticity. Cambridge: Cambridge Univ. Press.

MacDonald, K. B. (1983). Production, social controls and ideology: Toward a sociobiology of the phenotype. *Journal of Social and Biological Structures,* **6,** 297-317.

MacDonald, K. B. (1984). An ethological–social learning theory of the development of altruism in humans: Implications for human sociobiology. *Ethology and Sociobiology,* **5,** 97-109.

MacDonald, K. B., & Ginsburg, B. E. (1981). Induction of normal behavior in wolves with restricted rearing. *Behavioral and Neural Biology,* **33,** 133-162.

MacDonald, K. B., & Parke, R. D. (1984). Bridging the gap: Parent–child play interactions and peer interactive competence. *Child Development,* **55,** 1265-1277.

McKinney, W., Kleise, K., Suomi, S. J., & Moran, E. (1973). Can psychopathology be reinduced in rhesus monkeys? *Archives of General Psychiatry,* **29,** 630-634.

McKinney, W. T., Suomi, S. J., & Harlow, H. F. (1972). Repetitive peer separation in rhesus monkeys. *Archives of General Psychiatry,* **27,** 200-204.

Melzack, R., & Thompson, W. R. (1956). The effects of early experience on social behavior. *Journal of Comparative and Physiological Psychology,* **50,** 155-161.

Moss, H. A., & Susman, E. J. (1980). Longitudinal study of personality development. In O. Brim & J. Kagan (Eds.), *Constancy and change in human development.* Cambridge, MA: Harvard Univ. Press.

Novak, M. (1979). Social recovery of monkeys isolated for the first year of life: II. Long term assessment. *Developmental Psychology,* **15,** 50-61.

O'Conner, N. (1968). Children in restricted environments. In G. Newton & S. Levine (Eds.), *Early experience and behavior.* Springfield, IL: Thomas.

Parke, R. D., & Suomi, S. J. (1981). Adult male–infant relationships: Human and nonhuman primate evidence. In K. Immelmann, G. W. Balow, L. Petrinovich & M. Main (Eds.), *Behavioral development.* London: Cambridge Univ. Press.

Pfaffenberger, C. P., & Scott, J. P. (1959). The relationship between delayed socialization and delayed trainability in guide dogs. *Journal of Genetic Psychology* **95,** 145-155.

Plotkin, H. C., & Olding-Smee, F. J. (1981). A multiple-level model of evolution and its implications for sociobiology. *Behavioral and Brain Sciences*, **4**, 225-268.

Pringle, M. L. K. (1966). *Adoption facts and fallacies*. New York: Humanities Press.

Pringle, M. L. K., & Bossio, V. (1960). Early prolonged separation and emotional maladjustment. *Journal of Child Psychology and Psychiatry*, **1**, 37-48.

Quinton, D., & Rutter, M. (1976). Early hospital admission and later disturbances in behavior: An attempted replication of Douglas' findings. *Developmental Medicine and Child Neurology*, **18**, 447-459.

Rabb, G. B., Woolpy, J., & Ginsburg, B. E. (1967). Social relationships in a captive wolf pack. *American Zoologist*, **7**, 305-311.

Rathbun, C., DiVirglio, L., & Waldfogel, S. (1958). The restitutive process in children following radical separation from family and culture. *American Journal of Orthopsychiatry*, **28**, 408-415.

Rathbun, G. H., McLaughlin, H., Bennet, C., & Garland, J. (1965). Later adjustment following radical separation from family and culture. *American Journal f Orthopsychiatry*, **35**, 604-609.

Ruppenthal, G. C., Arling, G. A., Harlow, H. F., Sackett, G. P., & Suomi, S. J. (1976). A ten-year perspective on motherless-mother monkey behavior. *Journal of Abnormal Psychology*, **85**, 341-349.

Rutter, M. (1982). Epidemiological and longitudinal approaches to the study of behavioral development. In W. A. Collins (Ed.), *The concept of development. Minnesota symposia on child psychology*. Hillsdale, NJ: Erlbaum.

Sackett, G. P., Ruppenthal, G. C., Fahrenbruch, C. E., Hold, R. A., & Greenough, W. T. (1981). Social isolation rearing effects in monkeys vary with genotype. *Developmental Psychology*, **17**, 313-318.

Sameroff, A. J. (1975). Early influences: Fact or fancy? *Merrill–Palmer Quarterly*, **20**, 275-301.

Sameroff, A. J. (1983). Contexts of development: The systems and their evolution. In W. Kessen (Ed.), *History, theories and methods* (Vol. 1, *Carmichael's manual of child psychology*, P. Mussen, Ed.). New York: Wiley.

Scarr, S. (1976). An evolutionary perspective on infant intelligence: Species patterns and individual variations. In M. Lewis (Ed.), *The origins of infant intelligence*. New York: Plenum.

Scarr, S., & McCartney, K. (1983). How people make their own environments: A theory of genotype–environment effects. *Child Development*, **54**, 424-435.

Schnierla, T. C. (1957). The concept of development in comparative psychology. In D. B. Harris (Ed.), *The concept of development*. Minneapolis: The Univ. of Minnesota Press.

Scott, J. P. (1979). Critical periods in organizational processes. In F. Fauler & J. M. Tanner (Eds.), *Human growth* (Vol. 3). New York: Plenum.

Sigman, M., Cohen, S. E., & Forsythe, A. (1981). The relation of early infant measures to later development. In S. L. Friedman & M. Sigman (Eds.), *Preterm birth and psychological development*. New York: Academic Press.

Spencer-Booth, Y., & Hinde, R. A. (1971). Effects of brief separations from mothers on behavior of rhesus monkeys 6-24 months later. *Journal of Child Psychology and Psychiatry*, **12**, 157-172.

Sroufe, L. A. (1979). Socio-emotional development. In J. D. Osofsky (Ed.), *Handbook of infant development*. New York: Wiley.

Sroufe, L. A. (1984). Infant caregiver attachment and patterns of adaptation in preschool: The roots of maladaptation and competence. In M. Perlmutter (Ed.), *Minnesota symposia on child psychology*. NJ: Erlbaum.

Stern, D. (1977). *The first relationship*. Cambridge, MA: Harvard Univ. Press.

Stevenson-Hinde, J., Zunz, M., & Stillwell-Barnes, R. (1980). Behavior of one year old rhesus monkeys in a strange situation. *Animal Behavior*, **28**, 266-277.

Suomi, S. J., DeLizio, R., & Harlow, H. F. (1976). Social rehabilitation of separation induced depressive disorders in monkeys. *American Journal of Psychiatry*, **133**, 1279-1285.

Suomi, S. J., Eisele, C. D., Grady, S. A., & Harlow, H. F. (1975). Depressive behavior in adult monkeys following separation from family environment. *Journal of Abnormal Psychology*, **84**, 576-578.

Suomi, S. J., & Harlow, H. F. (1972). Social rehabilitation of isolate-reared monkeys. *Developmental Psychology*, **6**, 487-496.

Suomi, S. J., & Harlow, H. F. (1975). Effects of differential removal from group on the social development of the rhesus monkey. *Journal of Child Psychology and Psychiatry*, **16**, 149-164.

Thompson, W. R., & Heron, W. (1954). Exploratory behavior in normal and restricted dogs. *Journal of Comparative and Physiological Psychology*, **47**, 77-82.

Thompson, R. A., Lamb, M. E., & Estes, D. (1983). Harmonizing discordant notes: A reply to Waters. *Child Development*, **54**, 521-524.

Tizard, B. (1978). *Adoption: A second chance*. New York: Free Press.

Tizard, B., & Rees, J. (1975). The effect of early institutional rearing on behavior problems and affectional relationships. *Journal of Child Psychology and Psychiatry*, **16**, 61-73.

Uzgiris, I. (1980, May). *Changing patterns of infant environment interaction at various stages of development*. Paper presented to the symposium on biosocial factors and the infant who is at risk for developmental disbilities, University of Massachusetts Medical School, Worcester, MA.

Wachs, T. D. (1979). Proximal experience and early cognitive–intellectual development. *Merrill–Palmer Quarterly*, **25**, 3-41.

Wachs, T. P., & Gruen, G. G. (1982). *Early experience and human development*. New York: Plenum.

Waddington, C. H. (1957). *The strategy of the genes*. London: Allen.

Waters, E. (1983). The stability of individual differences in infant attachment: Comments on the Thompson, Lamb, and Estes' contribution. *Child Development*, **54**, 516-520.

Waters, E., Wippman, J., & Sroufe, L. A. (1979). Attachment, positive affect and competence in the peer group: Two studies in construct validation. *Child Development*, **50**, 821-829.

Werner, E. E., & Smith, R. S. (1982). *Vulnerable but invincible*. New York: McGraw–Hill.

Winick, M. M., Meyer, K. K., & Harris, R. C. (1975). Malnutrition and environmental enrichment by adoption. *Science (Washington, D.C.)*, **190**, 1173-1175.

Wohlwill, J. (1980). Cognitive development in childhood. In O. Brim & J. Kagan (Eds.), *Constancy and change in human development*. Cambridge, MA: Harvard Univ. Press.

Wolins, M. (1970). Young children in institutions. *Developmental Psychology*, **2**, 99-109.

Wolkind, J. N. (1974). The components of affectionless psychopathy in institutionalized children. *Journal of Child Psychology and Psychiatry*, **15**, 215-220.

Woolpy, J., & Ginsburg, B. E. (1967). Wolf socialization: A study of temperament in a wild species. *American Zoologist*, **7**, 356-363.

Zentall, S. S., & Zentall, T. R. (1983). Optimal stimulation: A model of disordered activity and performance in normal and deviant children. *Psychological Bulletin,* **94,** 446-471.

Zuckerman, M., Buchsbaum, M. S., & Murphy, D. L. (1980). Sensation seeking and its biological correlates. *Psychological Bulletin,* **88,** 187-214.

6

The Psychic Life of the Young Infant: Review and Critique of the Psychoanalytic Concepts of Symbiosis and Infantile Omnipotence

Thomas M. Horner

University of Michigan Medical Center, Ann Arbor

The subjective life of the young infant is examined in the light of classical psychoanalytic theory and of recent empirical studies of early infant behavior and development. The concepts of symbiosis and omnipotence are argued to be products of poetic but largely misguided reconstructions from adult experience, providing a questionable developmental foundation for contemporary psychodynamic theories of object relations.

The psychic life of the human infant—that is, its subjective dimensions—is an elusive topic of psychological inquiry, standing as a hinterland of contemporary academic infant psychology. In the field of infant psychiatry, however, where there is an emphasis on affective processes and communication, the phenomenology of infancy is a tacit but fundamental part of considering the infant's mental and behavioral status. Most clinicians accept the proposition that there is at least a rudimentary phenomenology of infancy—that infants feel and experience events in their day-to-day lives. Adults, particularly those who are involved in

Reprinted with permission from the *American Journal of Orthopsychiatry*, 1985, Vol. 55, 324–344. Copyright 1985 by the American Orthopsychiatric Association, Inc.

everyday contacts with infants, act *as though* there is a subjective domain, and there are processes by which adults, particularly primary caregivers, act selectively according to their understanding of the infant's subjectivity.[12, 68, 77, 105] Not everyone, however, would agree as to how the infant's subjective world is organized, nor would there be agreement as to the content of that subjectivity.

In psychoanalytic theory, three ideas concerning the qualitative, subjective dimensions of infant mental life have long stood at the forefront: *1)* a condition of nondifferentiation of self and other characterizes the earliest phases of infancy; *2)* the infant's predominant experience of its relationship with others is one of omnipotence, and *3)* this nondifferentiated condition is the basis of an intrinsic regressive pull throughout infancy as well as the whole of development.

Collectively these ideas are specific to what is widely termed, after Mahler,[95, 100] symbiosis and the differentiation subphase of the separation-individuation line of object-relational and self development. To be sure, as Mahler herself has pointed out, the ideas describe conditions of infancy that are extremely difficult if not impossible to verify or disconfirm.[99] Yet, they constitute a highly visible, influential segment of contemporary theory concerning early psychic experience and object-relational predispositions.

Infancy has been the focus of a number of recent reexaminations of psychoanalytic concepts of development.[27, 89, 130] The aims of this paper will be to trace briefly and to examine critically these conceptions of infant psychic life. In the end I will assert that they have little behavioral foundation (that is, identifiable behavior correlates) in the actual life and development of infants and that they are related to adult proclivities for idealizing infancy as an original condition of innocence and perfection. At the same time there is the adult's recognition of the extreme vulnerability of the infant with respect to the power of surrounding caregivers. Such proclivities, when examined, expose the adult's penchant for attributing to infants qualities of subjective life that are not, in the ultimate analysis, truly explanatory.

SYMBIOSIS AND OMNIPOTENCE IN INFANCY: HISTORICAL ROOTS IN PSYCHOANALYSIS

Freud, Ferenczi and M. Klein

Freud used the term symbiosis only once in his writings[4] but not to refer to phenomena associated with concepts listed above.[60] Benedek used the term as early as 1949 to characterize the early mother-infant unit.[4] Before that, Fromm used it to describe the developmental foundations of his social psychoanalytic theory of human adjustment.[50] He also described separation-individuation phenomena that are essentially the same as those later described by Mahler.

Others also within or in contact with the early psychoanalytic movement incorporated the basic tenets of infantile symbiosis and individuation into their developmental frameworks, even though these specific terms were not employed. Thus, Rank[118] made separation and individuation factors, including the creation of symbiotic modes of functioning to deal with the trauma of birth, the central tenet of his conceptual framework (see also Ferenczi, below). Piaget several times referred to nondifferentiation of self and others as a central feature of development.[116] Sullivan's prototaxic and parataxic modes of early infant experiences are drawn along similar lines.[131] Despite the clear historical divergences of these schools of thought, the common acceptance of the symbiotic, undifferentiated nature of early psychic life is unmistakable.

It is well documented that Freud contemplated infancy from his position as a parent.[21, 73] He had a penchant for reconstructing childhood phenomena from the standpoint of an archeologist of adult mental life. It is intrinsic to everything Freud wrote that he was a developmentalist, a trait Kaufmann has shown to have been largely influenced by Goethe.[75] Freud therefore quite naturally turned to the infant as a prototype of mental processes.[43,46,47] He averred that the infant's recognition of the object world is prompted by the rise of unavoidable experiences of pain (frustration). This formulation appears in a number of writings concerning early psychic mechanisms associated with the differentiation of the self and non-self.[43, 45] Freud's theory of reality testing, thought, and judgment pivoted in large part upon this conception of early psychic life.

Following Freud, Ferenczi[33] broadly outlined a series of steps taken by the child toward mature reality testing, emphasizing that primary feelings of omnipotence are embedded in the original psychic condition of nondifferentiation and that there is an innate regressive pull toward the original undifferentiated state:

> If ... the human being possesses a mental life when in the womb, although only an unconscious one—and it would be foolish to believe that the mind begins to function only at the moment of birth—he must get from his existence the impression that he is omnipotent. For what is omnipotence but the

feeling that one has nothing left to wish for. The fetus, however, could maintain this of itself, for it always has what is necessary for the satisfaction of its instincts, and so has nothing to wish for; it is without wants. (p. 219). . . The first wish-impulse of the child, therefore, cannot be any other than to regain this situation. (p. 221)

Historically, these ideas are predicated on Freud's principle of constancy, a principle holding the human organism to be, like a bird's egg, a closed biological system. Like Freud, Ferenczi also viewed the role of frustration and discrepancies between wish and reality (the "promptings" specified by Freud) to be the major impetus of the child's giving up magical-omnipotent thoughts and feelings over the course of its development.

While contemporary authorities dismiss or respectfully ignore much of Melanie Klein's work, basic tenets of infant psychic life that she incorporated into her thinking continue to reverberate in contemporary psychoanalytic theory of infant mental activity. They include the metapsychological constructions of good and bad objects and the strong notion that subjective-affective factors play a key role in the formation of self and ego structures as well as psychic conflict. The importance of Klein's contributions rests not with her extreme and unacceptable metaphorical dramatizations of infant subjective experience, anchored to the two poles of the paranoid-schizoid and depressive positions in object relations, but in her readiness to meet infant subjectivity on its own terms, that is, not solely as a reconstruction from adult material but as a domain of experience to be studied directly. The absence of language in infancy was not a deterrent to her pursuit of a suitable framework for conceptualizing infant psychic life. She believed that there are many details of early emotional development that can be gathered through modalities other than language. Thus, she asserted, if one is to understand the young infant it will be through empathic modalities ("a full sympathy with [the baby]") that are in many respects outside the domain of language.[83] Recent studies of affective life in infancy have demonstrated that empathic perceptual modalities on the part of the observer can be objective—that is, reliably used in ratings of behavior and affect.[52, 64]

The few actual behavioral vignettes that occur in her works suggest that Klein was attuned to interactional data that today would be used to counter the theories she expounded. Thus, in her essay "On Observing the Behavior of Young Infants," one finds references to the wakeful periods of focused positive involvements that occur between young infants and their caregivers, including not only eye-to-eye contact at the breast but also the young infant's interests in peek-a-boo activity.[83] (See Kleeman[80] in this regard.) Unfortunately, the concepts that emerged from Klein's pursuits found a vocabulary that essentially cast infant psychic life in terms of the grossly disturbed adult.

The theory of Klein and her associates[81, 119] incorporated the basic tenets of Freud and Ferenczi's model of the infant mind. The undifferentiated phase (merged objects) of development (autoeroticism) is retained, although, following Glover, Klein held firmly to the notion that early on (first three months of life) the infant experiences part-object relationships that are predicated on primitive distinctions between itself and not-self (*i.e.*, the breast)—hence the paranoid-schizoid position that she considered to be dominant during this period. Klein and her colleagues also held to the notion of infantile omnipotence. Finally, they took the unmodified view that the experience of self evolves primarily out of painful experiences: "It seems that at first the conscious idea of 'me' is largely colored by painful associations. Phantasy is then taken up as a refuge from the reality of 'me' " (p. 55).[119] Yet withal, they emphasized the important domain of subjective life in infants:

> Surely the [infant] *feels*, if it does not yet *know*, that it is at least "acquiring knowledge" of new sights and sounds, and so on, every day. We say "he recognizes me!" and it means "he has preserved his perception of me intact in his mind since he first took it in." And I think the baby too knows in this way that *he* is involved in the process. . . .[119]

This emphasis was later continued by Spitz (see below) and has continued, modified by extensive and systematic direct infant observational study, into important contemporary approaches to infant psychic life (see, for example, Emde[29]).

Loewald, Jacobson and Modell

While terms and collateral concepts have changed over the decades since Freud, the main presumptions and imagery concerning early stages of nondifferentiation, regression toward fusion states, and omnipotence have remained essentially unchanged in the developmental psychoanalytic literature.[38, 39, 40,71,78, 79, 93, 103, 128, 129] The writings all emphasize the basic compromise between the child's need to retain the symbiotic situation and opposing tendencies to loosen symbiotic ties largely by way of aggressive, narcissistic expansion, and independent ego function-ing.[71, 93] All stress the period of early infancy as being one of nondif-ferentiation. Jacobson[71] and Modell[104] viewed the early condition of nondifferentiation to be an abiding feature of object-relational devel-opment. Modell wrote, for example, that the "wish to merge, to fuse, to lose one's separateness" (pp. 61-62) is elemental to all love relationships. Tensions and conflicts associated with merging wishes and fears were central to Jacobson's codification of these object-relational principles.

According to Modell, the function of omnipotence is to deny (elimi-nate) separateness between self and object—to create an illusion of action upon the object from a distance. Such denial serves to protect the ego from feelings of loss.

> The object that is eaten is "all gone": it needs to be re-cre-ated... [I]nstinctual demands made upon parental objects, ... implicitly threaten the loss of the object. There-fore the danger of separation is not limited to the danger of actual, physical separation from the protecting parental ob-ject, but may also arise as a result of the fundamental ambi-valent instinctual wishes that the child experiences toward the parents.... We [sic] suggest that the capacity for magical thought mitigates the danger of catastrophic anxiety through the creation of an illusion of lack of separateness between the self and the object.... [This anxiety] is the motive of the institution of a magical, created environment that serves to mitigate the danger of the experience of total helplessness. (pp. 22-23)

Jacobson viewed complementary processes of symbiosis to be at work with respect to the mother's side of the early dyadic relationship. In this context she cited Benedek's[5] and Greenacre's[57] comments regarding the mother's emotional ties to the infant. These complementary processes were conceived as something to guard against. Drawing on the work of Olden[106, 107] and Mahler, Jacobson emphasized the need on the part of the mother to maintain a climate of essential differences between her own and her child's needs and roles, thereby insuring that the merging wishes on the part of the infant are not solidified.

Modell, however, objected to the use of the term *symbiosis* because "there is no compelling reason to assume that the object of this dyad is bound to the subject in an equivalent manner" (p. 41).[104] He stated that the concept of symbiotic object relationship is misleading in that it erroneously implies the existence of a particular emotional bond of the object to the subject. Curiously, he stated that the emotional attitude of the object to the subject may in fact be quite irrelevant; that is, a transitional object relationship on the part of the subject (*i.e.*, infant) may be established regardless of the attitude of the object.

Direct Psychoanalytic Applications to Infants: Spitz and Mahler

Spitz[127-129] and Mahler[96-100] systemically applied themselves on an extensive scale to direct observations of the infant-mother caregiving unit, introducing to psychoanalytic theory systematic observations of the communications, interactions, and general behavioral patterns of infants with their mothers.* The work of both of these individuals has transmitted the prevailing notions of initial self/other nondifferentiation and the collateral sense of omnipotence, giving, at least ostensibly, an empirical foundation to theory formerly based on reconstructions and clinical observations from adult psychic experience.

In the main, Spitz remained within the classical framework of psychoanalytic theory of object relations. With Hartmann, Spitz[128] addressed the phenomenological dimension of the self, and he attempted to account for it in his conceptualization of self development in infants. Unfortunately, some convolutions in his analysis of the early stages of the self resulted in a failure to resolve some of the problems connected with distinguishing self, ego, and awareness. Thus, he cryptically asserted that the infant's

> ever-increasing [external] cathectic investment finally compels the ego to become aware of the "I's" function in the unfolding object relations. Through this awareness of the ego the "I" achieves identity as the self. (pp. 120-121)[127]

Following previous theorists, Spitz subscribed to the view that the infant stands poised between progressive developmental forces away from the objectless (undifferentiated) condition of primary narcissism and regressive forces toward that condition and that there exists a coun-

---

* To be sure, direct observation of infants by psychoanalysts preceded the work of Spitz and Mahler (see for example, A. Freud;[41] Hoffer[66]). However, unlike their predecessors, Spitz and Mahler represent focal points for contemporary developments in the field of infant psychiatry, and so their respective works are emphasized here.

terpart tendency in the mother: "the equally conflicting strivings of the mother, to embrace and to remove" (p. 124).[128]

> Under normal circumstances, in the first few months, the mother's antithetic tendencies are in harmonious interaction with the antithetic tendencies in the child. With the increase in the child's autonomy the synchronicity of child and mother is subjected to ever more disturbances. Such asynchronous incidents, as well as the attempts from both sides to re-establish synchronicity, contribute greatly to the richness of the developing object relations. (p. 124)*

Like his predecessors, Spitz held to the view that inevitable frustrations in the infant's behavioral-affective commerce with the environment facilitate the differentiation of the self. But he enlarged the crucible of self/not-self differentiation in an important way when he emphasized the function of action in the development of self/other boundary representations:

> The clash between the child's will and that of the mother leads the child to recognize the limits of his will, his wishes, his fantasies about himself, and thus the boundaries of the self are narrowed and set up. (p. 139)

Finally, omnipotence, while infrequently mentioned by Spitz, was nevertheless a key part of his overall model:

> One may say without exaggeration that the self is fashioned from the atrophied remains of magic omnipotence. . . . This origin of the self, its linkage with magic omnipotence, will never be completely eradicated and can be traced even in the adult. Reality testing blocks the road of return to the omnipotent origin of the self. (p. 139)

Mahler's well-known theory of separation-individuation[95, 98, 100] epit-

---

* This point comprises one of Spitz's many original and lasting contributions to psychoanalytic approaches to infancy, his emphasis on the communication matrix with its emotional climate and the critical auxiliary ego functioning of the mother. Some contemporary psychoanalytic approaches to the study of early affect communication[26, 31] owe much of their impetus to Spitz's seminal work in these areas.

omized contemporary psychoanalytic approaches to early child development and psychopathology. For Mahler, the starting point in development is the period ("first few weeks of extrauterine life") of absolute primary narcissism, termed the stage of normal autism. Mahler characterized this period as one of virtual absence of object cathexis, except for instances where transient responses to external stimuli can be demonstrated. Re-evoking Freud's analogy of the bird's egg,[43] Mahler[100] depicted the phenomenology of this period as one in which

> . . . the infant seems to be in a state of primitive *hallucinatory disorientation* [my emphasis] in which need satisfaction seems to belong to his own "unconditional" omnipotent, *autistic* orbit. (p. 42)

In the second month and beyond,

> dim awareness of the need-satisfying object marks the beginning of the phase of normal symbiosis, in which the infant behaves and functions *as though* he and his mother were an omnipotent system—a dual unity within one common boundary. [It is] that state of undifferentiation, of fusion with mother, in which the "I" is not yet differentiated from the "non-I" and in which inside and outside are only gradually coming to be sensed as different. (p. 44)

In Mahler's theory, then, the mother-infant unit is viewed as the essential ego, an extension of Freud's concept of "purified pleasure ego"[45] and a direct application of Spitz's concepts of the auxiliary ego and "unified situational experience."[129]

Although not the totality of primary narcissism that characterizes the normal autistic phase, the symbiotic phase, according to Mahler, is essentially a condition existing "within the orbit of the omnipotent symbiotic dual unity" (p. 46).[99] The ego is now being "molded under the impact of reality, on the one hand, and of the instinctual drives, on the other" (p. 46).[100] The infant's inner sensations

> . . . form the *core*. They seem to remain the central crystalization point of the "feeling of self," around which a "sense of identity" [ego feeling;[32] identity theme[91]] will become established. . . . The sensoriperceptive organ—the "peripheral rind of the ego," as Freud called it—contributes mainly to the

self's demarcation from the object world. The two kinds of intrapsychic structures *together* form the framework for self-orientation. (p. 47)[126]

The child's movement through the four subphases of separation-individuation (differentiation; practicing; rapprochement; individuation and object constancy) entails a long series of behavioral transformations and achievements aimed toward differentiating the self and object from the original dual unity. In the first three years of life the stimultaneous or alternating *attraction to* (to combat separateness) and *threat of* remerging with the mother (and losing individuality) looms in the background of the infant's and young child's development. According to Mahler,[96] it is the basis of an entire life cycle of longing, derived from the original symbiotic motive, for the actual or fantasized ideal state of self—that perfect and blissful state of union between infant and mother. (See also Joffe and Sandler.[72] See again Modell, above. See also the recent experimental work of Silverman, Lachmann and Milich.[124]) Correlatively, there is the potential parental liability of overgratification or overfrustration, which could draw the child regressively or fixate it to a level of nondifferentiation. (See again Jacobson, above.) It is not uncommon in clinical presentations for these liabilities to be interpreted as central causes of severe early childhood disturbances,[6, 15, 53, 85, 98] and they are certainly part of the theoretical foundation upon which several contemporary psychoanalytic models of severe adult psychopathology are built.[79, 101, 122]

EPISTEMOLOGICAL FACTORS

Given the foregoing psychoanalytic material, it is pertinent to consider briefly the genetic epistemology of Piaget, since his view, generated from a wholly different orientation, seems to corroborate some of the psychoanalytic points that have been cited.

The child interview data amassed and reported by Piaget is compelling when one ponders the thesis that self and non-self are indistinct in the child's mind. Yet Piaget had in mind an ultimate formal logical distinction, not the practical and everyday distinctions made by young children between themselves and others. Thus, he averred that the self/other distinction did not occur until 11-12 years of age (p. 241),[116] and he held that not even by direct intuition could this distinction be made before then (p. 129).[116] These are, of course, positions contrary to psychoanalytic thought.

"The problem of the child's consciousness of self is extremely complex and it is not easy to treat it from a general standpoint"—so begins the section on consciousness of self in Piaget's early book, *The Child's Conception of the World*.[116]

> The child may be aware of the same contents of thought as ourselves but he locates them elsewhere. He situates in the world or in others what we seat within ourselves, and he situates in himself what we place in others. In this problem of the seat of the contents of mind lies the whole problem of the child's consciousness of self, and it is through not stating it clearly that what is in fact exceedingly complex is made to appear simple. . . . The consciousness of self rises in fact from the dissociation of reality as conceived by the primitive mind and not from the association of particular contents. That the child shows a keen interest in himself, a logical, and no doubt a moral, egocentricity, does not prove that he is conscious of his self, but suggests, on the contrary, that he confuses his self with the universe, in other words that he is unconscious of his self. (p. 125)
>
> . . . the child begins by confusing his self and the world—that is to say in this particular case, his subjective point of view and the external data—and only later distinguishes his own personal point of view from other possible points of view. In fact the child always begins by regarding his own point of view as absolute. (p. 126)

Piaget's references to the self here are essentially epistemological, largely centered on the capacity for *self-reflective* (observing ego) thought. As much as his writing on the subject contains references to particular confusions between self and external world, Piaget's perspective is always from the standpoint of the child's inability to *introspect* and to *conceptualize* the other's point of view in a situation.* In his thinking, Piaget borrowed from earlier psychologists, particularly Baldwin,[1] who spoke of an "ad-

---

* While there is no basis whatsoever for disputing the infant's inability to introspect it is not so clear that infants lack totally the rudimentary capacity to take another's point of view. Hoffman[67] has recently communicated some highly interesting examples of infants aged 15 and 20 months, respectively, who, by virtue of actions taken toward others, must have possessed elementary capacities for evaluating the other's point of view (see also Hoffman,[66] Borke,[7] and Lempers, Flavell and Flavell[86]).

ualistic" period in development in which perception and reality are not distinguished from one another. It is, however, a period in which, according to Baldwin, "an incipient perception of persons as different from things" does exist.[13]

Piaget's idea of how the self becomes differentiated in the child's mind from the external world is similiar to the view held by psychoanalysts, namely, that it is through contact with and frustration from the object world that differentiation takes place.[109, 116] Psychoanalysts have been concerned, of course, with frustrations that are connected with *drives* (need satisfaction) or, in Spitz's[137] view, affect-motivated actions. From Piaget's standpoint, frustration centers primarily on the clashes between *points of view* that arise from the imposition of the child's interpretations on others:

> It is by a series of disillusions and through being contradicted
> by others that [the child] comes to realize the subjectivity of
> feeling. (p. 127)[116]

Thus, it is through the experience of being thwarted, hence frustrated, by others' points of view that the child's cognition of self as distinct from reality emerges. Interestingly, Piaget's remarks concerning the self and the external world referred to the five- to eight-year-old child, an age range in which, in contradistinction to Piaget, psychoanalytic theorists consider self/object differentiations to be for the most part (see Jacobson[71]) established and functioning except in extreme psychopathological disorders.* (Observational studies of children's play during this age period in turn corroborate the psychoanalytic view.[139] All of Piaget's comments concerning the differentiation of self and external world, then, must be taken from the standpoint of his dealing strictly with self-reflective capacities. Thus, while findings from his interviews with children "point to the child's ignorance of the *fact* [my italics] of subjectivity"[116] they do not imply anything in the way of an absence of conscious *experiences* of subjectivity; nor do they imply an absence of an awareness of distinctions between self and other in everyday social intercourse.

---

* It is perhaps ironic that none of Piaget's major discussions concerning the mental activities of children in the first two years of life[111, 113,116] specifically raised the issue of self and other. In fact, none of them directly involve others, only things and actions on things. In actuality, the observations themselves are not incompatible with a dismantling of the idea of self/other fusion, omnipotence, etc., from the larger framework of psychoanalytic object relations theory. Yet, it is clear throughout his writings that he held to the theory, following Baldwin (see Piaget[109]), that the phenomenology of infancy is devoid of self-awareness (see also Piaget[115]).

It is well known that Piaget characterized the thinking of the young child as essentially egocentric, a term referring to the child's inferior position in logical and objective analysis. Egocentrism is not synonymous with self-interest although individuals characterized by such qualities are often egocentric in their thinking. Objectivity, according to Piaget,

> consists in so fully realizing the countless intrusions of the self in everyday thought and the countless illusions which result—illusions of sense, language, point of view, value, etc.—that the preliminary step to every judgment is the effort to exclude the intrusive self. (p. 34)[116]

Egocentrism ignores the existence of the self's impact on perceptions and thought, disregards the relativity of one's own perspective, and thus takes the subject's point of view as immediately real and absolute. According to Piaget,

> so long as thought has not become conscious of self [which is to say, conscious of the impact made by one's self in everyday thought and communication], it is a prey to perceptual confusions between objective and subjective, between the real and the ostensible; it values the entire content of consciousness on a single plane in which ostensible realities and the unconscious interventions of the self are inextricably mixed. (p. 34)[116]

Nevertheless, these qualities of children's thinking are evidently related to the absence of introspective capacities—that is, self-observing ego capacities—not to the failure to differentiate representations of the self and of objects. Young children know they are not the wind, the sun, their fathers, etc. and act, *except when pretending*, in accordance with this knowledge. However, since children assume that all other objects in the world act and feel as they do, they confer traits on them that are similar to what they experience of themselves. But this animalistic trait does not require the corollary assumption that children make or feel no actual distinction between themselves and others.

BEHAVIORAL FACTORS

The last two decades have witnessed a grand expansion of empirical investigatory interest in the human infant. New technologies, particularly videotaping, permit detailed (microanalytic) analyses of behavior sequences and interactive states and open new doors to the internal processing capacities of very young infants. Affect, once viewed as part of the passive discharge phenomena associated with drive fluctuations, now has transactional/communicative significance in the caregiving relationship, and Darwinian hypotheses along these lines are now being resurrected after a long period of relative dormancy.[26] The concept of the infant as a sometime interactive partner has replaced the notion of the infant as a passive-dependent figure (Mahler's[97] "passive lap baby") in an asocial caregiving context.[3, 10, 68]

In this section I will emphasize that very early on in development the infant is a true agent in its social relationships. This emphasis is supported by an accumulating array of observations and experimental studies of early communicative and interactive capacities in infants (*e.g.*, Lewis and Rosenblum,[89] Thoman,[133] and Kaye[77]). While they do not entirely dispose of many of the ambiguities characterizing early infant developmental phenomena, these studies nevertheless offer glimpses of early organizational and dynamic properties of infant mentation that not only do not require symbiotic conceptions of early object relations but also challenge the utility of such conceptions.

In this section, two questions will occupy the discussion of behavioral factors, each having to do with one of two aspects of separation theory reviewed thus far: *1)* Is the 3–6-month-old infant symbiotic? *2)* Does the infant feel omnipotent in its relations with others?

Is the 3–6-Month-Old Infant Symbiotic?

This question has a corollary question: Is the 0-3-month-old infant normally autistic? The questions go together because both refer to the premise that the young infant is incapable of making the fundamental distinctions critical to the differentiation of self from object. These questions will be considered with reference to infants' periods of wakefulness, leaving aside those periods when infants are asleep or do not sustain focused attention to surrounding events.

Peterfreund[108] has already exposed the terminological fallacy in the concept of *normal* autism. A number of studies have shown that the infant is capable, from neonancy onward, of alert visual interest in the face—or more precisely, in features of the face.* Brazelton[89] based a

---

* The bulk of formal research strongly suggests that the face of the parent is not perceived as a Gestalt until 3–4 months of age[16, 123] Yet, the capacity for feature analysis and extraction of information from the face is a conspicuous and documented set of visual factors from neonancy on.[16 62] The point underlying my comments about the 0–3-month-old infant is

significant part of his behavioral examination of the neonate on this premise, emphasizing the distinct tracking of the examiner's moving face. Haith's remarkable studies of neonatal visual perception indicate that far from being strictly reflexive—that is, obligatory to the stimulus—the neonate's "approach" to visual stimuli (and presumably faces as well) is an active, self-guided process of inspection and analysis.[62] Field et al[35] and Meltzoff[103] have separately reported findings that, while highly controversial from the standpoint of imputing actual imitative capacities to the newborn, take advantage of the quiet, wakeful states of facial interest commonly evident in healthy full-term newborns.

Contemporary theories of early infant cognition emphasize the importance of motor processes in the formation of mental representations of space and objects. (Piaget, of course, is a major proponent of this view.) Yet well-known and widely cited neurophysiological studies by Hubel and Weisel[70] (see also Colonnier,[17] Edelman and Mountcastle,[22] and Szengothai and Arbib[132]) provide evidence of probable innate feature analytic mechanisms in sensory perception that permit the organism to make basic perceptual distinctions. Their findings are compatible with another view of early mental representational processes, namely, that object representations are not solely derived from actions upon the object but from direct perceptions of the object.*

These neurophysiological and epistemological considerations provide an empirical foundation for conceiving of the very young wakeful infant as *oriented toward* external events in the surrounding world—capable, in other words, of direct perceptions of objects as existing apart from its own body. The organism is equipped to act not *as though* an external/internal distinction exists but on the basis of an ability to make an *actual* external/internal distinction. Thus, Ball and Tronick[2] have documented neonates' anticipations of impending collisions with approaching objects, and Wishart, Bower and Dunkeld[143] have shown through infrared photography that young infants would suddenly cease reaching for objects

---

not that the infants are visually drawn to (and visually alert to) the "faceness" of the parent but that they are alert to the facial *features* of the parent. Far from being phenomena that can only be exposed through the advanced technology of the infant behavior laboratory—the latter does, of course, allow for crucial refinements to be made at microtemporal levels—they are conspicuous phenomena in everyday contact with parents and their 0–3-month-old quietly awake infants.

* This is a distinct alternative to Piaget's constructivist account and it is the subject of a recent cogent theoretical discussion by Butterworth.[14] Butterworth draws on Gibson's theory[24, 54] of direct perception, which holds that perception does not depend on action patterns for mental constructs. The theoretical orientation, then, is one of "direct realism"[14] as opposed to the "indirect realism" of Piaget.

when the laboratory lights were extinguished. Recent observations of patterned visual-behavioral interests (pre-peek-a-boo-activity) made between 6½-17 weeks of an infant's development have suggested the ability to make external/internal representational distinctions.[68]

Very young infants prove capable of face-to-face engagements, and they are equipped as organisms to register the textural and spatial information that is required to make such representations at neurophysiological levels. It is likely, then, that almost from the very beginning the infant makes elementary body/nonbody distinctions that are the direct precursors of self/nonself distinctions. These body/nonbody distinctions call not for a theory of autism or symbiosis but rather for further elaborations of a theory of the body self[65] that is from the beginning imbued with primary self feeling, *i.e.*, a sense of presence in the perceived world of objects.*

Does the Infant Feel Omnipotent?

Does the infant feel all powerful? Doesn't the infant feel omnipotent when it is fed in response to its cries? The tacit assumption in these questions is that the infant feels an illusory omnipotence—illusory because objectively the infant is vulnerable, dependent, and helpless; omnipotent because things happen when the infant wants them to. But do infants ever *not* get what they want? Is a feeling of efficacy in the world—the feeling that one can make things happen, which is certainly a characteristic of the 3–6-month-old,[88, 113, 138] the same as the feeling of omnipotence? We have accumulated in our behavioral laboratory evidence that many attempts by babies to make things happen, both interactionally as well as nonsocially, fail. Trying to capture the mother's attention, trying to get out of a high chair, trying to reach an object that is just out of reach—all constitute instances wherein the feeling of efficacy is not forthcoming because the aim of the behavioral attempt is not achieved. The babies' reactions in Brazelton *et al.*'s study[11] of still-faced mothers constitute additional evidence that the infant whose intended interactions are thwarted is not in a position to feel omnipotent.

Freud was correct in ascribing a role to pain and frustration in the development of a sense of the limits in reality. Similar assertions can also

---

* There is, of course, a substantial psychoanalytic literature that addresses the topic of primary self (or ego) feeling (see, for example, Federn,[32] Greenacre,[57] Rose,[120, 121], Jacobson,[71] and most recently Pine[117]) but which does not deal with any of the issues I have raised in the service of correcting problems with symbiotic postulates.

be found in Piaget[116] and in some Soviet psychological writings (*e.g.,* Leowald[94]). But Freud did not dwell on experiences of a nonpainful, nonfrustrating, nonthwarting nature—experiences that also contribute to the acquisition of sensorimotor impressions of self, not/self, things-affected-by-self, etc. Too much is now known about the early intentional capacities of infants to fall back on a theory of symbiosis and omnipotence as explanatory or even descriptive of the infant's subjective experiences. The behavior of infants, preserved on videotape and calculated to the second,[3, 134, 135, 136] attests to the very young infant's active interests in the social world—and even to some differential behavior patterns according to who (father, mother, unfamiliar adult) the partner is.[20] Lewis and Brooks-Gunn[87] have described the distinct action-outcome pairings (cognitions) of this period which, despite an absence of permanence, could well be the basis of clear-cut sensorimotor self/other distinctions during the 3–4 month period and beyond. These are not concepts, of course, but percepts—proprioceptive in large part but also cross-modal (*i.e.,* visual-tactile, visual-proprioceptive, etc.). They do not achieve concept status *per se* until the child has gained the capacity for rudimentary self-observation and reflection, a capacity that is native to older childhood and adolescence. But the absence of a self-reflective capacity should in no way be used as the standard by which the capacity for self/other distinctions is judged, for they truly are of a different order of experience (see *Epistemological Factors,* above).

The characterization of infant subjectivity as a condition of felt omnipotence derives largely from the presumption of undifferentiated self/other representations during the symbiotic period. Naturally, if one is all and all is one, there must be an all-encompassing sense of existence. However, behavioral and subjective analyses of the infant (*supra*) suggest that the perceptual and affective worlds involve experiential distinctions, even though they are not a matter of self-knowledge *per se.* Following Piaget, the infant's actions upon objects may be viewed as the predominant vehicles through which these representational distinctions are constructed. *Intra*modal perceptual-behavioral experiences (*e.g., object seen/not seen, object palpated/not palpated*) and *inter*modal perceptual-behavioral experiences (object seen can be touched/not touched; object shaken can be heard [rattle]/not heard [teething ring]), each corresponding to early stages of sensorimotor development,[113] are both predicated on such distinctions.

The symbiotic foundation removed, it is difficult to mount a reasonable case for infantile omnipotence or grandiosity. True, in the play of children one frequently witnesses sequences and episodes of omnipotent contents, which are largely associated with the egocentric cognitions of children. Much of this kind of play derives from imitations of and, in older children and adolescents, identifications with adults; or from temporary excitements engendered by being powerful; or from the temporary abandonment of constraints imposed by external and internal limits; or from needs to counteract pervasive feelings of vulnerability, helplessness, or inferiority. There is, then, a capacity to *represent* and *feel* oneself as omnipotent within the bounds of play or pathologically suspended reality testing. This capacity, however, may well be an acquired one, whose *appearance* of innateness is inevitable given the child's cumulative experiences with adults in caregiving relationships that are suffused with the latter's power. The adult's experience of the child (and infant) is, in turn, a key factor in the ascription of omnipotence to the latter. This will be elaborated further in the next section.

SOURCES OF INFERENTIAL ERROR

There is poetry in the antithetical concept of a dual unity[100] or of "a self-object polarity, even when self and object representations are not yet differentiated" (p. 17)[79]. Poetry, which appeals to us as a medium for bringing the ineffable into relief against a background of nonverbal experience, bridges the verbalized and nonverbalized realms of experience. It is not surprising, therefore, that some of the most elegant depictions of infant psychic life in terms of symbiotic theory are indeed poetic.[74, 142]

The poetry in this case, however, does not necessarily capture the realities under scrutiny and may reflect more of the poet than the poetic object. Because the theory of symbiosis and omnipotence is formulated on the basis of psychic material drawn from adults as well as from direct observation of and interaction with infants, objective analyses of the phenomenological terrain of infancy must first deal with two sources of inferential error: *1*) errors involving *reconstructions* from adult psychic material and *2*) errors deriving from *ascriptive processes* in adults' perceptions of infants.

Reconstruction

Freud had a well-known penchant for archeological-evolutionary technique and analogy, according to which it was possible to reconstruct (archaeology) the past on the basis of presently observed structures and according to which early forms were germinal to later forms (evolution).

In a timely discourse on the processes of psychoanalytic inquiry and inference, Spence[125] has recently drawn into sharp focus some of the fallacies that attend reliance upon reconstruction as a tool of scientific reasoning. His thesis is that inference made from clinical data concerning past events in an individual's life, which are gathered from free associative or active recollection material, is better conceptualized as

> ... a *construction* ["creative proposition"] rather than as a *reconstruction* that is supposed to correspond to [an actual] something in the past. (p. 35)

Spence's discourse enlarged on the important distinction to be made between two kinds of truth, historical and narrative, in the conceptualization of relationships between past events and present circumstances. Drawing on cogent methodological critiques by Viderman[137] and Lock,[92] Spence carefully demonstrated why reconstruction of past history is an extremely tentative and illusory proposition. According to Spence, historical truths may ultimately be less important than narrative (constructed) truths to the individual's self-coherence. To the scientist and clinician concerned with infant phenomenology, the narrative truths derived from adult phenomenology must defer to the data of direct observation and inference, much as the historian faced with both primary documents and secondary sources will defer to the former.

To summarize Spence's reasoning, without recapitulating its careful and straightforward demonstrations,* *1*) the existence of formal correspondences between present circumstances and past events does not imply a causal relation between the two, and *2*) finding even partial correspondences is likely to be by chance (p. 151ff).[125] As Spence pointed out, strong observer bias undermines the possibility (let alone the feasibility) of making meaningful assessments of the chance factors operating in reconstructive inference processes. There is also the question of how specifically the reconstruction is to be formulated. Global reconstructions are much more likely to be confirmed than highly specific ones, particularly if they overlap with universal truths or conventional wisdom.

In the history of psychoanalytic theories concerning symbiotic, om-

---

* Spence illustrated, for example, how in case studies Freud and other analysts have sometimes hypothesized the occurrence of early events on the basis of manifest patient material and then taken the reconstructed events as facts upon which later events, as explained by them, were based.

nipotent, and regressive characteristics of infancy, much of what has been suggested to us about infant phenomenology is based on observations of adult psychopathology, particularly under primitive or regressed conditions. Spence's points expose the essential methodological flaws in deriving views of infancy from observations of the functioning of older children or adults.

Ascriptive Processes

Infants are natural projective screens for adults: embodying a host of individual (most often parental) and collective aspirations and trepidations, they are the most palpable link between the individual and immortality. The infant's position in life is therefore profoundly, if not cosmically, charged for the individual, and subject to the timeless ascriptions that flow from the mortal soul.

In "On Narcissism" Freud[44] wrote:

> The primary narcissism of children which we have assumed and which forms one of the postulates of our theories of the libido, is less easy to grasp by direct observation than to confirm by inference from elsewhere. If we look at the attitude of affectionate parents towards their children, we have to recognize that it is a revival and reproduction of their own narcissism, which they have long since abandoned. . . . Thus they are under a compulsion to ascribe every perfection to the child—which sober observation would find out occasion to do—and to conceal and forget all his shortcomings. Moreover, they are inclined to suspend in the child's favor the operation of all the cultural acquisitions which their own narcissism has been forced to respect, and to renew on his behalf the claims and privileges which were long ago given up by themselves. . . . At the most touching point in the narcissistic system, the immortality of the ego, which is so hard-pressed by reality, security is achieved by taking refuge in the child. Parental love . . . is nothing but the parents' narcissism born again, which, transformed into object-love, unmistakably reveals its former nature.

Thus, Freud was keenly aware of ascriptive processes underlying adult perceptions and interpretations of infant psychic life. Yet he opted for a view that the primal narcissism of infancy is *revived* in parenting rather than derived from adults' fantasies and ideals about infant psychic life. While parental narcissism as described by Freud is easily observable and, to a large extent, penetrable by means of psychoanalytic inquiry, its genesis need not be attributed *a priori* to the early forms and conditions of narcissism he postulated—that is, narcissism characterized by the absence of self/other distinctions (with its corollary regressive pulls) and omnipotence. Equally tenable, for example, is the hypothesis that parental ascriptions of narcissism and omnipotence to the psychic life of the infant are a function of the parents' deeper knowledge that the infant is in fact vulnerable to and largely helpless in the face of the powerful adult world surrounding it. A corollary hypothesis might be that narcissistic ascriptions made by parents are in fact idealizing defenses against hostility or potential aggression toward the child,[140] a factor in civilization well-documented by history.[19, 56, 60]

There are several infant traits common to everyday adult contacts and interactions with babies, and they bear directly on the ascription of omnipotence to infant subjectivity. Thus, infants are in a position to arouse many affects in adults that frequently favor perceptions of the former's omnipotence. First, the physiological-behavioral states of infants, particularly in the first few months of life, frequently change and thereby affect their manner of engagement. Correlatively, their attentional states are brief. They characteristically focus their attention from object to object; or, as numerous examples from our videotaped observations of infants show, attention may shift cyclically from autoactivity to interactivity. As anyone who interacts directly with infants knows, the baby always takes the lead in such circumstances. In fact, when one "forces" oneself on the infant, for example, either by constantly adjusting oneself in order to remain in the infant's visual field[34] or by intensifying the social stimulation of the baby (unpublished observations in our laboratory), infants visibly thwart the insistent partner through gaze aversion. As unsocialized beings, infants do not follow the rules that govern ordinary social intercourse. However, they seem to follow many simple interactive rules (routines) that are either innately endowed or acquired through interactions. It is a fact of everyday laboratory experience, easily replicable in the natural environment, that when adults violate these rules infants behave in ways geared toward "restoring" them.[136]

Second, through self-directed, egocentric pursuits, older infants and toddlers frustrate and thwart their adult caretakers. Persistence and insistence in matters of self-interest and a refusal to take the other's point of view (which is *not* the same as failing to differentiate the self and other), are familiar and sometimes aggravating traits in infants and toddlers, which lead occasionally to their being characterized as tyrannical.

Third, infants and toddlers require large amounts of attention and involvement from the caregiving environment. Matters of safety and protection, discipline and control, and basic affiliative needs on the part of the young child stand ready to press the vulnerable adult caregiver (*e.g.*, the socially isolated parent, the highly ambivalent parent, and the parent who has no other duties or personal outlets) into feeling enslaved by the child.

Finally, adults' own generative needs as beings conscious of their individual mortality may spiritually incline them to exalt the condition of infancy. The inffant as *tabula rasa,* fresh start, renewal of life, innocent creature—all convey basic existential themes that devolve from adults' contemplations of their own limits and finiteness in life.

Ascriptions are made throughout everyday intercourse with infants. Most are innocuous in substance and reflect shifting affects aroused in the course of stimulating, controlling, or prohibiting them.[76] Ascriptions may be idealizing or indicting in quality and serve to enhance or diminish the infant. In toxic forms, ascriptions become dangerous forces in the caregiving practices of parents and lead to abuse or other damaging events in the life of the infant. In both positive and negative forms, though, it is the adult's *experience* of the infant that is central, not an archaic condition of infancy that reasserts itself.*

CONCLUSION

Although more behavioral observational material could be adduced to counter the alleged utility of symbiotic theory, such data may still not amount to deductive proof. As Mahler and McDevitt[99] have recently stated:

> Whereas there is no conceivable method by which the validity
> of the hypothesis of a symbiotic phase of the mother-infant

---

* The point here is not that introjects derived from early childhood experiences do not operate to form adult outcomes (see the valuable insights of Fraiberg, Adelson and Shapiro[37] concerning the insidious role played by negative maternal introjects in the mothering of some infants), only that the outcome is not a derivation of an inherent pattern of infantile omnipotence.

dual unity can be proven, it is just as impossible, we think, to empathically or otherwise provide or militate for acceptance of the contrary hypothesis—namely, that the infant of a few weeks "knows" or even "feels" that it is his-self that reacts to stimuli emanating from the "other," or that he can in any way discern them from stimuli arising intrinsically within his own body. (p. 828)

Hypotheses that cannot be falsified are of little value to the scientist unless they have some heuristic value. Ironically, the chief heuristic value of symbiotic theory consists of providing a plausible set of syntheses concerning the etiology and subjective correlates of many conditions of adolescent and adult psychopathology, particularly borderline and psychotic conditions.[79, 102] Yet, symbiotic features of psychopathological, as well as normal, adult adjustment (and this includes rapprochement themes as well) cannot be argued to derive from earlier stages that, in circular fashion, have been essentially constructed out of the adult experience. The infant specialist must seriously question the value of symbiotic theory because its explanations and predictions of the infant's everyday behavior often seem less reliable than those based on simple description.

Theories serve two purposes in science. On the one hand, they organize and synthesize facts derived from systematic observation and inference. On the basis of such syntheses, hypotheses are formulated that either predict or lead to new facts or to new interpretations of old facts, and thus to new insights and new actions on behavioral events and situations. On the other hand, theories are used to speculate in areas where facts are few or absent. Such theories, while compelling for their apparent logic or their appeal to intuition or imagination, are, as Freud[48, 49] once characterized psychoanalytic instinct theory, mythologies: philosophical excursions awaiting empirical tests. One cannot escape the impression that the symbiotic theory of object relations grasps for a kind of philosophical rectitude when it emphasizes the intrinsic tension between oneness and separateness. But the remaining questions for symbiotic theory, with its corollary postulates of omnipotence and intrinsic regressive pulls toward self/object fusion, are: What does it predict (correlatively or causally)? To which behavioral data does it refer correlatively? To what internal events, in terms of the infant's and child's actual state of helplessness and naive experience of adults, do these traits actually apply in the infant's direct experience of the world?

REFERENCES

1. Baldwin, J. (1976). Thought and Things. (3 Vols.) (1906-11). AMS Press, New York.
2. Ball, N. and Tronick, E. (1971). Infant responses to impending collision: optical and real. Science 171:818-820.
3. Beebe, B. and Stern, D. (1976). Engagement-disengagement and early object experiences. *In* Communicative Structures and Psychic Structures, N. Friedman and S. Grand, eds. Plenum, New York.
4. Benedek, T. (1949). The psychosomatic implications of the primary unit: mother-child. Amer. J. Orthopsychiat. 19:642-654.
5. Benedek, T. (1959). Parenthood as a developmental phase. J. Amer. Psychoanal. Assn. 7:389-417.
6. Bergmann, A. (1971). "I and you": the separation-individuation process in the treatment of a symbiotic child. *In* Separation-Individuation, J. McDevitt and C. Settlage, eds. International Universities Press, New York.
7. Borke, H. (1972). Chandler and Greenspan's "Ersatz ego-centrism": a rejoinder. Devlpm. Psychol. 7:107-109.
8. Brazelton, T. (1973). Neonatal Behavioral Assessment Scale. Clinics in Developmental Medicine No. 50. Lippincott, Philadelphia.
9. Brazelton, T. (1979). Evidence of communication during neonatal behavioral assessment. *In* Before Speech. The Beginning of Interpersonal Communications, M. Bullowa, ed. Cambridge University Press, New York.
10. Brazelton, T. and Als, H. (1979). Four early stages in the development of mother-infant interaction. Psychoanal. Stud. Child 34:349-369.
11. Brazelton, T. et al. (1975). Early mother-infant reciprocity. *In* Parent-Infant Interaction, CIBA Foundation Symposium 33. Associated Scientific Publishers, New York.
12. Brinich, P. (1982). Rituals and meanings: the emergence of mother-child communication. Psychoanal. Stud. Child 37:3-13.
13. Broughton, J. (1981). The genetic psychology of James Mark Baldwin. Amer. Psychol. 36:396-407.
14. Butterworth, G. (1983). Structure of the mind in human infancy. *In* Advances in Infancy Research, Vol. II, L. Lippsitt, ed. Ablex, New York.
15. Call, J. (1983). Toward a nosology of psychiatric disorders in infancy. *In* Frontiers of Infant Psychiatry, J. Call, E. Galenson and R. Tyson, eds. Basic Books, New York.
16. Cohen, L., DeLoache, J. and Strauss, M., (1979). Infant visual perception. *In* Handbook of Infant Development, J. Osofsky, ed. John Wiley, New York.
17. Colonnier, M. (1966). The structural design of the neocortex. *In* Brain and Conscious Experience, J. Eccles, ed. Springer-Verlag, New York.
18. Cooley, C. (1902). Human Nature and the Social Order. Scribner's, New York.
19. De Mause, L., ed. (1974). The History of Childhood. Harper, New York.
20. Dixon, S., et al. (1981). Early social interactions with parents and strangers. J. Amer. Acad. Child Psychiat. 20:32-52.
21. Dyer, R. (1983). Her Father's Daughter: The Work of Anna Freud. Aronson, New York.
22. Edelman, G. and Mountcastle, U. (1979). The Mindful Brain: Cortical Organization and the Group Selective Theory of Higher Brain Function. MIT Press, Cambridge, Mass.
23. Edgecumbe, R. (1981). Toward a developmental line for the acquisition of language. Psychoanal. Stud. Child 36:71-103.

24. Elkisch, P. (1971). Initiating separation-individuation in the simultaneous treatment of a child and his mother. *In* Separation-Individuation, J. McDevitt and C. Settlage, eds. International Universities Press, New York.

25. Emde, R. (1980). Toward a psychoanalytic theory of affect. *In* The Course of Life: Psychoanalytic Contributions Toward Understanding Personality Development. Vol. I: Infancy and Early Childhood, S. Greenspan and G. Pollock, eds. National Institute of Mental Health, Washington, D.C.

26. Emde, R. (1980). Toward a psychoanalytic theory of affect, I: the organizational model and its propositions. *In* The Course of Life: Psychoanalytic Contributions Toward Understanding Personality Development. Vol. I: Infancy and Early Childhood, S. Greenspan and G. Pollock, eds. National Institute of Mental Health, Washington, D.C.

27. Emde, R. (1981). Changing models of infancy and the nature of early development: remodeling the foundation. J. Amer. Psychoanal. Assn. 29:179-219.

28. Emde, R. (1981). Searching for perspectives: systems sensitivity and opportunities in studying the organizing child of the universe. *In* Prospective Issues in Infancy Research, K. Bloom, ed. Erlbaum, Hillsdale, N.J.

29. Emde, R. (1983). The prerepresentational self and its affective core. Psychoanal. Stud. Child 38:165-192.

30. Emde, R. (1984). The affective self and its origin in infancy. Presented to the Department of Psychiatry, University of Michigan.

31. Emde, R., Gaensbauer, T. and Harmon, R. (1976). Emotional expression in infancy: a biobehavioral study. Psychol. Issues (Whole No. 37) 10(1):1-198.

32. Federn, P. (1952). *In* Ego Psychology and the Psychoses, P. Federn. International Universities Press, New York.

33. Ferenczi, S. (1950). Stages in the development of the sense of reality (1913). *In* Selected Papers of Sandor Ferenczi, Vol. 1. Basic Books, New York.

34. Field, T. (1977). Effects of early separation, interactive deficits, and experimental manipulations on infant-mother face-to-face interactions. Child Devlpm. 48:763-771.

35. Field, T. et al. (1982). Discrimination and imitation of facial expressions by neonates. Science 218:179-181.

36. Fraiberg, S. (1980). Clinical Studies in Infant Mental Health. Basic Books, New York.

37. Fraiberg, S., Adelson, E. and Shapiro, V. (1975). Ghosts in the nursery. J. Amer. Acad. Child Psychiat. 14:387-422.

38. Freud, A. (1981). Child analysis as the study of mental growth, normal and abnormal (1979). *In* The Writings of Anna Freud, Vol. VIII. International Universities Press, New York.

39. Freud, A. (1965). Normality and Pathology in Childhood: Assessments of Development. International Universities Press, New York.

40. Freud, A. (1969). The assessment of borderline cases (1956). *In* The Writings of Anna Freud, Vol. V. International Universities Press, New York.

41. Freud, A. (1973). Infants Without Families. International Universities Press, New York.

42. Freud, S. (1966). The Etiology of Hysteria (1896). Standard Edition of the Psychological Works of Sigmund Freud. Hogarth, London.

43. Freud, S. (1962). Formulations on the two principles of mental functioning (1911). Standard Edition of the Psychological Works of Sigmund Freud, Vol. 12. Hogarth, London.

44. Freud, S. (1957). On narcissism: an introduction (1914). Standard Edition of the

Psychological Works of Sigmund Freud, Vol. 14, Hogarth, London.

45. Freud, S. (1957). Instincts and their vicissitudes (1915). Standard Edition of the Psychological Works of Sigmund Freud. Vol. 14. Hogarth, London.
46. Freud, S. (1961). Negation (1925). Standard Edition of the Psychological Works of Sigmund Freud, Vol. 19. Hogarth, London.
47. Freud, S. (1961). Civilization and its discontents (1930). Standard Edition of the Psychological Works of Sigmund Freud, Vol. 21. Hogarth, London.
48. Freud, S. (1964). Why War? (1932). Standard Edition of the Psychological Works of Sigmund Freud, Vol. 22. Hogarth, London.
49. Freud, S. (1964). New Introductory lectures on psychoanalysis (1933). Standard Edition of the Psychological Works of Sigmund Freud, Vol. 22. Hogarth, London.
50. Fromm, E. (1941). Escape from Freedom. Holt, Rinehart and Winston, New York.
51. Frosch, J. (1964). The psychotic character: clinical psychiatric considerations. Psychiat. Quart. 38:81.
52. Gaensbauer, T. (1982). The differentiation of discrete affects. Psychoanal. Stud. Child 37:29-66.
53. Galenson, E. (1981). Evaluation for in-depth comprehensive treatment. Presented to the Training Institute of the National Center for Clinical Infant Programs (Indicators of Mental Health Disturbance in the First Eighteen Months of Life), Washington, D.C.
54. Gibson, J. (1950). The Perception of the Visual World. Houghton Mifflin, Boston.
55. Gibson, J. (1966). The Senses Considered as Perceptual Systems. Houghton Mifflin, Boston.
56. Gil, D., ed. (1979). Child Abuse and Violence, AMS Press, New York.
57. Greenacre, P. (1958). Early physical determinants in the development of the sense of identity. J. Amer. Psychoanal. Assn. 6:612-627.
58. Greenacre, P. (1960). Considerations regarding the parent-infant relationship. Inter. J. Psychoanal. 41:571-584.
59. Greenspan, H. (1982). Psychopathology and Adaptation in Infancy and Early Childhood. International Universities Press, New York.
60. Grubb, W. and Lazerson, M. (1982). Broken Promises: How Americans Fail Their Children. Basic Books, New York.
61. Guttman, S., Jones, R. and Parrish, S., eds. (1980). The Concordance to the Standard Edition of the Complete Psychological Works of Sigmund Freud. G. K. Hall, Boston.
62. Haith, M. (1980). Rules that Babies Look By: The Organization of Newborn Visual Activity. Erlbaum, Hillsdale, N.J.
63. Hartmann, H. (1950). Comments on the psychoanalytic theory of the ego. Psychoanal. Stud. Child 7:9-30.
64. Hiatt, S., Campos, J. and Emde, R. (1979). Facial patterning and infant emotional expression. Child Devlpm. 50:1020-1035.
65. Hoffer, N. (1950). Development of the body ego. Psychoanal. Stud. Child 5:18-23.
66. Hoffman, M. (1975). Developmental synthesis of affect and cognition and its implications for altruistic motivation. Develpm. Psychol. 11:607-622.
67. Hoffman, M. (1981). Perspectives on the differences between understanding people and understanding things: the role of affect. *In* Social Cognitive Development. Frontiers and Possible Futures, J. Flavell and L. Ross, eds. Cambridge University Press, New York.
68. Horner, T. (1985). Intentionality and the emergence of reality testing in early infancy. Psychoanal. Psychol. (in press)

69. Hubel, D. and Weisel, T. (1963). Shape and arrangement of columns in the cat's striate cortex. J. Physiol. 165:559-568.
70. Hubel, D. and Weisel, T. (1974). Sequence regularity and geometry of orientation columns in the montuey striate cortex. J. Compar. Neurol. 158:267-294.
71. Jacobson, E. (1965). The Self and the Object World. Hogarth, London.
72. Joffe, W. and Sandler, J. (1965). Notes on pain, depression, and individuation. Psychoanal. Stud. Child 20:394-424.
73. Jones, E. (1953). The Life and Work of Sigmund Freud, Basic Books, New York.
74. Kaplan, L. (1978). Oneness and Separateness: From Infant to Individual. Simon and Schuster, New York.
75. Kaufmann, W. (1980). Discovering the Mind, Vol. 3: Freud Versus Adler and Jung. McGraw-Hill, New York.
76. Kaye, K. (1980). The infant as a projective stimulus. Amer. J. Orthopsychiat. 50:732-736.
77. Kaye, K. (1982). The Mental and Social Life of Babies. University of Chicago Press, Chicago.
78. Kernberg, O. (1977). The structural diagnosis of borderline personality organization. *In* Borderline Personality Disorders. P. Hartcollis, ed. International Universities Press, New York.
79. Kernberg, O. (1980). Internal World and External Reality. Aronson, New York.
80. Kleeman, J. (1967). The peek-a-boo game: part 1—its origins, meanings, and related phenomena in the first year. Psychoanal. Stud. Child 22:239-273.
81. Klein, M. (1948). Infant analysis (1928). *In* Contributions to Psychoanalysis. Hogarth, London.
82. Klein, M. (1952). Some theoretical conclusions regarding the emotional life of the infant. *In* Development in Psychoanalysis, J. Riviere, ed. Hogarth, London.
83. Klein, M. (1952). On observing the behavior of young infants. *In* Development in Psychoanalysis, J. Riviere, ed. Hogarth, London.
84. Kohut, H. (1971). The Restoration of the Self. International Universities Press, New York.
85. Kupferman, K. (1971). The development and treatment of a psychotic child. *In* Separation-Individuation, J. McDevitt and C. Settlage, eds. International Universities Press, New York.
86. Lempers, J., Flavell, E. and Flavell, J. (1977). The development in very young children of tacit knowledge concerning visual perception. Genet. Psychol. Monogr. 95:3-53.
87. Lewis, M. and Brooks-Gunn, J. (1979). Social Cognition and the Acquisition of the Self. Plenum, New York.
88. Lewis, M. and Goldberg, S. (1969). Perceptual-cognitive development in infancy: a generalized expectancy model as a function of the mother-infant interaction. Merrill-Palmer Quart. 15:81-100.
89. Lewis, M. and Rosenblum, L., eds. (1974). The Effect of the Infant on his Caregiver. John Wiley, New York.
90. Lichtenberg, J. (1983). Psychoanalysis and Infant Research. Analytic Press, Hillsdale, N.J.
91. Lichtenstein, H. (1964). Narcissism and primary identity. Inter. J. Psychoanal. 45:49-56.
92. Lock, W. (1977). Some comments on the subject of psychoanalysis and truth. *In* Thought, Consciousness and Reality, J. Smith, ed. Yale University Press, New Haven.
93. Loewald, H. (1951). Ego and reality. Inter. J. Psychoanal. 32:10-18.

94. Luria, A. (1966). Human Brain and Psychological Process. Harper and Row, New York.
95. Mahler, M. (1963). Thoughts about development and individuation. Psychoanal. Stud. Child 18:307-324.
96. Mahler, M. (1967). On human symbiosis and the vicissitudes of individuation. J. Amer. Psychoanal. Assn. 15:740-763.
97. Mahler, M. (1972). On the first three subphases of the separation-individuation process. Inter. J. Psychoanal. 53:333-338.
98. Mahler, M. and Furer, M. (1968). On Human Symbiosis and the Vicissitudes of Individuation, Vol. 1. International Universities Press, New York.
99. Mahler, M. and McDevitt, J. (1982). Thoughts on the emergence of the sense of self, with particular emphasis on the body self. J. Amer. Psychoanal. Assn. 30:827-848.
100. Mahler, M., Pine, F. and Bergmann, A. (1975). The Psychological Birth of the Human Infant. Basic Books, New York.
101. Masterson, J. (1976). Psychotherapy of the Borderline Adult. Brunner/Mazel, New York.
102. Masterson, J. (1981). The Narcissistic and Borderline Disorders. Brunner/Mazel, New York.
103. Meltzoff, A. and Moore, M. (1977). Imitation of facial and manual gestures by human infants. Science 198:75-78.
104. Modell, A. (1968). Object Love and Reality. International Universities Press, New York.
105. Newson, J. (1979). Intentional behavior in the young infant. *In* The First Year of Life. Psychological and Medical Implications of Early Experience, D. Shaffer and J. Dunn, eds. John Wiley, New York.
106. Olden, C. (1958). Note on the development of empathy. Psychoanal. Study Child 13:505-518.
107. Olden, C. (1953). On adult empathy with children. Psychoanal. Study Child 8:111-126.
108. Peterfreund, E. (1978). Some critical comments on psychoanalytic conceptualization of infancy. Inter. J. Psychoanal. 59:427-441.
109. Piaget, J. (1927). La première année de l'enfant. Brit. J. Psychiat. 18:97-120.
110. Piaget, J. (1952). Language and Thought in the Child (1916). Routledge and Kegan Paul, London.
111. Piaget, J. (1954). The Construction of Reality in the Child (1937). Basic Books, New York.
112. Piaget, J. (1962). Play, Dreams and Imitation in Childhood (1951). Norton, New York.
113. Piaget, J. (1963). The Origins of Intelligence (1936). Norton, New York.
114. Piaget, J. (1968). Judgement and Reasoning in the Child (1928). Littlefield, Adams and Co., Totowa, N.J.
115. Piaget, J. (1968). The mental development of the child (1940). *In* Six Psychological Studies. Vintage, New York.
116. Piaget, J. (1976). The Child's Conception of the World (1929). Littlefield, Adams and Co., Totowa, N.J.
117. Pine, F. (1982). The experience of self. Psychoanal. Stud. Child 37:143-167.
118. Rank, O. (1929). Truth and Reality. Knopf, New York.
119. Riviere, J. (1952). Genesis of psychical conflict in earliest infancy. *In* Development in Psychoanalysis, J. Riviere, ed. Hogarth, London.
120. Rose, G. (1966). Body ego and reality. Inter. J. Psychoanal. 47:502-509.

121. Rose, G. (1964). Creative imagination in terms of ego "core" and boundaries. Inter. J. Psychoanal. 45:75-84.

122. Settlage, C. (1980). The psychoanalytic understanding of narcissistic and borderline personality disorders; advances in developmental theory. *In* Rapprochement: The Critical Subphase of Separation-Individuation, R. Lax, S. Bach and J. Burland, eds. Aronson, New York.

123. Sherrod, L. (1979). Social cognition in infants: attention to the human face. Infant Behav. Devlpm. 2:279-294.

124. Silverman, L., Lachmann, F. and Milich, R. (1983). The Search for Oneness. International Universities Press, New York.

125. Spence, D. (1982). Narrative Truth and Historical Truth. Norton, New York.

126. Spiegel, L. (1959). The self, the sense of self, and perception. Psychoanal. Stud. Child 14:81-109.

127. Spitz, R. (1955). The primal cavity. Psychoanal. Stud. Child 10:215-240.

128. Spitz, R. (1957). No and Yes: On the Genesis of Human Communication. International Universities Press, New York.

129. Spitz, R. and Coblinger, W. (1965). The First Year of Life: A Psychoanalytic Study of Normal and Deviant Development of Object Relations. International Universities Press, New York.

130. Stern, D. and Sander, L. (1980). New knowledge about the infant from current research: implications for psychoanalysis. J. Amer. Psychoanal. Assn. 28:181-198.

131. Sullivan, H. (1947). Conceptions of Modern Psychiatry. William Alanson White Foundation, Washington, D.C.

132. Szentagothai, J. and Arbib, M. (1975). The "module concept" in cerebral cortex architecture. Brain Res. 95:475-496.

133. Thoman, E., ed. (1979). Origins of the Infant's Social Responsiveness. Erlbaum, Hillsdale, N.J.

134. Trevarthen, C. (1977). Descriptive analyses of infant communicative behavior. *In* Studies in Mother-Infant Interaction, H. Schaffer, ed. Academic Press, New York.

135. Tronick, E., ed. (1982). Social Interchange in Infancy, Affect, Cognition and Communication. University Park Press, Baltimore.

136. Tronick, E., Als, H. and Adamson, L. (1979). The communicative structure of face to face interaction. *In* Before Speech: The Beginnings of Human Communication, M. Bullowa, ed. Cambridge University Press, Cambridge.

137. Vinderman, S. (1979). The analytic space: meaning and problems. Psychoanal. Quart. 48:257-291.

138. Watson, J. (1979). Perception of contingency as a determinant of social responsiveness. *In* Origins of the Infant's Social Responsiveness, E. Thoman, ed. Erlbaum, Hillsdale, N.J.

139. Whiteside, M., Busch, F. and Horner, T. (1976). From egocentric to cooperative play in young children: a normative study. J. Amer. Acad. Child Psychiat. 15:294-313.

140. Winnicott, D. (1958). Hate in the countertransference. *In* Collected Papers: Through Pediatrics to Psychoanalysis. Basic Books, New York.

141. Winnicott, D. (1965). Ego integration in child development (1962). *In* The Maturational Process and the Facilitating Environment. Hogarth, London.

142. Winnicott, D. (1967). Mirror-role of the mother and family on child development. *In* The Predicament of the Family: A Psychoanalytical Symposium, P. Lomas, ed. Hogarth, London.

143. Wishart, J., Bower, T. and Dunkeld, J. (1978). Reaching in the dark. Perception 7:507-512.

PART II: DEVELOPMENTAL ISSUES

7

Looking Out from the Isolator: David's Perception of the World

Mary A. Murphy

Baylor College of Medicine, Houston

Jacqueline B. Vogel

Texas Children's Hospital, Houston

David, who from September 1971 to February 1984 actively lived his life in a sterile isolator, was severely deprived of experience of the physical world. His difficulty with the concepts of space, depth, and size related clearly to his limited experience rather than to cognitive or visual-motor-perceptual deficits.

To write an article about David,* who from September 1971 to February 1984 actively lived his life in a sterile isolator, is painful. Although

Reprinted with permission from *Developmental and Behavioral Pediatrics,* 1985, Vol. 6, 118–121. Copyright 1985 by Williams & Wilkins Co.

David's gnotobiotic care was funded, in part, by USPH grant RR-00188, from the General Clinical Research Centers Branch, National Institutes of Health.

Developmental support for David was provided formally from age 3 years until his death by a multidisciplinary team based in the Meyer Center for Developmental Pediatrics and headed by Murdina M. Desmond, M.D.

* David was placed in a sterile isolator moments from birth because of severe combined immune deficiency. His care alternated between identical isolator systems at Texas Children's Hospital and at the home of his parents. Until age 8, 50% of his time was spent at the hospital in periods of 4 to 6 weeks. Then for 3½ years his time at home increased, varying from 6 weeks to 5 months; his last 9 months were spent mostly at the hospital. The space suit was used six times: four times within the hospital and twice for a brief trip to his home.

it has proved to be therapeutic in our mourning process, it is by no means the closure of our sadness. David described the authors as "best friends, Mary number one, Jackie number two." Our relationship spanned the greatest part of his life; we were with him when he left the isolator and at the time of his death. The very personal and private nature of our involvement allowed us unprecedented opportunity to observe a child develop in an environment so different and unusual that it is virtually impossible to comprehend.

David's unique perceptual development intrigued us from the beginning and seemed worthy of description. We are not offering a systematic case history, let alone a conceptual model. To have placed this child into a situation of experimental study would have destroyed our ability to support him emotionally. Our intimacy with David and the tragic circumstances of his life obviously preclude our ever being able to present him as a research subject. If our observations about David stimulate interest or even controversy about the way in which children in limiting environments grow and develop, then a closer look at these children would be a most fitting tribute to a very special and much-loved child.

HIS PHYSICAL WORLD

To understand the limits of David's knowledge of the world, his environment must be described. The isolator in which he lived consisted of a 6 × 8 × 6 ft high plexiglass room and three rectangular flexible plastic "bubbles." The largest bubble, 6 × 2 × 4½ ft, and the small supply bubble, 4 × 2 × 3 ft, were on a table; a 4 × 2 × 4 ft transport bubble was on a wagon. All of these were housed in a room on the third floor of the Texas Children's Hospital. Windows all along one side faced West. The opposite side had two doors opening into a hall. From the windows, David saw the doctor's parking lot, a two-story hospital annex, a traffic artery and, across the street, a variety of buildings. Directly opposite was a one-story bank, to his left a 14-story Holiday Inn, and to the right a five-story medical clinic. He could see the front as well as the roof of the bank and two sides of both the clinic and the Holiday Inn. To his left he could see the Holcomb-Fannin and Interfirst Bank buildings and the front of the more distant Shamrock-Hilton Hotel.

David's isolator system in his parents' home was identical to the one at the hospital, but his view of the world was from ground level. The playroom was parallel to and inches away from a large picture window. He could, in essence, sit or stand at the edge of the front yard.

Observations

The first author's (M.A.M.) involvement with David began during a visit to his home in September 1974, the month of his third birthday. Already, he had an excellent vocabulary and could identify virtually any geometric figure. He defined many objects or pictures by shape and described a tree as a brown rectangle and a green circle. He refused to believe that the green was given its color by leaves and was only convinced when he watched from the window as a branch with leaves was broken off and brought to him. He asked that a leaf be put beneath the clear plastic bottom of his isolator so that he could examine it.

On the second author's (J.B.V.) first visit, the 16th of July 1976, David's parting request was that she write the exact date and time of her return on his calendar. Since he functioned by clock and calendar, his mastery of time concepts was precocious. Even before he could actually tell time he used the clock. Probably few, if any, children have ever gazed at a clock so much. He was dependent upon people and things coming into his world, and lateness or changes in routine were stressful for him. He never seemed to lose his orientation to time. At 9:30 p.m., the night before he died, as weak and ill as he was, he had both of us scrambling to repair the television because *Star Trek* would be on at 10 p.m.

David's difficulty with space, depth, and size related clearly to his drastically limited and confined physical experience rather than to cognitive or visual-motor-perceptual deficits. He consistently performed in the superior range (age 8; WISC-R Performance IQ 126) on intelligence tests, and his school achievement test scores were always above his grade placement. Eye-hand coordination and dexterity skills were always excellent. At age 4 he had a sight vocabulary of at least 50 words.

At 5, he said, "Nothing in the whole world is as big as the hospital parking lot." He insisted that the buildings across the street had no backs. The two visible sides of the Holiday Inn and of the medical clinic he described as "flat," and the edge of a building was merely a line. The same was true of the bank roof and front. Neither drawings nor explanations convinced him that the buildings actually had four sides. Construction paper silhouettes pasted on a blue poster board were to David no different than his percept of the buildings and sky. To teach him the concept that the building has a front and back, M.A.M. built models. The first step was to draw each side that he could see. He described the window positions and determined when the drawings were correct. Then with sticks for reinforcement the sides were pasted together, duplicating the buildings. Finally, at age 6 he conceded that the buildings did have four sides. However, he still insisted they only had windows on one side. He asked someone to check for windows on the other side of the medical clinic, and, unfortunately for the teaching sessions, this building does have windows on one side only.

From age 5 on David frequently requested sketches of what could be seen from our windows at home: backyards, courtyards, streets. Attempts at a more complex drawing which showed a floor plan with front, back, and side yards frustrated him. "Don't bother about that, Jackie," he would say, "just draw what you can see from one window."

At 6 a "space suit" designed by NASA allowed David a limited opportunity to walk outdoors on two occasions. After he was outfitted, he was taken by a van to his home and enjoyed playing with a hose and water in his backyard. When a second excursion was planned, he again wanted to go into the backyard and sprinkle. When M.A.M. discussed this excursion with him beforehand, it became evident that he did not realize that his family's house had four walls. Its structure remained obscure to him even after detailed descriptions. For this reason, it was planned that he be allowed to walk completely around the house. Others involved in the excursion thought this ridiculous, since this very bright boy, of course, knew that houses had four sides.

David was familiar with the front yard because of his view of it from the window. When the van parked in front of his house, he got out and, surprisingly, started to walk across the street away from his front yard, saying, "I want to go in the backyard." When attempts were made to redirect him, he asserted adamantly, "No, no, I want to sprinkle in the back." Finally, on faith alone, he agreed to cross the front lawn to the backyard. After going completely around the house, his comment was, "Gee, Mary, you're right, the house is a box, and the backyard is where you said it was. You know everything!"

Similarly, he was confused and unsure about the different floors in the hospital itself. He understood that the rows of windows in the buildings across the street each represented a story, but he did not relate this knowledge to the hospital. He knew that M.A.M.'s office was on the first floor directly under him (he was on the third), because he had visited it, but until age 7 he was certain that no story existed between. Only an elevator stop on the second floor convinced him. As far as he was concerned, there were only three floors in the hospital: First, Third, and Seventh (J.B.V.'s office).

The Interfirst Bank and the Shamrock-Hilton Hotel are similar in height, both being approximately 16 stories high. The Shamrock-Hilton, however, is a much larger building in terms of cubic feet. Because David viewed it at a greater distance, it was impossible to convince him that the hotel was really the larger of the two structures and only appeared smaller due to the effect of distance. After counting the stories in the building he reluctantly agreed that they were the same height, but he could not comprehend the more complex issue of square footage or the amount of ground covered by the building. The linear perspective in his sketch (see Fig. 1) is correct, yet at 12 he firmly believed that the Shamrock-Hilton was the smallest building, when in reality it was the largest. He held to his trust in appearance.

At age 11 two weather circumstances, fog and rain as the sun set, did help to give David a vague percept of distance. On a foggy night when the Holiday Inn lights were brighter than the Interfirst Bank and the more distant Shamrock-Hilton Hotel lights were barely visible he said, "I think I understand what you were trying to get at with the little flashlight." One evening he related how he had watched rain approach the hospital, "I could see the parking lot get wet; as the rain came closer the sun moved back."

David knew at age 4 that it took 1 hour to drive from the hospital to his home, and he knew that it took 5 minutes for M.A.M. to drive from the hospital to her home. However, he could not relate distance to time. At age 7 he outlined a route on a road map from St. Louis to Houston and then to an address on a city map. But seeing locations of homes on a map did not help him to comprehend distance. M.A.M.'s attempts to construct a "map" with boxes for buildings and string for the road to his home were met with "No, no, that's not right. We can never do it as long as I'm in here and you're out there." It was only after the excursion in the space suit to his home, when shown were M.A.M. lived (en route to his house), that he began to associate time and distance. He said, "Mary, be sure to show me where you live on the way back," realizing that he needed a reference point both coming and going. When he was back at the hospital he said, "Now I understand why it takes you only five minutes to get here."

The vast expanse of the oceans eluded him, as became evident when M.A.M. told him when he was 11 of her plans to fly to Singapore. He located Singapore on the globe, and stated that it certainly was far away, about halfway around the earth. To her lament at having to fly 28 hours, his comment was, "Well, if you don't like flying that long, why don't you just drive over?" His advice after listening to explanations that driving across the States took days and that one cannot drive on oceans was, "take a ship." Cognitively, he was aware that Houston and Singapore were far apart and he reluctantly conceded, "You should probably just

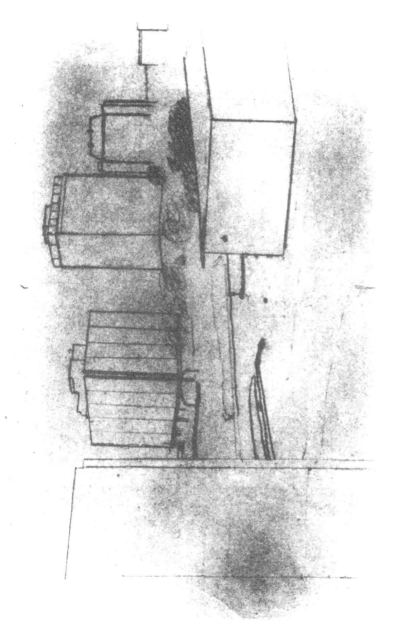

FIGURE 1. Sketched by David in December 1983. From left to right: Three-story Texas Children's Hospital wing, 10-story Holcomb-Fannin Building, 16-story Interfirst Bank, 16-story Shamrock-Hilton, top of Houston-Place. Right front: two-story hospital annex and the doctors' parking lot.

go ahead and fly." Clearly, the relationship of time and distance continued to remain a mystery to him.

The concept of bodies of water, lakes and rivers and pools, were virtually impossible for David to understand. Even more basic than David's problem with water was his belief that the ground's surface was like a sheet of paper. Trees had no roots, and, certainly, holes did not exist. J.B.V. undertook to explain trees and roots by bringing a plant in a pot of soil. He was allowed to pull up the plant and see the roots.

The underpass at Fannin and Holcombe Streets could not be explained to him despite many attempts. From his vantage point, he could only glimpse the top of the railing marking the beginning of the underpass. He would see cars on the one-lane frontage road continue at street level, while the cars in the center two lanes disappeared. Even photographs taken by J.B.V. from all sides of the underpass failed to clarify its structure or the practical function of an "underpass."

David showed little interest in photographs of landscapes but could analyze subtleties of abstract and surrealistic paintings for hours. Surprisingly, he inquired, "Why do you call those abstract? They are not abstract, they are real. This is a peaceful forest, and that one is *Hawaii Five-O*. See the waves, the beach, and seashells." On many occasions, attempts were made to enlarge David's understanding of the natural world by way of nature documentaries on television. Despite repeated encouragement, however, his interest in these films was minimal.

David preferred the "soaps" and situation comedies on television. One common element in these programs was that the action is all in one room. He liked the characters in *Little House on the Prairie*, which has many outdoor scenes, but he needed an interpreter. For example, when the horse and wagon went over a hill and out of sight, he did not understand why it disappeared. Learning by television can distort perception; for example, at age 8 he believed the cart was what "made the horse go." When watching a film with action, especially a Western, he would ask, "What happened, where is he?" or state, "Look up and watch, so you can tell me what's going on." He had no problem following action in outer space films and cartoons.

In February 1984, 2 weeks before his death, he was removed from his isolator to a regular room across the hall. His view was restricted to the hospital's second-story roof and wings. Until then he had always watched for M.A.M. to park her car in front of the hospital. He asked, "Mary, where are you parking now?" To the reply, "The same place," he said, "Well, I guess you just can't break a habit." As to the garage where J.B.V. parked, he had only a vague idea, since he never saw it.

Few people were aware that David's percepts did not agree with objective reality. He understood this problem and in conversion was quick to cover errors. His relationship with both of us was such that he could discuss the discrepancy between his observations and assumptions and our descriptions of the physical world. Having lost trust in his own perception, he needed to check out reality with us.

LITERATURE AND COMMENTS

Our observations of David's perceptual development suggest that neither looking at buildings, photographs, and television nor the use of the power of cognition is a substitute for experience. Phenomena must be experienced to be learned.

In the 18th century British empiricist Bishop Berkeley argued that judgments made about depth, distance, and space were based entirely on memories of past experiences. We would agree. The literature on visual spatial perception, especially experimental studies, is voluminous, yet a survey produced only a few articles that had any relevance to David's case.[1-6]

Two dominant theorists, Gibson and Piaget, stress the importance of interaction with environment. We cannot fit our observations into Gibson's[7] framework: visual perception is direct and does not require interpretation or experience; the organism's locomotion and behavior are continually controlled by detecting information from the environment. David's description of his world as "flat" is the exact opposite of Gibson's (p. 286) position:

> No one ever saw the world as flat patchwork of colors—no infant, no cataract patient, and not even Bishop Berkeley or Baron von Helmholtz, who believed firmly that the cues for depth were learned. The notion of a patchwork of colors comes from the art of painting, not from any unbiased description of visual experience.

Piaget's[8] theory that reality is constructed out of experience seems to hold the most promise in understanding David's perceptual development. Piaget's[9] passage could almost have been written by David:

> The sky seems to us a big spherical or elliptical cover on whose surface move images without depth which alternately interpenetrate and detach themselves: sun and moon, clouds, the

stars as well as the blue, black, or gray spots which fill the interstices. It is only through patient observations relating the movements of these images and the way they mask each ther, that we arrive at the kind of elaborating subjective groups. . . . At first, with regard to immediate perception, there exist neither conscious groups nor permanent solids (the celestial bodies seem to be reabsorbed in each other and not to hide behind one another), nor even depth.

"If we passed our lives fixed to a solid object, as do oysters to a rock, and were deprived of movement and manipulations, our projective estimates would no doubt be excellent, but size constancy would probably not develop."[10] Piaget's oyster and rock can be seen as analogous to David and his bubble.

REFERENCES

1. Foley, J. M., Held, R.: Visually directed pointing as a function of target distance, direction, and available cues. Percept. Psychophys. 12:263-267, 1972.
2. Fine, B. J., Kobrick: Individual differences in distance estimation: Comparison of judgments in the field with those from projected slides of the same scene. Percept. Mot. Skills 57:3-14, 1983.
3. Pick, A. D., Pick, H. L. Jr.: Culture and perception, in Carterette, E. C., Friedman, M. P. (eds): Perceptual Ecology. Handbook of Perception, Vol. 10. New York, Academic Press, 1978.
4. Deregowski, J. B.: Pictorial perception and culture. Sci. Am. 227:82-88.
5. Kennedy, J. M.: Perception, pictures, and the etcetera principle, in Mac Leod, R. B., Pick, H. L., Jr. (eds): Perception: Essays in Honor of James J. Gibson. Ithaca, NY, Cornell University Press, 1974.
6. Hochberg, J., Brooks, V.: The perception of motion pictures, in Carterette, E. C., Friedman, M. P. (eds.): Perceptual Ecology. Handbook of Perception, Vol. 10. New York, Academic Press, 1978.
7. Gibson, J. J.: The Ecological Approach to Visual Perception. Boston, Houghton Mifflin, 1979.
8. Piaget, J., Inhelder, J. L.: The Child's Conception of Space (translated by F. J. Langdon, J. L. Lunzer). London, Routledge & Kegan, 1956.
9. Piaget, J.: The Construction of Reality in the Child (translated by M. Cook). New York: Basic Books, 1954, pp. 144-145.
10. Piaget, J.: The Mechanisms of Perception (translated by G. N. Seagrim). New York, Basic Books, 1969, p. 228.

Part III
GENDER IDENTITY

The process by which a child develops a normal gender identity has been explained in the past by simple answers, such as an identification with the parent of the same sex and an absorption of the sex stereotype formulations of what constitutes masculine versus feminine behavior and attitudes. But serious studies of this issue indicate that the development of gender identity is a more complex process that is shaped by a number of influences. The first two papers in this section, the ones by Fagot and Huston, present complementary reviews of the research literature and current thinking on this important developmental topic.

Both Fagot and Huston emphasize that recent research studies indicate that the beginnings of gender identity can be noted at an earlier age than was previously assumed, even as early as 18 months. Fagot emphasizes the importance of the distinction between gender identity as a private subjective understanding and gender role as a public expression of this subjective understanding. Gender identity is learned very early in life and is very difficult to change, while gender-role behaviors can be modified or changed by a number of factors, such as age or cultural change. In a similar view, Huston points out that the Women's Movement has radically changed traditional sex typing. The girl who wants to be on the little league baseball team or play football is no longer automatically regarded as showing a denial of her "femininity," nor is a father's active child-caring activities or interest in cooking labeled as "unmasculine" as they would have been even in the recent past. Both articles review the complexities involved in the development of gender identity and the currently more sophisticated research approaches that promise to illuminate.

The paper by Harkness and Super highlights the influence of the cultural setting in gender-role development through a study of a community in western Kenya. In this community there is no gender segregation until about the age of 6 years, when a shift toward same-sex peer activities begins. But clearcut and different sex-role patterns do not become fixed until adult life, following ceremonial adolescent rites. The authors conclude that gender segregation is the product of "the social settings of daily life, parental theories of child behavior and the customary duties of children" operating as a system. They emphasize that it would be an error to attribute the pattern of gender segregation in America to personal growth alone and suggest that "a larger cultural perspective" would be profitable.

The papers by Coates and Person and by Green both report clinical studies of boys with the DSM-III diagnosis of gender identity disorder, which includes the persistent wish to be a girl and the display of traditional female stereotypical behavior. Such effeminate boys do not show abnormalities of external genitalia or sex chromosome pattern. The Coates and Person study concentrated on the psychiatric evaluation of their cases, with the finding that 84% showed behavioral disturbances, and a majority had significant difficulties in peer relationships and/or symptoms of separation anxiety disorder. The authors conclude that these findings suggest that extreme boyhood feminity is part of a pervasive disorder rather than an isolated finding. As they indicate, this formulation suggests directions for further research as to the nature of this disorder.

The paper by Green reports a followup of a group of 44 boys with gender identity disorder, with the finding that 30 of the 44 became bisexually or homosexually oriented. A comparison study of these 30 with the 14 who became heterosexual would be of great interest. Further clarification of this syndrome of gender identity disorder could undoubtedly result from a study of girls with the same disorder, with an analysis comparing the results of the male study.

The final paper by Gualtieri and Hicks tackles the knotty problem of why boys have a significantly higher incidence of neurodevelopmental and psychiatric disorders than do girls. The research literature is reviewed, and the various theories offered as explanations are subjected to a critical analysis. Gualtieri and Hicks then present their theory that the male fetus induces a state of maternal immunereactivity, which "evokes an inhospitable uterine environment." The authors admit that this theory is necessarily speculative, but present some suggestive supporting evidence from the existing literature and their own research. Their paper is noteworthy both for its comprehensive review of this baffling problem of selective male affliction in childhood and for the heuristic value of their own concept.

PART III: GENDER IDENTITY

8

Changes in Thinking about Early Sex Role Development

Beverly I. Fagot

University of Oregon, Eugene

How do we learn to recognize ourselves and to live as beings endowed with gender? This paper discusses changes in our answer to this question over the last 15 years. As our methods of study have changed, we have been forced to see the development of sex role as an increasingly complicated process. This paper documents two studies that were attempts to bring together two methodologies: cognitive development and social learning. In the first study, 180 children were tested using the R. G. Slaby and K. S. Frey (1975, Child Development, 46, *849-856) gender identification interview. The findings documented that children's gender understanding followed the sequence predicted by L. Kohlberg (1966, in E. Maccoby (Ed.),* The development of sex differences. *Stanford, CA: Stanford Univ. Press): identity, stability, and constancy. However, the child's level of gender understanding was unrelated to the adoption of sex-typed behaviors. In the second study, a second group of 64 children, 20 to 30 months of age, were tested for understanding of gender labels, gender identity, and sex-typed behaviors. Sex of playmates and boys' play with feminine toys were related to understanding of verbal gender labels. Reasons for continuing problems of interpretation in the sex role area are discussed.*

Reprinted with permission from *Developmental Review*, 1985, Vol. 5, 83–98. Copyright 1985 by Academic Press, Inc.

Data analyses were supported by BRSG Grant RR07980 awarded by the Biomedical Research Support Grant Program, Division of Research Resources, National Institutes of Health. The final writeup was completed on a postdoctoral fellowship (Grant 1 T32 MH 16955-01) through the Oregon Social Learning Center.

In science and out, a good question has consequences as well as answers. It stings us to thought as we try to loose the knot of its particular mystery, but it also changes the way we think about other questions and, sometimes, the way we lead our lives. *How do we learn to recognize ourselves and to live as beings endowed with gender?* When do we begin? At five? At three? At one? Who is the master/mistress of this art? Who teaches us? The family we inherit? The language we assume? The body we are born to? What is the cost if we stumble in this learning, or if we are tripped? Who must pay then? Who will pick us up when we fall? Clearly, the constant fact of gender and the inescapable consequences of that fact pose a very good question. What have we done with this question we have been given? Often we have ignored it, pretending that we could study personality without some understanding of sex role development, even though these roles are founded deep in the grammar with which we announce ourselves to the world. We study a neutered kind of cognition or social development, even though boys and girls obviously are not neuters and live in different worlds in which the same behaviors may have different consequences according to the perceived sex of the child.

When I first began to study sex differences, I started with the social learning viewpoint then current. I assumed that if I could understand the types of reinforcers received by children for sex-typed behaviors, I would understand sex role development. My early work concentrated on 4- and 5-year-old boys and girls, for it was fairly well accepted in the literature prior to 1961 that sex differences in children below the age of 4 were unstable. Freudians speculated that the identification process took place between 4 and 5, when we were too old for the crib, too young for the couch, but just the right age to remember (with a practitioner's help, of course). Two more modern approaches, modified learning theory and cognitive theory, led to the same opinion. Working within the terms of the former approach, Sears (1965) held that the child of either sex matched behaviors with the mother until such time as the father took a more active role with the boy, and then, at about 5, the male child could start matching behaviors with the father. Working within the latter approach, Kohlberg (1966) also suggested that real sex differences would emerge at around 5 years of age as a function of the cognitive understanding of gender identity. And where the theorists led the metricists followed, for the technique of measurement used in many of these early studies—the It test (Brown, 1956)—also led to the conclusion that a stable estimate of sex differences was not really obtained until the subject was about 5.

Today, we can see that there were three serious shortcomings in this early research. First, the children were too old. Second, it tended to subordinate investigation to theory and in the process to create a kind of Ptolemaic psychology dedicated to saving the appearances and the sanctity of the laboratory. Third, it tended to substitute for the complex reality of a single organic process—a child coming to know its sex—the simpler ideology of Developmental Psychology or of Cognitive Psychology or of Social Learning. Obviously, these failings are not without connection, so in working to correct one, we inevitably work on all. For example, it is now generally accepted that 3- and probably 2-year-old children show well-developed sex differences in their behavior. Have children suddenly become more sophisticated than they used to be? No, the indication is that children have not changed much at all. Data collected in 1963 on 3-year-olds are very similar to data collected in the 1970s (Fagot, 1977), but what has changed is the way the data are collected. More flexible theoretical approaches in social learning and in ethology have led to children being observed as they play in their natural environments. At first, findings from this research indicated that sex differences were present from age 3 (Clark, Wyon, & Richards, 1969; Fagot & Patterson, 1969). Then studies using similar techniques found stable sex differences as early as 18 months (Blurton-Jones, 1972; Etaugh, Collins, & Gerson, 1975). The earlier negative and inconsistent findings were due to the difficulties of obtaining reliable verbal responses to testing rather than to the lack of real sex differences in the younger children.

What are some of these differences and why do they merit study? Block (1983) grouped sex-related differences in each child into seven conceptual domains: aggression, activity, impulsivity, susceptibility to anxiety, achievement-related behaviors, self-concept, and social relationships. These categories can help us explain why there is so much evidence that boys and girls are at risk in different areas of their development and at different ages. Baumrind (1979), for example, pointed out that male insufficiencies in development are apparent by the age of 4 in the guise of less developed prosocial behaviors, so that boys are more aggressive, work less well at tasks, and often lack control over their impulses. Girls seem to show insufficiencies at a later age, displaying in their early teens lower self-esteem, a more diffuse self-concept, and an unwillingness to break away from dependent relationships. Similarly, Eme (1979) noted that sex differences are present in psychopathology from a very early age, and basically show a pattern of undercontrol of impulses for males and overdependency for females, and that boys run into difficulties at a much earlier age than girls.

The study of sex role development has been hindered by vocabularies that are only approximately shared, which leads to a coarsening of discriminations and can yield downright confusion. A careful distinction must be made between the development of cognitive categories concerning sex and the expectancy of one's sex. Money and Ekhardt (1972) made an important distinction between gender identity (as a private understanding) and gender role (as a public expression of this private understanding). We must not allow these two terms to blur, for it appears that gender identity is learned very early, and is extremely difficult to change, while gender role behaviors often change as a function of age (Maccoby & Jacklin, 1974), of particular stages of life, or of movement across cultures (Block, 1973). Huston (1983) carefully delineated the dimensions of sex role in terms of content and private and public expressions of such constructs. Her schema suggested that different investigators often give the same names to quite different content areas and constructs, and this should help us understand why results in the area often appear contradictory. In particular, self-perception, beliefs, and behavioral enactment are often simply subsumed under a label of sex typing, despite the fact that they may all be quite uncorrelated. We know something about the socialization of gender role behaviors or behavioral adoptions by family and peer groups, for these processes are highly visible and easy to study; we do not know how these variables affect gender identity, or even if they do.

Sex differences in child behavior do not begin to appear with any regularity until about the first birthday, and even then the differences are few in comparison with the similarities observed between such young boys and girls. Nor are all differences, once found, found again. One widely quoted study (Goldberg & Lewis, 1969) found several sex differences in the behavior of 1-year-olds when they were individually observed with their mothers during a "free play" situation. The infants' behavior corresponded to sex stereotypes of parents and to observations of sex differences in older children's behavior. However, most replication studies with children of this age have not found such extensive sex differences in style of play or behavior toward the mothers (Brookes & Lewis, 1974; Clarke-Stewart, 1973; Jacklin, Maccoby, & Dick, 1973). While sex differences in the behavior of infant boys and girls are minimal, by the time children approach their second birthday, there is substantial evidence for consistent differences that would appear to be an extension of those occasionally observed during the first year of life. For example, a frequent finding involves differences in the toy preferences of toddler girls and boys observed during play at home. Girls tend to play with soft toys and dolls, they dress up and dance, while boys tend to play with transportation toys and blocks, to manipulate objects actively, and to play more often with toys and household items forbidden by parents (Fagot, 1974, 1978; Fein, Johnson, Kosson, Stork, & Wasserman, 1975; Smith & Daglish, 1977). Also consistent with the expected or stereotyped social expressive orientation of girls and the object orientation of boys, girls tend to begin to talk earlier than boys (Schachter, Shore, Hodapp, R., Chalfin, & Bundy, 1978) and to use this ability to their advantage in problem situations such as the barrier frustration task (Feiring & Lewis, 1979).

Information provided by the child's environment is not always consistent and there may be fairly long intervals between presentations of similar events, yet children develop categories or gender schemata which allow them to classify behaviors, attitudes, and themselves as male or female. Parental interventions and environmental factors may punctuate the process of growth, but the child, too, must be studied in terms of its own developing capabilties so far as this is possible. The most popular technique during the 1970s was to focus upon the sequence in which the child comes to recognize gender. According to Eaton and Von Burgen's (1981) summary, *gender understanding* consists of four components that enter a child's cognitive repertoire in the following order: (1) *labeling* of self, then others as "boy" or "girl," (2) *stability*, the recognition that gender is permanent over time, (3) *motive*, knowledge that gender cannot change even if one wants it to, and (4) *constancy*, knowledge that gender (one's own and that of others) is invariant despite changes in activity, appearance, attire, and so on. Much of the work done so far has concentrated upon looking at whether this sequence of understanding holds true.

The work by Martin and Halverson (1981) and Bem (1981) is an attempt to apply information process theory to the child's understanding of gender. Both researchers suggest that understanding of gender is an attempt by the child to organize and structure social information. Both approaches suggest that children will develop a very differentiated schema for their own sex and a much less differentiated schema for the opposite sex. Carter and Patterson (1982) found that conception of gender, like understanding of other social conventions, became more flexible with age. They also suggested that gender is merely one aspect of the development of social–conventional thought. Cognitive research on sex role in the 1980s has attempted to look at sex role through more conventional information-processing approaches, while social learning and ethological research have concentrated upon the child's performance in the natural environment. It is now time to bring the two systems of research together to develop a more complete understanding of the child's attempt to understand the complexities of gender.

A normative study of cognitive gender understanding in children from 18 months to 5 years of age is presented in this paper. Several normative studies have been completed but the results have been somewhat con- tradictory as to age-related developments, because each has covered very small age ranges (Kuhn, Nash, & Brucken, 1978; Marcus & Overton, 1978; Slaby & Frey, 1975). In the longitudinal study presented in this paper, the development of gender constructs was examined to determine whether it follows the predicted sequences. A major purpose of the study was to examine the relationship between the child's construction of gen- der identity and the adoption of sex role behavior.

STUDY 1

Method

Subjects. The total sample for this study consisted of 180 children, 90 boys and 90 girls, whose ages ranged from 18 to 54 months old at the beginning of the study. The broad age range of the sample allowed observation of change at several levels of gender understanding and development. Subjects were blocked into 6-month age intervals for sta- tistical treatment of the group data. There were 15 children of each sex within each 6-month age interval. One hundred seventeen of these chil- dren were also observed in play groups while the testing took place, and were followed up and retested every 3 months for a period of 1 year.

The 117 children (59 boys, 58 girls) who were observed in play groups and followed for 1 year all attended play groups in the psychology department at the University of Oregon. The additional children at- tended child day-care centers which had a population of parents very similar to the psychology department groups. The socioeconomic back- ground of the children was varied, from professional to welfare families. Approximately one half of the mothers in this sample were employed or attended school, but this was not related to the social class of the family. Approximately half of the children were in various kinds of alternative care for 5 or more hours per day. The children were all Caucasian (white); 10 minority children were tested but not included in the results.

Behavior checklist.[1] A list of 34 child behaviors and 15 teacher and peer

---

[1] A coding manual for the behavior checklist can be obtained from the author.

reactions were used for this study. The child behaviors included activities such as rough-and-tumble play, build with small blocks, and dance, while the reactions included categories of behaviors such as hug and give physical affection, parallel play, and continue alone. The child behavior was always recorded first, then the reactor (if there was one), and then the reaction. For each observation there were always separate child behaviors and reactions.

Psychology department play group setting. The play groups consisted of 12 to 15 children, with an approximately equal number of boys and girls in each class. Two undergraduate students served as teachers throughout each term in each class. The large study has been in progress for 6 years, with each year divided into three 10-week terms corresponding to the university school year. The children for this study were observed during their first two terms of attendance in the project, with approximately 15 children observed each year. There were no consistent differences in play behaviors or in teacher or peer consequences among the different cohorts, so the children were combined into a single sample. The playroom was approximately 20×25 ft, equipped with standard preschool toys such as blocks, dolls, books, and transportation toys. Teachers were instructed to let the children choose their own activities and to interfere only when a child was obviously disturbed. The teachers did provide varied activities each day by placing toys on the tables or the floor for the children to choose, but no attempt was made to have each child sample all activities.

Observations. Observers were first trained using videotapes from children engaged in the play groups in previous terms. The tapes were precoded so that over the 2 years of the study all observers were checked against criterion tapes. None of the videotaped interactions are included as data in this study. Throughout each term of data collection, reliability spot checks were run at least once a week and sometimes three times a week. There was an average of 12 reliability checks in a term of data collection, with a range of 10 to 15.

The observers had to give exactly the same code number on each observation to be considered in agreement. Each spot check lasted approximately 15 min, which gave the observers time to code all children in the room three different times so that each set of coders working at the same time shared 120 or more observations. The pairs of observers all exceeded 90% agreement for the child behaviors (range = 91 to 98%) and 75% for the reactions (range 78 to 92%).

Procedures. Observers were in an observation room with a separate entrance and observed the children through a one-way mirror. Two hours of observation were completed during each play session. All children were observed each session using a scan sampling technique. Each child was observed in predetermined order for 2–5 s, and the child's behavior, the reactors, and the reaction were coded. Using this technique, each child in the play group was observed 12 times per hour for a total of 480 to 720 observations during the term. This technique gives a picture of the types of activities favored by the children in the group, and gives a pattern of peer and teacher reaction within the group.

Gender constancy task. The child was administered the gender constancy interview of Slaby and Frey (1975) with minimal changes. The interview consisted of a set of 14 questions. We also added the question used by Emmrich that combined motivation and a belief in the constancy of gender (If I had a magic wand, could I change you into a [child of the opposite sex])?

Definition of male, female, and neutral behaviors. Behaviors were categorized as male, female, or neutral in a previous study (Fagot, 1984), in which tests for sex differences in behavior were made for a separate sample of 180 children. At least 12 and as many as 80 h of observation per child were coded using the behavior checklist described above. Eight play activities showed significant sex differences (i.e., were more likely to be engaged in by one sex or the other as determined by *t* tests significant at the .01 level). Male-typical activities included rough-and-tumble play, transportation toys, large blocks, and carpentry play. Female-typical activities were doll play, dress up, art activities, and dance. The 10 following behaviors showed no significant sex differences and were designated as neutral behaviors: play in wagon, climb and slide, play with clay, play with design boards and puzzles, play with small blocks, play with puppets, play ball or frisbee, fantasy play, sing or listen to records, and look at books. This system was used to classify the behavior observed in the present study, so that scores for the play behavior categories were combined to yield male-typical, female-typical, and neutral behavior scores for each child.

Results

Gender Constancy. The percentage of boys and girls who answered both the question and its reverse correctly for each stage in the gender constancy task during their first interview are presented in Table 1. As can be seen, there was an age-related trend, with gender identity questions answered earlier than stability, and stability earlier than constancy. There were no sex differences in the number of boys and girls passing the items at each age category (sign test). The results replicate those by Slaby and Frey (1975) and Marcus and Overton (1978), who used slightly older samples, and Kuhn, Nash, and Brucken (1978).

Longitudinal results. Children were retested once a term during their attendance in the play groups so that their development over a time span could be plotted. The data from the longitudinal sample also fit the cognitive development predictions. Table 2 presents the results of children who received the gender constancy test over at least three different terms. Only six children, three boys and three girls, differed from the predicted sequence.

Relationship between sex preference and gender constancy. Sex role scores

TABLE 1
GENDER STAGE PASSED AT EACH AGE LEVEL

Age (months)	Total N	Own identity		Gender identity		Stability		Constancy	
		n	%	n	%	n	%	n	%
				Boys					
18–24	14	2	13	2	13	1	7	0	
25–30	15	7	47	4	27	0		0	
31–36	15	10	67	10	67	0		1	7
37–42	15	15	100	15	100	3	20	4	27
43–48	15	15	100	15	100	4	27	8	53
49–54	15	15	100	12	80	12	80	12	80
				Girls					
18–24	15	1	6	2	13	0		0	
25–30	15	2	13	2	13	1	7	0	
31–36	15	8	53	8	53	2	13	0	
37–42	15	11	73	11	73	4	27	4	27
43–48	15	15	100	15	100	6	40	6	40
49–54	15	15	100	15	100	15	100	15	100

TABLE 2
NUMBER OF CHILDREN IN EACH TYPE OF SEQUENCE OVER 1 YEAR

	Boys	Girls
Predicted sequence	37	40
− + − −	0	1
+ + − +	3	1
− − + −	0	1
None (no stage passed successfully)	19	15
Total	59	58

were the proportion of time spent in each sex-typed category normalized using arc sine transformations. The correlations between gender constancy scores and sex role scores were computed with age partialed out. There were no significant relationships for either boys or girls between sex role preference and gender constancy (girls, .10; boys, −.01). In other words, there was no linear relationship between the sex role score and the child's gender understanding. However, Kohlberg's (1966) theory predicts a curvilinear relationship. Children should start to show more sex-typed behavior once gender identity is established, and then should become increasingly sex typed as sex role is organized. However, once constancy is achieved, then the child should begin to try out different behaviors and could become less stereotyped.

When we look at children who achieve constancy, we see no change in their behavior. Those who were very stereotyped continue so, while those less stereotyped continue in their mode. Neither the group data nor the individual data help us to understand the relationship between the cognitive category and the adoption of behaviors. The nature of Slaby and Frey's task may contribute to these findings. First, they make verbal responses—though minimal—necessary. Second, the interview itself is confusing. For each discrimination, the child must produce the correct response and then negate the incorrect one. For example, in the attempt to avoid random and preseverative correct answers, the child is asked, "Is this a girl?" If the answer is "Yes," she/he is asked of the same figure, "Is this a boy?" Such questioning may disconcert young children, and perhaps lead them to think their first answer was wrong. Finally, the child is considered to have mastered a level only when *all* of the questions at that level are answered correctly; such stringent criteria may easily mask the beginnings of competence. While it appears likely that findings with regard to sequence in the acquisition of gender constancy are valid, the beginnings of the process are not illuminated by this line of work.

STUDY 2

Although there was no relationship between sex role behavior and gender constancy tasks in the first study, it still seemed reasonable that a child's understanding of "boy" and "girl" might influence the way she/he organizes his or her play behaviors. The Slaby–Frey interview is built to ensure that a child understands the concept under confusing conditions. In other words, the Piagetian model of pushing to the limits is used. Perhaps the organization is done earlier at a much simpler level.

Thompson (1975) included a nonverbal gender discrimination task in his investigation of gender labeling and sex role development in preschool children: subjects could identify pictures according to the label paired boy–girl, man–woman, man–lady, father–mother, mommy–daddy, brother–sister, he–she, him–her, and his–hers. At 24 months, children were correct on 61% of the noun pairs and 51% of the pronoun pairs; by 36 months these figures were 90 and 88%, respectively. In addition, subjects sorted pictures of children, including photographs of themselves, into separate containers: 24-month-olds classified their own pictures correctly 50% of the time, 36-month-olds 88%. Except for the brother–sister pairs, which elicited the most errors, it is not clear whether children responded differentially to pictures of adults and children, nor whether the discrimination task included reinforcement for correct responses (i.e., trained, rather than just assessed the ability in question). Some children may have begun to make gender discriminations regarding other people by the age of 2, but their ability to identify themselves as male or female was not evident. However, the beginning of this ability may develop before the child is able to communicate such knowledge and may even precede any conscious awareness of sex differences.

In the next study, the relationship among the child's ability to give gender labels and the adoption of sex-typed play and same-sexed friends is examined.

Method

Subjects. Sixty-four children, half boys and half girls, from 20 to 30 months of age were included in this study. Except that the mean age was younger, they did not differ from the children in the first study.

Procedure. The children were observed while participating in peer play groups. Scan samples were done in each group over a period of 4 weeks during which each child was observed. A very simple checklist of play with male and female toys (defined from previous study) and play with peer male, female, or both sexes was constructed. Each child was scanned 10 times on four different occasions for a total of 40 observations. From these observations it was possible to determine whether the children adopted behaviors typical to their sex (sex-typical behaviors), and their playmate choice. Two different measures of the child's understanding of sex and sex role were given to the child. One was similar to a task derived from Thompson (1975), where the child was asked to point to pictures as either a male or female (gender label). The second task was the interview devised by Slaby and Frey (1975) designed to test the child's understanding of gender identity, stability, and constancy. For this study, only the gender identity questions of the Slaby–Frey are examined. The children fall into three different groups. One group correctly identified 75% of the pictures (gave the appropriate gender label) and showed gender identity on the Slaby–Frey interview. Another group identified the pictures (gave the appropriate gender labels) but did not answer gender identity questions correctly. A third group answered neither gender labels above chance levels nor gender identity questions correctly. The mean age of the three groups was the same.

Results

The first question is, are there any differences among the three groups in the amount of time spent with same- and opposite-sex peers? Children of both sexes who answered the gender label questions correctly spent an average of 80% of their time in same-sex groups, while children who answered the gender label questions below that level spent about 50% of their time in same-sex groups (see Table 3). If playing with a member of the same sex is an attempt to match your behavior to someone you perceive as like you, then it appears that understanding of gender labels predicts playmate choices. The second question is, does the understanding of gender labels predict the choosing of sex-typical behaviors? Here the answer is more complicated. For girls, there was no difference among the three groups in the amount of time spent with male-typical and female-typical toys. For boys, there was no significant difference in amount of time spent with male-typical toys, but boys who did not have gender labels spent more time with female-typical toys than boys who

TABLE 3
STUDY 2: COMPARISON OF PLAY GROUPS' PLAY BEHAVIORS FOR
THREE GROUPS OF CHILDREN

Play behavior	No gender understanding		Gender labels		Gender labels and identity	
	Boys	Girls	Boys	Girls	Boys	Girls
Percentage of peer play with same-sex peers	55	49	82	78	78	80
Percentage all toys same-sex toys	11	9	13	10	14	15
Percentage all toys opposite-sex toys	10	10	4	9	5	8

did have such labels. In particular, boys without gender labels or gender identity played with dolls at about equal rates as girls, but this behavior was almost nonexistent in boys who showed some knowledge of gender labels.

DISCUSSION

The work in sex role development has diverged in two directions over the past 6 or 7 years. One group of researchers examined the construction of gender categories. There has been good progress made in understanding the different stages of cognitive understanding of gender. Cohen and Strauss (1979), for instance, have adapted the habituation paradigm to study the development of gender categories in children under a year. Martin and Halverson (1981) have employed a schematic processing model to explain the prevalence of sex stereotyping in young children. Work in social learning has documented just how prevalent sex-typed socialization is in the environment. Fagot (1978) demonstrated differential socialization of boys and girls in the home. Lamb and his colleagues (Lamb, Easterbrooks, & Holden, 1980; Lamb & Roopnarine, 1979) have shown how peer groups teach boys and girls different ways of behaving. Bem (1981, 1983) suggested that, while children do actively attempt to develop a gender schema during the first 3 years of life, parents should make every attempt to help them not overgeneralize such a schema.

However, just how the cognitive development of understanding of gender and the social information received interact is not clear. The two studies presented in this paper were an attempt to understand that relationship. While the first study gave fairly clear evidence that there is a consistent sequence of cognitive development, it did not help illuminate the relationship between that cognitive development and the adoption of sex role behaviors. It is my belief that this is because the measurement instrument was not developed to tap into the beginnings of gender understanding. The second study used a simplified procedure to measure the beginnings of gender understanding. By studying the beginnings of gender understanding, we began to see how adoption of sex role behaviors is related.

Perry and Bussey (1979) presented a modified social learning theory view of how imitation contributes to sex role development. They proposed that the child observes the different frequencies at which each sex performs certain behaviors in different situations. The child then employs the different frequencies as abstractions of what constitutes male-appropriate and female-appropriate behavior as models for imitative performance. It would seem reasonable to hypothesize that children also abstract information from the differential frequencies of reinforcement they receive for performance of different types of behavior. However, children also react to the category of respondent, so it is necessary to assume that the child has some concept of gender that would lend greater value to some individuals than others.

Why did not we see relationships between gender understanding and adoption of sex role behaviors in our earlier studies? I would like to argue that sex role behavior after very early awareness is a particularly good example of what Langer (1978) calls "automatic behavior" or "non-thinking behavior." This refers to behavior which is so overlearned that one does not have to "think" about what one is doing. The behavior occurs when one has overlearned the script, which is then enacted without engaging the rational thought processes. Most of what has been studied about sex role has dealt with subjects who have already invoked such "automatic processes." After behaviors are so overlearned and have become automatic, then relationships between cognitive variables and behavioral performance may be poor. However, in the period up until 3 years of age, when children are actively engaged in the construction of gender categories, we should see them attempting to behave in ways congruent with those categories. In our attempts to study such relationships in the first study, most children were beyond this construction phase. It is now my belief, still to be fully tested, that stronger relationships between behavioral adoption and categorization will take place between 12 and 36 months of age because children are actively trying out behaviors to match their developing gender categories.

In our lab we have developed a discrimination task (Leinbach, 1983) which allows us to examine children from 16 months of age concerning their knowledge of gender labels. I believe that when the child is constructing gender categories, all kinds of attempts to categorize the world by gender will be made. For instance, children who show the ability to categorize boys and girls, are more likely to choose same-sex playmates than children who do not yet have such knowledge (Fagot, 1983). In the Fagot study, techniques developed from the cognitive approach and observational technology developed from social learning were used to help understand an old finding, that of the rapid gender segregation we find in preschool-aged children.

However, there is still one aspect of sex role development which needs to be incorporated; that is, how does the process become so important to the child, or to put it in another way, how does the category of one's gender become so affect laden? With recent attempts to study the interface between cognition and affect, new methods are being developed which should help us study all aspects of sex role development rather than splitting our studies into artificial domains.

REFERENCES

Baumrind, D. (1979). *Sex related socialization effects.* Paper presented at the meetings of the Society for Research in Child Development. San Francisco.

Bem, S. L. (1981). Gender schema theory: A cognitive account of sex typing. *Psychological Review,* **88,** 354-364.

Bem, S. L. (1983). Gender schema theory and its implications of child development: Raising gender-aschematic children in a gender-schematic society. *Signs,* **8,** 598-616.

Block, J. H. (1973). Conceptions of sex role: Some cross-cultural and longitudinal perspectives. *American Psychologist,* **28,** 512-526.

Block, J. H. (1979). Socialization influences on personality development in males and females. In M. H. Parks (Ed.), *APA Master lecture series on issues of sex and gender.* Washington, DC: American Psychological Association.

Block, J. H. (1983). Differential premises arising from differential socialization of the sexes: Some conjectures. *Child Development,* **54,** 1335-1354.

Blurton-Jones, N. (Ed.). (1972). *Ethological studies of child behavior.* Cambridge: Cambridge Univ. Press.

Brookes, J., & Lewis, M. (1974). Attachment behavior in thirteen-month-old opposite sex twins. *Child Development,* **45,** 243-247.

Brown, D. C. (1956). Sex role preference in young children. *Psychological Monographs,* **70**(14, Whole No. 421).

Carter, D. B., & Patterson, C. (1982). Sex roles as social conventions: The development of children's conceptions of sex role stereotypes. *Developmental Psychology,* **18,** 812-824.

Clark, A. H., Wyon, S. M., & Richards, M. P. M. (1969). Freeplay in nursery school children. *Journal of Child Psychology and Psychiatry,* **10,** 205-216.

Clarke-Stewart, K. A. (1973). Interactions between mothers and their young children: Characteristics and consequences. *Monographs of the Society for Research in Child Development,* **38**(6-7, Serial No. 153).

Cohen, L. B., & Strauss, M. S. (1979). Concept acquisition in the human infant. *Child Development,* **50,** 419-424.

Eaton, W. O., & Van Burgen, D. (1981). Asynchronous development of gender understanding in preschool children. *Child Development,* **52,** 1020-1027.

Eme, R. F. (1979). Sex differences in childhood psychopathology: A review. *Psychological Bulletin,* **86,** 574-595.

Etaugh, C., Collins, G., & Gerson, A. (1975). Reinforcement of sex-typed behaviors of two-year-old children in a nursery school setting. *Developmental Psychology,* **11,** 255.

Fagot, B. I. (1974). Sex differences in toddlers' behavior and parental reaction. *Developmental Psychology,* **10,** 554-558.

Fagot, B. I. (1977). Consequences of moderate cross-gender behavior in preschool children. *Child Development,* **48,** 902-907.

Fagot, B. I. (1978). The influence of sex of child on parental reactions to toddler children. *Child Development,* **49,** 459-465.

Fagot, B. I. (1983, April 21-24). Recognition of gender and playmate choice. In L. Serbin

(Chair), *A cognitive–developmental approach to affiliation patterns: Children's awareness of and use of gender language and body type as social dimensions.* Symposium presented at Biennial Conference for Society for Research in Child Development, Detroit, MI.

Fagot, B. I. (1984). Teacher and peer reactions to boys' and girls' play styles. *Sex Roles,* **11,** 691-762.

Fagot, B. I., & Patterson, G. R. (1969). An in vivo analysis of reinforcing contingencies for sex-role behaviors in the preschool child. *Developmental Psychology,* **1,** 563-568.

Fein, G., Johnson, D., Kosson, N., Stork, L., & Wasserman, L. (1975). Sex stereotypes and preferences in the toy choices of 20-month-old boys and girls. *Developmental Psychology,* **11,** 527-528.

Feiring, C., & Lewis, M. (1979). Sex and age differences in young children's reactions to frustration: A further look at the Goldberg and Lewis subjects. *Child Development,* **50,** 848-853.

Goldberg, S., & Lewis, M. (1969). Play behavior in the year-old infant: Early sex differences. *Child Development,* **40,** 21-31.

Huston, A. C. (1983). Sex typing. In P. H. Mussen (Ed.), *Handbook of child psychology: Vol. 4. Socialization, personality, and social development.* New York: Wiley.

Jacklin, C., Maccoby, E., & Dick, A. (1973). Barrier behavior and toy preferences: Sex differences (and their absence) in the year-old child. *Child Development,* **44,** 196-200.

Kohlberg, L. (1966). A cognitive-developmental analysis of children's sex-role concepts and attitudes. In E. Maccoby (Ed.), *The development of sex differences.* Stanford, CA: Stanford Univ. Press.

Kuhn, D., Nash, S. C., & Brucken, L. (1978). Sex role concepts of two- and three-year olds. *Child Development,* **49,** 445-451.

Lamb, M. E., Easterbrooks, M. A., & Holden, G. A. (1980). Reinforcement and punishment among preschoolers: Characteristics, effects and correlates. *Child Development,* **51,** 1230-1236.

Lamb, M. E., & Roopnarine, J. (1979). Peer influences on sex role development in pre-schoolers. *Child Development,* **50,** 1219-1222.

Langer, E. J. (1978). Rethinking the role of thought in social interaction. In J. Harves, W. Ickes, & R. Kidd (Eds.), *New directions in attribution theory* (Vol. 2). Hillsdale, NJ: Erlbaum.

Leinbach, M. D. (1983, April 21-24). *Gender discrimination in toddlers' identifying pictures of male and female children and adults.* Paper presented at biennial conference for Society for Research in Child Development, Detroit, MI.

Maccoby, E. E., & Jacklin, C. N. (1974). *The psychology of sex differences.* Stanford, CA: Stanford Univ. Press.

Marcus, D. E., & Overton, W. F. (1978). The development of cognitive gender constancy and sex role preferences. *Child Development,* **49,** 434-444.

Martin, C. L., & Halverson, C. F. (1981). A schematic processing model of sex typing and stereotyping in children. *Child Development,* **52,** 1119-1134.

Money, J., & Ekhardt, A. A. (1972). *Man and woman, boy and girl.* Baltimore: Johns Hopkins Univ. Press.

Perry, D. G., & Bussey, K. (1979). The social learning theory of sex differences: Imitation is alive and well. *Journal of Personality and Social Psychology,* **37,** 1699-1712.

Sears, R. R. (1965). Development of gender role. In F. A. Beach, *Sex and behavior.* New York: Wiley.

Schachter, F. F., Shore, E., Hodapp, R., Chalfin, S., & Bundy, C. (1978). Do girls talk earlier?: Mean length of utterance in toddlers. *Developmental Psychology,* **14,** 388-392.

Slaby, R. G., & Frey, K. S. (1975). Development of gender constancy and elective attention to same-sex models. *Child Development,* **46,** 849-856.

Smith, P. K., & Daglish, L. (1977). Sex differences in parent and infant behavior. *Child Development,* **48,** 1250-1254.

Thompson, S. K. (1975). Gender labels and early sex-role development. *Child Development,* **46,** 339-347.

9

The Development of Sex Typing: Themes from Recent Research

Aletha C. Huston

University of Kansas, Lawrence

A conceptual framework for organizing the constructs and content areas included in research on sex typing is presented in this review of recent research on the development of sex typing. Two major themes are discussed. First, sex-typed play activities and interests emerge clearly in the first few years of life. Both play activities and peer preferences are sex typed earlier and more definitely than are personality traits and social behaviors such as aggression or dependency. It is suggested that researchers have underemphasized the importance of interests, activities, and peer associations while overemphasizing personality attributes as the core of sex typing. The second theme is that cognitions and concepts about sex typing are important in the acquisition of gender typing, but they are not sufficient by themselves for understanding the process by which sex-typed behavior is acquired. Children's sex-role concepts are sometimes related to their behavioral preferences, but other factors are also important influences on behavior.

During much of the 20th century, psychologists studied sex typing because their theories contained the assumption that acquisition of an

Reprinted with permission from *Development Review*, 1985, Vol. 5, 1–17. Copyright 1985 by Academic Press, Inc.

This article is based on an invited address to Divisions 35 and 7 of the American Psychological Association, August 1982. Preparation of the review was aided by a grant from the National Institute of Mental Health (MH 33082).

"appropriate" sex role was crucial for normal, healthy development. Theories and research were directed to learning how young boys could become masculine and young girls could become feminine. The Women's Movement and the resulting rejection of traditional sex roles by many people led to a conceptual about-face in the early 1970s. Many of the scholars who became interested in the subject were committed to the values of feminism. Their research was designed to learn about the negative consequences of traditional sex typing and about means for socializing children toward "androgyny" or away from socially prescribed sex roles. Partly because of the radical shift in social values, the topics and questions addressed in the research of the past 10 or 15 years have been quite different from those in preceding periods.

The purpose of this paper is to discuss some of the themes emerging from this recent research and to suggest some profitable directions for future studies (as well as some directions that should be avoided). A second purpose is to present an organizational framework for conceptualizing the domain of sex typing. This framework is intended primarily as a heuristic device for organizing and discriminating among various concepts presently used in the field.

CONCEPTUAL FRAMEWORK

I begin with the conceptual framework because it guides the analysis of themes in the research literature. One of the most important conceptual advances of the 1970s was the clear recognition that sex typing is multidimensional. Although others had proposed dimensional structures for understanding sex typing, Constantinople's (1973) review of measures for adults marked a point after which no reasonable scholar could again speak of "masculinity" or "femininity" as unitary constructs. Furthermore, the work of Bem (1974), Spence and Helmreich (1978), and others made it clear that bipolar conceptions were inadequate for understanding personality traits that are socially stereotyped as feminine and masculine.

The full implications of multidimensionality became apparent to me, however, when I began trying to integrate the sex typing literature for a major review (Huston, 1983). Very diverse characteristics of people are subsumed under the rubrics "sex role, sex typing, gender identity," and so on. The outcome of my struggle to make sense of the literature was a matrix based on two continua: content and construct. It appears in Table 1. It is intended primarily as a heuristic device, not with any claim that it represents factorially pure or unitary constructs.

The rows in the matrix are categories of content that have been in-

TABLE 1

A Matrix of Sex-Typing Constructs by Sex-Typed Content (All Entries Are Examples)

Content area	Construct			
	A. Concepts or beliefs	B. Identity or self-perception	C. Preferences, attitudes, values (for self or for others)	D. Behavioral enactment, adoption
1. Biological gender	A1. Gender constancy	B1. Gender identity as inner sense of maleness or femaleness. Sex role identity as perception of own masculinity or femininity	C1. Wish to be male or female or gender bias defined as greater value attached to one gender than the other	D1. Displaying bodily attributes of one gender (including clothing, body type, hair, etc.)
2. Activities and interests Toys Play activities Occupations Household roles Tasks Achievement areas	A2. Knowledge of sex stereotypes or sex role concepts or attributions about others' success and failure	B2. Self-perception of interests, abilities; or sex-typed attributions about own success and failure	C2. Preference for toys, games, activities; attainment value for achievement areas; attitudes about sex-typed activities by others (e.g., about traditional or nontraditional roles for women)	D2. Engaging in games, toy play, activities, occupations, or achievement tasks that are sex typed
3. Personal–social attributes Personality characteristics Social behavior	A3. Concepts about sex stereotypes or sex-appropriate social behavior	B3. Perception of own personality (e.g., on self-rating questionnaires)	C3. Preference or wish to have personal–social attributes or attitudes about others' personality and behavior patterns	D3. Displaying sex-typed personal–social behavior (e.g., aggression, dependence)

	A	B	C	D
4. Gender-based social relationships Gender of peers, friends, lovers, preferred parent, models, attachment figures	A4. Concepts about sex-typed norms for gender-based social relations	B4. Self-perception of own patterns of friendship, relationship, or sexual orientation	C4. Preference for male or female friends, lovers, attachment figures, or wish to be like male or female, or attitudes about others' patterns	D4. Engaging in social or sexual activity with others on the basis of gender (e.g., same-sex peer choice)
5. Stylistic and symbolic content Gestures Nonverbal behavior Speech and language patterns Styles of play Fantasy Drawing Tempo Loudness Size Pitch	A5. Awareness of sex-typed symbols or styles	B5. Self-perception of nonverbal, stylistic characteristics	C5. Preference for stylistic or symbolic objects or personal characteristics or attitudes about others' nonverbal and language patterns	D5. Manifesting sex-typed verbal and nonverbal behavior, fantasy, drawing patterns

Note. Reprinted, with permission, from Huston in P. H. Mussen (Ed.), *Handbook of Child Psychology* (4th ed.), 1983 copyright, John Wiley, New York.

cluded by some investigators in measures or conceptions of sex typing. *Biological gender* is self explanatory. *Activities and interests* include toys and play activities, occupations, household tasks, family roles, and areas of achievement. Much of what sociologists define as *sex roles* (in the technically precise use of that term) falls in this content category. *Personal–social attributes* include personality traits and social behaviors such as aggression, dominance, dependence, and gentleness. Most of the measures of androgyny and most psychological research fall in this content domain. The fourth area is *gender-based social relationships*. It includes the gender of one's friends, one's sexual partners, the persons one chooses to imitate, and the persons one selects as attachment figures, all of which have been used as indexes of sex typing. The common theme among all of these is that one's relation to another person is based on that person's gender. For young children, friendship patterns serve as a good example. Children are expected to form most of their friendships with members of their own gender. A child who plays consistently with the other gender is often thought deviant. In fact, one criterion for diagnosing "gender deviant" boys is that they prefer girls as playmates (Rekers, 1979). *Stylistic and symbolic contents* of sex typing include gestures and nonverbal behavior (Frieze & Ramsey, 1976; Rekers, Amaro-Plotkin, & Low, 1977) speech and language patterns (Fillmer & Haswell, 1977; Haas, 1979), symbolic patterns or attributes such as tempo, size, pitch, open vs closed, angular vs round (e.g., Franck & Rosen, 1949), and patterns of fantasy or play (Cramer & Hogan, 1975; Erikson, 1963; May, 1971).

The columns in the matrix represent constructs describing an individual's relation to the content categories. They include *concepts* or *beliefs* about what is sex typed in each domain, *identity or self-perception* of one's own attributes, *preference or attitudes* about your own or other people's sex-typed characteristics, and *behavioral enactment* demonstrating sex-typed behavior. This matrix serves as a reference point for the discussion of two major themes from the recent literature on children's sex typing.

CENTRAL CONTENT OF EARLY SEX TYPING

Activities and Interests

The first theme is that throughout development, play activities, interests, occupations, and family roles are sex typed earlier and more definitely than are personality and social behaviors. Yet, psychologists have emphasized personal–social attributes as the core of sex typing while often dismissing activities and interests as either obvious or trivial.

Before explaining what I think we can learn from recognizing the importance of activities and interests, let me document the statement that they are primary in development.

A large body of literature on children's sex-typed concepts has accumulated in the last 10 years, and the results are quite consistent. Sometime between ages 2 and 3, children learn to label themselves and others correctly as male or female. Almost as soon as they can produce these labels, they know the sex stereotypes for toys, clothing, tools, household objects, games, and work. Children who are just 2 years old respond at chance levels on questions about stereotypes, but by age 2½ several investigations have found better-than-chance responding when children were asked to classify objects and symbols of sex-typed activities and interests (Blakemore, LaRue, & Olejnik, 1979; Kuhn, Nash, & Brucken, 1978; Myers, Weinraub, & Shetler, 1979; Thompson, 1975; Venar & Snyder, 1966). By age 3 and beyond, children are clearly aware of the feminine and masculine connotations of many activities, interests, and adult occupations (Edelbrock & Sugawara, 1978; Falkender, 1980; Flerx, Fidler, & Rogers, 1976; Huston, 1983; Marantz & Mansfield, 1977; Masters & Wilkinson, 1976; Schau, Kahn, Diepold, & Cherry, 1980).

Parallel patterns occur in children's spontaneous play behavior or when they are asked to choose toys and games for themselves. By age 2, girls and boys play with sex-stereotyped toys more often than with toys stereotyped for the other gender (Fagot, 1974; Fein, Johnson, Kosson, Stork, & Wasserman, 1975; Weinraub & Leite, 1977). For example, in one series of studies, toddlers from ages 15 to 36 months were observed in a day care center during periods when toys selected to represent masculine, feminine, and neutral stereotypes were provided. Girls played more with the feminine toys and boys with the masculine toys (O'Brien, Huston, & Risley, 1983). Some of these children are too young to produce meaningful verbal labels about male and female, yet they show sex-typed toy choices.

By age 4 or 5, children also state highly stereotyped occupational preferences. If you ask them what they want to be when they grow up, the majority of preschool girls say teacher, nurse, secretary, or mother. Boys name a wider range of occupations, most of which fit a masculine stereotype (e.g., fireman, pilot) (Garrett, Ein, & Tremaine, 1977; Huston, 1983; Kleinke & Nicholson, 1979; Marantz & Mansfield, 1977; Nemerowicz, 1979; Papalia & Tennent, 1975; Thornburg & Weeks, 1975).

These patterns become ingrained early, even when parents and teachers make an effort to counteract them. I have heard numerous anecdotes from professional women that are similar to my own experience. When my daughter was 3½, she announced with certainty that women could not be doctors. I pointed out that I was a doctor and her aunt was a physician. She looked at me with suspicious belief.

Gender-Based Social Relationships

Along with sex-typed play activities in preschool come gender-based social relationships. Children are more responsive to peers of their own gender than to peers of the other gender as early as age 3. Jacklin and Maccoby (1978) found that unacquainted pairs of 33-month-old children interacted more when they were the same gender than when they differed. In preschool, and probably in other settings, sex segregation of the peer group is inextricably intertwined with sex-typed play activities. When boys and girls gravitate to different activities, then they play primarily with children of their own gender. Conversely, if children select same-sex playmates, they often find themselves in sex-stereotyped activities. If you like playing dolls, you will end up playing mostly with girls. Or, if you choose to play with girls, you will often find them in the doll corner. Thus, it seems that sex segregation of peers, which increases from preschool through middle childhood, is an integral part of the early pattern of sex-typed activities and interests (Eisenberg-Berg, Boothby, & Matson, 1979).

Personal-Social Attributes

Now let us turn to personal–social attributes. It is probably significant that investigators have rarely tried to ascertain children's knowledge about sex stereotypes in this domain before about age 5. When they have questioned preschool children, most investigators have found little awareness of socially prescribed feminine and masculine social behavior (Etaugh & Riley, 1979; Flerx et al., 1976; Katz & Rank, 1981; Kuhn et al., 1978). Between 5 and 11, children gradually acquire knowledge of sex stereotypes about traits such as aggression, crying easily, kindness, and dominance. Such stereotypes not only emerge much later developmentally than those for activities and interests, but they are leess definite (Best et al., 1977; Williams, Bennett, & Best, 1975). Children are less certain about the sex typing of kindness and independence than they are about doll play and love of trucks.

Children's personal–social *behavior* is also less clearly gender typed than play patterns and peer choices. Aggression is the only behavior in this domain for which sex differences consistently appear in early childhood. In 1974, Maccoby and Jacklin concluded that there was not definite evidence of mean sex differences for any other personality attribute. Although that conclusion has been challenged (e.g., Block, 1976), it is clear that sex differences in altruism, nurturance, independence, dependence, dominance, and the like, where they exist at all, are neither as pronounced nor as early developmentally as play patterns and peer choices.

In short, my first major theme is that, of all the content areas subsumed under the rubric of sex typing, psychologists have paid too little attention to activities and interests and to peer choices while overemphasizing personality attributes and social behavior. I do not mean to imply that the latter are unimportant, but that we have not given enough emphasis to the most obvious, earliest, and most well-documented differences in expectations and experiences of young girls and boys.

Research Implications

If we turned our attention to activities, interests, and peer groupings, what might we learn? I will suggest two directions for new research. There are undoubtedly many others. First, play activities themselves may cultivate patterns of behavior and teach cognitive or social skills. For example, Sherman (1967) and others have suggested that male sex-typed activities such as block play provide more opportunities to learn about spatial relationships than female-stereotyped play activities. A small body of empirical literature provides some support for this contention, but the evidence is far from conclusive (Huston, 1983; Newcombe, 1982).

A related line of research (Carpenter, 1983; Carpenter & Huston-Stein, 1980) is based on the hypothesis that sex-typed activities provide different amounts of structure or guidance about how to perform the activity. "Structure" in this work refers to the rules, guidelines, and parameters of an activity—what to do and how to do it. If an activity is structured by an adult, children look to the adult for guidance about what to do. They learn to be compliant and to seek recognition from adults. When they are in unstructured activities, they may create a structure for themselves. In so doing, they practice leadership, innovation, and initiative.

A second research direction that might arise from an emphasis on activities and interests is more intensive study of sex segregation and its consequences. Segregation of peer groups is such a prevalent pattern during the preschool and elementary years that we sometimes treat it as an ontogenetic "given." Yet the literature on school settings shows that the amount of sex segregated play varies greatly from one environment to another. For example, children in open school programs spend much less time playing exclusively with same-sex peers than those in traditional schools (Bianchi & Bakeman, 1978). Varying the room arrangement or varying where adults spend their time in the preschool can also alter the ratios of boys and girls in an activity (Serbin, Connor, & Citron, 1981). Careful investigations of the environmental structures and contingencies that increase or decrease sex segregated play would provide valuable information.

While sex segregation contributes to sex differentiated play patterns, it may also, under some circumstances, permit more flexibility in sex-typed behavior. For example, boys consider reading more masculine when they are in all male reading classes than in mixed sex classes (McCracken, 1973). Similarly, students in single-sex colleges more often take nontraditional majors than those in coeducational institutions (Block, 1981). More data on the outcomes of segregated and mixed settings might clarify these complex patterns.

COGNITIVE BASES OF SEX TYPING

The second major theme emerging from recent literature is the importance of cognitive variables in the acquisition of sex typing. Concepts or beliefs about sex appropriateness—that is, cognitions about sex typing—constitute the first construct heading in Table 1. Social psychology and the psychology of personality have been swept by the "cognitive revolution" in the past 15 or 20 years. Instead of explaining behavior primarily by motives and needs, many theorists have elaborated the ways in which people conceptualize and interpret their social worlds. In developmental psychology, this trend has often included an emphasis on cognitive–developmental changes as a basis for social cognition.

The major theoretical work applying Piagetian theory to sex typing was Kohlberg's (1966). Rejecting the psychoanalytic notion that motivational variables, such as a desire to identify with the parent, were the primary determinants of sex typing, he proposed that cognitions about gender *preceded* motivation to adopt same-sex attributes. Cognitions or concepts about social expectations for males and females were proposed as the major antecedents of sex-typed attitudes and behavior.

Not only were cognitions primary, according to Kohlberg, but they did not need to be taught in any deliberate fashion. Children spontaneously classify and categorize their worlds. Most developmental psychologists now agree with the view that children actively organize the stimuli and information they encounter. They are cognitive constructivists, not passive recipients of adult tuition. It is also agreed that gender is one of the earliest social categories learned although there is some disagreement about why gender is so fundamental. Are the physical differences between females and males so obvious that children in all cultures will learn to classify people as male and female (as Kohlberg argues), or do children learn that gender is important because their culture emphasizes it as Bem (1981) contends? Whatever the reasons, in most known cultures, children do spontaneously categorize the world according to gender, and they proceed to fill in those categories with information about the work, play activities, clothing, hair styles, and behavior which are associated with females and males in their own societies. They acquire the information from many sources—what they observe directly, what is portrayed in fiction and media, and what they are told. No one needs to teach concepts about gender directly; children construct them on their own.

The cognitive emphasis has generated a great deal of research on children's concepts about gender, most of which provides empirical support for the basic propositions of the theory. Recent formulations, based on schema theories (Bem, 1981; Martin & Halverson, 1981), have elaborated the constructive nature of concepts about sex typing. Children not only categorize their social environment by gender and learn the stereotypes associated with females and males in their culture, they use the schemas created by this cognitive activity to select and interpret new information as they receive it. They assimilate new information to existing concepts. As a result, gender schemas can lead them to ignore information that does not fit the schema or to distort perceptions to make them more consistent with the schema.

This process is illustrated dramatically in several studies in which children were shown pictures or films of people performing stereotypic or counterstereotypic behavior actions. When children see counterstereotypic behavior, they often fail to recall it or they distort their recollection to make the behavior more consistent with sex stereotypes. For example, in two studies by different investigators, children saw toy commercials in which child actors played with stereotyped or counterstereotyped toys. When asked afterward whether the children in the commercial were boys or girls, about half of the children who had seen the counterstereotyped advertisements recalled the sex of at least one child actor incorrectly. Almost all children who saw the stereotyped versions recalled the actors' genders accurately (Atkin, 1975; Frey & Ruble, 1981). Similar distortions occurred when children saw one of four films depicting a doctor and nurse. The four versions contained all possible combinations of males and females playing the two roles. When children were shown photographs of the actors and asked whether each was a doctor or nurse, all who had seen the male doctor and female nurse answered correctly. Only 22% of those who saw the female doctor and the male nurse identified both roles accurately (Cordua, McGraw, & Drabman, 1979).

Age Trends

The cognitive–developmental focus has also led to an expansion of the age range during which we are aware that important learning about sex typing occurs. Virtually all theorists in recent years have moved away from the psychoanalytic emphasis on the first 5 years as the formative period for sexual identity. Particularly as theorists like Block (1973) have tried to specify how people move beyond traditional bifurcated sex roles to androgynous patterns, continuing change and development during the entire life span have been increasingly emphasized.

Not only does change continue beyond the preschool years, but the direction of that change is not linear. In his initial formulation, Kohlberg proposed that children's sex role concepts would become more flexible in middle childhood as concrete operational thinking emerged. That hypothesis receives some support when questions abut sex stereotypes are posed in a way that permits children to say a behavior is equally appropriate for girls and boys. In some studies, children are simply asked whether behaviors are more typical of females or males. When they are forced to choose, older children generally give more stereotyped responses than younger ones. But, if they have a third choice—is it more appropriate for males, females, or equally appropriate for both?—there is an increasing tendency from about 5 or 6 on for children to say that activities or behaviors are equally appropriate for both genders. As children move into middle childhood, they are increasingly able to break away from the either–or absolutism of preschool children's thought (Garrett et al., 1977; Huston, 1983; Kleinke & Nicholson, 1979; Marantz & Mansfield, 1977; Meyer, 1980; Nemerowicz, 1979).

The increase in flexibility about sex typing parallels more general increases in children's understanding that social conventions are culturally relative and changeable. This pattern was demonstrated in a study of children from kindergarten to eighth grade. They were asked about sex stereotypes and about social conventions involving table manners. For sex-typed activities, they were asked who usually engaged in an activity (stereotyped knowledge), whether girls or boys *can* engage in that activity, and whether there might be a country somewhere where this activity would be appropriate only for the gender opposite the stereotype (flexibility). Older children knew sex stereotypes better, but they were also more aware of exceptions and of cultural relativity. The same developmental pattern occurred for social conventions about table manners—older children knew the conventions, but were also aware that they could be changed (Carter & Patterson, 1982).

These findings suggest that changes in children's sex stereotypes may be easier to communicate when children are in middle childhood than in the preschool years. It may imply that children are more cognitively ready for interventions designed to teach nontraditional concepts about gender after they have achieved some flexibility in social cognitive processing than before.

Cognition and Behavior

Cognitive developmental theory also contains the premise that concepts and cognitions are the major *determinants* of sex-typed preferences and behavior. That is, they play an important causal role. In the framework of Table 1, the theory implies that concepts and beliefs should have an impact on the other constructs—self-perception, preferences, and behavior. In my judgment the evidence for the causal role of cognitions is not strong. If cognitions are major determinants of other constructs then (1) cognitions ought to *precede* behavioral sex typing, (2) at least after the first few years of life, cognitions ought to be correlated with preferences, identity, and behavior, and (3) changes in concepts or stereotypes ought to produce changes in self-perception, preference, or behavior.

First, cognitions do not necessarily precede sex-typed behavior and preferences developmentally. As noted earlier, children demonstrate sex-typed toy choices by age 2 before they demonstrate even a clear differentiation of males and females. Of course, it is possible that we are simply unable to measure cognitions when children are basically preverbal, but it seems unlikely that such young children are guided by concepts of gender appropriateness. It seems more reasonable to conclude that concepts and behavior develop in parallel or simultaneous fashion. Fagot (1982) suggested in a recent paper that the two may develop rather independently until middle childhood. Sex-typed behaviors are learned, according to her hypothesis, through direct reinforcement, punishment, and modeling in the preschool years at the same time concepts about sex stereotypes are acquired. Only later do children use cognitions about sex typing and parental values as guides for behavior. In any case, the available data indicate that sex-typed behavior and preferences emerge at least as early, if not earlier, than cognitions about sex appropriateness.

Second, the relations between cognitions and identity, preference, or behavior are not strong. On the whole, people with very pronounced sex stereotypes have somewhat more pronounced sex-typed preferences or behavior than individuals with more flexible cognitions, but the correlations are usually modest. For example, children who stereotype reading as feminine and math as masculine have more sex-typed achievement goals than those who do not accept such stereotypes (Boswell, 1979; Crandall, 1978; Dwyer, 1974; Stein, 1971). Of course, even when correlations exist, one cannot be sure of causal direction. Stereotypes could arise from one's preferences or one's behavior as well as being causal agents.

Another source of evidence bearing on the correlations between cognition and behavior comes from the different developmental paths followed by girls and boys. Both males and females learn more and more about social definitions of masculinity and femininity as they get older. At any age, however, boys usually have more pronounced stereotypes than girls. Girls usually show more flexibility in their sex-typed concepts—that is, they view more activities and behaviors as equally appropriate for both sexes than boys do. There are some sex differences in sex-typed cognitions, but both genders follow the same developmental curves (Huston, 1983).

Sex-typed *preferences*, by contrast, follow very different developmental curves. Males generally show a monotonic increase with age in masculine preferences and identity. The older they are, the more they express male sex-typed preferences and the more they perceive themselves as masculine (at least until adolescence). Girls *move away* from feminine preferences and identity during the age period from about 5 or 6 until adolescence. In this age range, girls often show declining preferences for feminine activities and interests, and they become increasingly interested in masculine activities (Brown, 1956; Huesmann, et al., 1978; Huston, 1983; Huston-Stein & Higgins-Trenk, 1978; Kohlberg & Zigler, 1967; Sutton-Smith, Rosenberg, & Morgan, 1963). The few developmental studies of self-perception using the children's Personal Attributes Questionnaire or similar measures show the same trend. Older girls perceive themselves as more masculine than younger ones (Hall & Halberstadt, 1980). This pattern appears in studies carried out in the 1920s, the 1950s, and 1960s. It is not merely an artifact of recent consciousness about the evils of sex stereotyping (see Huston, 1983).

Third, changes in cognitions do not necessarily produce changes in identity, preference, or behavior. There is little evidence presently available, but it cannot be assumed, for example, that changes in stereotypes will produce changes in behavior. Many intervention efforts in the past few years have been aimed at changing children's sex stereotypes. People have assumed without evidence that changing stereotypes will change behavior. One of the most widely cited examples is Guttentag and Bray's (1976) study described in their book, *Undoing Sex Stereotypes.*

Another large-scale intervention effort was the television series, *Freestyle,* which was designed to present nontraditional career interests and behavior patterns to children in the age range from 9 to 12. After seeing 13 half-hour programs in their classrooms, children responded to measures of stereotypes, attitudes, and behavioral intentions (e.g., would you join a basketball team?). The program was reasonably successful in changing children's concepts about what was appropriate for females and males, but produced fewer changes in attitudes and behavioral intentions (Johnston & Ettema, 1982). I do not mean to suggest that we should stop trying to teach nontraditional concepts about gender, but we should not expect such concepts to carry the full weight of bringing about changes in attitudes and behavior.

CONCLUSIONS

Two major themes have been presented. The first is the importance of activities and interests and of peer associations in the early acquisition of sex typing. Children learn sex-typed play activities, occupations, family roles, and interests earlier and more definitely than they learn personality traits or social behaviors. Along with play activities goes sex segregation of the peer group. Researchers need to focus more attention on these content areas ˜whether they are interested primarily in describing the process or in bringing about change. Some of the most effective ways of teaching nontraditional behavior to preschool children may involve making changes in home and school settings that bring about less sex-stereotyped divisions of play activity and more mixed-sex peer activity. The work of Serbin and Connor (see Serbin, 1980; Serbin et al., 1981) employing careful experimental manipulations and observations of behavior is an example of how productive such research can be.

The second theme is that cognitions and concepts about sex typing are important elements in the acquisition of gender typing, but they are not sufficient by themselves for understanding the process of sex typing or for producing change. Children actively construct concepts and schemata about their social worlds. Cognitive developmental changes permit (but do not guarantee) increasing flexibility with age in children's thinking about gender. At the same time, one should exercise considerable caution in assuming that concepts and cognitions are the major causal variables influencing other aspects of sex typing. Self-perceptions, preferences, and behavior are often relatively independent of concepts and are affected by many other variables in addition to the individual's belief about what is appropriate for each gender.

Finally, a methodological note. Few researchers take multidimensionality seriously. One of the major weaknesses in this field is that people use one measure of sex typing, often without being explicit about why they chose it or what aspect of sex typing it measures. The cumulative impact of the research in the area is seriously weakened because different studies include diverse measures that are noncomparable. The 20 cells in Table 1 all have logically possible entries, and there are empirical studies that fall in most of them. How does one compare a study using the Personal Attributes Questionnaire with one using a Toy Preference Index? Individual studies should include multiple measures of multiple constructs and/or content areas to permit a comprehensive understanding of the processes involved. Hetherington's studies of father absence (Hetherington, 1966, 1972) and divorced families (Hetherington, Cox, & Cox, 1982) are examples of this approach. They included behavioral observations, preference tests, peer choices, and self-perception measures—a variety of methods and content areas. Developmental psychologists have made enormous conceptual and empirical strides in understanding one of the most basic components of human development. Continued gains in knowledge depend on making the methods and design of research match the sophistication of theory and available concepts.

REFERENCES

Atkin, C. (1975). *Effects of television advertising on children. Second year experimental evidence.* Michigan State University, Department of Communication.
Bem, S. L. (1974). The measurement of psychological androgyny. *Journal of Consulting and Clinical Psychology,* **42,** 155-162.
Bem, S. L. (1981). Gender schema theory: A cognitive account of sex-typing. *Psychological Review,* **88,** 354-364.
Best, D. L., Williams, J. E., Cloud, J. M., Davis, S. W., Robertson, L. S., Edwards, J. R.,

Giles, H., & Fowles, J. (1977). Development of sex-trait stereotypes among young children in the United States, England, and Ireland. *Child Development, 48,* 1375-1384.

Bianchi, E. D., & Bakeman, R. (1978). Sex-typed affiliation preferences observed in preschoolers: Traditional and open school differences. *Child Development, 49,* 910-912.

Blakemore, J. E. O., LaRue, A. A., & Olejnik, A. B. (1979). Sex-appropriate toy preference and the ability to conceptualize toys as sex-role related. *Developmental Psychology, 15,* 339-340.

Block, J. H. (1973). Conceptions of sex role: Some cross-cultural and longitudinal perspectives. *American Psychologist, 28,* 512-526.

Block, J. H. (1976). Issues, problems, and pitfalls in assessing sex differences: A critical review of *The Psychology of sex differences. Merrill–Palmer Quarterly, 22,* 285-308.

Block, J. H. (1981). *Gender differences and implications for educational policy.* Unpublished manuscript, University of California at Berkeley.

Boswell, S. L. (1979, March). *Sex roles, attitudes and achievements in mathematics: A study of elementary school children and Ph.D.'s.* Paper presented as part of a symposium of *Gender Differences in Participation in Mathematics.* Paper presented at the Society for Research in Child Development, San Francisco.

Brown, D. G. (1956). Sex role preference in young children. *Psychological Monographs, 70,* Whole No. 421.

Carpenter, C. J. (1983). Activity structure and play: Implications for socialization. In M. B. Liss (Ed.), *Children's play: Sex differences in the acquisition of social and cognitive skills.* New York: Academic Press.

Carpenter, C. J. & Huston-Stein, A. (1980). Activity structure and sex-typed behavior in preschool children. *Child Development, 51,* 862-872.

Carter, D. B., & Patterson, C. J. (1982). Sex roles as social conventions: The development of children's conceptions of sex-role stereotypes. *Developmental Psychology, 18,* 812-824.

Constantinople, A. (1973). Masculinity-femininity: An exception to a famous dictum? *Psychological Bulletin, 80,* 389-407.

Cordua, G. D., McGraw, K. O., & Drabman, R. S. (1979). Doctor or nurse: Children's perceptions of sex typed occupations. *Child Development, 50,* 590-593.

Cramer, P., & Hogan, K. A. (1975). Sex differences in verbal and play fantasy. *Developmental Psychology, 11,* 145-154.

Crandall, V. C. (1978, August). *Expecting sex differences and sex differences in expectancies.* Paper presented at the annual meeting of the American Psychological Association, Toronto.

Dwyer, C. A. (1974). Influence of children's sex role standards on reading and arithmetic achievement. *Journal of Educational Psychology, 66,* 811-816.

Edelbrock, C., & Sugawara, A. I. (1978). Aquisition of sex-typed preferences in preschool-aged children. *Developmental Psychology, 14,* 614-623.

Eisenberg-Berg, N., Boothby, R., & Matson, T. (1979). Correlates of preschool girls' feminine and masculine toy preferences. *Developmental Psychology, 15,* 354-355.

Erikson, E. H. (1963). *Childhood and society* (2nd ed.). New York: Norton.

Etaugh, C., & Riley, S. (1979). Knowledge of sex stereotypes in preschool children. *Psychological Reports, 44,* 1279-1282.

Fagot, B. I. (1974). Sex differences in toddlers' behavior and parental reaction. *Developmental Psychology, 10,* 554-558.

Fagot, B. (1982). Adults as socializing agents. In T. Field, A. Huston, H. Quay, L. Troll, & G. Finley (Eds.), *Review of human development.* New York: Wiley.

Faulkender, P. J. (1980). Categorical habituation with sex-typed toy stimuli in older and younger preschoolers. *Child Development,* **51,** 515-519.

Fein, G., Johnson, D., Kosson, N., Stork, L., & Wasserman, L. (1975). Sex stereotypes and preferences in the toy choices of 20-month-old boys and girls. *Developmental Psychology,* **11,** 527-528.

Fillmer, H. T., & Haswell, L. (1977). Sex-role stereotyping in English usage. *Sex Roles,* **3,** 257-263.

Flerx, V. C., Fidler, D. S., & Rogers, R. W. (1976). Sex role stereotypes: Developmental aspects and early intervention. *Child Development,* **47,** 998-1007.

Franck, K., & Rosen, E. (1949). A projective test of masculinity–femininity. *Journal of Consulting Psychology,* **13,** 247-256.

Frey, K. S., & Ruble, D. N. (1981, April). *Concepts of gender constancy as mediators of behavior.* Paper presented at the biennial meeting of the Society for Research in Child Development, Boston.

Frieze, I. H., & Ramsey, S. J. (1976). Nonverbal maintenance of traditional sex roles. *Journal of Social Issues,* **32**(3), 133-142.

Garrett, C. S., Ein, P. L., & Tremaine, L. (1977). The development of gender stereotyping of adult occupations in elementary school children. *Child Development,* **48,** 507-512.

Guttentag, M., & Bray, H. (1976). *Undoing sex stereotypes. Research and resources for educators.* New York: McGraw–Hill.

Haas, A. (1979). Male and female spoken language differences: Stereotypes and evidence. *Psychological Bulletin,* **86,** 616-626.

Hall, J. A., & Halberstadt, A. G. (1980). Masculinity and femininity in children: Development of the Children's Personal Attributes Questionnaire. *Developmental Psychology,* **16,** 270-280.

Hetherington, E. M. (1966). Effects of paternal absence on sex-typed behaviors in Negro and white preadolescent males. *Journal of Personality and Social Psychology,* **4,** 87-91.

Hetherington, E. M. (1972). Effects of father absence on personality development in adolescent daughters. *Development Psychology,* **7,** 313-326.

Hetherington, E. M., Cox, M., & Cox, R. (1982). Effects of divorce on parents and children. In M. E. Lamb (Ed.), *Nontraditional families: Parenting and child development.* Hillsdale, NJ: Erlbaum.

Huesmann, R., Fischer, P., Eron, L., Mermelstein, R., Kaplan-Shain, E., & Morikawa, S. (1978, September). *Children's sex-role preference, sex of television model, and imitation of aggressive behaviors.* Paper presented at the third biennial meeting of the International Society for Research on Aggression, Washington, D.C.

Huston, A. C. (1983). Sex Typing. In P. H. Mussen & E. M. Hetherington (Eds.), *Handbook of child psychology.* (Vol. 4, 4th ed.) *Socialization, personality, and social behavior.* New York: Wiley.

Huston-Stein, A., & Higgins-Trenk, A. (1978). Development of females from childhood through adulthood: Career and feminine role orientations. In P. B. Baltes (Ed.), *Lifespan development and Behavior* (Vol. 1, pp. 258-296). New York: Academic Press.

Jacklin, C. N., & Maccoby, E. E. (1978). Social behavior at 33 months in same-sex and mixed-sex dyads. *Child Development,* **49,** 557-569.

Johnston, J., & Ettema, J. S. (1982). *Positive images: Breaking stereotypes with children's television.* Beverly Hills, CA: Sage.

Katz, P. A., & Rank, S. A. (1981, April). *Gender constancy and sibling status.* Paper presented at the biennial meeting of the Society for Research in Child Development, Boston.

Kleinke, C. L., & Nicholson, T. A. (1979). Black and white children's awareness of de facto race and sex differences. *Developmental Psychology,* **15,** 84-86.

Kohlberg, L. (1966). A cognitive developmental analysis of children's sex-role concepts and attitudes. In E. E. Maccoby (Ed.), *The development of sex differences* (pp. 82-172). Stanford, CA: Stanford Univ. Press.

Kohlberg, L., & Zigler, E. (1967). The impact of cognitive maturity on the development of sex-role attitudes in the years 4 to 8. *Genetic Psychology Monographs, 75,* 89-165.

Kuhn, D., Nash, S. C., & Brucken, L. (1978). Sex role concepts of two- and three-year-olds. *Child Development, 49,* 445-451.

Maccoby, E. E., & Jacklin, C. N. (1974). *The psychology of sex differences.* Stanford, CA: Stanford Univ. Press.

Marantz, S. A., & Mansfield, A. F. (1977). Maternal employment and the development of sex-role stereotyping in five- to eleven-year-old girls. *Child Development, 48,* 668-673.

Martin, C. L., & Halverson, C. F., Jr. (1981). A schematic processing model of sex typing and stereotyping in children. *Child Development, 52,* 1119-1134.

Masters, J. C., & Wilkinson, A. (1976). Consensual and discriminative stereotypy of sex-type judgments by parents and children. *Child Development, 47,* 208-217.

May, R. R. (1971). A method for studying the development of gender identity. *Developmental Psychology, 5,* 484-487.

McCracken, J. H. (1973). Sex typing of reading by boys attending all male classes. *Developmental Psychology, 8,* 148.

Meyer, B. (1980). The development of girls' sex-role attitudes. *Child Development, 51,* 508-514.

Myers, B. J., Weinraub, M., & Shetler, S. (1979, September). *Preschoolers' knowledge of sex role stereotypes: A developmental study.* Paper presented at the meeting of the American Psychological Association, New York.

Nemerowicz, G. M. (1979). *Children's perceptions of gender and work roles.* New York: Praeger.

Newcombe, N. (1982). Sex-related differences in spatial ability: Problems and gaps in current approaches. In *Spatial abilities: Development and physiological foundations.* New York: Academic Press.

O'Brien, M., Huston, A. C., & Risley, T. (1983). Sex-typed play of toddlers in a day care center. *Journal of Applied Developmental Psychology, 4,* 1-10.

Papalia, D. E., & Tennent, S. S. (1975). Vocational aspirations in preschoolers: A manifestation of early sex role stereotyping. *Sex Roles, 1,* 197-199.

Rekers, G. A. (1979). Psychosexual and gender problems. In E. J. Mash & L. G. Terdal (Eds.), *Behavioral assessment of childhood disorders.* New York: Guilford.

Rekers, G. A., Amaro-Plotkin, H. D., & Low, B. P. (1977). Sex-typed mannerisms in normal boys and girls as a function of sex and age. *Child Development, 48,* 275-278.

Schau, C. G., Kahn, L., Diepold, J. H., & Cherry, F. (1980). The relationships of parental expectations and preschool children's verbal sex typing to their sex-typed toy play behavior. *Child Development, 51,* 266-270.

Serbin, L. A. (1980). Sex role socialization: A field in transition. In B. Lahey & A. Kazkin (Eds.), *Advances in clinical child psychology* (Vol. 3). New York: Plenum.

Serbin, L. A., Connor, J. M., & Citron, C. C. (1981). Sex-differentiated free play behavior: Effects of teacher modeling, location, and gender. *Developmental Psychology, 17,* 640-646.

Sherman, J. A. (1967). Problems of sex differences in space perception and aspects of intellectual functioning. *Psychological Review, 74,* 290-299.

Spence, J. T., & Helmreich, R. L. (1978). *Masculinity and femininity: Their psychological dimensions, correlates, and antecedents.* Austin, TX: Univ. of Texas Press.

Stein, A. H. (1971). The effects of sex-role standards for achievement and sex-role preference on three determinants of achievement motivation. *Developmental Psychology,* **4,** 219-231.

Sutton-Smith, B., Rosenberg, B. G., & Morgan, Jr., E. F. (1963). Development of sex differences in play choices during preadolescence. *Child Development,*34, 119-126.

Thompson, S. K. (1975). Gender labels and early sex role development. *Child Development,* **46,** 339-347.

Thornburg, K. R., & Weeks, M. O. (1975). Vocational role expectations of five-year-old children and their parents. *Sex Roles,* **1,** 395-396.

Venar, A. M., & Snyder, C. A. (1966). The preschool child's awareness and anticipation of adult sex roles. *Sociometry,* **29,** 159-168.

Weinraub, M., & Leite, J. (1977, April). *Knowledge of sex-role stereotypes and sex-typed toy preference in two-year-old children.* Paper presented at the meeting of the Eastern Psychological Association, Boston.

Williams, J. E., Bennett, S. M., & Best, D. L. (1975). Awareness and expression of sex stereotypes in young children. *Developmental Psychology,* **11,** 635-642.

10

The Cultural Context of Gender Segregation in Children's Peer Groups

Sara Harkness and Charles M. Super

Harvard University and Judge Baker Guidance Center

Recent American research has explored developmental trends in gender segregation of children's peer groups. It is important to differentiate, however, systematic trends in children from systematic changes in their environments. Observational data are presented from 152 rural Kenyan children ages 18 months to 9 years. There is no gender segregation in peer groups until around age 6, at which time changes in settings, parental expectations, and customary duties result in an increase in the proportion of same-sex peers. Even within this pattern, however, there is some evidence that children do not interact more with same-sex peers, given their greater presence. A contrast is drawn with the adult pattern of gender segregation and emphasis is given to the importance of culture and development as interactive systems.

Reprinted with permission from *Child Development*, 1985, Vol. 56, 219–224. Copyright 1985 by the Society for Research in Child Development, Inc.

A preliminary version of this paper was presented in J. Rubenstein (Chair), *Gender segregation in the peer group: Social and affective consequences*, a symposium conducted at the biennial meeting of the Society for Research in Child Development, Detroit, April 1983. The research reported here was supported by the Carnegie Corporation of New York, the William T. Grant Foundation, the Spencer Foundation, and the National Institute of Mental Health (grant no. 33281). All statements made and views expressed are the sole responsibility of the authors.

The contribution of peer relations to the socialization of children has recently received increased attention in the developmental literature. Hartup (1983, p. 103), in his comprehensive review, asserts, "In most cultures, the significance of peer relations as a socialization context is rivaled only by the family." One is hard pressed to think of a culture in which this is *not* the case; in fact, current scientific interest in peer relations reverses a long-standing bias in western psychology that overemphasized the role of parents, especially the mother, as socialization agents.

Among the characteristics of children's peer groups as contexts for social learning, the tendency of boys and girls to associate preferentially with members of their own sex has frequently been noted. Hartup (1983, p. 109) states, "Children of all ages associate more frequently with members of their own sex and like them better." Recent research has suggested that this tendency appears early in the opening years of life. In middle childhood and early adolescence, according to Hartup, the tendency toward behavioral dimorphism becomes so pronounced that "no observer would question the fact that children avoid the opposite sex in middle childhood and adolescence" (p. 110).

As with other aspects of children's social development, the influence of contextual factors on the nature and extent of sex segregation in children's peer groups is difficult to separate from ontogenetic factors, especially in a monocultural research tradition. Most of the observations on children's peer behavior have been carried out in settings characterized by large groups of same-age children—that is, in schools. Since school experience in American culture is closely tied to age, there is a danger, as we have discussed elsewhere (Harkness, 1980; Super & Harkness, in press), that the stucture of development may be confused with the structure of the environment.

Although the role of the environment in producing regularities in the development of children's behavior may not be salient when all the research has been carried out within limited and familiar contexts, its importance becomes more evident when the behavior is observed in a different culture. Comparisons with other cultures are especially valuable when they lead to further questioning about the functions served for the developing child by particular kinds of behavior in particular settings.

This report presents evidence on gender segregation in children's peer groups in a rural community of Kenya. Gender segregation during the first 9 years of life is examined in culturally characteristic settings and is discussed in relation to both developmental and cultural issues.

METHOD

The data reported here were collected during 3 years of research on child development and family life in the community of Kokwet, a Kipsigis settlement in the western highlands of Kenya. Like many other East African highland peoples, the Kipsigis are patrilineal and traditionally engaged in hoe agriculture and cattle herding; more recently, communities like Kokwet have adapted to the modern economy through cash and dairy farming, while still retaining many features of traditional life. The community of Kokwet consists of 54 households established on land repatriated from the British at national independence in 1963. Although as a government-sponsored "settlement scheme" Kokwet is intentionally modern in some agricultural practices, the community remains traditional in many significant respects; at the time of our research (1972–1975), most adults had little or no schooling, few men worked at salaried jobs away from the homesteads, cows were still used for the customary brideprice, polygymy was the preferred form of marriage for many, and virtually all adolescents still chose to undergo the traditional circumcision ceremonies.

Many features of child life in Kokwet, as elsewhere, are derived from the economic and social organization of adult life. The work of mothers in Kokwet includes farming on the family fields, as well as gathering firewood and bringing water from the river, preparing food, and being responsible for the care of the children. Fathers are in charge of the cows, plowing the fields when new crops are to be planted, major repairs around the property, and the important political business of the community.

Children also are essential contributors to the economic well-being of the household. Large families are preferred, and family size averages over six children for each mother. Children help in taking care of younger siblings, watching the cows, weeding the gardens, running errands, and many other chores. One striking aspect of these childhood tasks is the age at which children are expected to carry out important responsibilities. It is not unusual, for example, to see a child of three chasing a calf out of the garden. The children responsible for taking care of babies are usually about 8–10 years old and may be as young as 5 or 6. The general scene, then, is one in which life for all members of the family centers around the homestead, and all are participants in work as well as sociability and leisure.

Within this cultural setting, a large corpus of observations of children's social behavior was collected. Running records of naturally occurring

behavior in the home were written and later coded according to a modification of the system developed by the Whitings (see Whiting, 1980).

Sample

There were 152 children selected from a recent census to be representative of variation within the community and balanced on sex and
age (from 18 months to 9 years); a majority of children in Kokwet were
included.

Procedure

Observations were carried out by a trained local observer who went
to the homesteads four times (9 AM, 11 AM, 3 PM, and 5 PM) on different
days. (Two cases were incomplete, yielding a total of 606 observation
sessions.) Each observation lasted 30 min, and during this time the children and families were asked to carry out normal activities. Thus the
observer would accompany the children as they went to the river and
fields, as well as sit unobtrusively in the hut to observe the children's
activities there. In the relatively fluid, mostly outdoor setting of daily
life, this procedure seemed comfortable to all concerned and the recorded behaviors and activities are consistent with casual observations
throughout 3 years of residence in the community. Recording consisted
of writing in narrative form every individual behavior (e.g., draw with
stick in dirt), social act (e.g., ask mother for food), or social activity (e.g.,
sitting quietly with sister) by the focal child, and every response from
others (e.g., mother gives food) or social act (e.g., sister tells brother to
come help) directed toward the focal child. Aspects of the immediate
social context, such as the cast of characters present, the location, and
the ongoing activities, were also noted. Brief excerpts from the running
records are available elsewhere (Harkness & Super, in press).

Coding was carried out by American assistants who were trained in
interpreting the Kipsigis material. Each social act, response, or social
activity was scored as one of nearly one hundred kinds of goal-directed
behavior directed by specified "actors" toward "target" persons.

Analysis

To describe the composition and interaction patterns of children's
peer groups, the actors, targets, and others present were categorized by

sex and age level (infancy to 2.9 years, 3 to 5.9 years, and 6 to 8.9 years). Two-way analysis of variance (age × sex) was then used to address two main questions. First, did boys and girls at any age level form peer groups in which one sex or the other predominated? The dependent measure was calculated as the percentage of males (vs. females) of the same age level surrounding each child in the observed group. Second, did boys and girls at any of these age levels preferentially choose children of one sex or the other as targets of social interaction, given whatever distribution of peers existed? The dependent measure in this analysis was the percentage of acts directed by each child to male (rather than female) children of the same age level; the percentage of male peers present was subtracted to adjust for available targets and nondifferential behavior should thus yield an average score of 0. In addition, the cast of characters present was analyzed in terms of relationships between the target child and peers (whether family members or neighbors) and whether the mother was present or not.

RESULTS

The behavior observations show children involved in a variety of activities, including many chores as well as social play, in and around their living compounds. The number of people present normally varied from five to eight, usually members of the child's immediate family, half-siblings, or neighbors, including infants as well as adults. Thus the potential "targets" for children's social behavior span a wide age range as well as including both sexes.

In the analysis of the percent of males in children's peer groups in relation to age and sex of the actor, a main effect of sex was found, $F(1,315) = 4.31, p < .04$. This proved secondary, however, to an interaction between sex and age, which had a more powerful effect on peer group composition, $F(2,315) = 10.32, p < .0001$. As indicated in Table 1, the proportion of male peers present was very similar for boy and girl actors in the two younger age categories, but diverged sharply for the 6–9-year-olds. Further analysis at each age level confirms that the sex difference in gender composition of peer group is reliable only at the oldest age. (Reanalysis using an arcsine transformation of the percentage did not alter the results, nor did analysis with nonparametric methods.)

The second analysis, on the choice of targets within the peer group, showed no significant main effects or interactions; neither boys nor girls

TABLE 1

PERCENTAGE OF MALES PRESENT AND PERCENTAGE OF MALE TARGETS IN
PEER GROUP, BY SEX

AGE AND SEX OF FOCAL CHILD	PEERS, PERCENTAGE MALE		TARGETS, PERCENTAGE MALE	
	Mean	SD	Mean	SD
0–3 years:				
Male	44.9	46.8	20.0	44.7
Female	44.8	47.4	25.0	46.3
3–6 years:				
Male	33.3	44.9	34.9	47.2
Female	42.0	45.5	50.7	49.3
6–9 years:				
Male	67.4	45.5	72.2	46.1
Female	24.6	39.9	15.6	35.3

of any age category differentially chose children of one sex or the other
as targets of social interaction. Thus the trends for choice of targets by
boys and girls at each age level, not adjusted for the availability of targets,
parallel the trends in the sex ratio of those present (Table 1). Although
there was a high proportion of instances in which only one peer was
present (and thus there was no opportunity for choice), examination of
the smaller number of cases with choices suggests the overall finding is
accurate.

Age differences were found in the relationships between the target
children and their peers. In all the age groups the most likely peer was
from the same homestead—that is, a sibling or half-sibling (Table 2).

TABLE 2

RELATIONSHIP OF TARGET CHILD TO PEERS FOR THREE AGE GROUPS

AGE GROUP OF FOCAL CHILD	RELATIONSHIP OF PEER					
	From Same Homestead		From Adjacent Homestead		From Distant Homestead	
	No.	%	No.	%	No.	%
0–3 years	35	52	12	18	20	30
3–6 years	143	65	50	23	27	12
6–9 years	67	53	28	22	31	25

NOTE.—$\chi^2(4) = 14.67$, $p = .005$.

Among the 3–6-year-olds, the next most likely peer comes from an adjacent homestead. For the oldest children, this is not the case, and the peer is equally likely to come from a more distant household. The youngest children are also often found with peers from a nonadjacent homestead, but this seems to be part of a different pattern of social contacts. Mothers often take their very young children with them on visits around the community, but they do not take older children. Thus, the presence of a peer from a nonadjacent household could be because of a visiting mother with baby or the target child itself being observed while with the mother on a visit. Hence, in the oldest age group, but not the youngest, peers from nonadjacent households are likely to result from the children's own choice of companions.

DISCUSSION

Social life for the infant in Kokwet does not start out primarily in an isolated dyad, as is the case for large numbers of American babies. Rather, from the beginning the young Kipsigis baby is usually found in a social group that includes the mother, several siblings, and half-siblings. The average number of companions in Kokwet was observed to be 6.7 during the first year, compared with 1.8 in an American community (Super, 1982). The infant's social group in Kokwet is not differentiated by sex except for the near absence of adult males. The present data indicate that the pattern of mixed sexes in the peer group continues into middle childhood.

This pattern stands in marked contrast to Kipsigis customs of gender segregation in adulthood. The separation of men and women is inaugurated in the adolescent circumcision ceremonies, where groups of boys or girls undergo the public ordeal of circumcision or clitoridectomy, followed by a period of communal seclusion under the care and tutelage of a same-sex elder. The circumcision rites are the ceremonial focal point of the acquisition of culture for the Kipsigis, and they mark the beginning of a new life-stage in which men and women are expected to live separately from each other in many ways. As adults with their own families, women will spend much of their working time with other women in the fields while the men tend to the cattle or to the business of the community. At home, men will maintain separate huts for entertaining their male friends and for sleeping except when visiting their wives. Even meals are served separately to men, while women eat with the children.

Thus, it seems that the relatively late and mild emergence of gender segregation in children's peer groups in Kokwet, when contrasted with the American pattern, cannot be explained either by a unitary factor of culture or development. Although the cultural ethos of gender segregation in adulthood is one of the most salient aspects of Kipsigis culture, it does not seem to operate in childhood, where the majority of time is spent in mixed-sex and mixed-age groups. The age pattern and extent of gender segregation in children's peer groups in Kokwet also does not seem to fit the kind of developmental model that could be derived from research in American settings.

To explain the patterning of gender associations in any cultural context, whether Kokwet or American, intermediate variables must be identified. One of these appears to be the immediate social setting. Luria and Herzog (1983) have noted the influence of setting on children's choice of peers in a recent study with American school-age children. Their observations of children in school showed a high degree of gender segregation; at home in their own neighborhoods, on the other hand, less gender segregation was reported. In Kokwet, children through the age span studied were observed in the same settings—the family homesteads—but their relationships to these settings were undergoing a process of change resulting from the interaction between their own development, as perceived by their caretakers, and the culturally defined roles and expectations of children at different ages.

The Kipsigis case highlights what is also true of the American situation: the intermediate variable of setting is not independent of the larger cultural system in which children participate. The emergence of gender segregation in children's peer groups in the 6–9-year-olds in Kokwet can be related to several general changes in parental ethnotheories of child development and the customary duties of children that influence the structuring of settings in daily life.

The local view of child development in Kokwet sees in the years around 6 the emergence of several important abilities and personal qualities (Super, 1983; Super & Harkness, 1983). Central among them is *ng'omnotet,* universally translated as "intelligence" but applied especially to personal and interpersonal skills that enable one to maintain a sense of direction in one's behavior oriented to larger goals and values. Mothers are careful in keeping track of where their younger children are and with whom. Around the age of 6 years, as they become *ng'om,* children are thought to need less immediate supervision, and a mother might feel comfortable leaving the homestead for several hours knowing that the child will exercise judgment about both activities and companions.

Around the same time, it is customary in Kokwet for children to be assigned substantial household duties and to be expected to carry them out without the immediate presence of a parent. Girls at this age, for example, may spend much of their day taking care of an infant sibling. Both boys and girls are assigned to watching the cows, although there is a tendency for boys to be more often found in this activity, in keeping with its cultural labeling as a male domain. Children who are perceived as *ng'om* by their parents may also be asked to take a message to another homestead in the community or to walk a mile or two to the local store to buy sugar or soap.

Children respond to the greater freedom and greater responsibility given them in middle childhood by choosing their own companions to share work and play. Two girls from nearby homesteads may spend much of the day together caring for their younger siblings. Boys may find a buddy to help watch the cows and have a good game of tag or climb a tree together in the meantime. Having become *ng'om*, children at this age also begin to become aware of the sex typing of activities in adult life. In their free time, boys may play together building in the mud by the stream, while girls play house.

Thus the social settings of daily life, parental theories of child behavior, and the customary duties of children operate as a system, the "developmental niche" (Harkness & Super, 1983; Super & Harkness, in press). Culture, in Whiting's (1980) phrase, is a "provider of settings"; it also provides customs and ethnotheories that are systematically related. The organism and niche are mutually adapted, as Lewontin (1978) has illustrated with a biologist's array of examples. Children play an active role in exploiting and manipulating their niche; in the present context, we see the older children structuring their environments through the exercise of preferential patterns of association. Just when and how such gender segregation appears is the joint product of the individual and the culturally constructed niche. It would be erroneous to attribute the developmental pattern of gender segregation found by scientists in America to phenomena of personal growth alone, even modified in expression by settings. The data presented here suggest a larger cultural perspective to be profitable, for the relationship between culture and individual development is active and interactive in both directions.

REFERENCES

Harkness, S. (1980). The cultural context of child development. In C. M. Super & S. Harkness (Eds.), *New directions for child development: Vol. 8. Anthropological perspectives on child development* (pp. 7–14). San Francisco: Jossey-Bass.

Harkness, S., & Super, C. M. (1983). The cultural construction of child development: A framework for the socialization of affect, *Ethos, 11*, 221-231.

Harkness, S., & Super, C. M. (in press). Child-environment interactions in the socialization of affect. In M. Lewis & C. Saarni (Eds.), *The socialization of emotions*. New York: Plenum.

Hartup, W. W. (1983). Peer relations. In P. H. Mussen (Series Ed.), E. M. Hetherington (Vol. Ed.), *Handbook of child psychology*. Vol. **3:** *Socialization, personality, and development* (pp. 103-196). New York: Wiley.

Lewontin, R. C. (1978). Adaptation. *Scientific American,* **239**(3), 212-235.

Luria, Z., & Herzog, E. (1983, February). Gender segregation in play groups: A matter of where and when. In J. Rubenstein (Chair), *Gender segregation in the peer group: Social and affective consequences*. Symposium conducted at the biennial meeting of the Society for Research in Child Development, Detroit.

Super, C. M. (1982). Infants' daily experience and attention to faces. *Infant Behavior and Development,* **5,** 234 (abstract).

Super, C. M. (1983). Cultural variations in the meaning and uses of children's "intelligence." In J. B. Deregowski, S. Dziurawiec, & R. C. Annis (Eds.), *Expiscations in cross-cultural psychology* (pp. 199-212). Lisse, The Netherlands: Swets & Zeitlinger.

Super, C. M., & Harkness, S. (1963, December). Parental theories of children's intelligence and personality. In K. Anderson-Levitt (Chair), *Folk theories of childhood: The impact of cultural notions of adult-child interactions*. Symposium conducted at the annual meeting of the American Anthropological Association, Chicago.

Super, C. M., & Harkness, S. (in press). Looking across at growing up: The expressions of cognitive growth in middle childhood. In E. Gollin (Ed.), *Developmental plasticity: The social context of development*. New York: Academic Press.

Whiting, B. B. (1980). Culture and social behavior: A model for the development of social behavior. *Ethos,* **8,** 95-116.

11

Extreme Boyhood Femininity: Isolated Behavior or Pervasive Disorder?

Susan Coates

Childhood Gender Identity Project
Roosevelt Hospital, New York

Ethel Spector Person

Columbia University Center for Psychoanalytic
Training and Research, New York

Twenty-five extremely feminine boys with DSM-III diagnosis of gender identity disorder of childhood were evaluated for the presence of behavioral disturbances, social competence and separation anxiety. Using the Child Behavior Checklist created by Achenbach and Edelbrock in 1983, 84% of feminine boys were reported to display behavioral disturbances usually seen in clinic-referred children. Sixty-four percent of the sample had difficulties with peers that were comparable to those of psychiatric-referred boys. Sixty percent of the sample met the criteria for diagnosis of DSM-III separation anxiety disorder. Only one child in the sample fell within the normal range on all three

Reprinted with permission from the *Journal of the American Academy of Child Psychiatry,* 1985, Vol. 24, 702-709. Copyright 1985 by the American Academy of Child Psychiatry.

This research was supported by a National Institute of Health Biomedical Research Support Grant 1-S07-RR05840 to Dr. Susan Coates. Special thanks are due to Dr. John Fogelman, Director of Child and Adolescent Psychiatry at Roosevelt Hospital for his generous support of this project. We gratefully acknowledge the assistance of several staff members, including Penny Donnenfeld, Sonia Marantz, Dr. Bernd Meyenburg, Toby Miroff, Dr. Nancy Schultz and Robert Sherman.

*of these parameters. Results suggest extreme boyhood femininity is not
an isolated finding, but part of a more pervasive psychological disturbance. Additional clinical findings support this contention.*

The following is the first of a series of reports on 25 extremely effeminate boys who met the DSM-III criteria for gender identity disorder
(GID) of childhood and were referred for treatment and study by the
Childhood Gender Identity Project of the Child and Adolescent Psychiatry Department at the St. Luke's-Roosevelt Hospital Center. The
goals of this project are (1) to provide clinical care for severely gender
confused children, (2) to investigate the natural history of boyhood femininity and its antecedents, and (3) to clarify psychodynamic issues as
they emerge in in-depth psychotherapy.

To date, studies of boys referred to gender identity units have focused
largely on establishing descriptions, exploring demographic variables
and charting the natural history of extreme boyhood femininity. Few
studies have focused either on the behavioral and emotional correlates
of effeminacy or the early experiences of the child in his family matrix.
In contrast, this project is designed to do both.

Most researchers agree that effeminate boys display the following characteristics: they express the wish to be a girl, claim that they will grow
up to be a girl, or both; they show a marked interest in girls' activities
such as playing with dolls and enjoy play-acting the role of girls; they
like dressing up in girls' clothes and exhibit an intense interest in cos-
metics, jewelry and high heeled shoes; and they prefer girls as friends
(Bates et al., 1973, 1974; Green, 1974, 1976; Rosen et al., 1977; Zucker,
1982).

Significantly, research reveals that effeminate boys are not different
from controls either in external genitalia or in karyotype (Green, 1976;
Rekers et al., 1979).

In the most extensive demographic study reported in the literature
(60 boys), Green (1976) found that femininity was unrelated to ethnic
background, religion or educational level of either parent, the mother's
age at the time she gave birth, or the number of years between the next
oldest and next youngest child.

Long-term follow-up studies are few in number and difficult to interpret. The clearest of these was reported by Money and Russo (1979).
Of 11 boys diagnosed with prepubertal gender-identity discordance, 5
were available for follow-up. At the time of the follow-up, all were in
their twenties and all 5 considered themselves homosexual or predom-

inantly so. Follow-up studies by Green (1979), Lebowitz (1972) and Zuger (1978) have been done at the time of adolescence, but this is too early an age to gauge outcome, since major shifts and consolidations in identity and sexuality occur during adolescence. Even so, these studies report from 37 to 75% atypical outcome in gender identity and sexual orientation.

It is clear from the data that boyhood femininity is correlated with an increased incidence of homosexual object choice in later life, atypical gender behavior, or both. However, we are presently unable to predict the development of heterosexuality, homosexuality, transvestism or transsexuality as these boys, treated or untreated, reach adulthood.

One of the critical issues in the study of these boys has been the question of whether extreme femininity is a behavioral pattern that is unrelated to other emotional difficulties in the child and in this sense is an isolated finding, or whether it is etiologically associated with other pervasive personality difficulties.

Stoller (1975), with regard to his sample of effeminate boys, explicitly states, "These mothers do not cripple the development of ego functions in general or even body ego, except in regard to this sense of femaleness. . . . None of these boys has shown the slightest evidence of psychosis or precursors of psychosis" (p. 54). Stoller thus appears to view extreme boyhood femininity as an isolated finding that is not inextricably connected to more pervasive psychopathology. (Note: Stoller does not distinguish extreme boyhood femininity from childhood transsexualism. He believes that the sample of boys he studied were a special sample of very young transsexuals. We do not share his assumption since there is no way to make this diagnosis in childhood.) Most systematic studies, however, have failed to confirm Stoller's contention. Three studies from the UCLA Gender Identity Unit suggest gender-referred boys have more concomitant behavioral disturbances than a control group and are pervasively behaviorally disturbed. ("Gender-referred" boys, in the UCLA studies, refers to all boys referred to their gender unit. Their sample was not limited to DSM-III diagnosed GID boys.) The samples from these three studies are overlapping and do not represent separate groups of children. In one study based on parental reports, 15 gender-referred boys scored significantly higher on a behavior disturbance factor than controls. Items in this factor included "acts defiant when given orders," "has temper tantrums," "restless and overactive," and "cries easily" (Bates et al., 1973).

In a second study of 29 gender-referred boys, clinical evaluation material was rated by staff clinicians on 88 items derived from clinical literature, theory and experience with the families. One of the four-factor analytically derived item scales combined items descriptive of an inhibited, fearful child, and items descriptive of an inhibiting, protective family environment. Effeminate boys scored higher on this factor than controls (Bates et al., 1974).

In a third study, 13 gender-referred boys were compared to both normal and clinical controls. The clinical controls were mainly diagnosed as conduct and personality disorders. Mothers rated the boys on the Gender Behavior Inventory for Boys (Bates et al., 1973). Both the gender-problem and clinical boys were rated by their mothers as marginally higher on the behavioral disturbance factor than normal controls. Behavior disturbance did not differ in the two clinical groups. The authors conclude: ". . . gender-problem boys evidence a general personality or behavioral disorder rather than simply a narrow set of deviant gender-attitudes or gender behavior tendencies" (Bates et al., 1979).

The Clarke group in Toronto (Bradley et al., 1980) compared a combined group of effeminate boys and masculine girls to psychiatric controls and found no differences in the Child Behavior Checklist (Achenbach, 1978; Achenbach and Edelbrock, 1979). Thus, gender-referred children in their sample were as behaviorally disturbed as their psychiatric controls. Results from both the UCLA and Clarke group provide growing evidence that boyhood femininity occurs in the context of behavioral disturbance.

Rosen et al. (1977) claim that the majority of gender-confused boys suffer from an "abnormal amount of depression and social conflict resulting from peer rejection, isolation, and ridicule of their feminine behavior" (p. 96).

Other clinical reports suggest that feminine boys have difficulty with their peers. They are often scapegoated, ridiculed and treated with verbal abuse by their cohorts (Green, 1974; Rekers et al., 1977). Research studies have found feminine boys to have a minimal interest in competitive athletic activities (Green, 1976) and to have less athletic competence than their peers (Bates et al., 1979). Systematic studies of general social competence have not yet been reported in the literature.

There are several limitations of the previous studies of behavior disturbances and peer relationships in cross-gender boys. First, all of these studies have used subjects with varying degrees of femininity, including both those who would and would not qualify for a DSM-III diagnosis of GID, making it difficult to compare one study to the other. In the studies by Bates et al. (1973, 1979), only a narrow range of behavior disturbances was investigated, while Bates et al. (1974) based their ratings on case reports rather than on direct standardized assessments. Although the Clarke group used a comprehensive and standardized behavior disturbance scale, they included gender cases of varying degrees of severity (children who both qualified and did not qualify for the DSM-III diagnosis of GID). Furthermore, both sexes were combined in their data analyses, which may have obscured some important differences between the sexes.

The present study attempts to rectify these difficulties first by limiting the study to boys who were diagnosed as DSM-III GID. This both restricts and defines the sample more clearly. Secondly, a comprehensive and standardized behavioral scale was used. Third, a standardized social competence scale was used to assess a broader spectrum of social competence than has been studied previously.

Another goal of this study has been to assess separation anxiety in GID boys. This rationale is based on clinical studies of adults with extreme gender problems who reveal a high incidence of separation anxiety (Ovesey and Person, 1973, 1976; Person and Ovesey, 1974a, 1974b).

The study predicted that GID boys would exceed normal children and be comparable to other clinic-referred children in behavioral disturbances and that they would show less social competence than normal boys and be comparable to clinic-referred children. It also predicted an increased incidence of separation anxiety compared with that anticipated in a normal population.

METHOD

Boys were referred to the Childhood Gender Identity Project if they showed behavioral signs of femininity. The sources of referral were psychiatrists, psychologists, social workers, pediatricians and teachers. Referrals came primarily from local public and Catholic schools that knew of the Childhood Gender Identity unit. Children were initially referred for evaluation and treatment. Five children were first seen in the Child and Adolescent Psychiatry department for presenting problems other than gender identity disorder and were only subsequently referred to the gender unit when a gender disorder came to light as a major issue. Initial diagnosis of these five children included overanxious, dysthymic, adjustment and conduct disorders. Six children were referred privately to Dr. Coates for gender problems and these children were referred to the gender unit for evaluation. One was referred from the Roosevelt Pediatric department and one from another outpatient child psychiatry unit. Out of a total number of approximately 40 referrals, 25 boys were accepted for study. All those excluded failed to meet the criteria for DSM-III diagnosis of GID. All of the 25 boys accepted did meet the criteria. All who were accepted for study participated in the study. All of these boys persistently expressed the wish to be a girl; all displayed female stereotypical behavior, while 40% repudiated their male anatomy. There were no intersexed children in this sample. External genitalia were normal in all boys except one who had unilateral cryptorchidism.

At the time of referral, as Table 1 shows, the boys in this study ranged in age from 4 to 14 years, the average being 7.4; 48% of the sample was white, 40% Spanish and 12% black. The high percentage of Spanish families reflects the racial patterns of the catchment area of the hospital.

On the Four-Factor Index of Social Status (Hollingshead, 1975) assessed by education and occupation, this sample ranged from 11 to 66 on the socioeconomic scale. The average was 34. Five children were only children. Of the remainder, 8 were first born and 11 were last born.

The range of Full Scale Wechsler IQ in this sample was 60–137, the average being 103. Only one child scored in the retarded range.

Procedures

Each child was seen for 5 or 6 sessions which included a psychiatric evaluation, extensive psychological testing and an observation of free play.

Mothers were seen for 2 or 3 sessions to obtain information on the history of the gender problem, to gather an extensive developmental history, and to rate the presence of behavioral problems in the child. At

TABLE 1

Sample Characteristic of Gender Identity Disorder (GID) Boys (N = 25)

Ethnic groups (N):	
White	12 (48%)
Hispanic	10 (40%)
Black	3 (12%)
Age (yr):	
Mean	7.4
Range	4–14
Social status (Hollingshead):	
Mean	34
Range	11–66

the end of this clinic evaluation, families were invited to participate in an extensive research study of the mothers and fathers that focused on their lives during the first 3 years of their sons' lives. These data are not dealt with in this report, but will be reported subsequently.

Assessment Methods

Each child was administered psychological testing that included the WPPSI or WISC-R, Draw-a-Person, Rorschach, Thematic Apperception Test and Sex-typed Animal Preference Test. School achievement and learning disability tests were administered when it was deemed clinically appropriate.

Developmental history was explored with the mothers through a structured interview that is rated for presence, absence and frequency of behaviors. These interviews focused on the child's perinatal experience, medical history, temperament, separation experience, behavior problems and gender development during the first 5 years of life.

The Child Behavior Checklist (CBCL) (Achenbach and Edelbrock, 1983) was administered to the mothers (and jointly to the fathers when present) during the initial evaluation, usually at the end of the first session or in the second.

The CBCL includes 118 behavior problems rated by the child's parents on a three-point response scale. A total score reflects the degree of overall behavioral disturbance. Behavior problem scales were derived by factor analysis of the item intercorrelations based on a clinic referred population, for ages 4–5, 6–11 and 12–16 (Achenbach and Edelbrock, 1983). Norms for these factor-based scales were derived from nonclinical standardization samples. The CBCL also includes three social competence scales encompassing the parent's reports of their child's participation and performance in areas designated as (1) Activities, (2) Social, and (3) School. The Activities subcluster assesses participation in sports and jobs; the Social subcluster, involvement with friends and organizations; the School subcluster, overall performance in school. A total score reflects the degree of the child's social competence in all three areas.

The presence of separation anxiety was evaluated using the DSM-III criteria for separation anxiety. This evaluation was based on the evaluation interview with the child and the interview with the mother.

Mothers were assessed using the Rorschach, Beck Depression Inventory, and the Gunderson Diagnostic Interview for Borderlines. In addition they received a structured interview that focused on their relationships with their own parents, on their relationship to their child during the first 3 years of life and on their own psychological status during the child's first 3 years of life. The results of the mothers' psychological assessment have been reported by Marantz (1984).

The results of the CBCL and of the interviews concerning separation anxiety will be reported in this paper. Since funding for a control group was not available, the analysis of the CBCL scales involved comparison with normative data. This required partitioning of the total sample into the age groups 4–5 (N = 11), 6–11 (N = 10) and 12–14 (N = 4). In addition, pertinent clinical findings will be reported.

RESULTS

CBCL Scores

On the CBCL, 21 of the 25 boys had a total behavior problem score in the clinical range (90th percentile or above: Table 2). Only 4 children scored in the normal range. Thus, 84% of the GID boys were as behaviorally disturbed as the majority of boys referred to psychiatric clinics in general. The behavior problem scales on which at least 50% of the

TABLE 2
Child Behavior Checklist (CBCL) Results

Total Behavior Problem Score	Normal Range ≤90th Percentile	Clinical Range >90th Percentile	Comparison with GID sample
CBCL standard samples:			
Nonclinical	90%	10%	0.001[a]
Clinical	26%	74%	NS[b]
Boys with GID (N = 25)	16%	84%	
Total Social Competence Score	>10th Percentile	≤10th Percentile	
CBCL standard samples:			
Nonclinical	90%	10%	0.01[a]
Clinical	43%	57%	NS[b]
Boys with GID (N = 25)	36%	64%	

[a] Binomial test using the CBCL standards as population values; 1-tailed.

[b] One-sample χ^2 using the CBLC standards for the calculations of expected values; 2-tailed.

boys scored in the clinical range (defined as scores above the 98th percentile) were: for ages 4–5, social withdrawal, depressed, immature and sex problems; for ages 6–11, schizoid, depressed, uncommunicative, obsessive-compulsive and social withdrawal; for ages 12–16, all nine factors (somatic complaints, schizoid, uncommunicative, immature, obsessive-compulsive, hostile-withdrawal, delinquent, aggressive and hyperactive). (The items with the highest loadings on the sex problems factor are: (1) wishes to be the opposite sex and (2) acts like opposite sex. Thus the name "sex problems" is misleading and fails to reflect the cross-gender nature of the behaviors that are rated.) With regard to Social Competence, 64% of the boys had a total score in the clinical range (10th percentile or lower). On the Activities scale, 24% scored in the clinical range (below the 2nd percentile); on the Social scale, 48%, and on the School scale, 43%.

The overall results of the School scale may be misleading. The finding of 43% of the boys falling in the clinical range is based on a restricted sample. This scale does not apply to children under age 6. Thus, the scale was not rated for 11 boys. In our older boys, ages 12 and above, 3 out of 4 cases were in the clinical range in the School scale. If one calculates the rate of school problems for the two samples separately, only 22% of the 6–11-year-olds scored in the clinical range and 80% of the older boys scored in the clinical range. We believe that the older boys are a more extreme sample. First, their continued wish to be a girl and intense female stereotypical interests have continued unabated since early childhood. This is not the usual pattern reported in the literature. In particular, the expressed wish to be a girl usually stops in middle childhood (Zucker, 1982). We believe that this subsample is a more extreme subgroup not only in terms of gender disturbance but also in terms of behavioral disturbance and, therefore, is not representative of the GID population as a whole.

Clinical Findings

Separation Anxiety. A major clinical goal of our work has been to document the frequent coexistence of separation anxiety and effeminate behavior. Separation anxiety was evident in a large number of our cases. Out of 25 children, 15 (60%) met the DSM-III criteria for separation anxiety disorder at the time of the examination. Six children had no indications of separation anxiety and 4 showed fewer criteria than required to meet a DSM-III diagnosis. Of the separation anxious group,

8 of the 15 were currently or had been school reluctant, school avoidant or both.

Behavioral manifestations of separation anxiety were observed in the initial evaluations of the child and in ongoing psychotherapy and were elicited by history in interviews with the mothers. Many of the boys had difficulty leaving their mothers in the waiting room and several of the younger children could not be separated from their mothers without becoming severely agitated.

Mothers reported that their boys ceaselessly shadowed them around the house, refused to sleep in a bedroom by themselves and had major difficulties when left alone even for short periods of time. Several boys worried that their mothers would be killed in a catastrophe while she was away from them. One mother reported that her child had tantrums whenever she spoke on the phone to another person.

Early in their psychotherapy, these boys displayed profound anxiety and rage when issues of being left by their mothers arose. In addition, rage often emerged dramatically in psychotherapy at the end of therapy sessions. Some children would bite, kick and scream at the end of sessions; one child regularly threatened to jump out the window as soon as his therapist told him his session would soon be over. Others would attempt to cope with the separation by "flipping" into a female role. This solution seemed to ward off the anxiety generated by the separation from the therapist. For some children, the prospect of separation from the mother created such severe anxiety that they had to be treated with the mother present in the room.

According to parental report and our own observation, three children showed no evidence of even age appropriate separation anxiety. One child was brought by his mother for a research appointment for herself that she knew would take 6 hours and would not include her son. She was clearly accustomed to leaving him for hours alone and proceeded to leave him in a room alone nearby. He remained by himself for hours making no protest whatsoever. Two of the children with no manifestation of separation anxiety developed severe manifestations after they were in psychotherapy and had begun to become affectively involved.

Of the six children who displayed no separation anxiety at all, three had histories of chronic asthma. This surprising finding raised the question of whether asthma served to bind their separation anxiety or whether asthma itself was a predisposing factor to boyhood femininity. In addition, two children who were separation anxious also had a history of asthma. Thus, in this small sample of children, 5 out of 25 (20%) had histories of chronic asthma.

Peer Relations. Both the parents and the boys themselves report that they are isolated from their peers. They rarely have male friends and rarely engage in athletic pursuits or in rough-and-tumble play. Most often they have friendships with girls, but these relationships are not described as close and most often do not last long. School-aged effeminate boys usually befriend girls who will allow them to participate in traditional girls' activities. Several of the boys in our study described themselves as being lonely, noting that no one liked them and that they did not like themselves either.

During adolescence, they suffer even further disruption in their peer relations. They are frequently treated abusively by being taunted, called "sissy" or "faggot." Many boys refuse to go to gym class because they are humiliated by their incompetence at athletics and by exposing their bodies to other males while changing in the locker room.

These findings (taken in conjunction with Social Competence data) suggest greater peer problems in adolescence, as would be anticipated with the increasing social disapprobation as well as the problem of emerging sexuality. But because age trends reported here are based on cross-sectional data we are unable to determine whether this represents a true developmental trend or sampling fluctuation. Longitudinal follow-up of the sample would help to clarify this.

Depression. None of the children in our study met the criteria for a DSM-III major depressive episode at the time of referral to our unit. One child had been hospitalized for suicidal gestures some years earlier. At least one other boy had a history of suicidal gestures. Seven children had histories of suicidal ideation.

As we have already noted, however, on the Child Behavior Profile, at both age levels that have a depressive factor (age 4–5 and 6–11), over 50% of our sample fell within the clinical range.

Several mothers reported that their sons repeatedly expressed the feeling of hating themselves. One boy said to his mother "I hate myself. I don't want to be me. I want to be someone else. I want to be a girl." Other self-deprecatory ideation was reported by mothers and by their sons as well. Many boys expressed a sense of being inadequate and unable to do things competently. Others referred to themselves as stupid, dumb, and ugly.

Although this study has not focused on depression as a central issue, we believe that enough evidence for depression emerged in our sample to warrant further systematic evaluation.

Personality Integration. Despite their gender confusion, peer isolation and other behavior problems, separation anxiety and depression, the boys seldom displayed either gross impairment in reality testing or psychotic functioning. In two cases, however, the children had transitory delusional episodes. One child feared for a short period that he would be taken over by the devil and would start attacking others as a result of this transformation. During these episodes, he would not sleep with the window open for fear that the devil would enter through the window and invade his body. This anxiety increased whenever his mother left him at home alone. Despite his severe emotional upset during these episodes, he continued to function adequately in school and other structured situations. The second boy had a delusion that the spirit of a particular woman had entered and taken over his body. His family took him to a spiritualist who attempted to exorcise the spirit of the woman. When this failed he began psychotherapy and his delusion disappeared some months later.

These boys functioned relatively well (adaptively) on psychological tests, if the tests were structured (Coates and Tuber, 1985; Tuber and Coates, 1985). On unstructured tests they displayed major ego impairments. On the Rorschach test, content indicating primitive object relations and boundary disturbances characteristic of impaired personality integration were commonly seen.

Thus, while there is evidence for personality disorder, these boys do not fall within the psychotic range.

Summary of Findings. If one compares individual children across three parameters (the total behavior problem score of the CBCL, the total Social Competence score of the CBCL and the absence or presence of DSM-III diagnosis of separation anxiety), all but one child scored in the clinical range on at least one of them: 51% scored in the critical range in all three parameters, 24% on two and 24% on one.

CONCLUSIONS AND DISCUSSION

The question must be raised as to whether our sample is representative of GID boys in general. While we have no absolute way of ascertaining its representativeness, we are impressed by the fact that 20 of the 25 referrals were made because of effeminancy, not because of social or behavioral disturbances which emerged in the course of our research. Even so, we are not in a position to know how frequently extreme boyhood femininity occurs without accompanying behavioral disturbance and as a result does not come to the attention of mental health workers.

The large number of Spanish referrals to our unit is a reflection of the ethnic balance in the Roosevelt Hospital catchment area. The proportion of upper-middle-class children is atypically large for the Roosevelt Child and Adolescent Psychiatry department and reflects the fact that several of the cases were private referrals to Dr. Coates who were in turn referred to the childhood gender unit for evaluations. Inspection of scatter plots revealed no ethnic patterns for any of the subgroups. In terms of demographic proportions, the sample is not representative of New York City or even the hospital population. For this reason the study must be considered exploratory.

The fact that the CBCL was given after the families were initially interviewed may have resulted in a warm-up effect, the result of which may have been that families reported more problems than they would have to total strangers. Although this may have elevated scores to some degree, we doubt that it has produced a major distortion in our results. Clinical interviews and ongoing psychotherapy provided a more elaborate picture of these childrens' behavioral difficulties supporting the questionnaire data.

We believe that our findings confirm our major hypotheses. GID boys appear to exceed normal children in behavioral disturbance and separation anxiety and they are less socially competent. Our data suggests that extreme boyhood femininity occurs in the context of a more pervasive psychological disorder, and that it is not a single or isolated finding. We believe the data speaks for itself regarding this contention and supports a growing body of research indicating that extreme boyhood femininity is typically assocated with significant behavioral disturbance. (It can be argued that the results on behavioral disturbance, social competence and separation anxiety have been artifically inflated by the inclusion of 5 children who were originally referred to a child psychiatry unit for behavioral problems other than extreme femininity. If one reanalyzes the data omitting these 5 boys (one of which was the retarded boy) the following results emerged. On the behavior problem checklist 75% of the boys were in the clinical range. On the Social Competence scale 65% were in the clinical range and 60% met the criteria for a DSM-III diagnosis of separation anxiety. Thus our hypotheses remain corroborated.)

A significant finding has been to correlate a high incidence of separation anxiety with GID. A higher percentage of GID boys had a diagnosable separation anxiety disorder than we can estimate to be the upper limits for normal boys. Orvaschel and Weissman (1985) report that "no epidemiologic data are available regarding anxiety disorders in children." However, they report the classical epidemiologic study of Lapouse and Monk (1978) who found that 41% of the children between the ages of 6–12 had a fear of "anyone in the family getting sick, having an accident or dying," which may be viewed as an item related to separation anxiety. In a cross-sectioned survey of preschool children from two Danish municipalities, Kastrup (1976) found fear of separation in 12% of boys. We can estimate that these are upper limits for indicators of separation anxiety. In all likelihood DSM-III-defined separation anxiety must be considerably lower than these upper limit estimates. Even so, our sample had a higher percentage of separation anxiety disorder than those reported in these epidemiological studies.

Several of the children in our study began cross-dressing for the first time on the heels of a precipitous actual separation from their mother. In psychotherapy with these children, clues as to the meaning of the relationship of their cross-gender behavior to separation anxiety symptoms have emerged. A number of children appear to use cross-gender behavior and dressing as an attempt to restore a fantasy tie to the physically or emotionally absent mother. In imitating "Mommy" they confuse "being Mommy" with "having Mommy." This symptom appears to allay, in part, the anxiety generated by the loss of the mother.

Because Stoller (1975) predicated mother-son symbiosis as the etiologic agent in extreme boyhood femininity, one might say that our research findings of separation anxiety could be predicted by his theoretical formulations. But nothing could be further from the case. Although Stoller believes that if the mother extends a blissful symbiosis with her infant son for too long, the result is femininity in the little boy, he regards this femininity as a product of imprinting. In his formulation, imprinting produces a conflict-free feminine core gender identity, so that these little boys feel themselves to be females in the face of demonstrable male anatomy.

Thus, although his formulation might intuitively seem to suggest that one would see evidence of separation anxiety in effeminate boys, Stoller himself posits that imprinting is nonconflictual. He does not believe that imprinting of a feminine identity affects other aspects of personality development. His contention has been criticized on theoretical grounds by Mahler (1975), and on clinical grounds by Person and Ovesey (1974a, 1974b), Socarides (1975), and Weitzmann et al. (1970).

Moreover, our research on the family matrix (to be reported subsequently) indicates that separation anxiety more often results from actual separation trauma or a distant, disturbed mother-child interaction rather than from any blissful symbiosis.

Insofar as this sample shows correspondence to retrospective histories gleaned in the studies of adult groups of cross-gender disorders, they most closely resemble those derived in studies of cross-dressing homo-sexuals (Ovesey and Person, 1973; Person and Ovesey, 1984) or those elicited in a group of extremely effeminate adolescent homosexuals (Bieber et al., 1962). (In particular, Ovesey and Person posited separation anxiety as a necessary but not sufficient condition for the development of severe cross-gender pathology as seen in adults.) However, it would be a mistake to assume the congruence of these groups, as erroneous as it is to assume that one can study the childhood of transsexuals by studying effeminate boys. The correspondence between these groups remains unknown and indicates one of the lines of longitudinal inves-tigation that should be undertaken.

We also believe that the finding that 40% of our sample did *not* evi-dence separation anxiety is extremely important. It suggests that the pathways leading to boyhood femininity are disparate. This particular finding may suggest an important subdivision in antecedents to feminine behavior.

While there is some agreement in the literature that effeminate boys suffer depression and peer problems, there are two opposing explana-tions to account for these findings: either they are secondary to the pain of social ostracism and being labeled deviant, or they are more intrin-sically associated with the gender confusion and may even be prerequisite to the development of effeminancy.

As for the argument that the associated behavioral difficulties, depres-sions and separation-anxiety should be *exclusively* attributed to social ostracism, we find this position far from convincing. In the younger age ranges, the child is primarily at home, where social disapproval is not even an issue. In fact, Green (1974) points to family *reinforcement*, not disapproval, and yet we see that many very young effeminate boys suffer from severe separation anxiety and constantly shadow their mothers. It seems clear that although social ostracism and labeling as deviant almost certainly compound the psychological problems for this group of chil-dren as they grow older, the time sequence demonstrates the integral coexistence of psychopathology with extreme boyhood femininity.

In sum, we agree with investigations from the UCLA and Clarke gender units that have found extreme childhood effeminacy to be a part of a pervasive disorder rather than an isolated finding. However, it is still far from clear what the implications are for adult personality or-ganization. Furthermore, these conclusions apply only to those instances of boyhood femininity of such magnitude that they fall within the DSM-III criteria for diagnosing childhood gender-identity disorder.

In terms of future research, our findings point to a need for more systematic studies of a wide spectrum of diagnostic disorders in GID boys to determine whether separation anxiety is a major predisposing factor in its development and/or whether other disorders may play a significant role as well. Our findings suggest that while separation anxiety is important in one large subgroup, the sample may consist of different subtypes with different underlying structures.

REFERENCES

Achenbach, T. M. (1978). The Child Behavior Profile; I. Boys aged 6–11. *J. Consult. Clin. Psychol.*, 46:478-488.

———————— (1979). The Child Behavior Profile; II. Boys aged 12–16 and girls aged 6–11 and 12–16. *J. Consult. Clin. Psychol.*, 47:233-233.

———————— (1983). *Manual for the Child Behavior Checklist and Revised Child Behavior Profile*. Queen City Printers Inc.

Bates, J. E., Bentler, P. M. & Thompson, S. K. (1979). Gender deviant boys compared with normal and clinical control boys. *J. Abnorm. Child Psychol.*, 7:243-259.

———————— & Thompson, S. K. (1973). Measurement of deviant gender development in boys. *Child Develpm.*, 44:591-598.

———— Skilbeck, W. M., Smith, K. V. R. et al. (1974). Gender role abnormalities in boys: an analysis of clinical ratings. *J. Abnorm. Child Psychol.*, 2:1-16.

Bieber, I., Dain, H. J., Dince, P. R. et al. (1962). *Homosexuality: A Psychological Study of Male Homosexuals*, New York: Basic Books.

Bradley, F., Doering, R., Zucker, K., Finegan, J. & Gonda, G. M. (1980). Assessment of the gender/disturbed child: a comparison to sibling and psychiatric controls. In: *Childhood and Sexuality*, ed. J. Sampson. Montreal: Editions Etudes Vivantes, pp. 554-568.

Coates, S., & Tuber, S. (1985). Representations of object relations in the Rorschach's of feminine boys. In: *Primitive Mental States and the Rorschach*, ed. P. Lerner & H. Lerner. New York: International Universities Press (in press).

Green, R. (1974). *Sexual Identity Conflict in Children and Adults*. New York: Basic Books.

———— (1976). One-hundred feminine and masculine boys: behavioral contrasts and demographic similarities. *Arch. Sex. Behav.*, 5:425-446.

———— (1979). Childhood cross-gender behavior and subsequent sexual preference. *Amer. J. Psychiat.*, 36:106-108.

Hollingshead, A. B. (1975). Four-Factor Index of Social Status. Unpublished manuscript (available from the Dept. of Sociology, Yale University, New Haven, CT 06510).

Kastrup, M. (1976). Psychic disorders among pre-school children in a geographically delimited area of Aarhus County, Denmark. *Acta Psychiat. Scand.*, 54:29-42.

Lapouse, R., & Monk, M. A. (1978). An epidemiologic study of behavior characteristics in children. *Amer. J. Public Hlth.*, 48:1134-1144.

Lebowitz, P. S. (1972). Feminine behavior in boys: aspects of its outcome. *Amer. J. Psychiat.*, 128:1283-1289.

Mahler, M. (1975). Discussion of healthy parental influences on the earliest development of masculinity in baby boys. *Psychoanal. Forum*, 5:244-247.

Marantz, S. (1984). Mothers of extremely feminine boys: child rearing practices and psychopathology. Doctoral dissertation, New York University.

Money, J., & Russo, A. J. (1979). Homosexual outcome of the discordant gender identity/role in childhood: longitudinal follow-up. *J. Pediat. Psychol.*, 4:29-41.

Orvaschel, H., & Weissman, M. M. (1985). Epidemiology of anxiety disorders in children: a review. In: *Anxiety Disorders in Children*, ed. R. Gittelman. New York: Guilford Press (in press).

Ovesey, L., & Person, E. S. (1973), Gender identity and sexual psychopathology in men: a psychodynamic analysis of homosexuality, transsexualism and transvestism. *J. Amer. Acad. Psychoanal.*, 1:53-72.

———— ———— (1976). Transvestism: a disorder of the sense of self. *Int. J. Psychoanal. Psychiat.*, 5:219-236.

Person, E., & Ovesey, L. (1974a). The transsexual syndrome in males; I. Primary transsexualism. *Amer. J. Psychother.*, 28:4-20.

———— ———— (1974b). The transsexual syndrome in males; II. Secondary transsexualism. *Amer. J. Psychother.*, 28:174-193.

———— ———— (1984), Homosexual cross-dressers. *J. Amer. Acad. Psychoanal.*, 12:167-186.

Rekers, G. A., Bentler, P. M., Rosen, A. C. & Lovaas, O. I. (1977). Child gender disturbance: a clinical rationale for intervention. *Psychother. Theory Res. Pract.*, 14:1-8.

———— Crandall, B. F., Rosen, A. C. & Butler, P. M. (1979). Genetic and physical studies of male children with psychological gender disturbances. *Psychol. Med.*, 9:373-375.

Rosen, A. C., Rekers, G. A. & Friar, L. R. (1977). Theoretical and diagnostic issues in child gender disturbances. *J. Sex Res.*, 13:89-103.

Socarides, C. (1975). Discussion of healthy parental influences on the earliest development of masculinity in baby boys. *Psychoanal. Forum*, 5:241-243.

Stoller, R. J. (1975), *Sex and Gender; Vol. II. The Transsexual Experiment*. New York, Jason Aronson.

Tuber, S., & Coates, S. (1985), Interpersonal phenomena in the Rorschach's of feminine boys. *Psychoanal. Psychol.*, 2:251-265.

Weitzmann, E. L., Shamoian, C. A. & Golosow, N. (1970). Identity diffusion and the transsexual resolution. *J. Nerv. Ment. Dis.*, 151:295-302.

Zucker, K. J. (1982), Childhood gender disturbances; diagnostic issues. *This Journal*, 21:274-280.

Zuger, B. (1978). Effeminate behavior in boys in childhood: ten additional years of follow-up. *Comp. Psychiat.*, 19:363-369.

12

Gender Identity in Childhood and Later Sexual Orientation: Follow-Up of 78 Males

Richard Green

State University of New York at Stony Brook

Two groups of males were evaluated on parameters of gender identity, initially in boyhood and later in adolescence or young adulthood. One group was composed of 66 clinically referred boys whose behaviors were consistent with the diagnosis of gender identity disorder of childhood. The other group consisted of 56 volunteers selected on the basis of demographic matching. Two-thirds of each group were reevaluated for sexual orientation; 30 of the 44 who previously had shown extensive cross-gender behavior and none of the 34 in the comparison group were bisexually or homosexually oriented.

Several retrospective studies link boyhood cross-gender behavior with late adolescent and adult homosexual orientation. Saghir and Robins (1) found that 65% of 89 homosexual men and only 3% of 35 heterosexual men recalled a "girl-like" syndrome, which was characterized by

Reprinted with permission from the *American Journal of Psychiatry*, 1985, Vol. 142, 339–341. Copyright 1985 by the American Psychiatric Association.

Supported by NIMH grants MH-31739 and MH-26598, grants from the Playboy Foundation, and grant G-69-471 from the Foundations' Fund for Research in Psychiatry.

Robert Stoller helped initiate and has sustained this project since 1968. Katherine Williams has directed many facets of project management since 1974. Thelma Guffan, Carol Sancimo, and Virginia Bentley helped with subject scheduling, correspondence, and transcript typing.

an aversion to playing with boys, an aversion to boys' games and activities, and an interest in playing with dolls. A larger study by Bell et al. (2) of 575 homosexual and 284 heterosexual men found that the most significant correlate of adult homosexuality recalled from boyhood was "gender noncomformity," which was characterized by a preference for girls' rather than boys' activities and cross-dressing. Harry (3), who conducted an even larger study (1,400 homosexual and 200 heterosexual men) found that significantly more homosexual than heterosexual men recalled being called "sissy," being social loners, wanting to be girls, playing with girls, and cross-dressing. This association between boyhood nonerotic behaviors and adulthood erotic behaviors is also supported by cross-cultural research. Whitam (4) studied homosexual and heterosexual men in Brazil and Guatemala as well as in the United States; homosexual men in the three cultures more often recalled an interest in toys typically preferred by girls, cross-dressing, a preference for girls' games and activities, and being regarded as a "sissy."

The potential fallacies of retrospective recall include inaccuracies produced by the eroding influence of time and conscious and unconscious needs to selectively recall events to construct a coherent developmental theory of the self or to present the self in a socially acceptable manner. To overcome such limitations, this study was prospective. Two groups of subjects were initially evaluated in childhood and then reevaluated during adolescence and/or young adulthood. During childhood, extensive data were gathered on the child's sex-typed behaviors, his relationships with other children, and his relationship with his parents. The parents were also extensively evaluated.

METHOD

One group of families (N = 66) was clinically or self-referred and contained boys with extensive cross-gender behavior. The other (N = 56) was composed of demographically matched paid volunteers. Matching variables were age, gender, and sibling sequence of the child and race, religion, educational level, and marital status of the parents.

The age range of the boys at initial evaluation was 3½–11 years. The average age was 7½. Seventy-four percent of the families were maritally intact, 6% were separated, 18% were divorced, and 2% had no legal father. Seventy-nine percent were white, 8% were black, 8% were Hispanic, and 6% were a mix of ethnic groups. Thirty-seven percent were Protestant, 25% were Catholic, 19% were Jewish, and 14% had no religion. With respect to the educational level of the fathers, 31% had partially or fully completed high school, 40% partially or fully completed college, and 27% had some postcollege work. With respect to sibling order, 15% of the boys were only children, and the remaining 85% had a random assortment of younger and older brothers and sisters.

Boyhood behaviors were recorded via multiple-choice questionnaires, designed by me and completed by parents, and audiotape semi-structured parent interviews, designed and conducted by me. The two groups of boys showed a markedly different behavioral pattern at initial evaluation. One group showed extensive interest in cross-dressing, preferentially role-played as females, frequently played with female-type dress-up dolls, had a primarily female peer group, expressed the wish to be girls, and avoided rough-and-tumble play and sports; today most if not all would be diagnosed as having gender identity disorder of childhood (*DSM-III*). The other group, while occasionally showing some of these behaviors, did not have the behaviors in combination or frequency to warrant that diagnosis. An extensive tabular description of demographic and behavioral features of the two samples of families can be found elsewhere (5), as can verbatim behavioral descriptions of some of the boys with cross-gender behavior, as given by their parents (6).

Most of the families of both groups of boys have been periodically reevaluated. The frequency of reevaluation ranged from every 18 months to 11 years to not at all. An attempt was made to schedule families for reevaluation at about 18-month intervals; however, some families were temporarily lost to or temporarily refused to return for follow-up, and other families are currently lost to or refuse to return for follow-up. Reevaluation into at least early adolescence has been possible for about two-thirds of both samples (44 families in the cross-gender group and 34 families in the comparison group).

Sexual orientation at follow-up was determined by semi-structured audiotape interviews conducted by me. Questions for assessing sexual orientation on the dimension of fantasy included masturbation fantasies, erotic nocturnal dream imagery, and genital responsivity to visual erotica (pornography). An average of responses to questions for the three variables was used in assigning a score for sexual orientation. The percentage of times that masturbatory fantasies included males or females, that nocturnal erotic dream imagery included males or females, and that the subject experienced penile tumescence in response to pornographic pictures of males or females was transformed into a designation on a 7-point continuum of sexual orientation.

A sexual behavior orientation score was given for a pattern of behaviors, i.e., a sequence of repeated experiences with a single partner or a sequence of single experiences with transient partners. The number of interpersonal genital experiences leading to orgasm with males or females was used to designate a point on the 7-point continuum of sexual orientation.

Interview procedures were the same for both groups of subjects. Sexual orientation was coded on a 7-point continuum, derived from the work of Kinsey et al. (7), from 0 (exclusive heterosexuality) to 6 (exclusive homosexuality) where 1 = predominant heterosexuality with incidental homosexuality, 2 = predominant heterosexuality with more than incidental homosexuality, and 3 = equal amounts of heterosexuality and homosexuality, etc. A person who has a rating of 2 or higher may be categorized as bisexual to exclusively homosexual. To transform the interview responses to a Kinsey score, the score on the 7-point continuum of sexual orientation would be a proportional distance between 0 and 6. For example, if 85% of masturbatory fantasies involved males and 15% involved females, here the score would be 5.

The sexual orientation data were divided into fantasy and behavior for two reasons: 1) because of the age of the respondents, there may be data for fantasy only, and 2) fantasy and behavior scores may differ substantially within a subject.

RESULTS

The ages at initial evaluation and follow-up and sexual orientation scores on fantasy and behavior of the 44 boys with earlier extensive cross-gender behavior are given in table 1: 30 (68%) had scores in the 2–6 range (bisexual to homosexual) for fantasy, and 24 of these 30 (80%) had scores in the 2–6 range for behavior. By contrast, none of the 34 boys in the demographically matched contrast group, aged 13–23 years at follow-up, were in the bisexual or homosexual range on either dimension; two comparison subjects were rated 1 on fantasy and 0 on behavior.

Combination scores for fantasy and behavior (when enough information was reported to provide a basis for rating both) were computed for subjects who previously showed extensive cross-gender behavior. These scores were divded into three categories: 0–1 (heterosexual range), 2–4 (bisexual range), and 5–6 (homosexual range). There were 14 boys (32%) in the 0–1 category, 11 (25%) in the 2–4 category, and 19 (43%) in the 5–6 category.

TABLE 1. Age at First Evaluation and Follow-Up and Follow-Up Sexual Orientation Scores of 44 Males Who Manifested Extensive Cross-Gender Behavior During Boyhood

Subject	Age (years)		Sexual Orientation Score	
	First Evaluation	Follow-Up	Fantasy	Behavior
1	8	18	0	—
2	7	13	0	—
3	10	19	0	0
4	4	14	0	—
5	9	22	2	2
6	8	20	6	6
7	10	21	5	5
8	7	14	0	—
9	6	19	5	4
10	5	15	0	—
11	6	17	6	—
12	8	17	2	—
13	5	15	1	—
14	7	21	5	5
15	10	23	6	6
16	7	16	1	0
17	4	16	5	—
18	4	16	5	4
19	8	21	2	2
20	6	18	0	—
21	6	20	6	6
22	8	18	4	—
23	10	20	5	5
24	10	20	6	6
25	7	16	0	0
26	8	19	6	6
27	6	20	2	6
28	6	23	4	—
29	5	14	0	1
30	6	18	6	4
31	8	20	4	4
32	5	18	0	0
33	7	18	5	6
34	10	21	4	3
35	6	19	5	4
36	10	22	4	4
37	7	21	6	6
38	5	17	0	0
39	4	18	4	—
40	5	14	0	—
41	8	21	5	5
42	10	21	5	5
43	8	20	4	4
44	5	19	5	5

DISCUSSION

This longitudinal study of two groups of boys demonstrates that the association between extensive cross-gender behavior in boyhood and homosexual behavior in adulthood, suggested by previous retrospective reports, can be validated by a prospective study of clinically or family-referred boys with behaviors consistent with the gender identity disorder of childhood. However, not all boys with extensive cross-gender behavior evolved as bisexual or homosexual men. No boys in the comparison group evolved as bisexual or homosexual, which may be a reflection of the low rates of this orientation in the general population (about 10%) (7) combined with the relatively small sample studied; there is also the possibility that the majority of that 10% derives from a small subsample of boys who show extensive cross-gender behavior (none of whom were found in the comparison group).

During the course of the study, 12 of the boys in the cross-gender group were involved in formal psychotherapy, including behavior modification, group therapy, individual psychotherapy, and family therapy (6, 8). The rates of bisexual/homosexual orientation in this treated group were comparable to that of the entire group. The frequency of follow-up interviews was also not associated with sexual orientation scores. There was no difference in the proportion of bisexual/homosexual to heterosexual persons between those interviewed more than once between prepuberty and young adulthood and those not seen from prepuberty until follow-up in young adulthood (8).

Other reports from this project will describe the relationship between parent-child and parent-parent variables associated with the development of extensive cross-gender behavior, boyhood and family characteristics associated with later sexual orientation scores, and other psychological features of the men at follow-up. Extensive descriptions of the boys and their parents, with verbatim interviews conducted during the boys' childhood, adolescence, and adulthood and descriptions by these men of their current sexual orientation, are also forthcoming (8).

REFERENCES

1. Saghir, M., Robins, E.: Male and Female Homosexuality: A Comprehensive Investigation. Baltimore, Williams & Wilkins, 1973.
2. Bell, A., Weinberg, M., Hammersmith, S.: Sexual Preference: Its Development in Men and Woman. Bloomington, Indiana University Press, 1981.
3. Harry, J.: Gay Children Grown Up. New York, Praeger, 1982.

4. Whitam, F. The prehomosexual male child in three societies: the United States, Guatemala, Brazil. Arch. Sex. Behav. 9:87-99, 1980.
5. Green, R.: One hundred ten masculine and feminine boys: behavioral contrasts and demographic similarities. Arch. Sex. Behav. 5:425-446, 1976.
6. Green, R.: Sexual Identity Conflict in Children and Adults. New York, Basic Books (London, Gerald Duckworth), 1974.
7. Kinsey A., Pomeroy, W., Martin, C.: Sexual Behavior in the Human Male. Philadelphia, W.B. Saunders, 1948.
8. Green, R.: "Sissy" Boys to "Gay" Men: A Fifteen Year Prospective Study. New Haven, Yale University Press (in press).

13

An Immunoreactive Theory of Selective Male Affliction

Thomas Gualtieri and Robert E. Hicks

University of North Carolina, Chapel Hill

Males are selectively afflicted with the neurodevelopmental and psychiatric disorders of childhood, a broad and virtually ubiquitous phenomenon that has not received proper attention in the biological study of sex differences. The previous literature has alluded to psychosocial differences, genetic factors and elements pertaining to male "complexity" and relative immaturity, but these are not deemed an adequate explanation for selective male affliction. The structure of sex differences in neurodevelopmental disorders is hypothesized to contain these elements: (1) Males are more frequently afflicted, females more severely; (2) disorders arising in females are largely mediated by the genotype in males, by a genotype by environment interaction; (3) complications of pregnancy and delivery occur more frequently with male births; such complications are decisive and influence subsequent development. We hypothesize that there is something about the male fetus that evokes an inhospitable uterine environment. This "evocative principle" is hypothesized to relate to the relative antigenicity of the male fetus, which may induce a state of maternal immunoreactivity,

Reprinted with permission from *The Behavioral and Brain Sciences,* 1985, Vol. 8, 427-441. Copyright 1985 by Cambridge University Press.

The authors wish to acknowledge the contributions of the following to the preparation of this manuscript: Susan Council, Sue Ellis, Morris Lipton, James Mayo, and Debra Patterson.

Work was supported in part by grants from the National Institute of Child Health and Human Development (HD 07201) and from the National Institute of Mental Health (MH 33127).

leading either directly or indirectly to fetal damage. The immuno-reactive theory (IMRT) thus constructed is borrowed from studies of sex ratios and is the only explanation consistent with negative parity effects in the occurrence of pregnancy complications and certain neu-rodevelopmental disorders. Although the theory is necessarily specu-lative, it is heuristic and hypotheses derived from it are proposed; some are confirmed in the existing literature and by the authors' research.

Males are selectively afflicted with virtually every neurologic, psychiatric, and developmental disorder of childhood (see Table 1). There are conditions, of course, like anencephaly and dysraphism, which are commoner in females (Glucksmann 1978; Nakano 1973); but for the most important neurodevelopmental disorders—mental retardation, autism, hyperactivity, dyslexia, epilepsy, dysphasia, cerebral palsy, and conduct disorders—the sex differential works unequivocally to male disadvantage (Butler & Bonham 1963; Nichols & Chen 1981; Rutter 1970). This phenomenon is largely unexplained. Though the biology and psychology of sex differences has been an attractive area of recent scientific concern, the issue of selective male affliction seems to have generated neither broad interest nor systematic research.

In its ubiquity and breadth, the phenomenon compels an explanation that is couched, somehow, in the biology of sex differences. Although it is not unlikely that sex differences in parental handling or societal attitudes may have a role in the development or identification of at least some of the behavioral and emotional disorders of childhood (Rutter 1970), the role sex differences in adult perceptions of children, referral and labeling processes, and tolerance of deviant behaviors may actually play in the development of psychiatric disorders in children with normal brain development has yet to be determined. Boys are believed to be more vulnerable than girls to certain kinds of family disharmony (Rutter 1970) and other psychosocial stressors. (Cadoret & Cain 1980), but the reason for this is not understood. However, psychosocial theories are hardly germane to the problem of selective male affliction with severe neurodevelopmental disorders like epilepsy, autism, and mental retardation.

It has been suggested that the genetic endowment of the male comprises sufficient cause for male "inferiority" (Childs 1965; Ounsted & Taylor 1972; Rutter 1970). The Y chromosome is considerably smaller than the X and also relatively inert, thus giving the female a "4–5% quantitative superiority in genetic material" (Childs 1965). This disparity means that the homogametic sex (female) is diploid with respect to many loci, whereas the heterogametic sex (male) must always be haploid. Because there are loci on the X chromsome that control functions apart from reproductive sex, males are necessarily the victims of whatever uncompensated dosage effects may exist (Childs 1965). X linkage has been proposed to account for greater male variability for virtually all biological traits, including mental functioning (Lehrke 1978). Untoward X-linked recessive genes will be expressed in males but not in heterozygous females, and the occurrence of X-linked disorders of development is not infrequent. However, they are not sufficiently frequent to account for the breadth and ubiquity of the phenomenon of selective affliction. Most of the conditions in Table 1 are not X linked, and the large majority do not show a pattern of inheritance that characterizes specific chromosomal abnormalities.

The effect of the Y-chromosome message has been described by Ounsted and Taylor (1972, p. 257) as catalytic; that is, it serves to "modify any genome." Females express neither the fullest advantages nor the worst disadvantages of their genome. Their characteristics are said to be "less scattered," whereas males suffer the "extremes of viable disadvantage and the greatest advantage" (Ounsted & Taylor 1972, p. 258). Thus, male inferiroity is said to be the consequence of greater genetic variability for "the majority of measurable characteristics" (Wing 1981).

According to Ounsted and Taylor, the increased variability expressed in males is at least in part a consequence of the function of the Y chromosome in regulating the pace of development. "Transcription of expressed genomic information in males occurs at a slower ontogenetic pace; the operation of the Y chromosome is to allow more genomic information to be transcribed" (Ounsted & Taylor 1972, p. 245). Whether or not the pace of development is regulated by the Y chromosome—there is, to the author's knowledge, no direct evidence that it is—it is an incontestable fact that development and maturation occurs more slowly in males (Taylor, 1969). At every developmental stage, the male is less mature than the female (D. C. Taylor 1969). A newborn girl is the physiological equivalent of a 4-to-6-week old boy, and physiological maturity is achieved two years later in boys than in girls (Hutt 1972). In general, immature organisms are more susceptible to damage than mature ones (Rutter 1970), and the developing male is more susceptible to the information he extracts from his genome and the environment (Taylor & Ounsted 1972). Thus, relative immaturity means that males are more vulnerable to environmental factors for a longer period of time; these may be intrauterine, peri- or postnatal, psychosocial, or biol-

Table 1. *Male–female differences in developmental neuropsychiatry and obstetrics*

Disorder	Sex ratio	Reference
A. *Pediatric psychiatry*		
Hyperkinetic syndrome	300	(Butler & Bonham 1963; Trites et al. 1979)
Conduct disorders	270	(Rutter 1970; Trites et al. 1979)
	200–900	(Zerssen & Weyerer 1982)
Childhood schizophrenia	170	(Kramer 1978)
Early onset schizophrenia	160	(Samuels 1979; Flor-Henry 1974)
Process schizophrenia	150	(Flor-Henry 1974; Allon 1971)
Suicide		(Schaffer & Fisher 1981)
Referrals to child psychiatry clinics	200	(Taylor & Ounsted 1972)
Admission to child psychiatric service	213	(Gualtieri 1983)
B. *Pediatric neurology*		
Seizure disorders		
All ages	120	(Taylor & Ounsted 1972)
Neonatal convulsions	116	(Taylor & Ounsted 1972)
Childhood seizures	140	(Taylor & Ounsted 1972)
Infantile spasms	210	(Taylor & Ounsted 1972)
Temporal lobe epilepsy	132	(Taylor & Ounsted 1972)
Febrile seizures	140	(Taylor & Ounsted 1972)
In mentally retarded children	170	(Corbett, Hannis & Robinson 1975)
Cerebral palsy	150–260	(Wing 1981; Taylor & Ounsted 1972)
Subacute schlerosing panencephalitis	220	(Taylor & Ounsted 1972)
Encephalitis (echo type 9)	220	(Sabin, Krombiegel & Wigand 1958)
Abnormal neurological exam at one year of age	114	(Singer et al. 1968)

C. *Developmental disorders*		
Severe mental retardation	130	(Abramowicz et al. 1975)
Down's syndrome	128–260	(Tsai & Beisler 1983; Burgio et al. 1981)
Speech and language disorders	260	(Ingram 1959)
Stuttering	400	(Reinisch et al. 1979)
Learning difficulties	219	(Nichols & Chen 1981)
Dyslexia	430	(McKinney & Feagans 1983)
Autism	400	(Ingram 1964)
D. *Obstetrics perinatal*		
Spontaneous abortion	120–140	(McMillen 1979)
Toxemia	109–171	(Toivanen & Hirvonen 1970)
Placenta praevia	120	(Ounsted 1972)
Abruptio placentae	206	(Ounsted 1972)
Antepartum hemorrhage	140–210	(Rhodes 1965)
Intra-partum anoxia	130	(Butler & Bonham 1963)
Pulmonary infection	250	(Butler & Bonham 1963)
Hyaline membrane disease	180	(Butler & Bonham 1963)
Pulmonary hemorrhage	210	(Butler & Bonham 1963)
Cerebral birth trauma	180	(Butler & Bonham 1963)
Apgar 6	130	(Singer et al. 1968)

The sex ratio is expressed, by convention, as the number of males divided by the number of females, multiplied by one hundred, or $(N_m/N_f)100$.

ogic. The classical and often cited example of the untoward clinical sequelae of prolonged immaturity was reported by Taylor and Ounsted (1971). The interval of susceptibility to convulsive seizures originating in the temporal lobe as a consequence of cerebral injury is considerably longer in the male infant.

The complement to prolonged maturation is increased complexity; the male human is said to be a more complex organism than the female and his brain is a more complex organ. The male brain is more completely lateralized (McGlone 1980), it is heavier (Dekaban & Sadowsky 1978), its oxygen requirements are higher (Hutt 1972), and it is an androgenized female brain (Reinisch, Gandelman & Spiegel 1979). If male brain development is more complicated and prolonged, "there are likely to be more opportunities for errors to occur" (Reinisch et al. 1979, p. 221). However, it is not explicit precisely how these errors come about, or precisely what they are, at least on a physiologic basis. By the same token, the immaturity hypothesis fails to describe any specifics about the information the developing child extracts from his genome or his environment, or how this process unfolds.

Male vulnerability is, of course, hardly limited to congenital disorders, and no review of the topic can afford to overlook the general pattern of male vulnerability at every age to accident and disease. (The notable exceptions are the autoimmune diseases and, of course, diseases of the female reproductive organs [Rutter 1970; Vessey 1972].) The higher mortality of males is reflected in the sex ratio ((male/females) × 100). Although the primary sex ratio (i.e. at conception) is probably around 120 (estimated range 110–170), male fetuses are more prone to spontaneous abortion and stillbirth, and by the end of gestation the (secondary) sex ratio falls to about 105 (McMillen 1979). By the end of childhood, the sex ratio drops to unity, a consequence of increased male mortality from accidents and childhood diseases (Reinisch et al. 1979). The relative vulnerability of males is a lifelong phenomenon, and overall the population of the United States is 51% female (Reinisch et al. 1979).

It is not likely, however, that this general, lifelong pattern of male vulnerability can be molded to accommodate a single, parsimonious, and unifying theory, or at least one that would make sense or generate testable hypotheses. The range of problems to which males succumb is simply too broad; each is probably the consequence of a host of different intervening variables. The specific area of concern here, the neurodevelopmental disorders of childhood, also encompasses a broad and diverse range of problems, but the topic is more tractable, and one that may well be open to intelligent theory.

It is fair to say that most of the foregoing ideas about selective male affliction may succeed as explanations or as seminal ideas, but they fail as theories; their capacity to generate testable hypotheses seems to have been extremely limited. Like Butler, we conclude that "the explanation for most of these striking [sex] differences is not understood" (Butler & Bonham 1963, p. 268). Many of the ideas have merit and are incorporated into the theory that is developed herein. However, by themselves, they leave an "unexplained residue . . . of staggering proportions" (Medawar 1963, p. 321).

THE STRUCTURE OF SEX DIFFERENCES

> In general, the morbific processes, mild and grave, attack the females with greater intensity than the males (Ciocco 1940, p. 204)

While females are less prone to affliction with neurodevelopmental problems, when such conditions do arise in the female, a severer form is usually manifest (Taylor & Ounsted 1972). This principle appears to hold for most of the pathologic conditions in which it has been tested. For example, although males are more frequently found to be mentally retarded, at the lowest levels of IQ the proportion of females is relatively higher (Taylor & Ounsted 1972). Autistic children are more commonly males, but at the lowest IQ levels the number of autistic females is proportionately higher (Lord, Schopler, & Revicki 1982; Lotter 1974; Tsai & Beisler 1983; Tsai, Stewart, & August 1981; Wing 1981). The mortality rate of institutionalized retardates (Forssman & Akesson 1970) and of Down's children (Fabia & Drolette 1970) is higher in females and the mortality rate of females with cerebral palsy is also higher (Ingram 1964; Schlesinger, Alaway & Peltin 1959). Females are less prone to epilepsy, but they are more prone to the morbid sequelae of febrile seizures (Taylor & Ounsted 1972) and to the development of epileptic psychosis (Flor-Henry 1969; Slater, Beard & Glithero 1963; D. C. Taylor 1969; Taylor & Ounsted 1972). In order to understand why this is important, it is essential to consider the structure of male–female differences as they relate to the disorders in question, and especially as they relate to the occurrence of perinatal problems.

In the neurodevelopmental disorders, sex differences cause a dissociation between the elements of frequency, or incidence, and intensity, or severity. As a general rule, males are more frequently afflicted and females more severely impaired when they are afflicted. An additional sex-based dissociation is that the occurrence of neurodevelopmental disorders in females seems to be mediated primarily through genetic channels, and that their disorders may be, as a consequence, more specific, whereas in males, the disorders are mediated largely through the occurrence of perinatal problems, and are less specific and more diverse in their manifestation. There is strong evidence suggesting this.

The occurrence of pure type dyslexia is more frequent in girls (Pennington & Smith 1983) and it is possible to fit a genetic model to learning disabilities in girls but not boys (Lewitter, DeFries & Elston 1980). The clinical picture of autistic children with positive family histories of developmental dysfunction is more homogeneous than that of those with negative family histories (August, Stewart & Tsai 1981). The range of IQ in autistic males is wider (Wing 1981). Autistic girls are more likely than boys to have family histories of cognitive and language dysfunction (Tsai & Beisler 1983) and members of the families of dyslexic girls (Decker & DeFries 1980) and of girls with conduct disorders (Robins 1966) are more frequently afflicted. The clinical presentation of a disorder that is largely mediated by the genotype is likely to be more specific, whereas the behavioral and developmental sequelae of early brain damage are known to be relatively nonspecific (Graham & Rutter 1968).

The same pattern is suggested by studies of the genetics of schizophrenia. For example, the concordance for schizophrenia in monozygous (MZ) twins is higher for females than males (Rosenthal 1962). Schizophrenic mothers of children who become schizophrenic tend themselves to have had an earlier onset of the disorder than mothers of children who do not become schizophrenic (Mednick 1970), and the births of their children are characterized by relative difficulty (Mednick 1970; Mednick, Mura, Schulsinger & Mednick 1971). However, severity of the maternal illness is associated with the level of schizophrenia only in high-risk daughters and not in sons (Gardner 1967; Sobel 1961); perinatal complications, on the other hand, are more likely in high risk sons than in daughters (Mednick, Schulsinger, Teasdale, Schulsinger, Venables & Rock 1978). There is a significant relation between perinatal complications and the later development of schizophrenia in high-risk boys but not in girls (Mednick, Schulsinger, Teasdale, Schulsinger, Venables & Rock, 1977). The daughters of schizophrenic mothers are likely to be schizophrenic if they have any disorder at all, whereas the sons exhibit a more diverse range of psychopathology, especially sociopathy and criminal behavior (Mednick et al. 1978). What this suggests is that "schizophrenia in females is more genetically determined and that schizophrenia in males has a heavier environmental weight" (Mednick et al.

1977, p. 181). When the high risk daughters of schizophrenic mothers develop schizophrenia, it is largely (though not entirely) determined by their genotype; the sons develop schizophrenia or other severe psychiatric disorders, and this is mediated by a genotype by environment interaction. The environmental effect is keenly felt by male fetuses during pregnancy and parturition.

Schizophrenia is not properly counted among the neurodevelopmental disorders, although a cogent case could probably be made that it ought to be, especially the form of schizophrenia with early onset, which occurs more commonly in males, responds poorly to treatment, is often associated with demonstrable neuropathic changes, and follows a dementing course (Weinberger, Cannon-Spoor, Potkin & Wyatt 1980).

We have recently described a similar structure in the sex differences that occur in developmentally handicapped children (Hicks & Gualtieri 1984). In a retrospective review of 223 developmentally handicapped children referred for evaluation at the University of North Carolina within a given year, the majority of patients were, as expected, male (78%). In terms of IQ and SQ (social quotient), however, females were more severely impaired (Table 2A). For both males and females, there was found to be a positive linear relationship between the occurrence of newborn problems (e.g., hypoxia, jaundice) and IQ (F_{linear} [1,166] = 5.255, P = .025) and SQ (F_{linear} [1,185] = 4.715, P = .025), and between the occurrence of neurological problems in the first year of life (e.g., seizures, dystonia) and IQ (F_{linear} [1,168] = 11.907, P = .001) and SQ (F_{linear} [1,188] = 10.713, P = .001). Newborn problems and first-year neurological problems were associated (Pearson X^2 = 24.295, P = .0001). There was a positive relationship between newborn problems and low birthweight (F_{linear} [1,204] = 8.087, P = .005) as well as with delivery complications (Pearson X^2 = 21.7, P = .0002). Both newborn problems (F_{linear} [1,172] = 8.521, P < .01) and neurological problems were associated with pregnancy complications (F_{linear} [1,174] = 15.147, P < .001). However, pregnancy complications were significantly more common with male fetuses (Table 2B). On the other hand, a family history of neurodevelopmental disorders was more frequent in females (Table 2C). The severity of affliction was worse for females, and their genetic background was loaded. Male fetuses were more frequently afflicted, they experienced a higher rate of pregnancy complications, and their genetic background was less decisive (Hicks & Gualtieri 1984).

The structure of sex differences occurring in the neurodevelopmental disorders of childhood consists of four elements: Males are more commonly afflicted. When females are afflicted, the manifestation of the condition is more severe. In females, such disorders are largely influenced by the genotype and as a consequence, the manifestation is more specific. In males, the occurrence of neurodevelopmental disorders is mediated by a genotype by environment interaction; pre- and perinatal problems play a more important role and their manifestation is more diverse.

Such a pattern is consistent with a model that posits a spectrum or a continuum of liability. Liability to a neurodevelopmental disorder is a function of a number of genes acting in concert, and these polygenes are presumed to be normally distributed within the population (Carter 1965). The essential part of this model is a differential threshold for

Table 2. *The structure of sex differences*

A. Females are more severely impaired than males

		Males	Females
IQ	Mean	55.3	41.2
	S.D.	+23.7	+21.5
	N	139	35

$F(1,172) = 10.18, P = .002$

		Males	Females
SQ	Mean	63.0	52.9
	S.D.	+24.2	±18.9
	N	154	40

$F(1,192) = 6.0, P = .015$

B. Proportion of each sex classified by number of problems in pregnancy

	\multicolumn{3}{c}{Pregnancy problems}		
	None	One	More than one	N
Boys	.058	.234	.708	171
Girls	.283	.130	.587	46
				217

Pearson $\chi^2 = 19.785, P = .0001$

C. Proportion of each sex classified by family history of neurodevelopmental disorders

	Relatives affected	Relatives not affected	
Male proband	21	146	167
Female proband	11	31	42
	32	177	209

Pearson $\chi^2 = 4.798, P = .05$

expression of the phenotype for males and females. For females, a substantial genetic load is required for expression; for males a lower quantity of untoward genes is required. This threshold of liability model was originally proposed by Carter to account for sex differences in the occurrence of certain congenital malformations (Carter 1965) and the model has also been advanced with respect to dyslexia (Lewitter, DeFries & Elston 1980) conduct disorder and sociopathy (Cloninger, Christiansen, Reich & Gottesman 1978), stuttering (Garside & Kay 1964), left handedness (Hicks & Kinsbourne 1981), autism (Tsai & Beisler 1983), pyloric stenosis (Carter 1965), and cleft lip and palate (Woolf 1971).

The threshold for expression of neurodevelopmental problems in males may be lower by virtue of their proclivity to encounter serious and damaging pre- and perinatal difficulties. It is not necessary to postulate an increased level of vulnerability to such difficulties for males, although this may be the case, simply because the very occurrence of pregnancy complications in male fetuses is substantially more frequent (Butler & Bonham 1963; Nichols & Chen 1981; Singer, Westphal & Niswander 1968). The male fetus is much more likely to encounter intrauterine difficulties like toxemia (Toivanen & Hirvonen 1970b), abruptio placentae (Rhodes 1965), placenta praevia (Ounsted 1972), prematurity (Niswander & Gordon 1972), and miscarriage (McMillen 1979). It is well known that severe pre- and perinatal problems may cause or aggravate developmental problems, and that less severe gestational events like occasional bleeding are significantly associated with subsequent neurological, behavioral, and developmental problems (Nichols & Chen 1981). The increased frequency with which males encounter an inhospitable uterine environment or a difficult passage compromises brain development and lowers their threshold of liability to neurodevelopmental problems.

The natural question here is why male fetuses are more prone to pre- and perinatal difficulties. Males are heavier in utero and at birth (Butler & Bonham 1963), and larger fetuses are more prone to certain kinds of obstetrical and perinatal problems, but when birth weight is controlled, such problems are still more common in males (Singer et al. 1968). There seems to be something about the male fetus that evokes an untoward uterine environment.

MATERNAL INSUFFICIENCY AND NEGATIVE PARITY EFFECTS

Selective male affliction is hypothesized to arise as a consequence of a lower threshold for expression of a deviant phenotype, and the threshold is lowered through the mediation of complications during pregnancy and delivery. These occur more frequently with male fetuses, and "the female conceptus is better adapted to survive in the maternal uterine environment than the male" (Loke 1978, p. 164). An evocative principle is called for: What is it about the male fetus that causes such trouble? Fetal size is not a suitable answer, but what may be?

There are two plausible alternatives: an endocrine effect or an antigenic effect. The former is a compelling idea, because a male fetus causes intermittent elevation of maternal levels of testicular androgens (Mizuno, Lobotsky, Lloyd, Kobayashi & Murasawa 1968), and the balance among androgenic, progestational, and estrogenic hormones is known to affect fetal brain development (Maccoby, Doering, Jacklin & Kraemer 1979) and the gestational health of the mother (Siiteri, Febres, Clemens, Chang, Gondos & Stites 1977). The endocrine aspects of pregnancy and fetal brain development, however, are extraordinarily complex, even ambiguous, and the state of the science is not amenable, in our opinion, to a ready explanation of the phenomenon of selective affliction. In addition, immediately below, we describe data that are incompatible, in our opinion, with an endocrinologic viewpoint.

The idea of male antigenicity is also interesting and is considered at greater length below. It is necessary, first, to turn two additional areas of study that have important bearing on the occurrence of perinatal complications; these are the issues of maternal insufficiency, and the existence of parity effects in disorders of development. Together, they suggest that successive pregnancies are not independent events, but that there exists a kind of "memory" in the phenomenon of reproduction. The fate of one pregnancy influences, even predicts, the outcome of the next.

The terms "maternal insufficiency" (Costeff, Cohen, Weller & Kleckner 1981), "uterine inadequacy" (Ahern & Johnson 1973), and "reduced optimality" (Gillberg & Gillberg 1983) refer to the tendency of some mothers to experience an unusual degree of pre- and perinatal complications, including bleeding, toxemia, prematurity, difficult delivery, miscarriage, and perinatal death. As described above, the adequacy of a child's intrauterine environment exercises a substantial long-term influence on his neurological and cognitive development (Joffe 1969). Maternal insufficiency is an important risk factor in developmental disorders like autism (Aarkrog 1968; Gillberg & Gillberg 1983; Tsai & Beisler 1983; Tsai et al. 1981), mental retardation, mild and severe (Costeff, Cohen & Weller 1983; Drillien 1968; Hagberg, Hagberg, Lewerth & Linberg 1981; Lilienfield & Pasamanick 1956), minimal brain dysfunction (MBD) (Nichols & Chen 1981; Gillberg & Rasmussen 1982), and childhood psychoses (Funderburk, Carter, Tanguay, Freeman & Westlake 1983), among others. There may be a dosage effect because signs of uterine inadequacy occur more frequently and in greater number in severer disorders like autism than in MBD. It is also interesting that the signs of uterine inadequacy associated with certain disorders such as autism are not necessarily those that directly induce cerebral hypoxia (Gillberg & Gillberg 1983).

Central to the concept of maternal insufficiency is the idea of tendency. Although any woman can have an isolated bad pregnancy, there are some who are unusually prone to bad pregnancies. This tendency is at least in part genetically determined; for example, the tendency to give birth prematurely is familial (Keller 1981), there is a maternal genetic effect on the birth weight of cousins (Robson 1955), and the aunts and sisters of mentally retarded children have more mental retardation, miscarriage, stillbirth and neonatal death in their families than the uncles and brothers of mentally retarded children have in theirs (Ahern & Johnson 1973). Daughters from toxemic pregnancies are affected themselves with toxemia more often than those from control groups (Chesley, Annito & Cosgrove 1968).

Because of familial uterine inadequacy, a troubled pregnancy does not occur as an independent event. The nature of one pregnancy is capable of predicting the nature of another. The low birth weight of the first child is the most powerful predictor of low birth weight in the second (Bakketeig 1977), the percentage of premature infants increases with the previous number of premature births (Placek 1977), previous fetal, peri- or neonatal deaths predict similar deaths in subsequent pregnancies (Niswander & Gordon, 1972). And there is, again, an element of non-specificity, since previous fetal loss predicts prematurity, and previous prematurity predicts fetal loss (Niswander & Gordon 1972; Placek 1977). The first factor that operates here is the mother's constitutional insufficiency, which is genetic and probably speaks to a common underlying mechanism; the second factor is pre- or perinatal damage, and the effects of this on the fetus are nonspecific.

A demonstration of how reproductive inefficiency of mothers of developmentally impaired children may be related to fetal antigenicity is provided by Costeff, Cohen, Weller, and Kleckner (1981) who compare the incidence of complications of pregnancy, labor, and infancy in 87 mentally retarded children ("undifferentiated phenotype") of consanguinous matings with 161 (idiopathic) mentally retarded children of nonconsanguinous matings. Complications were significantly more common in the latter group. Consanguinous matings, in which antigenic differences are minimized, were not associated with obstetrical or perinatal complications. The authors speculated that "maternal [reproductive] inefficiency [i.e., obstetrical difficulties] may well reflect some so far unidentified factor [which also causes] fetal brain damage" (Costeff et al. 1981, p. 489).

Beyond the genetic memory of inherited uterine inadequacy is another kind of memory that is expressed in the parity effect. The parity effect refers to systematic change in some measurable characteristic of offspring with increasing birth order or pregnancy order. Here again, there is a common pattern: the incidence of the complications of pregnancy and delivery, prematurity, miscarriage, fetal and neonatal deaths increases with birth order; later born are at greater risk (Niswander & Gordon 1972). Parity effects are also observed in at least some of the neurodevelopmental disorders, for example, mental retardation (Belmont, Stein & Wittes 1976), MBD (Badian 1984; Nichols & Chen 1981; Schrag 1973) and autism (see below, "The primiparity effect"). A retarded, hyperactive, or learning disabled child is more frequently later born.

Maternal insufficiency has a predictable negative effect on pregnancies occurring within an extended family. The effects of maternal insufficiency within a family seem to be mediated however, by the parity effect, with an increasingly negative impact on successive pregnancies. This incremental phenomenon is a form of nongenetic memory. It suggests an immunologic aspect; some kind of sensitization process is at work. What could be inherited as maternal insufficiency is, in fact, a genetic proclivity to react immunologically to fetal antigen. The ensuing maternal immune attack against the fetus would appear to the clinician as a complication of pregnancy and as a sign of an inadequate uterine environment.

Selective male affliction, or at least a portion of it, is mediated through complications of pregnancy and childbirth, which occur more frequently in male offspring. An evocative principle was postulated to characterize the male fetus and to render the occurrence of such complications more likely. The phenomenon of maternal insufficiency suggests a genetic element at play on the mother's side. The existence of negative parity effects is compatible with an antigenic but not an endocrine explanation of the phenomenon on the fetal side. The evocative principle, therefore, is deduced to be the unique antigenic character of the male fetus.

THE EXISTENCE OF AN EVOCATIVE PRINCIPLE: THE ANTIGENIC CHARACTER OF THE MALE FETUS

The identification of a male-specific antigen, termed H-Y, was originally made in connection with the Eichwald-Silmser effect (see below,
"The primiparity effect"). The expression of H-Y antigen probably derives from a monomorphic gene locus (Ohno 1979). The original hypothesis was that H-Y antigen is specified by a gene located on the Y
chromosome (Goodfellow & Andrews 1982), but Wolf (1981) presented
evidence to suggest that the structural gene for H-Y antigen is autosomal
and that its expression is regulated by an X-linked repressor and a Y-
linked inducer. Whatever the genetic origin of H-Y antigen, there is no
disagreement over issues of ubiquity or specificity. H-Y antigen has been
shown to be conserved to the extreme throughout vertebrate evolution
(Ohno 1979). Having performed an extensive series of H-Y antibody
absorption tests, Wachtel, Koo, and Boyse (1975) demonstrated that
male cells of all mammalian species tested, including man, absorbed out
the male-specific cytotoxicity of H-Y antibody, whereas no cross reacting
materials were found on female cells. H-Y antigen is ubiquitously expressed in every somatic cell type of the mammalian male (Ohno 1979).
It is first expressed in preimplantation male embryos at the eight cell
stage (Krco & Goldberg 1976). An exact and invariant function seems
to have been assigned by evolution to H-Y antigen, and as far as mammals
are concerned, it is believed to lie in the determination of primary (gon-
adal) sex; H-Y is an absolute prerequisite, though it is not necessarily
sufficient, for testicular organization (Ohno 1979).

Although H-Y is the prime candidate to account for the hypopthesized
antigenicity of the male fetus, it is a minor histocompatibility antigen,
and its effects may be exercised in clinically important ways only through
a cumulative effect with other antigens, including those of the ABO
(Toivanen & Hirvonen 1970a), Rh (Renkonen & Timonen 1967; Scott
& Beer 1973) and human lymphocytotoxic antigen (HLA) systems
(Goulmy, Termijtelen, Bradley & van Rood 1977; Johansen, Festenstein
& Burke 1974; Loke, 1978). Alternatively, maternal–fetal immunoreactivity could be mediated in males whose mothers are sensitized to other
antigens but not to H-Y, or in females, who do not express H-Y antigen,
by virtue of an X-linked antigenic system (e.g. H-X, Xg^a) (Berryman
& Silvers 1979; Loke 1978) that may have clinical importance.

Sex differences in antigenicity were first described in the so called
Eichwald–Silmser effect: male skin grafts survive less well in female
animals than do male-to-male, female-to-male, or female-to-female al-

lografts (Eichwald & Silmser 1955). Trophoblast grafts from female concepti survive longer than male trophoblasts (Borland, Loke & Oldersnaw 1970); most choriocarcinomas arise from female concepti (Scott 1976) and those which arise from male concepti are notably less aggressive (Loke 1978).

There is clinical evidence that male fetuses are more antigenic than females. Immune complexes are found more frequently in the cord blood of male newborns (Farber, Cambiaso & Masson 1981); runt disease and Rh disease occur more commonly in males (Beer & Billingham 1973; Scott & Beer 1966); toxemia, which is probably an autoimmune disorder, is more common when the fetus is male, and the sex ratio increases proportionately with the severity of the disease (Toivanen & Hirvonen 1970b) (see Figure 1).

Antigenic differences between zygote and mother are thought to confer an implantation advantage (Kirby, McWhirter, Teitelbaum & Darlington 1967). Trophoblastic invasion of the uterine decidua may be more extensive if the fetus is antigenically dissimilar to the mother, a mechanism that seems to promote genetic diversity. The male zygote, by virtue of its greater antigenic dissimilarity, is the beneficiary of this putative implantation advantage (Brent 1971). Thus, the special anti-

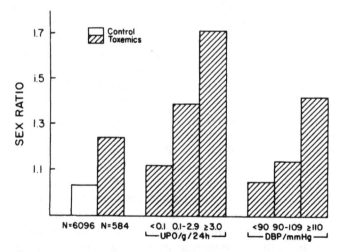

Figure 1.   Preponderance of males in toxemia of pregnancy, from Toivanen & Hirvonen (1970b). UPO refers to urinary protein output; DBP to diastolic blood pressure; both are measures of the severity of toxemia, which increases with the sex ratio, on the ordinate.

genic character of the male fetus was first studied in connection with studies of the sex ratio. The secondary sex ratio, or sex ratio at birth, favors males in every human society that has been studied; the mean value for the United States is about 105 (Novitski 1977). The primary sex ratio, that is the sex ratio at conception, although difficult to measure, is even more favorable: around 120 (McMillen 1979). As if to compensate for selective male affliction, nature has produced an excess of boys to begin with. The implantation advantage of antigenic dissimilarity has been proposed to account for this initial male advantage. Thus, the advantage enjoyed by males in the primary and secondary sex ratio has been attributed to their unique possession of H-Y antigen.

Sex differences in antigenicity may confer a growth advantage as well as an implantation advantage (Clarke & Kirby 1966; Ounsted & Ounsted 1970). Fetuses which are antigenically dissimilar to their mothers are likely to be larger (Clarke & Kirby 1966), and the greater the antigenic dissimilarity, the greater the fetal growth rate (Ounsted & Ounsted 1970). Male embryos, of course, grow faster than females; a baby boy is about 150 grams heavier than a girl at term. The sex ratio of large-for-dates infants is 150 whereas that of small-for-dates infants is 63 (Ounsted 1972).

Placental weight is correlated with birth weight (Sedlis, Berendes, Kim, Stone, Weiss, Deutschberger & Jackson 1967), and mammalian placentation also seems to be under some sort of immunologic control (Jones 1968). In animal studies, antigenic dissimilarity is often found to promote placental growth (D. A. James 1965). The placental size of male fetuses is larger (Ounsted 1972). Interesting also in light of the presumed autoimmune origin of the disorder is the fact that increased placental size is associated with the development of toxemia (Gleicher & Siegel 1980).

Just as understanding the structure of sex differences influences one's appreciation of how males and females come to be afflicted by different pathways, so the sex ratio itself may influence one's respect for antigenicity as a causative agent in males, for at least some neurodevelopmental disorders. A telling example is the fact that the sex ratio decreases with parity; with increasing birth order, fewer boys are born (Novitski & Sandler 1956). There is a parallel between the sex ratio and selective affliction because in both there is a male preponderance, and in both parity effects are observed, and in both an argument in favor of male antigenicity and maternal immunoreactivity is raised.

An antigenic explanation for the secondary sex ratio, implantation, placentation, and fetal growth suggests that maternal sensitization to male antigens occurs and affects subsequent pregnancies. The sex ratio decreases with parity, whereas birth weight and placental size increase (Niswander & Gordon 1972; Novitski & Sandler 1956; Vernier 1975; Warburton & Naylor 1971). There is a nice balance here: the original implantation advantage enjoyed by the male zygote may be offset in subsequent pregnancies by the development of humoral antibodies or cell-mediated immune response in the mother. HLA antibodies, for example, develop in some mothers in response to pregnancy; with successive pregnancies, the number of HLA positive mothers increases (a ceiling seems to be reached at parity three or four) (Burke & Johansen 1974; Doughty & Gelsthorpe 1976). The sex ratio declines with parity in HLA positive mothers; in mothers who fail to develop HLA titres, the sex ratio actually increases with parity (Johansen & Burke 1974). (See Figure 2.) The model has a certain elegance; an early positive effect of immunoreactivity, which serves to promote genetic diversity, is balanced by a later negative effect which seems to favor in large sibships the birth of the less expensive (female) sex.

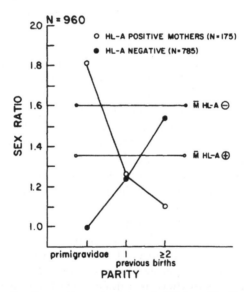

Figure 2. Sex ratio and maternal HLA antibodies, from Johansen, Festenstein & Burke (1974). In mothers who develop HLA antibodies, the sex ratio declines with parity; the opposite is true of HLA negative mothers. The mean (M̄) sex ratio of HLA positive mothers is lower than that of HLA negative mothers (horizontal lines).

If male fetuses are more antigenic, they should be more likely to sensitize mothers, and the impact of this should be felt in subsequent pregnancies in changes in placentation and the sex ratio. In fact, predictions based on the antecedent brother effect seem to hold up. Placental size increases with parity in all male sibships but not in all female sibships; mixed sibships fall in between (Vernier 1975). The sex ratio declines with parity if all antecedent siblings are male; it increases if all antecedent siblings are all female (Gualtieri, Hicks & Mayo 1984b; Renkonen, Mäkelä & Lehtovaara 1962) (See Figure 3).

It appears the parity effect on the sex ratio is mediated through an antecedent brother effect. This effect has also been observed with respect to the occurrence of pregnancy complications in the past history of autistic children. We have reviewed the medical records of 209 autistic children evaluated at the Medical School at the University of North Carolina. In 167 autistic boys, there was a significant relationship between the occurrence of pregnancy complications and the antecedent birth of brothers but not of sisters (see Table 3). Pregnancy complications were more common in autistic boys who had older brothers, but not in autistic boys who had older sisters. The number of autistic girls was too small to permit a complementary analysis, however.

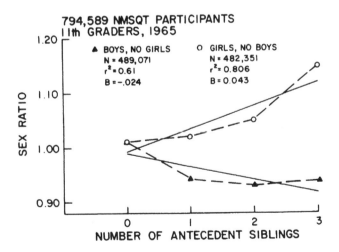

Figure 3.   Sex ratio by sex of antecedent siblings, from Gualtieri, Hicks & Mayo's (1984b) reanalysis of Breland's (1974) data.

Table 3. *Antecedent brother effect on complications of pregnancy, 167 autistic boys*

		Antecedent brothers		
		None	One	
Complications	none	12	2	14
of pregnancy	one	31	8	39
	more than one	71	43	114
		114	53	167

χ^2 for linear trend = 5.815, P = .015

		Antecedent sisters		
		None	One	
Complications	none	8	6	14
of pregnancy	one	32	7	39
	more than one	79	35	114
		119	48	167

χ^2 for linear trend = 0.005, N.S.

MATERNAL IMMUNE ATTACK

The concurrent evolution of viviparity and the ability to render an immunologic response to foreign antigens raised certain problems for the fetus. (Medawar 1963, p. 324).

Pregnancy is associated with the development of circulating maternal antibodies directed against the histocompatibility antigens of the fetus simultaneously with the specific inhibition of immune reactivity against the fetus as a graft. (Simmons 1971, p. 407)

The mechanisms by which the fetus is protected against the circulating antibodies and effector lymphocytes of the mother have been of considerable interest to transplantation biologists, oncologists, and other scientists, who have reviewed the topic (Bernard 1977; Billingham 1964; Simmons 1971). It is sufficient here to say that the mechanisms by which the fetus as an allograft is protected from maternal immune attack are still imperfectly understood (Simmons 1971); when they are, someday, they will doubtless prove to be marvels of biology. But they do not always work. The system, whatever it is, can break down. Fetal antigens and cells enter the maternal circulation and maternal antibodies and effector lymphocytes enter the fetal circulation (Adinolfi 1976; Adinolfi, Beck,

Haddad & Seller 1976; Barnes & Tuffrey 1971). A cell-mediated immune response can develop in mothers during pregnancy; it may increase in intensity with gestation and increase even more so with succeeding pregnancies (Burke & Johansen 1974; Doughty & Gelsthorpe 1976; Johansen & Burke 1974; Terasaki, Mickey, Yamazaki & Vredevoe 1970).

For HLA, maternal lymphocytotoxic antibody production increases with the first three or four pregnancies and then levels off (Doughty & Gelsthorpe 1976). It has been hypothesized that if certain kinds of cytotoxic antibodies reach critical levels in the maternal circulation, they will exceed the number of available binding sites on the placenta and enter the fetal circulation (Doughty & Gelsthorpe 1974). Other fetal antigens may also play a role; for example, the ABO system may also contribute to maternal immune sensitivity, and ABO incompatibility between mother and fetus is known to contribute to increased fetal wastage (Cohen & Mellitts 1971).

In the British Perinatal Study (Butler & Bonham 1963), perinatal mortality data relative to maternal ABO typing was available for 14,730 pregnancies. As predicted by the IMRT, perinatal mortality increased more sharply with parity in O type mothers, who are more likely to react to fetal red blood cell antigens than A, B, or AB mothers. The slope of the perinatal mortality–parity regression line was significantly steeper for O mothers: O = 16.9, A = 13.2, B = 12.7, AB = 12.9 (Gualtieri, Hicks & Mayo 1984a). (See Figure 4.) Thus, ABO antigens as well as sex-linked antigens may induce maternal immunoreactivity.

There appears to be substantial interindividual variation in the maternal immune response (Lawler, Ukaejoofo & Reeves 1975). In one study, only 15% of pregnancies were characterized by the development of maternal HLA antibodies (Doughty & Gelsthorpe 1974). Medawar has shown that antigenic incompatibility is necessary but not sufficient to cause Rh disease. Rh disease is also more likely to afflict males (Loke 1978; Medawar 1963); isoimmunization is necessary, but not sufficient, to produce hemolytic anemia in the newborn (Medawar 1963). Figure 5 captures the wide range of reactivity that may exist between maternal and fetal lymphocytes (Lawler et al. 1975). Maternal immunoreactivity is more likely in some women and it is more likely when the fetus is male. In light of the genetic nature of maternal insufficiency, it would be interesting to know whether maternal–fetal immunoreactivity follows a similar genetic pattern.

There are known pathologic consequences of maternal immune attack on the fetus, for example, Rh disease and runt disease, as mentioned

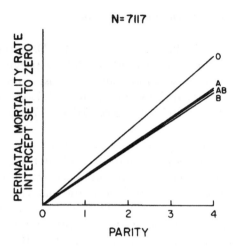

Figure 4. Perinatal mortality and maternal blood groups from Butler & Bonham (1963). See also Gualtieri, Hicks & Mayo (1984b).

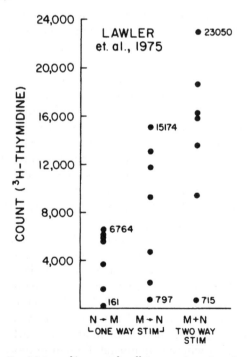

Figure 5. Maternal/neonatal cell interactions in mixed lymphocyte cultures, from Lawler, Ukaejoofo & Reeves (1975). One-way stimulation refers to live neonatal (N) cells admixed with killed maternal (M) cells, and vice-versa. Two-way stimulation (M + N) refers to two populations of live cells.

above. ABO incompatibility between mother and fetus is associated with an increased perinatal mortality (Cohen & Mellitts 1971). Other examples include autoimmune thrombocytopenia and autoimmune hemolytic anemia, myasthenia gravis, thyroiditis, and the lupus erythematosis (LE) phenomenon and cardiomyopathy in children of mothers with systemic lupus erythematosis (SLE) (Beer & Billingham 1973; Brent 1971; Bresnihan, Grigor, Oliver, Leiskomia & Hughes 1977; Kitzmiller 1978). In the latter condition, transplacental transfer of antinuclear antibody from mother to fetus occurs (Beck & Rowell 1963).

The autoimmune diseases are extremely interesting to consider in this context, because they are the only diseases to which both sexes are vulnerable that are more common in females; they are characteristically diseases of young women in their reproductive years (Kitzmiller 1978). Autoimmune disorders are also good examples of how maternal immunoreactivity can afflict the fetus. Some autoimmune disorders, like rheumatoid arthritis, tend to remit during pregnancy, while others, like SLE, often arise during pregnancy (Bresnihan et al. 1977; Kitzmiller 1978). In autoimmune hemolytic anemia, the disorder may remit post partum, only to arise again with a subsequent pregnancy (Kitzmiller 1978). Increased fetal loss through spontaneous abortion is seen in SLE, schleroderma, autoimmune hemolytic anemia, and autoimmune thrombocytopenic purpura. Fetal wastage is increased in SLE mothers even before the disease is clinically manifest (Kitzmiller 1978). Lymphocytotoxic antibody titres are higher in SLE mothers who have had spontaneous abortions than in mothers who had normal live births (Bresnihan et al. 1977). Toxemia is more common in mothers with SLE (Kitzmiller 1978). And, based on our review of an admittedly sparse literature, more girls than boys are born to mothers with SLE.

BRAIN AS THE TARGET OF IMMUNE ATTACK

The brain may be an immunologically privileged site in some respects, but immune attack on nervous tissue does occur in conditions like multiple sclerosis, polyneuropathy and spongiform encephalopathy (Abramsky, Lisalc, Silberger & Pleasure 1977; Dalakas & Engel 1981; Hauser, Dawson, Lehrich, Beal, Kevy, Propper, Mills & Weiner 1983; Sotelo, Gibbs & Gadjusek 1980). The heyday of taraxein is over (McPherson 1970), but neurobiologists continue to pursue the possibility of autoimmune mechanisms in the genesis of some forms of schizophrenia (Abramsky & Litvin 1978).

Brain tissue is antigenic (Foster & Archer 1979). It shares antigens with other tissues, including histocompatibility antigens, organ specific antigens, and antigens present on tissue cells (Foster & Archer 1979; Roszkowski, Plaut & Lichtenstein 1977). There are brain antigens specific to neurons and oligodendroglia (Poduslo, McFarland & McKahanon 1977); there are antigens specific to cells in functional groups (Williams & Schupf 1977) or anatomic areas (Blessing, Costa, Gefen & Rush 1977); there are antigens specific to subcellular components of neural tissue (Sotelo et al. 1980). Antibodies to brain antigens can act as teratogens when injected into pregnant animals (Brent 1971). Rats and guinea pigs immunized to nerve growth factor (NGF) develop anti-NGF antibodies which attack fetal nervous tissue in utero when the animals are bred (Johnson, Gorin, Brandeis & Pearson 1980). The immature blood–brain barrier is not capable of protecting the developing brain from damage by maternal antibodies or effector lymphocytes (Adinolfi 1976; Adinolfi et al. 1976).

It is not our purpose to review the vast research areas having to do with the immunoprotection of pregnancy or the immunopathology of the brain. Nor can we describe the precise immunopathic mechanisms that mediate maternal attack and induce neuropathic changes in the fetus. Nor can we specify whether H-Y antigen alone is involved, or whether there are other important antigens in the male at particular points in time during gestation, nor whether incompatibility in other antigen systems, like HLA and ABO, may also play a role, and if so, whether the reaction that ensues is additive or multiplicative. These are grounds for speculation and basic research. Sufficient to guide the argument are these conclusions, which are fair and conservative: fetal immunoprotection is not invariant or complete; breakdowns in the system do occur, with occasional pathologic consequences to the fetus, occurring along a continuum of severity; the brain, especially the fetal brain, is not invulnerable to immune attack; and in laboratory animals at least, maternal antibodies can damage the developing nervous tissue of the fetus.

The idea that male antigenicity or maternal immunoreactivity may exert a negative influence on the neurological development of children has been suggested on previous occasions by Adinolfi (1976), Foster and Archer (1979), Loke (1978), Rubenstein (1982), and Singer, Westphal, and Niswander (1968). The hypothesis has usually been advanced on the basis of indirect evidence, to explain, for example, the prevalance of pregnancy complications in males (Singer et al. 1968) or the negative parity effect on IQ (Foster & Archer 1979). Adinolfi based his argument on the immaturity of the fetal blood–brain barrier (Adinolfi et al. 1976), the detection of maternal specific antibodies in the cerebro-spinal fluid (CSF) of infants tested during the first week of life (Thorley, Holmes, Kaplan, McCracken & Sanford 1975), and supporting data from pre-clinical experiments (Admolfi 1976). There is additional direct evidence, but not much.

Bonner, Terasaki, Thompson, Holve, Wilson, Ebbin, and Slavkin, 1978 reported cytotoxic antibodies in the sera of 574 parous women; 25% had cytotoxins after their first pregnancy and 50% after the sixth. Children with congenital anomalies are more likely to be born to mothers who have developed cytotoxic antibodies. Harris and Lordon (1976) reported that mothers with lymphocytotoxic antibodies were more likely to show signs of maternal insufficiency (pre-eclampsia, fetal distress, carbohydrate intolerance, unexplained fetal death, intrauterine growth retardation, congenital anomaly and premature labor) than mothers with no lymphocytotoxic antibodies. Bardawil et al. (1962) reported that a group of 20 women with repeated miscarriage manifested rapid rejection of skin grafts from husbands four times more frequently than grafts that were made from unrelated donors (Loke 1978). In a mixed lymphocyte reaction paradigm, the percentage of transformed cells was discovered to be lower in normal fertile couples and higher in infertile couples; a dosage effect was observed in women who had had repeated miscarriage (Halbrecht & Komlos 1976; Omaha & Kadotani 1971). Finally, in two papers from the Soviet Union, it was reported that mothers with "antibrain antibodies" were more likely to give birth to children with developmental or neurological disorders (Burbaeva 1972; Kolyaskina, Boehme, Buravlev & Faktor 1977).

THE IMMUNOREACTIVE THEORY

Selective male affliction with the neurodevelopmental disorders may be related to male vulnerability to environmental stressors, to the genetic endowment of the male, or to his complexity and relative immaturity. In our opinion, these hypotheses are strong and compelling but insufficient. They do not explain the male fetus's proclivity to encounter complications in pregnancy and childbirth. It is argued, with some support, that pregnancy complications mediate the occurrence of neurodevelopmental disorders more strongly in male offspring. The incidence of such complications in males leads to the postulation of an evocative principle, which may be hormonal or antigenic. The first alternative is extremely attractive but it is not consistent with the occurrence of parity effects in fetal loss and in at least some developmental disorders.

The antigenicity of the male fetus is consistent with the negative parity effect. The proposition that the male is especially antigenic and that some mothers are immunoreactors finds convincing support in the literature. The antigenicity of the male is probably related to the sex-linked H-Y antigen, although the contribution of other antigen systems cannot be discounted.

Maternal immune attack on the fetus is well known in a number of pathologic conditions and when it occurs, it is the male who is more severely afflicted. Brain tissue is antigenic, the immature blood–brain barrier affords only slight protection from maternal immune attack, and maternal antibodies are sometimes found in the infant's CSF. Congenital anomalies, infertility, and complications of pregnancy may occur in mothers with elevated antibody titres more frequently than in mothers with low or absent titres.

The argument is based on indirect evidence for the most part, although there is some direct supporting evidence. The relative paucity of direct support is not surprising. Although the theory of maternal–fetal immunoreactivity was first applied to studies of the sex ratio by Renkonen, Makela, and Lehtovaara in 1962, only a few scientists have even raised the question with respect to selective male affliction. Furthermore, the argument presented above relies heavily on the structure of sex differences in the occurrence of schizophrenia, and this dimorphic pattern has not been widely tested in clinical samples of developmentally handicapped children. When we did test the idea, it held up (see above, "Structure of sex differences"). Finally, it is unfortunate that most scientists who undertake studies of pregnancy complications and developmental disorders do not analyze their data taking sex of the proband into consideration.

The fundamental premise of the immunoreactive theory is that pregnancy is an immunological phenomenon characterized by a state of maternal tolerance. But fetal immunoprotection is relative, not absolute, and the system can break down. There is substantial interindividual variation in maternal–fetal immunoreactivity, but on the average, male fetuses are more antigenic than females, and maternal attack on the male embryo is more likely, especially if the mother has been sensitized by previous male pregnancies. Finally, maternal immunologic attack can be directed against fetal brain antigens.

Immunoreactivity is by no means a global explanation for all of the neuropathic disorders of childhood. The phenomenon may be robust but at the same time relatively weak and difficult to discern, especially in small clinical samples. Furthermore, the precise nature of the immunologic reaction cannot be described: whether it involves cell-mediated or humoral antibodies, whether a specific antigen, like H-Y, is responsible, or whether a number of fetal antigens or a combination thereof may be involved. Some fetal antigens may be short-lived and impossible to detect postnatally.

We are aware that there is disagreement surrounding at least some of the facts upon which the theory is based. Parity estimates can be inaccurate, for example, since early abortions are easily missed (Metrakos & Metrakos 1963). Not every investigator has agreed that placentation is promoted by antigenic similarity (Jones 1968), or that the sex ratio decreases with antecedent brothers (McLaren 1962), or that toxemia is an autoimmune disorder (Gleicher & Siegel 1980). H-Y antigen is a fascinating new development in the study of sexual differentiation, but it is very difficult to measure (Goodfellow & Andrews 1982); nor is there any direct evidence that H-Y antigen is present on neural cell membranes in humans (Johnson, Bailey & Mobraaten 1981). There are, not surprisingly, alternative (and occasionally credible) explanations for virtually every natural or clinical phenomenon that has been described thus far or is described below. Still, it is our opinion that the theory has an appeal, and perhaps also a certain usefulness.

HYPOTHESES ENGENDERED BY THE THEORY

The immunoreactive theory and the structure of sex differences on which it is based are particularly interesting in light of the hypotheses they engender. It is likely that many of the hypotheses presented below can be tested in existing data sets.

Parity Effects

The immunoreactive theory is derived, in part, from the demonstration of negative parity effects in at least some of the developmental disorders. But it does not require, nor does it predict that parity effects will be found for all psychiatric, neurologic, and developmental disorders. The birth order–parity literature with respect to specific psychiatric and neurologic disorders (e.g. schizophrenia, epilepsy, alcoholism) is extensive but inconsistent, and there are serious methodological difficulties in executing a definitive parity study in clinical populations.

Because birth order effects are relatively slight, large numbers of subjects are required to detect them (Birtchnell 1971). Birth order studies rarely compare their findings to a general population control group, and the statistical analysis that is most often used, the Greenwood–Yule method, is not without its critics (McKeown & Record 1956). Birth order effects are sensitive to changes in the birth rate, numbers of marriages, and family size in the general population; a decrease in family size, for example, may lead to an overrepresentation of early birth ranks in small sibships and an increase in later birth ranks in large sibships (Price & Hare 1969). To consider sibling position irrespective of the size or composition of the sibship in which it occurs is probably unjustifiable (Birchnell 1971). Additional sources of bias that can compromise the findings of a birth order study include the analysis of incomplete sibships, differential survival by birth rank, differential migration to sources of ascertainment of patients (i.e., places such as clinics where patients are identified) (Hare & Price 1969) and the fact that birth order is not necessarily the same as pregnancy order (Metrakos & Metrakos 1963). Parity studies of psychiatric disorders may be compromised by the fact that death, divorce, separation or other causes of early parental loss cannot prevent the conception of the last child in a family. Accordingly, the likelihood of parental deprivation having occurred during early childhood will always be greater for later born than for earlier born persons (Delint 1966).

The Primiparity Effect

The deleterious effects of primiparity may obscure a birth order effect. Primiparas are more prone to obstetrical complications, such as dystocia and toxemia. Subfertile women will be overrepresented among primiparas. A woman whose first child is defective has a number of strong reasons to limit the size of her family. Congenital rubella and infantile autism are examples of disorders in which relative risk is greatest for first borns (Deykin & MacMahon 1980; Schoenbaum, Biano & Mack 1975); thereafter, however, a parity effect appears to emerge. A U-shaped distribution of pathologic events with parity has also been described in association with fetal loss after 20 weeks gestation, stillbirths, and neonatal death (Ernst & Angst 1983).

In Figures 6 and 7, the relative risk of rubella and autism is plotted against birth order. First borns are at greatest risk, but for ensuing birth orders there is a clear parity effect. One way to measure the relationship between parity and risk for these disorders is orthogonal polynominal analysis of variance. When this method is applied to the data contained in Deykin & MacMahon (1980) and Schoenbaum et al. (1975), it is found that the quadratic relation (i.e. risk declines from birth order 1 to 2;

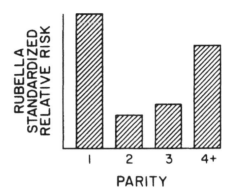

Figure 6.   Rubella and parity effects, from Schoenbaum, Biano & Mack (1975).

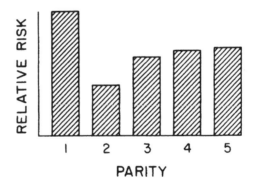

Figure 7.   Autism and parity effects, from Deykin and Mac-Mahon (1980).

increases thereafter) captures substantially more of the variance in the sample than the linear relation. (Rubella: r^2 *[linear]* $= 0.04$, F [1,106] $= 143.5$; r^2 *[quadratic]* $= 0.93$, F [1,106] $= 1423.3$; analysis of difference between slopes by Fischer's r to z transform, $z = 13.04$ [150]. Autism: r^2 *[linear* $= 0.05$, F [1,455] $= 45.86$; r^2 *[quadratic]* $= 0.46$, F [1,455] $= 417.3$; difference, $zRR = 4.07$ [151].) The proper analysis of a birth order effect has to take this primiparity effect into consideration.

Sex Differences in Parity Effects

Parity effects are more interesting to examine with an eye to specific hypotheses (Ernst & Angst 1983). If, for example, the question has to do with relative male vulnerability to a negative birth order effect, study of parity effects is enlightening. For example, the authors' reanalysis of data from the Second National Health Survey, 1963–65 (Roberts & Engel 1974), shows that males are more vulnerable to parity effects than females. The National Health Survey was an epidemiologically sophisticated population survey of 7,119 American children age 6–9 (Roberts & Engel 1974). One part of the survey was an IQ estimate derived from vocabulary and block design subtests of the Wechsler Intelligence Scale for Children. In this survey, clear parity effects on IQ were found; however, the parity effect was felt more sharply by boys than girls (see Figure 8). The slope of the regression line of IQ on birth orders is -2.34

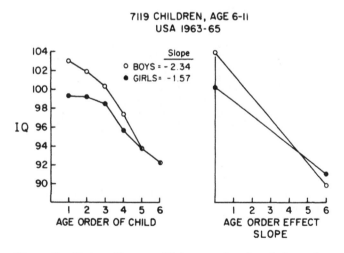

Figure 8.   Parity effects on IQ by sex of proband, from the National Health Survey, USA, 1963–65.

for boys and -1.57 for girls. (Orthogonal polynomial regression analysis, sex $\times$ birth order [*linear*], $F [1,7117] = 239.13, p < .005$. After we had made this analysis, Steelman and Mercy published the same data set using multiple regression analysis, and demonstrated the same effect [Steelman & Mercy 1983].)

Our reanalysis of IQ data published in two additional studies confirms the relative susceptibility of male offspring to negative birth order effects. In 1965, Reed and Reed published *Mental retardation. A family study*, an extraordinary and unique collection of pedigree analyses on 289 residents of an institution for the mentally retarded in Minnesota. Actual IQ scores were available for 258 probands, 118 boys and 140 girls. These were regressed against birth order. The correlation between IQ and birth order for boys was negative ($r = -0.45, p > .001, slope = -1.5$) whereas for girls the correlation was actually positive ($r = 0.48, p < .001, slope = 1.4$) (difference between slopes. $F [1,256] = 37.075, p < .0005$).

The data are even more striking in a more homogeneous group of mentally retarded children who had all been born prematurely. These data were reanalyzed from Moore's 1965 study of 137 mentally retarded residents of the Arizona Children's Colony. The correlation between birth order and degree of retardation was again negative for boys ($N = 63, r = -0.85, p .001, slope = -0.74$) and positive for girls ($N = 71, r = 0.93, p < .001, slope +0.30$) ($F [1,126] = 11.22, p < .001$).

It is clear that there is more to parity effects than a simple birth order analysis yields. The sex of the proband is a relevant variable, but it is not usually considered in birth order studies of cognitive development or of neuropsychiatric disorders.

If parity effects are greater on the male fetus, one should expect to see the birth of developmentally handicapped boys earlier in the sibship. The data of Reed and Reed (1965) and of Moore (1965) provide at least some support for this prediction. The mean birth rank for 137 boys in Reed and Reed was 3.3 (± 2.4) and for 152 girls, 3.7 (± 2.5). In Moore, the mean birth rank for boys ($N = 63$) was 3.1 (± 3.0) and for girls ($N = 71$) 3.3 (∓ 2.5). Although neither result was significant at the 0.05 level, both were in the predicted direction.

Another way to look at parity effects is to examine the sex ratio–parity interaction in special populations. Sex ratio decreases with parity in the general population, but the decrement is very small (slope $= -0.001$ [Novitski & Sandler 1956]). The IMRT predicts that the sex ratio–parity regression line will be steeper in developmentally impaired populations because of increased occurrence of maternal immunoreactivity. A comparison of sex ratio–parity lines is given in Figure 9 for three populations:

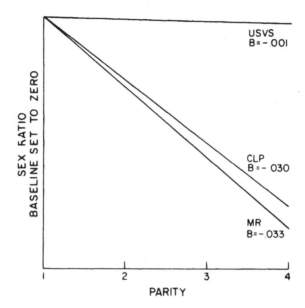

Figure 9.   Sex ratio and parity, normal and handicapped populations from Novitski & Sandler (1956); Reed & Reed (1965); and Woolf (1971). USVS = United States Vital Statistics, i.e., census data. CLP = cleft lip and palate; MR = mentally retarded.

the general population from the 1946–52 U.S. vital statistics (Novitski & Sandler 1956), a sample of 496 patients with congenital cleft lip–palate (Woolf 1971), and 880 siblings and probands from Reed and Reed's MR study (1965). The regression lines are substantially steeper, by a factor of 30, in the two disordered samples.

Yet another way to analyze parity effects in light of the IMRT is to test the hypothesis that with increasing birth order, offspring should increasingly come to resemble their mothers. Having been sensitized by several previous pregnancies, mothers ought to "prefer" antigenically similar zygotes. This hypothesis is guided, of course, by the fact that the sex ratio decreases with parity; that is, relatively more girls are born later in the sibship. Judging from the very small sex-ratio effect, however, we think that only a very large data base will yield a proper answer to this question.

An atheoretical approach to parity effects in psychiatric illness or neurodevelopmental disorders, executed in relatively small and possibly biased samples, is not likely to yield useful information. Within the context of a specific hypothesis, however, such as relative male–female vulnerability or the IMRT, the study of birth order effects can be both interesting and enlightening.

Parity Effects and IQ

In 1874 Francis Galton noted a disproportionate number of firstborn children among fellows of the Royal Society. Galton was the first modern scientist to suggest that primogeniture conferred a unique and selective advantage on intellectual development. The modern variant is found in studies of parity or birth order effects on intelligence. It is reasonably well established that IQ scores of first borns are higher, and that IQ decreases with birth order (Belmont & Marolla 1973), even when maternal age is controlled. This finding has usually been explained in psychosocial terms: parents spend more time with their first-born children, they play with them more, they talk to them more, they expect more of them (Altus 1966; Galton 1874; Zajonc 1976). The family environment of later borns is necessarily shared and diminished. This is an intuitive explanation, and one that is given to empirical examination; however, attempts to confirm the hypothesis have not been notably successful (Ernst & Angst 1983; Grotevant, Scarr & Weinberg 1977). For example, socioeconomic advantage and early stimulation mitigates, but does not abolish parity effects on IQ (Zajonc 1983). The family–environment argument, or confluence model, (Zajonc 1976) predicts that closer spacing of siblings will compound the parity effect; in fact, spacing effects on intellectual development have not been found to exist in developed countries, where close spacing does not lead to maternal undernutrition (Belmont, Stein & Zybert 1978; Grotevant et al. 1977).

Negative parity effects are found not only for IQ and academic achievement, which may be amenable to psychosocial explanation, but also for specific learning disabilities (Badian 1984; Schrag 1973), mental retardation (Belmont, Stein & Wittes 1976), perinatal mortality (Niswander & Gordon 1972), and height (Belmont, Stein & Susser 1975) which clearly are not. Parity effects have even been observed in newborns (Waldrop & Bell 1966). The IMRT represents an alternative, biological explanation for negative parity effects in general, and it is particularly germane to parity effects on intellectual development.

The Antecedent Brother Effect

The IMRT predicts that parity effects on later born boys will be greater if antecedent siblings are boys. In such cases, mothers may be sensitized to H-Y antigen, or to other sex-linked antigens. This sensitization can compromise the development of subsequent male fetuses. The idea is borrowed from studies of the sex ratio and of placentation relative to antecedent brothers. The antecedent brother hypothesis can be tested by comparing relative parity effects on any neurodevelopmental measure in males with antecedent brothers against males with antecedent sisters. Crossed comparisons can also be made with females who have antecedent brothers or sisters.

In a study of college entrance examination scores in 1013 students, secondborn males were found to score lower than firstborn males, whereas secondborn females scored the same as or higher than firstborn females. Boys with older sisters scored higher than boys with older brothers. The data in this paper, however, were not sufficient to allow a statistical reanalysis (Rosenberg & Sutton-Smith 1969).

Additional statistical support for the antecedent brother hypothesis is available, however, in Breland's study of 794,589 eleventh grade students who took the National Merit Scholarship Qualifying Test in 1965 (Breland 1974). In our reanalysis of these data, four family configurations were compared: males with antecedent brothers, males with antecedent sisters, females with antecedent brothers, and females with antecedent sisters. Negative parity effects are seen for all four groups, but the sharpest negative parity effect is observed in boys with antecedent brothers (Gualtieri, Hicks & Mayo 1984b).

These two data sets contain selected populations, college bound high-school students and college freshmen, who are not representative of the population as a whole. The fact that these students were at least 16 years old means that psychosocial factors may have played a role in the development of younger children from same sexed sibships, but we are not aware of a convincing psychosocial explanation for such an effect.

The antecedent brother hypothesis could conceivably be tested in large populations relative to any intellectual, developmental, or neuropathic measure. It could also be tested in deviant populations: In mentally retarded children, for example, the hypothesis predicts that increased severity or retardation will occur in males who have antecedent brothers compared to males who have antecedent sisters. The antecedent brother effect may also play a role in some other hypotheses derived from the IMRT.

Subfertility

If maternal immunoreactivity is related to development disorders, one may expect to see relative infertility in the families of developmentally disabled children. Relative infertility can be measured indirectly by family size or directly by the length of time required for unprotected mothers to conceive. In fact, relative infertility has been found in mothers of children with mental retardation (Wallace 1974), Down's syndrome and cerebral palsy (Tips, Smith & Mayer 1964), epilepsy and congenital anomalies (Drillien 1968), learning problems (Nichols & Chen 1981), and low birth weight (Wilson, Parmelee & Huggins 1963). This effect is even more pronounced when the disordered child is male (Wallace 1974). There is, as a rule, a longer period of relative infertility after the birth of male children (Wyshak 1969).

The IMRT predicts not only that relative infertility should characterize mothers of developmentally disabled children, but also that the phenomenon should be more apparent when the disabled child is a male. This prediction is supported by at least one study of children with febrile seizures (Bernard 1977). A reanalysis of Reed and Reed (1965) reveals that mentally retarded males tend to come from smaller families (males, mean family size 6.1, females 7.0, $t = 2.12$, $P = 0.02$, one-tailed test). Maternal immunoreactivity may contribute to the birth of a fetus who is developmentally retarded and may also lower fertility thereafter.

Studies of maternal subfertility and reproductive inefficiency support the IMRT, but further studies with much larger samples ought to be done.

Additional Hypotheses

The IMRT predicts that antigenic dissimilarity would increase the likelihood of maternal immune attack upon the fetus. When a developmentally handicapped child is born into a large sibship, it is hypothesized that he will be more likely to differ from his mother in measurable antigenic characteristics such as HLA or ABO. It is also predicted that there will be a tendency for later born sibs to resemble their mothers more closely in terms of the same antigenic characteristics. It is also proposed that antigenically dissimilar matings will be prone to produce female offspring. These hypotheses are based, of course, on the premise that H-Y and other antigen systems exercise an additive effect. They could conceivably be tested in the data banks that are maintained by tissue transplant services when typing records are maintained on families.

The IMRT is premised on the idea of an immunoreactive subgroup of mothers. It predicts that such immunoreactive mothers will exhibit an increased incidence of infertility and maternal insufficiency. It is possible that such women may be identified by the presence of allergic or autoimmune disorders. The occurrence of maternal insufficiency in women with autoimmune disease has been reviewed above. We propose that allergic and autoimmune disorders will occur more commonly in the mothers of developmentally handicapped children, in their families, and in the children themselves.

In fact, parents of developmentally disabled children frequently complain of their children's proneness to allergies. Although this has never received much attention from clinicians or researchers, recent studies have shown patterns of abnormal immunoresponsivity in children with infantile autism and Down's syndrome (Fialkow 1966; Stubbs 1976; Stubbs & Crawford 1977; Weizman, Weizman, Szekely, Wijsenbeek & Levni 1982). The IMRT predicts that mothers of such children would include a substantial number of immunoreactive individuals, and this factor could contribute to their children's disabilities. In support, abnormal levels of immunoreactivity have been reported in the families of children with Down's syndrome (Fialkow 1966). Geschwind's recent report of an increased occurrence of auto-immune disorders in left handers and their families is also consistent with this line of thinking, although in that study no distinction was made between familial and pathological sinistrals (Geschwind & Behan 1982). The latter would be expected to exhibit the trait more strongly. It is not unreasonable to suggest that a genetic disposition to autoimmune or allergic disorders might be associated with heightened maternal immunoreactivity, and non-right handedness may simply be one more clinical consequence thereof.

Clinicians who work with developmentally handicapped children occasionally come upon families who exhibit this pattern: the first child is normal, the second, learning disabled, and the third, retarded or autistic. Such families represent an ideal immunoreactive subgroup for further investigation. Mothers whose children follow such a pattern would be expected to be especially immunoreactive and might also be expected to have strong families histories of immunoreactive disorders. Hypotheses concerning specific kinds of immune activity connected with maternal–fetal attack would best be tested in such a subgroup.

Finally, a farfetched idea, but one which is intriguing and irresistible to us in light of the foregoing: there appears to be a unique and truly remarkable association between the sex of the fetus and schizophrenia occurring in pregnancy. In 1967, Shearer, Davidson, and Finch reported that only female children were born to women who conceived within one month before or after an acute schizophrenic episode. This finding was later confirmed by M. A. Taylor (1969) who also reported four stillbirths (all males), two perinatal deaths (both male) and six severe birth defects (five of six male) in mothers who became psychotic during the second or third month of pregnancy. It was suggested that there is a factor in acutely psychotic mothers that is especially toxic to the male embryo (Shearer et al. 1967). This element could be hormonal, but, in light of some recent autoimmune theories of schizophrenia, it could also be immunologic. Perhaps the element is the initiation of an acute hyperimmune state provoked by the fetus, leading to maternal attack not only against fetal tissue, but also against her own brain tissue. Of course there is no direct evidence to support the idea. But it is not outlandish to suggest that hypotheses germane to the IMRT might be profitably tested in schizophrenics, at least in schizophrenics with early onset or evidence of neuropathic damage.

SUMMARY

The IMRT draws from a diverse array of sources to present a possible etiology for many cases of neurodevelopmental impairment. It is concerned with the problems of selective male affliction, maternal insufficiency, the structure of sex differences, and negative parity effects on intellectual development. The strongest appeal of the theory lies neither in its internal consistency nor in its success in bringing together obscure and seemingly unrelated findings, but in its ability to engender testable hypotheses. Many of these are affirmed in the literature or by preliminary investigations derived from existing data. The theory suggests two interesting routes for further investigation: the antecedent brother effect and the study of immunoreactive subgroups. We strongly suggest that studies of parity effects, pre- and perinatal complications, maternal insufficiency, and family genetic background relative to intellectual development take the following elements into considerations; the sex of the proband and of antecedent siblings, and the family proclivity to autoimmune and to allergic disorders.

If the theory were supported by research along the lines suggested above, hypotheses concerning specific immunologic mechanisms might be developed. Such research might yield strategies for the prevention of some of the neurodevelopmental disorders of childhood.

REFERENCES

Aarkrog, T. (1968) Organic factors in infantile psychoses: Retrospective study of 46 cases subjected to pneumoencephalography. *Danish Medical Bulletin* 15:283–88.

Abramowicz, H. K. & Richardson, S. A. (1975) Epidemiology of severe mental retardation in children: Community studies. *American Journal of Mental Deficiency* 80:18–39.

Abramsky, O., Lisalc, R. P., Silberger, D. H. & Pleasure, D. E. (1977) Antibodies to oligodendroglia in patients with multiple sclerosis. *New England Journal of Medicine* 297:1207–11.

Abramsky, O. & Litvin, Y. (1978) Autoimmune response to dopamine-receptor as a possible mechanism in the pathogenesis of Parkinson's disease and schizophrenia. *Perspectives in Biology and Medicine* 22:104–14.

Adinolfi, M., Beck, S. E., Haddad, S. A. & Seller, M. J. (1976) Permeability of the blood—SCF barrier to plasma proteins during foetal and perinatal life. *Nature* 259:140–41.

Ahern, F. M. & Johnson, R. C. (1973) Inherited uterine inadequacy: An alternative explanation for a portion of cases of defect. *Behavior Genetics* 3:1–12.

Allon, R. (1971) Sex, race, socioeconomic status, social mobility, and process-reactive ratings of schizophrenics. *Journal of Nervous and Mental Disease* 153:343–50.

Altus, W. D. (1966) Birth order and its sequellae. *Science* 151:44–49.

August, G. J., Stewart, M. A. & Tsai, L. (1981) The incidence of cognitive disabilities in the siblings of autistic children. *British Journal of Psychiatry* 138:416–22.

Badian, N. (1984) Reading disability in an epidemiologic context: Incidence and environmental correlates. *Journal of Learning Disabilities* 17:129–36.

Bakketeig, L. S. (1977) The risk of repeated preterm or low birth weight delivery. In: *The epidemiology of prematurity*, ed. D. M. Reed & F. J. Stanley. Urban and Schwarzenberg.

Bardawil, W. A., Mitchell, G. W., McKeogh, R. P. & Marchant, D. J. (1962) Behavior of skin homografts in human pregnancy. 1. Habitual abortion. *American Journal of Obstetrics and Gynecology* 84:1283–95.

Barnes, R. D. & Tuffrey, M. (1971) Maternal cells in the newborn. *Advances in Biosciences* 6:457–73.

Beck, J. S. & Rowell, N. R. (1963) Transplacental passage of antinuclear antibody. *Lancet* 1:134–5.

Beer, A. E. & Billingham, R. E. (1973) Maternally acquired runt disease. *Science* 179:240–45.

Belmont, L., Stein, Z. A., & Susser, M. W. (1975) Comparisons of associations of birth order with intelligence test score and height. *Nature* 255:54–55.

Belmont, L., Stein, Z. A. & Wittes, J. A. (1976) Birth order, family size and school failure. *Developmental Medicine and Child Neurology* 18:421–30.

Belmont, L., Stein, Z. & Zybert, P. (1978) Child spacing and birth order: Effects of intellectual ability in two-child families. *Science* 202:995–96.

Bernard, O. (1977) Possible protecting role of maternal immunoglobulins on embryonic development in mammals. *Immunogenetics* 5:1–15.

Berryman, P. L. & Silvers, W. K. (1979) Studies on the H-X locus of mice. *Immunogenetics* 9:363–67.

Billingham, R. E. (1964) Transplantation immunity and the maternal-fetal relationship. *New England Journal of Medicine* 270:667–72.

Birtchnell, J. (1971) Mental illness in sibships of two and three. *British Journal of Psychiatry* 119:481–87.

Blessing, W. W., Costa, M., Gefen, L. B. & Rush, R. A. (1977) Immune lesions of noradrenergic neurons in rat central nervous system produced by antibodies to dopamine-B-hydroxylase. *Nature* 167:368–69.

Bonner, J. J., Terasaki, P. L., Thompson, R., Holve, L. M., Wilson, L., Ebbin, A. J. & Slavkin, H. C. (1978) HLA phenotype frequencies in individuals with cleft lip and/or cleft palate. *Tissue Antigens* 12:228–32.

Borland, R., Loke, Y. W. & Oldersnaw, P. J. (1970) Sex differences in trophoblast behavior on transplantation. *Nature* 228:572.

Breland, H. (1974) Birth order, family configuration and verbal achievement. *Child Development* 45:1011–19.

Bresnihan, B., Grigor, R. R., Oliver, M., Leiskomia, R. M. & Hughes, G. R. V. (1977) Immunological mechanism for spontaneous abortion in systemic lupus erythematosis. *Lancet* 5:1025–07.

Burbaeva, G. S. (1972) Antigen characteristics of the human brain. *Soviet Neurology and Psychiatry* 5:110–18.

Burgio, G. R., Fraccaro, M., Ticpolo, L. & Wolf, U. (1981) *Trisomy 21*. Springer-Verlag.

Burke, J. & Johansen, K. (1974) The formation of HL-A antibodies in pregnancy: The antigenicity of aborted and term fetuses. *Journal of Obstetrics and Gynaecology of the British Commonwealth* 81:222–28.

Butler, N. R. & Bonham, D. G. (1963) *Perinatal mortality*. Livingstone.

Cadoret, R. J. & Cain, C. (1980) Sex differences in predictors of antisocial behavior in adoptees. *Archives of General Psychiatry* 37:1171–75.

Carter, C. O. (1965) The inheritance of common congenital malformations. *Progress in Medical Genetics* 4:59–84.

Chesley, L. C., Annito, J. E. & Cosgrove, R. A. (1968) The familial factor in toxemia of pregnancy. *Obstetrics and Gynecology* 32:303–11.

Childs, B. (1965) Genetic origin of some sex differences among human beings. *Pediatrics* 35:798–812.

Ciocco, A. (1940) Sex differences in morbidity and mortality. *Quarterly Review of Biology* 15:59–92.

Clarke, B. & Kirby, D. R. S. (1966) Maintenance of histocompitability polymorphisms. *Nature* 211:999–1000.

Cloninger, C. R., Christiansen, K. O., Reich, T. & Gottesman, I. I. (1978) Implications of sex differences in the prevalences of antisocial personality, alcoholism, and criminality for familial transmission. *Archives of General Psychiatry* 35:941–51.

Cohen, B. H. & Mellitts, E. D. (1971) Blood group incompatibility and immunoglobulin levels. *Johns Hopkins Medical Journal* 128:318–31.

Corbett, J. A., Harris, R. & Robinson, R. G. (1975) *Epilepsy in mental retardation and developmental disorders*, vol. 7. Brunner/Mazel.

Costeff, H., Cohen, B. E., Weller, L. E. & Kleckner, H. (1981) Pathogenic factors in idiopathic mental retardation. *Developmental Medicine and Child Neurology* 23:484–93.

Costeff, H., Cohen, B. E. & Weller, L. E. (1983) Biological factors in mild mental retardation. *Developmental Medicine and Child Neurology* 25:580–87.

Dalakas, M. C. & Engel, W. K. (1981) Chronic relapsing (dysimmune) polyneuropathy: Pathogenesis and treatment. *Annals of Neurology* 9 (Suppl.):134–35.

Decker, S. N. & DeFries, J. C. (1980) Cognitive abilities in families of reading-disabled children. *Journal of Learning Disabilities* 13:517–522.

Dekaban, A. S., & Sadowsky, D. (1978) Changes in brain weights during the span of human life. *Annals of Neurology* 4:345–56.

Delint, J. E. E. (1966) The position of early parental loss in the etiology of alcoholism. *Alcoholism Zagreb* 2:56–64.

Doughty, R. W. & Gelsthorpe, K. (1974) An initial investigation of lymphocyte antibody activity through pregnancy and in eluates prepared from placental material. *Tissue Antigens* 4:291–98.

Doughty, R. W. & Gelsthorpe, K. (1976) Some parameters of lymphocyte antibody activity through pregnancy and further eluates of placental material. *Tissue Antigens* 8:43–48.

Drillien, C. M. (1968) Studies in mental handicap. 2. Some obstetric factors of possible aetiological significance. *Archives of Diseases in Childhood* 43:283–94.

Eichwald, E. J. & Silmser, C. R. (1955) *Transplanatation Bulletin* 2:148–49.

Fabia, J. & Drolette, M. (1970) Life tables up to age 10 for mongols with and without congenital heart disease. *Journal of Mental Deficiency Research* 14:235–42.

Farber, C., Cambiaso, C. L. & Masson, P. L. (1981) Immune complexes in cord serum. *Clinical and Experimental Immunology* 44:426–32.

Fialkow, P. J. (1966) Autoimmunity and chromosomal aberrations. *American Journal of Human Genetics* 18:93–108.

Flor-Henry, P. (1969) Psychosis and temporal lobe epilepsy—a controlled investigation. *Epilepsia* 10:363–95.

Flor-Henry, P. (1974) Psychosis, neurosis and epilepsy: Developmental and gender related effects. *British Journal of Psychiatry* 124:144–50.

Forssman, H. & Akesson, J. O. (1970) Mortality of the mentally deficient: A study of 12,903 institutionalized subjects. *Journal of Mental Deficiency Research* 14:276–94.

Foster, J. W. & Archer, S. J. (1979) Birth order and intelligence: An immunological interpretation. *Perceptual and Motor Skills* 48:79–93.

Funderburk, S. J., Carter J., Tanguay, P., Freeman, B. J. & Westlake, J. R. (1983) Parental reproductive problems and gestational hormonal exposure in autistic and schizophrenic children. *Journal of Autism and Developmental Disabilities* 13:325–32.

Galton, F. (1874) *English men of science: Their nature and nurture.* MacMillan.

Gardner, C. G. (1967) Role of maternal psychopathology in male and female schizophrenics. *Journal of Consulting Psychology* 31:411–13.

Garside, R. F. & Kay, D. W. K. (1964) The genetics of stuttering. In: *The syndrome of stuttering,* ed. G. Andrews & M. M. Harris. Heinemann.

Geschwind, N. & Behan, P. (1982) Left-handedness: Association with immune disease, migraine and developmental learning disorder. *Proceedings of the National Academy of Sciences of the United States of America* 79:5097–5100.

Gillberg, C. & Gillberg, I. C. (1983) Infantile autism: A total population study of reduced optimality in the pre- and peri-, and neonatal period. *Journal of Autism and Developmental Disabilities* 13:153–66.

Gillberg, C. & Rasmussen, P. (1982) Perceptual, motor and attentional deficits in seven-year-old children: Background factors. *Developmental Medicine and Neurology* 24:752–770.

Gleicher, N. & Siegel, I. (1980) The immunologic concept of EPH-gestosis. *Mount Sinai Journal of Medicine* 47:442–53.

Glucksmann, A. (1978) *Sex determination and sexual dimorphism in mammals.* Wykeham.

Goodfellow, P. N. & Andrews, P. W. (1982) Sexual differentiation and H-Y antigen. *Nature* 295:11–13.

Graham, P. & Rutter, M. (1968) Organic brain dysfunction and child psychiatric disorder. *British Medical Journal* 3:695–700.

Grotevant, H. D., Scarr, S. & Weinberg, R. A. (1977) Intellectual development in family constellations with natural and adopted children: A test of the Zajonc and Markus model. *Child Development* 48:1699–1703.

Gualtieri, C. T. (1983) Unpublished data.

Gualtieri, C. T., Hicks, R. E. & Mayo, J. P. (1984a) ABO incompatibility and parity effects on perinatal mortality. Submitted.

Gualtieri, C. T., Hicks, R. E. & Mayo, J. P. (1984b) Influence of sex of antecedent siblings on human sex ratio. *Life Sciences* 34:1791–94.

Gualtieri, C. T., Hicks, R. E. & Mayo, J. P. (1984c) Parity effects on intellectual development are influenced by sex of antecedent siblings. Submitted.

Hagberg, B., Hagberg, G., Lewerth, A. & Linberg, V. (1981) Mild mental retardation in Swedish school children. 2. Etiologic and pathogenetic aspects. *Acta Paediatrica Scandinavica* 70:445–52.

Halbrecht, I. & Komlos, L. (1976) E-rosette-forming lymphocytes in mother and newborn. *Lancet* 1:544.

Hare, E. H. & Price, J. S. (1969) Birth order and family size: Bias caused by changes in birth rate. *British Journal of Psychiatry* 115:647–56.

Harris, R. E. & Lordon, R. E. (1976) The association of maternal lymphocytotoxic antibodies with obstetric complications. *Obstetrics and Gynecology* 48:302–04.

Hauser, S. L., Dawson, D. M., Lehrich, J. R., Beal, M. F., Kevy, S. V., Propper, R. D., Mills, J. A. & Weiner, H. L. (1983) Intensive immunosuppression in progressive multiple sclerosis. *New England Journal of Medicine* 308:173–80.

Hicks, R. E. & Gualtieri, C. T. (1984) The structure of sex differences in developmental handicap. Submitted.

Hicks, R. E. & Kinsbourne, M. (1981) Fathers and sons, mothers and children: A note on the sex effect on left-handedness. *Journal of Genetic Psychology* 139:305–06.

Hutt, C. (1972) Neuroendocrinological, behavioral and intellectual aspects of sexual differentiation in human development. In: *Gender differences: Their ontogeny and significance*, ed. C. Ounsted & D. C. Taylor. Churchill Livingstone.

Ingram, T. T. S. (1959) Specific developmental disorders of speech in childhood. *Brain* 82:450–67.

Ingram, T. T. S. (1964) *Paediatric aspects of cerebral palsy.* Livingstone.

James, D. A. (1965) Effects of antigenic dissimilarity between mother and foetus of placental size in mice. *Nature* 205:613–14.

Joffe, J. M. (1964) *Prenatal determinants of behavior.* Pergamon Press.

Johansen, K. & Burke, J. (1974) Possible relationships between HL-A antibody formation and fetal sex. *Journal of Obstetrics and Gynaecology of the British Commonwealth* 81:781–85.

Johansen, K., Festenstein, H., & Burke, J. (1974) Possible relationships between maternal HL-A antibody formation and fetal sex: Evidence for a sex-linked histocompatibility system in man. *Journal of Obstetrics and Gynaecology of the British Commonwealth* 81:781–85.

Johnson, L. L., Bailey, D. W. & Mobraaten, L. E. (1981) Genetics of histocompatibility in mice. 4, Detection of certain minor (non-Hz) H antigens in selected organs by the popliteal node test. *Immunogenetics* 14:63–71.

Jones, W. R. (1968) Immunologic factors in human placentation. *Nature* 218:480.

Keller, C. A. (1981) Epidemiological characteristics of preterm births. In: *Preterm birth and psychological development*, ed S. L. Friedman & M. Sigman. Academic Press.

Kitzmiller, J. L. (1978) Auto immune disorders: Maternal, fetal and neonatal risks. *Clinical Obstetrics and Gynecology* 21:385–96.

Kolyaskina, G. I., Boehme, D. I., Buravlev, V. M. & Faktor, M. I. (1977) Certain aspects of the study of the brain of the human embryo. *Soviet Neurology and Psychiatry* 10:24–31.

Kramer, M. (1978) Population changes and schizophrenia, 1970–1985. In: *The nature of schizophrenia: New approaches,* ed. L. Wynne, R. Cromwell & S. Mathysse. Wiley.

Krco, C. J. & Goldberg, E. H. (1976) H-Y (male) antigen: Detection in 8-cell embryos. *Science* 193:1134–35.

Lehrke, R. G. (1978) Sex linkage: A biological basis for greater male variability in intelligence. In: *Human variation,* vol. 1, ed. R. T. Osborne, C. E. Noble & N. Weyl. Academic Press.

Lewitter, F. I., DeFries, J. C. & Elston, R. C. (1980) Genetic models of reading disability. *Behavior Genetics* 10:9–30.

Lilienfield, A. M. & Pasamanick, B. (1956) The association of maternal and fetal factors with the development of mental deficiency. 2. Relationship to maternal age, birth order, previous reproductive loss and degree of maternal deficiency. *American Journal of Mental Deficiency* 60:667–69.

Lord, C., Schopler, E. & Revicki, D. (1982) Sex differences in autism. *Journal of Autism and Developmental Disabilities* 12:317–30.

Lotter, V. (1974) Factors related to outcome in autistic children. *Journal of Autism and Childhood Schizophrenia* 4:263–77.

McGlone, J. (1980) Sex differences in human brain asymmetry: A critical survey. *Behavioral and Brain Sciences* 3:215–63.

McKeown, T. & Record, R. G. (1956) Maternal age and birth order as indices of environmental influence *American Journal of Human Genetics* 8:8–23.

McKinney, D. & Feagans, L. (1983) Unpublished data.

McPherson, C. F. C. (1970) Immunochemical approaches to the study of brain function and psychiatric diseases. *Canadian Psychiatric Journal* 15:641–45.

Mednick, S. A. (1970) Breakdown in individuals at high risk for schizophrenia: Possible predispositional perinatal factors. *Mental Hygiene* 54:50–63.

Mednick, S. A., Mura, E., Schulsinger, F. & Mednick, B. (1971) Perinatal conditions and infant development in children with schizophrenic parents. *Social Biology* 18:103–13.

Metrakos, J. D. & Metrakos, K. (1963) Is pregnancy order a factor in epilepsy? *Journal of Neurology, Neurosurgery, and Psychiatry* 26:451–57.

Mizuno, M., Lubotsky, J., Lloyd, C. W., Kobayashyi, T. & Murasawa, Y. (1968) Plasma androstenedione and testosterone during pregnancy and in the newborn. *Journal of Clinical Endocrinology and Metabolism* 28:1113–42.

Moore, B. C. (1965) Relationship between prematurity and intelligence in mental retardates. *American Journal of Mental Deficiency* 70:448–53.

Nakano, K. K. (1973) Anencephaly: A review. *Developmental Medicine and Child Neurology* 15:383–400.

Nichols, P. L. & Chen, T. C. (1981) *Minimal brain dysfunction: A prospective study.* Erlbaum.

Novitski, E. (1977) *Human genetics.* Macmillan.

Novitski, E. & Sandler, L. (1956) The relationship between parental age, birth order and the secondary sex ratio in humans. *Annals of Human Genetics* 21:123–31.

Ohama, K. & Kadotani, T. (1971) Lymphocyte reaction in mixed wife-husband leukocyte cultures in relation to infertility. *American Journal of Obstetrics and Gynecology* 109:477–79.

Ohno, S. (1979) *Major sex-determining genes.* Springer-Verlag.

Ounsted, C. & Taylor, D. C. (1972) The Y chromosome message: A point of view. In: *Gender differences: Their ontogeny and significance,* ed. C. Ounsted & D. C. Taylor. Churchill Livingstone.

Ounsted, C. & Ounsted, M. (1970) Effect of Y chromosome on fetal growth rate. *Lancet* 2:857–58.

Ounsted, M. (1972) Gender and intrauterine growth. In: *Gender differences: Their ontogeny and significance*, ed. C. Ounsted & D. C. Taylor. Churchill Livingstone.

Pennington, B. F. & Smith, S. D. (1983) Genetic influences of learning disabilities and speech and language disorders. *Child Development* 54:369–87.

Placek, P. (1977) Maternal and infant health factors associated with low infant birth weight: Findings from the 1972 National Natality Survey. In: *The epidemiology of prematurity*, ed. D. M. Reed & F. J. Stanley. Urban and Schwarzenberg.

Poduslo, S. E., McFarland, H. F. & McKahanon, G. M. (1977) Antiserums to neurons and to oligodendroglia from mammalian brain. *Science* 197:270–72.

Price, J. S. & Hare, E. H. (1969) Birth order studies: Some sources of bias. *British Journal of Psychiatry* 115:633–46.

Reinisch, J. M., Gandelman, R. & Spiegel, F. S. (1979) Prenatal influences on cognitive abilities: Data from experimental animals and human genetic and endocrine studies. In: *Sex-related differences in cognitive functioning*, ed. M. A. Wittig & A. C. Petersen. Academic Press.

Renkonen, K. O. & Timonen, S. (1967) Factors influencing the immunization of Rh-negative mothers. *Journal of Medical Genetics* 4:166–68.

Rhodes, P. (1965) Sex of the fetus in antepartum hemorrhage. *Lancet* 2:718–19.

Roberts, J. & Engel, R. (1974) Family background, early development and intelligence of children 6–11 years. United States Data from the National Health Survey. DHEW Publ. # (HRA) 75–1624, Department of Health, Education and Welfare. P. H. S., Rockville, Md.

Robins, L. (1966) *Deviant children grown up*. Williams and Wilkins.

Robson, E. B. (1955) Birth weight in cousins. *Annals of Human Genetics* 19:262–68.

Rosenberg, B. G. & Sutton-Smith, B. (1969) Sibling age spacing effects upon cognition. *Developmental Psychology* 1:661–68.

Rosenthal, D. (1962) Familial concordance by sex with respect to schizophrenia. *Psychological Bulletin* 59:401–21.

Roszkowski, W., Plaut, M. & Lichtenstein, L. M. (1977) Selective display of histamine receptors in lymphocytes. *Science* 195:383–85.

Rubenstein, A. (1982) An immunologic hypothesis concerning some congenital diseases and malformations. *Medical Hypotheses* 9:417–19.

Rutter, M. (1970) Sex differences in children's response to family stress. In: *International yearbook of child psychiatry*, ed. E. J. Anthony & C. Kupernik. Wiley.

Sabin, A. B., Krumbiegel, E. R. & Wigand, R. (1958) Echo type 9 virus disease. *Journal of Diseases of Children* 96:197–219.

Samuels, L. (1979) Reply to Lewine. *Schizophrenia Bulletin* 5:5–10.

Schlesinger, E. R., Alaway, N. C. & Peltin, S. (1959) Survivorship in cerebral palsy. *American Journal of Public Health* 49:343–49.

Schoenbaum, S., Biano, S. & Mack, T. (1975) Epidemiology of congenital rubella syndrome: The role of maternal parity. *Journal of the American Medical Association* 233:151–55.

Schrag, H. L. (1973) Program planning for the developmentally disabled: Using survey results. *Mental Retardation* 11:8–10.

Scott, J. R. (1976) Immunological aspects of trophoblast neoplasia. In: *Immunology of human reproduction*, ed. J. S. Scott & W. K. Jones. Grune & Stratton.

Scott, J. R. & Beer, A. E. (1973) Immunologic factors in first pregnancy Rh immunisation. *Lancet* 1:717–18.

Sedlis, A., Berendes, H., Kim, H. S., Stone, D. F., Weiss, W., Deutschberger, J. & Jackson,

E. (1967) The placental weight-birthweight relationship. *Developmental Medicine and Child Neurology* 9:160–71.

Shaffer, D. & Fisher, P. (1981) Suicide in children and adolescents. *Journal of the American Academy of Child Psychiatry* 20:545–65.

Shearer, M. L., Davidson, R. T. & Finch, S. M. (1967) The sex ratio of offspring born to state hospitalized schizophrenic women. *Journal of Psychiatric Research* 5:349–50.

Siiteri, P. K., Febres, F., Clemens, L. E., Chang, R. J., Gondos, B. & Stites, D. (1977) Progesterone and maintenance of pregnancy: Is progesterone nature's immunosuppressant? *Annals of the New York Academy of Sciences* 286:384–97.

Simmons, R. L. (1971) Viviparity, histocompatibility and fetal survival. *Advances in Biosciences* 6:405–19.

Singer, J. E., Westphal, M. & Niswander, K. R. (1968) Sex differences in the incidence of neonatal abnormalities and abnormal performance in early childhood. *Child Development* 39:103–12.

Slater, E., Beard, A. W. & Glithero, E. (1963) The schozophrenia-like psychoses of epilepsy. *British Journal of Psychiatry* 109:95–112.

Sobel, D. E. (1961) Children of schizophrenic patients: Preliminary observations on early development. *American Journal of Psychiatry* 118:512–17.

Sotelo, J., Gibbs, C. J. & Gadjusek, D. C. (1980) Auto antibodies against axonal neurofilaments in patients with Kuru and Creutzfeld-Jakob disease. *Science* 210:190–93.

Steelman, L. C. & Mercy, J. A. (1983) Sex differences in the impact of the number of older and younger siblings on IQ performance. *Social Psychology Quarterly* 46:157–62.

Stubbs, E. G. (1976) Autistic children exhibit undetectable hemagglutination-inhibition antibody titres despite previous rubella vaccination. *Journal of Autism and Childhood Schizophrenia* 6:269–74.

Stubbs, F. G. & Crawford, M. L. (1977) Depressed lymphocyte responsiveness in autistic children. *Journal of Autism and Childhood Schizophrenia* 7:49–55.

Taylor, D. C. (1969) Differential rates of cerebral maturation between sexes and between hemispheres. *Lancet* 2:140–42.

Taylor, D. C. & Ounsted, C. (1971) Biological mechanisms influencing the outcome of seizures in response to fever. *Epilepsia* 12:33–45.

Taylor, D. C. & Ounsted, C. (1972) The nature of gender differences explored through ontogenetic analyses of sex ratios in disease. In: *Gender differences: Their ontogeny and significance*, ed. C. Ounsted & D. C. Taylor. Churchill Livingstone.

Terasaki, P. I., Mickey, M. R., Yamazaki, J. N. & Vredevoe, D. (1970) Maternal-fetal incompatibility. *Transplantation* 9:538–43.

Thorley, J. D., Holmes, R. K., Kaplan, J. M., McCraken, G. H. & Sanford, J. P. K. (1975) Passive transfer of antibodies of maternal origin from blood to cerebrospinal fluid in infants. *Lancet* 1:651–53.

Tips, R. L., Smith, G. & Meyer, D. L. (1964) Reproductive failure in families of patients with idiopathic developmental retardation. *Pediatrics* 33:100–05.

Toivanen, P. & Hirvonen, T. (1970a) Placental weight in human foeto-maternal incompatibility. *Clinical and Experimental Immunology* 7:533–39.

Toivanen, P. & Hirvonen, T. (1970b) Sex ratio of newborns: Preponderance of males in toxemia of pregnancy. *Science* 170:187–88.

Trites, R. L., Dugas, E., Lynch, G. & Gerguson, H. B. (1979) Prevalence of hyperactivity. *Journal of Pediatric Psychology* 4:179–88.

Tsai, L. Y. & Beisler, J. M. (1983) The development of sex differences in infantile autism. *British Journal of Psychiatry* 142:373–78.

Tsai, L., Stewart, M. A. & August, G. (1981) Implications of sex difference in the familial transmission of infantile autism. *Journal of Autism and Developmental Disorders* 11:165–73.

Vernier, M. C. (1975) Sex-differential placentation. *Biology of the Neonate* 26:76–87.

Vessey, M. P. (1972) Gender differences in the epidemiology of non-neurologic disease. In: *Gender differences. Their ontogeny and significance*, ed. C. Ounsted & D. C. Taylor. Churchill Livingston.

Wachtel, S. S., Koo, G. C. & Boyse, E. A. (1975) Evolutionary conservation of H-Y (male) antigen. *Nature* 254:270–72.

Waldrop, M. F. & Bell, R. D. (1966) Effects of family size and density on newborn characteristics. *American Journal of Orthopsychiatry* 36:544–50.

Wallace, S. J. (1974) The reproductive efficiency of parents whose children convulse when febrile. *Developmental Medicine and Child Neurology* 16:465–74.

Warburton, D. & Naylor, F. (1971) The effect of parity on placental weight and birth weight: An immunological phenomenon. *American Journal of Human Genetics* 23:41–54.

Weinberger, D. R., Cannon-Spoor, E., Potkin, S. G. & Wyatt, R. J. (1980) Poor premorbid adjustment and CT scan abnormalities in chronic schizophrenia. *American Journal of Psychiatry* 137:1410–13.

Weizman, A., Weizman, R., Szekely, G. A., Wijsenbeek, H. & Levni, E. (1982) Abnormal immune response to brain tissue antigen in the syndrome of autism. *American Journal of Psychiatry* 139:1462–65.

Williams, C. A. & Schupf, N. (1977) Antigen-antibody reactions in rat brain sites induce transient changes in drinking behavior. *Science* 196:328–30.

Wilson, M. G., Parmelee, A. H. & Huggins, M. H. (1963) Prenatal history of infants with birth weights of 1500 grams or less. *Journal of Pediatrics* 63:1140–50.

Wing, L. (1981) Sex ratios in early childhood autism and related conditions. *Psychiatry Research* 5:129–37.

Wolf, V. (1981) Genetic aspects of H-Y antigen. *Human Genetics* 58:25–28.

Woolf, C. M. (1971) Congenital cleft lip: A genetic study of 496 propositi. *Journal of Medical Genetics* 8:65–84.

Wyshak, G. (1969) Intervals between births in families containing one set of twins. *Journal of Biological and Social Sciences* 1:337.

Zajonc, R. B. (1976) Family configuration and intelligence. *Science* 192:227–36.

Zajonc, R. B. (1983) Validating the confluence model. *Psychological Bulletin* 93:457–80.

Zerssen, D. V. & Weyerer, S. (1982) Sex differences in rates of mental disorders. *International Journal of Mental Health* 11:9–45.

Part IV
SOCIOCULTURAL ISSUES

The drive for desegregation of schools rests on the premise and evidence that segregated schools are damaging to the self-esteem and self-image of black children. This premise was basic to the 1954 Supreme Court decision that labeled school segregation as unconstitutional.

The paper by Gloria Powell starts by pointing out that this premise has been challenged by a number of recent studies, including several of her own. In the present report she examines this issue more extensively by a comparison of black and white children in three northern and three southern cities. Her total sample included 4088 children who were rated on a self-concept scale and a sociofamilial questionnaire. Surprisingly (at least to us), the black children in segregated southern schools scored higher than all the other groups. She identifies as the basic reason for this finding the fact that in the southern communities 90% of all the school personnel lived in the same communities in which they worked, and participated in the same community and political activities as the parents and the students. In the northern schools, by contrast, most of the teachers, whether black or white, had prevailing, demeaning white middle-class expectations of their black students and had no common community relationships with them. Black parents and students were "Worlds Apart" from their teachers. Powell then spells out the implications of these findings for dealing with the self-defeat, cynicism, and alienation of black students in large metropolitan areas—indeed, one of our country's major social problems.

The paper by Krell deals with therapeutic efforts made with survivors of the Nazi Holocaust who experienced unspeakable horrors as children. Most of these child survivors, who were located as adults, initially felt that they had little to contribute but agreed to be interviewed. But they did have much to tell, as could be expected. The author reports that the interviews had significant therapeutic value in enabling these survivors to integrate traumatic fragments into a "whole," which had the purpose of leaving a legacy for history and education. The interviews also gave them the opportunity to integrate, as adults, the complex childhood events that helped shape their personalities and lives. Most have displayed an extraordinary degree of resilience and adaptability in their subsequent lives, which the author documents impressively. But how few have survived to have this opportunity to lead a successful adult life!

Chivian and his coworkers report a comparison of the responses of 293 Soviet children on the subject of nuclear weapons with the attitudes of 201 age-matched California youngsters. The study had a number of limitations which the authors list, but their findings are still important. The Soviet children learned the facts of nuclear war earlier in life than did the American children, and their information appeared to be more detailed and accurate, as obtained through regular systematic programs in school and the Soviet mass media. The American children, by contrast, obtained their information sporadically through the media or in the relatively few schools that offered courses on this subject. The Soviet children were more optimistic than the American group that nuclear war could be avoided, but both groups had little hope for surviving a nuclear war. The authors conclude by quoting a major American TV news commentator's opinion regarding the attributes of Soviet children, which was completely at odds with their finding. They end with the very pertinent question as to "How much else that we have been presented with as factual about Soviet society—and in particular about the attitudes and knowledge of the Soviet people with regard to nuclear war—is equally without foundation."

Hsu and his associates report a study from Hawaii that compared the patterns of Japanese-American and Caucasian families by rating videotapes of structured family interactions. They document a number of significant differences between the two groups in a number of areas. They evaluated the differences as cultural in origin and emphasized the need for recognition of specific healthy family patterns in different cultural groups. Otherwise, as so often happens, such differences that deviate from the mainstream pattern, familiar to an examiner, will easily be mislabeled as pathological.

The final paper in this area reports a collaborative study of the cognitive performance and academic achievement of American children in Minneapolis, Japanese children in Sendai, and Japanese and Chinese children in Taipei, Taiwan. The importance of this study lies in the many accounts of a high level of academic achievement of Asian-American children, as well as the superior performance of Japanese children in international studies of achievement in mathematics and science. What accounts for this phenomenon? The present report addresses this question by a careful, thorough study. Their findings do not support the hypothesis that there is an intrinsic difference in cognitive ability between Asian and American children. Rather, the authors conclude, the differences must be related to their experiences at home and at school.

14

Self-Concepts Among Afro-American Students in Racially Isolated Minority Schools: Some Regional Differences

Gloria J. Powell

Neuropsychiatric Institute
UCLA Center for Health Sciences

Four thousand eighty-eight black and white children in three northern and three southern cities were tested using the Tennessee Self-Concept Scale and a sociofamilial questionnaire to determine the effects of school desegregation on self-concept development. The black children in segregated southern schools scored higher than all the other groups. Other regional and racial differences are noted and discussed in the context of the historical differences between black communities in the North and South in terms of community cohesiveness.

The data on the self-concepts of Afro-American students in three nonsouthern cities are actually the replication of an extensive study of the effects of school desegregation on the self-concepts of Afro-American students in three southern cities which began in the early 1970s (Powell, 1973; Powell and Fuller, 1970, 1972). The subjects in the southern study included 1720 white (945) and Afro-American (775) junior high school students from 22 schools. Five were segregated white schools, 6 were segregated Afro-American schools, and 11 were desegregated

---

Reprinted with permission from the *Journal of the American Academy of Child Psychiatry*, 1985, Vol. 24, 142–149. Copyright 1985 by the American Academy of Child Psychiatry.

schools. The major finding from the data analysis of the southern schools showed that Afro-American students in segregated or racially isolated minority (RIM) schools scored significantly higher on the Tennessee Self-Concept Scale (TSCS) than Afro-American students in desegregated schools. Although there were significant findings regarding southern white students (Powell, 1973; 1982), the intent of this report is to focus on the variables for self-concept and self-esteem of Afro-American children in RIM schools. The study contravened previous beliefs about the damaged self-percept of Afro-American youth (Dreger and Miller, 1960, 1968; Hauser, 1971, 1972), although other studies (Rosenberg and Simmons, 1972; Soares and Soares, 1969, 1972) have confirmed the findings of the Powell-Fuller study. Such data contradict the premise upon which the Warren court based the 1954 decision on de jure segregation.

In *Simple Justice*, Kluger (1976) writes:

> Such considerations apply with added force to children in grade and high schools. To separate them from others of similar age and qualifications solely because of their race generates a feeling of inferiority as to their status in the community that may affect their hearts and minds in a way unlikely ever to be undone. Segregation, with its detrimental effects on colored children, has a still more severe impact when it has the sanction of the law; for the policy of separating the races is usually interpreted as denoting the inferiority of the Negro group. A sense of inferiority affects the motivation of a child to learn. Segregation with the sanction of the law, therefore, has a tendency to retard the educational and mental development of Negro children . . . (pp. 704-705).

In view of such data in juxtaposition with previous studies on the damaged self-percept of Afro-American children as well as the implications for social policy and educational planning, the study was then replicated in three cities outside of the southeastern region in which de jure segregation was not an issue, although de facto desegregation was. The three cities included a large northeastern city, a mid-size midwestern city, and a large western city. It should be noted at the outset that the three southern cities were not comparable in all respects to each other or to the nonsouthern cities. As Pettigrew (1975) pointed out, the nature of school desegregation research has been that the researcher goes where he or she is welcomed and not always where he or she would want to go. However, in the long run the contrasts in the six cities in terms of size, population mix, the history of public school education in general, and the patterns of school desegregation and race relations in each particular city have enriched the findings and broadened the significance of such research.

The RIM schools in the inner city ghettoes of our large northern cities have become of increasing concern to educators, politicians, social scientists, and mental health professionals as the reports of violence, delinquency, underachievement, high rates of unemployment among youth, mental health and social problems proliferate. One cannot help but wonder how southern youth in segregated schools report feelings of psychological well-being in the face of the pathology reported among Afro-American students in racially isolated minority schools. Does the changing self-percept of southern Afro-American students to one of positive self-esteem extend to Afro-American students elsewhere? What are the special circumstances that mediate positive self-concept and high self-esteem among Afro-American students in segregated or racially isolated minority schools? These questions served as the focus of the investigation of self-concept among Afro-American students in the three nonsouthern cities with de facto segregated RIM schools.

It is well known that self-concept scores are consistent with self-reported acceptance of others, self-reported depression, and self-reported anxiety (Wylie, 1978). Thus the mental health implications of self-concept among Afro-American students in RIM schools present compelling reasons for further investigation in this area.

METHOD

The research protocol was identical to the design for the southern investigation in which at least one segregated white school, one segregated Afro-American school, and three desegregated schools with varying percentages of Afro-American students were selected. In the majority of the cases the schools were public schools. However, several parochial schools in the south and one private school in the western city were included to enlarge the sample of middle-class and upper-class Afro-American subjects. This was not necessary or possible in all of the six cities.

Subjects

The subjects were 2,368 students from three cities outside of the south—a western city, a midwestern city, and a northeastern city. The students were all from junior high schools and included 1,236 Afro-American students and 1,132 white students, ranging in age from 11 to 16 years. In all, there were 524 Afro-American students who were attending five segregated or RIM schools and 712 Afro-American students who were attending nine desegregated schools. Among the RIM schools, one was in the large western city, two were in the large northeastern city, and two were in the midwestern city.

Among the white students there were 680 attending desegregated schools and 388 attending 3 predominantly segregated schools (less than 5% Afro-American or other minority group enrollment).

Procedures

Self-concept scale. All students were given the Tennessee Self-Concept Scale (TSCS) which consists of 100 items which are multidimensional in description of the self-concept. The scale has been widely used and was standardized on a group of subjects ranging in age from 11 years old to 67 years old (Fitts, 1965). The scale was devised on a phenomenological system which asks the subject to rate him/herself in terms of (a) who he/she is (identity), (b) how he/she feels about the self (self-satisfaction or self-esteem), and (c) what he/she does (behavior). Within these three major dimensions the subjects were also asked to rate themselves in five subcategories which included the physical self, the moral-ethical self, the personal self, the family self, and the social self, thus creating a matrix of the self-percept or self-concept in 15 areas of the self as experienced and perceived. These self-descriptions coincide with Allport's (1963) seven aspects of selfhood. These aspects comprise the self as felt and known during the process of self-concept development, which begins during infancy with stage one, the sense of bodily self, and proceeds through six other developmental stages consisting of the sense of continuing self-identity, self-esteem and pride, the extension of self, the self-image, the self as a rational coper, and the self as a propiate striver, which begins in adolescence.

The Tennessee Self-Concept Scale has enumerable scores, both clinical and empirical. The scores that will be reported here will consist of the following:

1. Total Positive Score (TP). The mean norm is 345.37. A TP score above or equal to the mean norm indicates that the subject feels positively about him or herself. A lower score indicates a more negative self-concept or self-perception (see Table 3).

2. The Self-Criticism Score (norm mean = 35.34), which is the degree

of defensiveness and the ability to accept negative statements about the self.

3. The Variability Score (norm mean = 48.53) measures the amount of consistency from one area of self-perception to another. It is highly correlated with personality integration. Well-integrated people generally score below the norm mean but above the first percentile—e.g., above a score of 26.

4. The total positive scores for (a) identity (mean norm = 127.10), (b) self-satisfaction (mean norm = 103.67), and (c) behavior (norm mean = 115.01) will also be noted.

Sociofamilial questionnaire. The students were also asked specific questions about their aspirational attitudes toward school, family background, as well as some general questions regarding psychiatric symptoms. It is important to note that there were no questions or statements about racial identification or racial attitudes on the TSCS or the questionnaire.

School and community interviews. School personnel in each of the participating schools were interviewed regarding student attitudes and performance, classroom problems, race relations, community relations, parent involvement, and the progress of school desegregation in their communities. Similar questions were addressed to community leaders as well as broader social and community issues.

Data analysis. The data were analyzed using programs available in the Statistical Package for the Social Sciences (version 7.0, 1979). Analysis variance (program ANOVA) was performed using a two-tail test for determining level of significance beyond the probability of 0.05. Multivariate analysis of variance was used to determine f values for each of the cities and to determine the level of significance between cities and between regions. Correlational analyses were done to determine significance of the independent variables of sex, educational attainment of parents, occupational status of parents, family structure, and region of the country on the TSCS scores.

RESULTS

Comparison of TSCS Scores of Southern and Nonsouthern RIM Schools

The total positive self-concept mean score for the 999 Afro-American students (335.08) was lower than the TSCS norm group (345.57), but higher than the mean score obtained from eight studies of junior high school students tested on the TSCS (329.45) (Thompson, 1972). According to Thompson, junior high school students are inconsistent in

TABLE 1

TSCS Scores of Afro-American Students in RIM Schools[a]

Mean Scores	Southern Cities (N = 437)			Nonsouthern Cities (N = 562)			Total Mean Score
	City A (N = 94)	City B (N = 206)	City C (N = 131)	Mid-West City (N = 168)	Western City (N = 136)	N.E. City (N = 258)	Six Cities (N = 999)
TP mean	343.93	351.33	353.74[b]	333.20	316.92[b]	311.16[b]	335.08
S.D.	45.22	39.04	36.59	32.71	31.35	42.85	37.96
SC mean	33.81[c]	34.62	35.94	37.38[c]	36.44	35.58	35.63
S.D.	6.53	6.28	6.72	6.28	5.79	6.25	6.31
V mean	55.42	54.51	58.20[d]	52.03	57.48	51.54[d]	54.87
S.D.	13.29	13.28	13.73	3.89	14.38	13.87	12.07
TP Identity mean	117.56	120.64[e]	118.36	114.98	116.17	105.39[e]	115.51
S.D.	15.48	16.22	14.02	16.03	13.23	15.87	15.14
TP Self-satisfaction	108.65	111.28	115.07[f]	105.18	98.56[f]	100.31[f]	106.51
S.D.	21.94	10.53	16.58	17.22	13.43	17.76	16.24
TP Behavior mean	117.44	119.12	119.48[g]	113.02	102.16[g]	105.81[g]	113.84
S.D.	15.54	36.61	16.35	13.16	11.49	17.05	18.37

[a] Statistical significance is expressed between the highest mean score and the lowest mean scores.

[b] $f = 40.26$, $p < 0.0001$.

[c] $f = 5.73$, $p < 0.0001$.

[d] $f = 8.06$, $p < 0.0001$.

[e] $f = 27.57$, $p < 0.0001$.

[f] $f = 75.73$, $p < 0.0001$.

[g] $f = 19.62$, $p < 0.0001$.

their self-reports, have TP self-concept mean scores below the norm for the TSCS, and have behavior mean scores which are lower than the mean scores for identity and self-satisfaction (see Tables 1 and 3).

The RIM students from the six cities differ in that their mean scores for behavior and self-satisfaction are very similar to the norm mean, but their identity mean score is significantly below those for the norm group and other junior high school samples. It is particularly noteworthy that the RIM students have higher self-esteem than other junior high school students as indicated by their high mean self-satisfaction score. However, their high variability mean scores indicate considerable inconsistency with that of other junior high school samples. Such variability may indicate some difficulties in personality integration, which is expected in this age group.

A comparison of the TSCS mean scores of the 437 Afro-American students in RIM schools in the southern cities to those of the 562 students in similar schools in nonsouthern cities reveals many significant differences (see Table 2). The southern RIM students score significantly higher than the nonsouthern RIM students on total positive self-concept mean scores as well as on mean scores for identity, self-satisfaction, and behavior. It is interesting to note, however, that southern and nonsouthern RIM students have identity mean scores below the norm mean and junior high school mean (see Tables 2 and 3).

TABLE 2

TSCS Mean Scores in RIM Schools in Three Southern and Three Nonsouthern Cities[a]

TSCS Mean Scores	Southern Cities (No. of students = 437)	Nonsouthern Cities (No. of students = 562)	*f* Value
TP mean	349.65	320.09	0.014
S.D.	40.27	35.64	0.135
SC mean	34.78	36.47	0.135
S.D.	6.48	6.11	
V mean	56.04	53.68	11.58
S.D.	13.40	10.71	
Identity mean	118.84	112.18	73.49
S.D.	15.20	15.04	
Self-satisfaction mean	111.64	101.35	104.78
S.D.	16.34	16.34	
Behavior mean	118.66	107.10	76.06
S.D.	22.63	13.90	

[a] $p < 0.0001$ for all scores.

TABLE 3

TSCS Mean Scores for Normal Group and Junior High School Samples

TSCS Scores	Mean Scores for Normal Group	Mean Scores for Junior High School Students[a] (N = 1918)
TP	345.57	325.45
SC	35.54	36.31
V	48.53	54.70
Identity	127.10	122.21
Self-satisfaction	103.67	97.87
Behavior	115.01	105.00

[a] *W. Thompson Correlates of Self-Concept.* (Dede Wallace Center, Monograph VI). Nashville, Counselor Recordings and Tests, 1972.

With the exception of the identity mean score, the TSCS mean scores of the nonsouthern RIM students resemble those of other junior high school students. In contrast, the southern RIM students have TSCS scores more similar to the norm group with the exception of the mean scores for variability, which is much higher than the norm group mean, and identity, which is much lower than the norm group mean.

Although there are significant differences among RIM students in southern and nonsouthern cities, an examination of mean scores of RIM students in each of the six cities show many similarities among groups of students and wide differences among other groups of students that do not always follow regional differences that have been noted (see Table 4).

The graph in Table 4 demonstrates some striking features or patterns of TSCS mean scores among the cities. For instance, on four of the TSCS mean scores the western and northeastern cities have the lowest mean scores, which fall within a very narrow range of each other. Secondly, the northeastern city has the lowest mean scores for all measures of self-concept analyzed, with the exception of self-criticism. The third pattern is that the students in the midwestern city tend to score higher on the TSCS measures than the students in the other nonsouthern cities and in four instances in close range to the mean scores for southern city A—e.g., identity, behavior, self-satisfaction, and total positive. The fourth pattern that emerges is that students in southern cities B and C tend to score within the same high range in many areas of self-concept.

As Tables 2 and 4 demonstrate, there are significant differences between the mean scores of the one and/or two lowest scoring nonsouthern city and/or cities and the highest scoring southern city in every instance except self-criticism, in which case students in southern city A have the lowest mean score (33.81) and students in the midwestern city have the highest mean score (37.38). The differences in the mean scores between students in the lowest scoring city (usually nonsouthern) and those in the highest scoring city are statistically significant ($p < 0.0001$) (see Table 2).

In noting the similarities and differences in the scoring patterns among students in the different cities, it should be noted that southern students tend to have lower self-criticism scores than nonsouthern students, although students in the southern city C and the northeastern city score similarly in this regard. Additionally, although all the RIM southern and nonsouthern students score below the norm group mean and the junior

TABLE 4

Patterns of TSCS Mean Scores among the Six Cities

Total Positive

N.E.	West	Mid-West	So. A	So. B	So. C
311	317	333	344	351	354

Self-Criticism

So. A	So. B	N.E.	So. C	West	Mid-West
33.8	34.6	35.6	35.9	36.4	37.4

Variability

N.E.	Mid-West	So. B	So. A	West	So. C
51.6	52.0	54.5	55.4	57.4	58.2

Identity

N.E.	Mid-West	West	So. A	So. C	So. B
105	115	116.2	117.6	118.4	120.6

Self-Satisfaction

West	N.E.	Mid-West	So. A	So. B	So. C
98.6	100.3	105.2	108.7	111.3	115.1

Behavior

West	N.E.	Mid-West	So. A	So. B	So. C
102.2	105.8	113.0	117.4	118.1	119.5

high school mean on the identity items of the scale, four of the cities (two southern and two nonsouthern) cluster together (see Table 4). However, the students in the southern RIM schools tend to have higher mean identity scores (118.84) than those in RIM schools in nonsouthern cities (112.18) (see Table 2). Indeed, the greatest difference in mean identity scores is between the northeastern city (mean score 105.39) and southern city B (mean score 120.64) ($p < 0.0001$) (see Table 2).

Family Background Data

The data from the questionnaire on educational attainment of parents and occupational status of parents for southern and nonsouthern RIM students are given in Table 5. Occupational status of mothers and income levels of parents are omitted because more than 30% of the students in the south and 45% of the students in the other nonsouthern cities failed to respond. Income levels of parents were also included, but the students had not responded consistently.

TABLE 5

Educational Attainment and Occupation of Parents

A. Educational Attainment of Parents

	Southern Cities			Nonsouthern Cities		
	High school	Some college	College	High school	Some college	College
Father	55.6%	9.6%	16.6%	50%	5%	7%
Mother	63.3%	7.3%	14.6%	58%	8%	5%

B. Occupational Status of Father

	Professional/ Managerial	Technician/ Trade	Laborer	ND[a]
Southern cities	14.6%	54.3%	12%	19.1%
Nonsouthern cities	11%	50%	23%	26%

C. Employment Status of Mother and Marital Status of Parents

	Mother Works	Parents Together	Parents Separated/ Divorced
Southern cities	57.6%	75%	20.3%
Nonsouthern cities	39%	63%	37%

[a] No data available.

DISCUSSION

Self-concept has always been considered a significant variable in human behavior and psychological well-being. Maslow (1968) postulated that people who are more self-actualizing are more able to realize their true potentialities and to function in a more creative and effective manner. Indeed, the person who has a clear, consistent, positive, and realistic self-concept will generally behave in healthy, confident, constructive, and effective ways (Fitts et al. 1971; Rogers, 1961, 1969). Schools have come to realize that the promotion of positive self-concepts may play a major role in the prevention of school failure and promotion of achievement (Gurin and Epps, 1975; Purkey, 1970). Although the central role in identity formation begins with identification with parents, by early adolescence with the formation of the private world of the self, teacher's attitudes toward the student may become important to identify information and may be more significant than teaching techniques, materials, and new machines.

It is important to remember that during early adolescence the definitions of the self either as part of one's culture or separate from one's culture becomes the central tasks at this time. Schools may impede this process by treating it as irrelevant to the educational process or schools can facilitate these crucial tasks. The data indicate that they are crucial to the process.

For preadolescent children the likelihood that family experiences will be an important source of self-esteem is very high (Coopersmith, 1967). Also, preadolescents make little distinction about self-worth in different areas of experience; rather, such distinctions are made within the general appraisal of self-worth (Coopersmith, 1967). For the adolescent his or her entire system of self-appraisal is in flux and is more susceptible to changes in the environment, especially political, social, and cultural changes. In the struggle for independence, the adolescent will attempt to evaluate and even to incorporate some of the changing values he or she is encountering. Consequently, the socialization process of the adolescent is crucial in understanding his/her self-concept process.

The theoretical construct for the theme of the damaged self-percept of Afro-Americans has been based on the belief that the psychocultural aspects of the dominant white culture transports the Afro-American individual to a marginal, inferior, and circumscribed position, ultimately leading to the development of a fragile, split, inadequately functioning self (Mosby, 1972). The conceptualizations and conclusions are not new. The interpretations made by Kardiner and Ovesey (1968) in 1951 regarding the psychodynamic inventory of Afro-American personality basically concluded that the caste situation resulted in the basic destruction of self-esteem.

There are many problems in most of the studies on self-concept development in Afro-American children that have made it difficult to reach some basic conclusions about the self-percept of the Afro-American child, not the least of which have been (a) different definitions of self-concept, (b) different aspects of self-perception that are measured, (c) different methods of measuring self-concept, (d) the use of many non-standardized scales, (e) difficulties in sampling techniques, and (f) the confusion of racial attitudes and/or racial awareness studies with those of self-concept. In spite of these difficulties, it can be concluded after an extensive review of the literature on self-concept development (Powell, 1984a) and self-concept in segregated and desegregated schools (Powell, 1984b) that the majority of the studies fall equally into three categories: (a) those reporting no difference in self-concept between white and Afro-American children, (b) those reporting that Afro-American children have higher self-esteem than white children, and (c) those reporting lowered self-concept in desegregated but not integrated schools.

Self-Concept Among Afro-American Junior High School Students in Southern RIM Schools

The RIM schools in the three southern cities' studies have been able to utilize the schools' resources and inputs to facilitate self-concept development during a critical stage of development when the self-concept is in flux and to match the culture of the minority community with the culture of the school. This process has been a less difficult one for Afro-American schools in the South than for those outside the South for several historical reasons.

During the days of "separate but equal" schools and de jure segregation, although the purse strings were held by a white school board and broad policies regarding education of Afro-Americans were determined by them, the actual functioning of the school and content of the curriculum were determined not by the principal of the school, but in many southern communities by an Afro-American superintendent of schools. The content of the curriculum (the goals and purposes of the educational process) was determined by the faculty with the approval of the parents. The schools were a vital part of the cohesive Afro-American community and educators were highly respected individuals within those communities. Education was the road to true freedom from oppression (Lightfoot, 1978). In describing the characteristics of nine such Afro-American high schools which produced a disproportionate number of the Afro-American Ph.D.'s in the 1950s and 1960s, the common denominators of these schools were listed as: (a) dedication to education, (b) commitment to children, (c) faith that it was possible to achieve, (d) structural settings with emphasis on discipline and respect, (e) the outstanding characteristics and abilities of the principals, and (f) mixed social class status of the student body (Sowell, 1976). Prominent graduates of these schools have noted that these schools took Afro-American children from economically and culturally limited backgrounds and gave them both the education and self-confidence to advance later in life. Other noted graduates have observed that teachers promoted the idea of self-worth of the individual—e.g., they always called the students "Mr." and "Miss"—emotionally important titles in a segregated South. Most important, the teachers, counselors, and principals served as role models for the students.

Such were the characteristics of the Afro-American segregated schools which participated in this study, several of which are noted for some of their outstanding graduates.

In the South the world of the home and the world of the school were not "worlds apart." They belonged to the same community with similar goals and ideologies (Lightfoot, 1978). The extensive interview data with the teachers, counselors, and principals of these schools, as well as with community people and those designated as community leaders, indicated the historical cohesiveness of southern Afro-American communities and their commitment to "black consciousness, achievement, and identity" (Gurin and Epps, 1975) and the transmission of the traditional culture values within the school.

Erikson (1968) has espoused that, in order for the young person to reach that inner core of unification and identity, the mores and values of the home must be readily reinforced in the immediate environment or community. He has also stressed the importance of readily identifiable adult models which the young person can incorporate into his sense of self. The cohesive Afro-American communities in the South provided the reinforcement of the cultural values of the home and provided the role models. The dissonance between home and school was not there to create the pervasive apathy and alienation described by so many of the teachers interviewed in the nonsouthern RIM schools. The southern RIM students are less critical of themselves but not defensively so. They have maintained their self-esteem and are satisfied with their performance and behavior. Their mean scores for identity and variability are closer to the mean scores for other junior high school students and may reflect the state of flux in identity and personality integration process which heralds the period of early adolescence.

As noted in previous research (Wylie, 1978), SES, educational attainment of father, occupational status of father, or family stability were not important correlates of self-concept. Thus, we are left with other qualitative factors of their schools and communities that have been discussed to explain the high self-concept, high self-esteem, and satisfaction with performance and behavior among this group of Afro-American students.

Self-Concept among Afro-American Junior High School Students in Nonsouthern RIM Schools

The TSCS mean scores of the nonsouthern students are very similar to those of other junior high school students except for the mean identity score, which is lower (mean score = 112.18 for nonsouthern Afro-American students, mean score = 122.21 for other junior high school students). However, the marked difference in the six TSCS mean scores of nonsouthern RIM students and southern RIM students is a significant finding. SES and family stability are not significant variables for self-concept for southern or nonsouthern RIM students.

While the northeastern and western RIM schools were very similar in many ways, the midwestern RIM schools were less similar to those in the other two cities. First of all, the northeastern and western cities had large, diverse minority populations and a higher percentage of RIM schools within their school districts. The midwestern city was not as large as the other two nonsouthern cities and had a much smaller and less diverse minority group population. Indeed, the Afro-American population of this city was less than 10%. Second, the faculties at the midwestern RIM schools were 98% Caucasian, while the faculties at the RIM schools in the other two nonsouthern cities were more than 90% Afro-American.

The major similarity that all of the nonsouthern schools had that was so different from the southern schools was that none of the teachers, counselors, or principals lived in the same communities where they worked. In the southern cities, 90% of all the school personnel lived in the same communities in which they worked. They attended the same churches as their students, belonged to the same social clubs as the students' parents, and participated in the same community and political activities as the parents and the students.

The interview data from the teachers who taught in the nonsouthern RIM schools are particularly noteworthy in terms of the prevailing low expectations teachers had of their students, their disregard for parents, and their negative attitudes about the Afro-American communities where the schools were located. With few exceptions, most of the teachers, white and Afro-American, had prevailing white, middle-class expectations for their students. The consequences of such attitudes have been described at length by Kozol (1967), Rist (1975), and most recently Lightfoot (1978), who analyzes the relationships between Afro-American families and schools in a book entitled, *Worlds Apart*, the title of which in and of itself describes the destructive process which such attitudes breed. Lightfoot (1978) notes that the conflicts between Afro-American communities and white-controlled, middle-class schools have focused on parents' and teachers' different views of the educational needs of Afro-American children, curriculum, and teaching methods. Each perceives the other as uncaring about children and devaluing the educational process. Parents and students perceive teachers as demeaning and degrading the intellectual, spiritual, and cultural norms of their students (Glasgow, 1980). Such dissonance between the schools and the communities they purport to serve, between parents and teachers, and finally between teachers and students leads to apathy, underachievement, custodial teaching, disillusionment, and alienation.

Rutter et al. (1979) found that the most effective schools in terms of achievement, attendance, student participation beyond school requirements, and low levels of delinquency were those with a high degree of consensus on goals and enforcement of rules. The school's expectations are clear. This theme is reiterated in Bond's (1970) study of high schools that produced a disproportionate percentage of Afro-American Ph.D.'s and in Sowell's (1974, 1976) study of "Patterns of Black Excellence" and was clearly evident in the southern RIM schools in this study.

Newmann (1981), in enumerating the ways in which student alienation can be reduced, stresses that schoolwork that is "incongruent with a student's cultural commitments can assault self-esteem" (p. 555). He also advocates extension of the student-teacher relationship beyond the 50 minutes to learn a single subject and the engagement of students and teachers in a range of activities and the study of more than one subject. The extension of student-teacher contact beyond the traditional 50-minute hour helps develop trusting relationships and a greater sense of community, mutual caring, and responsibility. For early adolescents these kinds of school milieus are crucial for the development of self-concept, the incorporation of role models, and the establishment of educational and occupational goals. The creation of communality within the school engages the student in a working/learning process that stimulates social integration and collective identity. The communality within the school cannot be achieved for the Afro-American student unless his cultural heritage norms and values and the collective commitment to that heritage are also incorporated into the working/learning process.

CONCLUSION

The initial aims of this study were (1) to investigate the effects of school desegregation on the self-concept of young Afro-American adolescents, (2) to try to replicate the findings of high self-concept and high self-esteem among segregated southern Afro-American students, and (3) to understand that phenomenon.

What has emerged from the data is how schools, parents, and the community can enhance self-concept development and ultimately educational attainment of Afro-American students regardless of the type of school—i.e., RIM or desegregated. In spite of the caste system in the South, Afro-American schools, parents, and communities developed a social and cultural milieu within their schools and communities that fostered self-concept and self-esteem as well as individual and collective achievement. Although the RIM junior and senior high schools in the large urban metropoles have become fortresses of cynicism, self-defeat, and alienation, the data on self-concept in segregated southern junior high schools indicate that this need not be the case, and that self-actualization can occur among Afro-American youth even in Afro-American schools.

REFERENCES

Allport, G. W. (1963), *Pattern and Growth in Personality*. New York: Holt, Rinehart & Winston.

Bond, H. M. (1970), The Negro scholar and professional in America. In: *The American Negro Reference Book*, ed. J. P. Davis. Englewood Cliffs, N.J.: Prentice-Hall.

Coopersmith, S. (1967), *The Antecedents of Self-Esteem*. San Francisco: W. H. Freeman.

Dreger, R. M. & Miller, K. S. (1968), Comparative psychological studies of Negroes and whites in the United States: 1959-1965. *Psychol. Bull.*, 70 (Suppl.):1-58.

——— ——— (1960), Comparative psychological studies of Negroes and whites in the United States. *Psychol. Bull.*, 57:361-402.

Erikson, E. H. (1968), *Identity: Youth and Crisis*. New York: W. W. Norton.
Fitts, W. H. (1965), *Manual for Tennessee Self-Concept Scale*. Nashville, Tenn.: Counselor Recordings and Tests.
—— Adams, J. L., Radford, G., Richard, W. C., Thomas, B. K., Thomas, M. M. & Thompson, W. (1971), *The Self-Concept and Self-Actualization* (Monograph No. 3). Nashville, Tenn.: Dede Wallace Center.
Glasgow, D. G. (1980), *The Black Underclass: Poverty, Unemployment, and Entrapment of Ghetto Youth*. San Francisco: Jossey-Bass.
Gurin, P. & Epps, E. (1975), *Black Consciousness, Identity, and Achievement: A Study of Students in Historically Black Colleges*. New York: John Wiley & Sons.
Hauser, S. T. (1971), *Black and White Identity Formation: Studies in the Psychosocial Development of Lower Socioeconomic Class Adolescent Boys*. New York: Wiley-Interscience.
—— (1972), Black and white identity development: aspects and perspectives. *J. Youth Adolesc.*, 1:113-130.
Kardiner, A. & Ovesey, L. (1968), *The Mark of Oppression: Explorations in the Personality of the American Negro*. Cleveland: Meridian Books.
Kluger, R. (1976), *Simple Justice*. New York: Knopf.
Kozol, J. (1967), *Death at an Early Age*. Boston: Houghton Mifflin.
Lightfoot, S. L. (1978), *Worlds Apart: Relationships between Families and Schools*. New York: Basic Books.
Maslow, A. H. (1968), *Towards a Psychology of Being*, Ed. 2. Princeton, N.J.: Van Nostrand Co.
Mosby, D. P. (1972), Toward a theory of the unique personality of blacks—a psychocultural assessment. In: *Black Psychology*, ed. R. L. Jones. New York: Harper & Row.
Newman, F. M. (1981), Reducing student alienation in high schools: implications of theory. *Harvard Educ. Rev.*, 51:546-564.
Pettigrew, T. F. (1975), Trends in research on racial discrimination. In: *Racial Discrimination in the United States*, ed. T. F. Pettigrew. New York: Harper & Row.
Powell, G. J. (1973), *Black Monday's Children: The Psychological Effects of School Desegregation on Southern School Children*. New York: Appleton-Century-Crofts.
—— (1982), A six-city study of school desegregation and self-concept among Afro-American junior high school students: a preliminary study with implications for mental health. In: *The Afro-American Family: Assessment, Treatment, and Research Issues*, ed. B. Bass, G. Wyatt & G. J. Powell. New York: Grune & Stratton.
—— (1984a), Coping with adversity: the psychologic development of Afro-American children. In: *The Psychosocial Development of Minority Group Children*, ed. G. J. Powell, J. Yamamoto, A. Morales & A. Romero. New York: Brunner/Mazel.
—— (1984b), School desegregation: the psychological, social, and educational implications. In: *The Psychosocial Development of Minority Group Children*, ed. G. J. Powell, J. Yamamoto, A. Morales & A. Romero. New York: Brunner/Mazel.
—— & Fuller, M. (1970), Self-concept and school desegregation. *Amer. J. Orthopsychiat.*, 40:303-304.
—— —— (1972), The variables for positive self-concept among young southern black adolescents. *J. Nat. Med. Assn.*, 43:72-79.
Purkey, W. W. (1970), *Self-concept and School Achievement*. Englewood Cliffs, N.J.: Prentice-Hall.
Rist, R. C. (1975), Student social class and teacher expectation: the self-fulfilling prophecy in ghetto education. In: *Challenging the Myths: The Schools, The Blacks, The Poor. Harvard Educational Review*. (Reprint Series No. 5), pp. 70-111.

Rogers, C. R. (1961), *On Becoming a Person*. Boston: Houghton-Mifflin.
—— (1969), *Freedom to Learn*. Columbus, Ohio: Charles Merrill.
Rosenberg, M. & Simmons, R. (1972), *Black and White Self-Esteem: The Urban School Child*.
    Rose Monograph Series. Washington, D.C.: American Sociological Association.
Rutter, M., Maughan, B., Mortimer, P., Ouston, J. & Smith, A. (1979), *Fifteen Thousand
    Hours: Secondary Schools and Their Effects on Children*. Cambridge, Mass.: Harvard
    University Press.
Sewell, W. H. & Hauser, R. M. (1975), *Education, Occupation, and Earnings: Achievement in
    the Early Career*. New York: Academic Press.
Soares, A. T. & Soares, L. M. (1969), Self-perception of culturally disadvantaged children.
    Amer. Educ. Res. J., 6:31-45.
—— —— (1972), The self-concept differential in disadvantaged and advantaged stu-
    dents. *Proceedings of the Annual Convention of the American Psychological Association*, 7:195-
    196.
Sowell, T. (1974), Black excellence: the case of Dunbar high school. *The Public Interest*,
    4:11-18.
—— (1976), Patterns of black excellence. *The Public Interest*, 43:26-58.
Thompson, W. (1972), *Correlates of Self-concept*. (Monograph VI. Counselor Recordings
    and Tests). Nashville, Tenn.: Dede Wallace Center.
Wylie, R. C. (1978), *The Self-Concept; Vol. II. Theory and Research on Selected Topics*, (revised
    edition). Lincoln, Nebr.: University of Nebraska Press.

15

Therapeutic Value of Documenting Child Survivors

Robert Krell

Health Sciences Centre Hospital
University of British Columbia, Vancouver

As a child survivor/psychiatrist who is preoccupied with the implications of the Holocaust, the author has been involved in documentation projects to secure eyewitness accounts of that time. For the great majority of survivors who have participated, the taping proved a therapeutic experience through integration of traumatic fragments into a "whole" with a purpose, that of leaving a legacy for history and education. The child survivors particularly have not related their stories and, as a consequence, continue to bear a great psychologic burden. Documentation affords the opportunity to integrate, as adults, the complex childhood events which helped shape their personalities and lives.

Jewish survivors of the Nazi Holocaust are few in number. In recent years they have been rediscovered, discussed, and documented. Several of the survivors have organized gatherings in Israel and in Washington, D.C., in 1981 and 1983, respectively. At each of these gatherings, the children of survivors, the so-called "Second Generation," have figured prominently as the bearers of the parental legacy to remember, to educate, and to help prevent another such tragedy.

Reprinted with permission from the *Journal of the American Academy of Child Psychiatry*, 1985, Vol. 24, 397–400. Copyright 1985 by the American Academy of Child Psychiatry.

I happen to be a member of the first generation (as a child in hiding) as well as of the second generation (my parents survived in hiding independently). So I, too, have struggled with the memories and consequences of an oppressive past and a lingering remembrance of danger and terror. But not until recently have I been aware of belonging to a group of people, rather unique and not too visible—the child survivors.

The books by Friedländer (1979) and Moskovitz (1983) have paved the way to an awareness of this group of children who have mostly remained hidden within the larger group of Holocaust survivors. It is the child survivors who bring into focus the true meaning of genocide which, by definition, requires the deaths of children. After all, it is they who bear the potential for continuing their kind. Kosinski (1965) captures for his readers a sense of the odds against a Jewish child surviving the Holocaust. Child survivors of the Holocaust were robbed of childhood and/or adolescence. They were denied all that which is considered to be essential to normal development—parental nurturance, adequate nourishment, a sense of security and predictability. For as long as 6 years for some, they were alone in forests, in hiding places, and even in concentration camps.

The child survivors from concentration camps were very few. A child was not considered useful for labor and was therefore destroyed immediately. Remarkably, some did survive the death camps. Others walked from Poland to Shanghai. Some fought as partisans.

In psychoanalytical literature, the importance of even one critical life event is known to exert its power on development. What of these numerous critical events, singly sufficient to change the course of one's life, all brought to bear simultaneously and unremittingly for years on end? Should all child survivors not be mad, psychotic, destroyed, incapable of living life, of working, of loving, of parenting?

DOCUMENTING EYEWITNESS ACCOUNTS

In 1976, I had begun to audiovisually tape the eyewitness accounts of survivors. The survivors are aging and it was with great urgency that a project was initiated in 1980 to capture more accounts from Canadian survivors. A National Holocaust Documentation Project was funded by the Ministry of Multiculturalism and the Canadian Jewish Congress (1980). Shortly thereafter, a regional taping project was undertaken in Vancouver, B.C. (Krell, 1984). The National Project produced over 70 tapes, and the local project nearly 60 tapes to date.

Although the focus was initially on the elderly survivor, a number of child survivors had been scheduled for taping. Where the "older" survivor told us that 2 hours of interviewing was far too little for their stories which would require days or weeks to tell, the child survivors said they remembered little, did not experience much, and that in any case, the experience paled in comparison to the "real survivors" like those from the death camps. However, most agreed to participate if questions were asked to guide them, but they invariably apologized for having little to contribute.

The experience of our documentation team proved otherwise.

DEFINITION OF A CHILD SURVIVOR

For our purposes, we defined a child survivor as any Jewish child who survived in Nazi-occupied Europe by whatever means, whether in hiding, or as a fighter, or in the camps. To be considered a child, the survivor should have been no older than 16 at the end of the war. Children born in 1929 would have been 10 years old at the outbreak of war in Poland, 11 in Holland and Belgium, and 15 in Hungary. The age of disruption for all those aged 16 in 1945, therefore depended on the country of origin and citizenship and the timing of the Nazi occupation.

The child born in Hungary in 1929 would have had 15 years of relative calm before the catastrophe descended. Such older children remember family, tradition, and friends.

The child born in Poland in 1929 would have had 10 years before the Holocaust and 6 years to survive rather than 1. Any child born later in the 1930s would have had diminishing opportunities to establish family ties, develop a value and belief system, and have the opportunities for experiencing nurturing and safety. Those born in the late 1930s and hidden away may indeed have no recall of parents, language, or home. Some child survivors do not know their date of birth, their country of origin, or their first language.

It is in this world of total deprivation that some child survivors must reconstruct a past in order to live a present. On the slimmest of threads, new lives were built (Hogman, 1983).

This raises a fundamental question. What is left when a child has everything, absolutely everything, taken away—food and nurturance, parents and grandparents, shelter and safety? And what happens if by chance that child survives? Some say, all that is left is a child and a story. When everything is gone, a story remains. It should not surprise us that Eliach (1983), a child survivor, would write a book of tales, or that Wiesel (1972), an adolescent survivor, describes himself as a teller of stories.

For within this ghostly nation of child survivors, each is simply only a child with a story. Anne Frank told such a story through her diary. She did not survive but her story captured the imagination of a world of readers, in part perhaps because it is a story of hope and optimism. She could not record her death. A few others who did not write diaries did survive. But their stories are still unknown. Here is one.

Before the audiovisual taping began, Helen said, "What I have to tell you is not very important, but I've heard what you do and I agree with it. Help me with questions and I'll try to answer." When initially contacted, she was not reluctant about giving an account of what happened to her. She did, however, express the feeling that her story might not be too important, having been "only a child" during the war. Helen was born in 1931 in the Ukraine.

Helen described family life. Her father had been a professional soldier who, after marriage, ran a store with her bright, emancipated mother. She had a brother 3 years older. It was not a religious home so much as Zionist. She recalls talk of Trumpeldor, Weizman, and Jabotinsky. She remembers open markets, the public park, sitting with her mother on a park bench making a crown of flowers, her mother's perfume.

In September 1939 when she was 8 years old, her father went to war and was back after 3 days. Eastern Poland was now Russian. There were discussions of going to Siberia but the decision was made to go to Lvov (Lemberg) where father's family lived.

With the appearance of the first German patrols, mother said, "This is the end of us." It was 1942. Within weeks, they were in a ghetto, a wall was being built, her father incarcerated in the labor camp Janowska. Helen took parcels to him at great risk. She witnessed atrocities and heard screams. Mother told her not to go out because, "They are catching children for soap factories."

She was smuggled out of the ghetto to her birthplace to live with an aunt. There, hidden in an attic, she witnessed the roundup of local Jews and public hangings, including that of her own family doctor. She was passed on to a Ukrainian woman in exchange for goods. The woman displayed the jewelry, the villagers suspected she was hiding someone, and Helen was evicted. She then hid with a Jewish family of three in the bullrushes by the river. They shared their food with her.

Two Ukrainian peasants happened by and disguised her as a child of the local mountain people, some of whom died in a flood. She became the orphan Marushka, went to church and became an observant Catholic. She composed a prayer of her own: "Dear God of the Jews, I am doing this not to offend you. I am doing it to survive." And she did. She worked on the farm and tended the animals.

At liberation, her family gone, she made her way to Bratislava, then Prague. At first preparing to go to Palestine, Helen instead immersed herself in books and education. After many more adventures she sailed with a group of orphans to Canada and was adopted by a family in Regina, Saskatchewan. She ran away and was placed with a second family, more compassionate and understanding.

Helen told her new family what happened to her. They were the only ones with the patience to listen. No one else had until the present taping. At one point Helen and one other child survivor were said to be "the nice survivors. They don't go around talking about it." She felt they were driven into silence except with other survivors, "And in any case, who am I to tell my story? Some people were in Auschwitz."

Helen is happily married to a man who was not a victim of the Holocaust. Her son is 26 and her daughter 23. She states she did not know what to do with them. Being an avid reader, she was well-aware of the problems of some children of survivor parents: "I was desperately trying not to raise neurotic children of a survivor. But no one could tell me how and whether it was better to talk or not to talk about it."

She chose to tell her children bits and pieces of her story with a few more messages of what she felt they must know. She felt they must never forget and must not let their children forget. They must know there were righteous gentiles. And they must try to understand the feeling of horror. When asked what helped her to survive, she states: 1) A very private belief in God, a God with whom I had ongoing conversations; 2) survival techniques, a modus operandi to escape detection in hiding places and in haystacks; and 3) "I numbed myself. I flattened my emotions to keep my equilibrium. I have learned to feel tragedies not too strongly nor for that matter, joy."

THE THERAPEUTIC IMPACT

While the taping projects were initiated for the purpose of preserving historical accounts for future educational use, they conveyed as well a wealth of information regarding adaptive and coping strategies of children under unimaginable stress. Of particular interest are the differences in postwar adaptation between the adult survivor and the child survivor.

The older survivor is more likely to retain a sense of pride in survivorhood. While recognizing the primary role of chance and fate, the older survivor more readily recalls an instance of personal initiative which may account for survival. The older survivor has a past, a legacy of memories. In their postwar years, scattered about the world, they frequently associated with others who had experienced their kind of upbringing, perhaps even in the same geographic region. Adult survivors banded together in communities within communities. Many were married in displaced persons camps, frequently to another survivor. Love was not always so important as having known the same families, having lived in the same town, and having shared similar memories. Many children were born in displaced persons camps (Krell, 1979).

In contrast, the younger survivor finds little pride and no dignity in survivorhood. As children, they experienced degradation and humiliation from their Christian neighbors, particularly other children. They were made to feel different. All were forcibly separated from their loving families or given away in order to have the chance to survive. The younger the child at the onset of war, the fewer the memories for a foothold on life. In their turbulent postwar world, they too were scattered about, most finding refuge in adoptive or foster families. As a result they did not live within survivor communities, nor did they wish to do so.

More than anything, they wished to be normal. Of 21 Canadian child survivors interviewed for the documentation project, 18 are married, 2 remain single, and only 1 is divorced. Of those who are married, 3 have spouses who are themselves child survivors. The other 15 married Canadians, 13 to Jews and 2 to Gentiles. All 15 credit their marital partners with contributing to their stability in what most describe as "a reasonable semblance of normal life." Family life is treasured and the marriages, within contemporary standards, are stable indeed. Normality is attained, at least in part, through the existence of a solid family unit of which the child survivor is a part.

Child survivors, when offered the opportunity, have an acute awareness of what helped them to survive physically and emotionally, then and now. Throughout their ordeals, most sensed a special relationship, either with their parents or to God. They describe their adaptability in chameleon-like terms. They were able to sense change and adapt readily to new surroundings and provide what was demanded of them by adults. This adaptability has lasted for many into adulthood. Some child survivors speak of their ability to compartmentalize issues, extracting the affect, and dealing rationally with emotion-laden concerns. All possess a considerable intellect in addition to a set of intuitive skills which are often staggering.

As an example of their resilience, roughly half of the aforementioned child survivors caught up on 6-10 years of interrupted schooling, in 2 years or less, in a foreign language. Most are university educated, goal-oriented and successful, aggressive in pursuing their objectives, and understandably preoccupied with the welfare of their own children. The details of these initial observations deserve another paper. Suffice it to say that the telling of their story has changed the perspective of some of the child survivors who have participated to date. While providing the eyewitness accounts so important to history, and for future education, the child survivor experiences personal well-being, and a sense of closure. I believe this is due to the following: 1) There is a growing recognition by the child survivor of the importance of their experience and awareness that they are listened to very carefully; 2) in the process of telling their story, they inevitably discover accounts of personal courage, self-sacrifice, and a sense of accomplishment against overwhelming odds; 3) remembering often brings to the surface insight into various peculiar habits which earlier were considered strange or even crazy and which were obvious and normal consequences of their unique experiences; 4) through relating the chronological sequence of events, there is an integration of disparate fragments of a fragmented past; and 5) even child survivors who initially claimed they had no story felt an intense need to leave a personal legacy to their children and to future generations.

Hence their responses to a questionnaire sent to participants in the audiovisual project. In response to "How do you feel about having done the taping?" one stated, "It is a necessary task. I feel that in doing so I have fulfilled my duty to those who perished." To the question "Did the taping make you feel worse in any way over the past months?" came the answer, "Worse? No. I regard the taping as a catharsis." And another stated, "No. Except that I recently dreamed of my parents, of a tearful separation with them. I am convinced that the telling of my story is a most therapeutic undertaking."

The fact that documentation has a potentially therapeutic dimension is of comfort to us who feared that perhaps it might unleash the demons of remembrance to haunt the already haunted. And there is comfort also, and possibly encouragement in Wiesel's (1965) words: "Rejected by mankind, the condemned do not go so far as to reject it in turn. Their faith in history remains unshaken, and one may well wonder why. They do not despair. The proof: they persist in surviving—not only to survive, but to testify. The victims elect to become witnesses."

REFERENCES

Canadian Jewish Congress—National Holocaust Documentation Project. (1980), 1590 Avenue Docteur Penfield, Montreal, P.Q., Canada.

Eliach, Y. (1982), *Hasidic Tales of the Holocaust*. New York: Oxford University Press.

Friedländer, S. (1979), *When Memory Comes*. New York: Farrar, Straus & Giroux.

Hogman, F. (1983), Displaced Jewish children during World War II: how they coped. *J. Hum. Psychol.*, 23:51-66.

Kosinski, J. (1965), *The Painted Bird*. New York: Bantam Books.

Krell, R. (1979), Holocaust families: the survivors and their children. *Comprehen. Psychiat.*, 20:560-568.

——— (1984), Vancouver Holocaust Documentation Project. Information package for obtaining eyewitness accounts for history and education (unpublished).

Moskovitz, S. (1983), *Love Despite Hate: Child Survivors of the Holocaust and Their Adult Lives*. New York: Schocken Books.

Wiesel, E. (1972), *Souls on Fire: Portraits and Legends of Hasidic Masters*. New York: Random House.

——— (1965), *One Generation After*. New York: Avon Books.

16

Soviet Children and the Threat of Nuclear War: A Preliminary Study

Eric Chivian and John E. Mack
Harvard Medical School

Jeremy P. Waletzky
George Washington School of Medicine

Cynthia Lazaroff
US-USSR Youth Exchange Program

Ronald Doctor
California State University, Northridge

John M. Goldenring
Loyola Marymount University, Los Angeles

This study, the first undertaken by Western researchers with Soviet children on the subject of nuclear weapons, compared the questionnaire responses of 293 Soviet youngsters with those of 201 age-matched Californians. Interviews were conducted to supplement the questionnaire findings. Similarities and differences between the two samples are discussed in the context of how young people today perceive the threat of nuclear war.

Barely two years after the conclusion of World War II, the Purdue University Division of Educational Reference[24] polled 10,000 high school students throughout the United States and found that almost half be-

---

Reprinted with permission from the *American Journal of Orthopsychiatry*, 1985, Vol. 55, 484–502. Copyright 1985 by the American Orthopsychiatric Association, Inc.

lieved the United States would fight in another war within five years, while two-thirds expected the U.S. to become involved in another war within 25 years. The poll was conducted prior to the Soviet Union's first atomic bomb test explosion in 1948.

About 15 years after this initial survey of young people in the nuclear age, several studies prompted by the Berlin Wall and Cuban missile crises assessed the awareness and beliefs of American children and adolescents about nuclear weapons and the chances of war.[1,3,9,12,26,36] A majority of those polled spontaneously referred to nuclear weapons and war[3,12] and almost 50% believed a war possible or likely.[1,26] In a 1963 questionnaire study of 12- 14-year-old boys at a public school in Tennessee, for example, almost 60% worried "some, a lot, or all of the time" about a war starting, and 70% expected war within the next 20 years.[36] The pessimism about the future recorded in these early studies resulted in speculation that the threat of war in general, and nuclear war in particular, was having a destructive influence on developmental processes in normal, well functioning American children.[12,26]

Another 15 years passed before the next investigations about children and the threat of nuclear war. Awareness of this issue seemed, like the testing of nuclear weapons, to have gone underground. Then, in 1977, the American Psychiatric Association formed a task force to look at the "Psychosocial Aspects of Nuclear Developments." Between 1978 and 1980, questionnaires were administered to approximately 1000 grammar and high school students, ages 10 to 18, in Boston, Los Angeles, Baltimore, and Philadelphia, and more detailed responses were obtained through questionnaires and discussions with 100 students (15–18 years old) in the greater Boston area. In this study,[5] more than 50% of one sample surveyed thought a nuclear war was possible (with a substantial number of these thinking it likely). A great majority of another sample did not believe that they, their city, or their country would survive a nuclear attack, and many reported that the possibility of nuclear war had affected their plans for marriage or having children. The interviews revealed marked uncertainty, anxiety, and a sense of hopelessness and helplessness about the future. There was also much sadness, cynicism, and bitterness among these young people, based on the belief that adults were not protecting them. These responses caused a principal investigator in the American Psychiatric Association study to express concern about the possibility that:

> These young people are growing up without the ability to form stable ideals, or the sense of continuity upon which the development of stable personality structure and the formation

of serviceable ideals depend. We may find we are raising generations of young people without a basis for making long-term commitments . . .[19]

Other recent investigations, both questionnaire and interview studies,[2, 8,14–16,18] have supported these findings—that many American children are aware of the threat of nuclear war and live in fear of it. Further, there is evidence that preoccupation with this issue among children in the U.S. has increased markedly over the last several years. In 1975, 7% of approximately 19,000 17–18-year-olds polled in 130 schools around the nation said "often" when asked how frequently they worried about the chance of nuclear war; in 1982, the corresponding figure was over 31%.[4] These figures demonstrating an increasing concern are echoed in recent adult surveys.[23,33]

In the last few years, studies in Western Europe have demonstrated that children's worry about war is not just an American phenomenon. In 1981, the Institute of Peace Research at the University of Groningen in the Netherlands conducted a survey with 13–14-year-olds in the city of Groningen. Most of the children polled thought a nuclear war would occur and would destroy their city; almost half thought they would not survive.[10] In West Germany, recent public opinion polls have shown that approximately 50% of young people between the ages of 18 and 24 expect the world to be destroyed by nuclear war.[25] In February 1983, among more than 5000 randomly selected Finnish 12–18-year-olds, the threat of war was their most frequently mentioned fear when they were asked to list their three foremost hopes and fears.[27] (Of interest in this study was that the younger children were more likely than the older children to mention fear of war first, with almost 70% of the 12-year-olds doing so, and a greater percentage of girls in each age group than boys reporting having felt strong fears of war during the month prior to the survey.)

There are similar findings from a variety of surveys of youth in Canada,[28] the United Kingdom,[7] Sweden,[17] Belgium,[20] and New Zealand,[31] but to our knowledge there have been no studies assessing the fear of nuclear war among children from the Soviet Union, either by Soviet or Western scientists. It was this lack of comparative information about Soviet children that prompted the present study.

STUDY DESIGN

In November 1982, one of the authors (EC) asked Yevgueni Chazov, the Soviet Union's leading cardiologist and chief physician of the medical unit treating the Politburo, to assist us in setting up a study to measure Soviet children's responses to the threat of nuclear war. Having just seen videotapes of American school children interviewed on this subject,[8] and having acknowledged that he felt moved by their distress, he agreed. During the next several months, a formal proposal was made and approved by Gosteleradio (Soviet state TV and radio). It contained the following requests: 1) that our American team be permitted to interview Soviet children over a broad age range, asking what they knew about nuclear weapons and how this information affected them; 2) that we be allowed to bring our own translator; 3) that the children not be prepared for these interviews beforehand or prompted during them; and 4) that Soviet TV crews videotape our interviews, but that all the unedited, uncensored tapes be brought back to the United States for editing. (It should be noted that the professional and personal relationships between American and Soviet physicians in the organization International Physicians for the Prevention of Nuclear War made this cooperative research effort possible.) To supplement the recorded interviews and to provide quantitative data, we adapted a questionnaire on the subject of nuclear war developed by two of the authors (JG, RD), and translated it into Russian for use with the Soviet children. This questionnaire had been given to more than 900 American students in 1983.[14]

Four of the authors (EC, JEM, JW, CL) visited two Pioneer camps in mid-summer 1983, one near Moscow and the other in the Caucasus, on the Black Sea. Practically all children in the Soviet Union between the ages of 10–15 join the Pioneers and attend one of the more than 50,000 camps scattered around the Soviet Union. The camp near Moscow, called Gargarin after the Soviet astronaut, had approximately 350 children whose parents worked at a domestic airport near Moscow. Children are eligible to attend this camp if their parents are members of the airport's trade union. Thus they represent a broad cross-section socioeconomically and academically. Orlyonok, the camp in the Caucasus, had 2800 children divided into five subcamps. Run by the state, this camp selected children from throughout the Soviet Union who had won various academic, athletic, artistic, or citizenship competitions in their districts. One of the main competitions was the Fireman's Contest, rewarding those children who had demonstrated skills in climbing ladders or running over obstacle courses, or who had the best fire safety records. At the time of our visit, ten children had saved people's lives in fires. Although Orlyonok children represented Soviet elite by virtue of their intelligence, skill, and achievement, as at Gargarin their parents came from a broad socioeconomic range. In most cases both parents worked—as factory and construction workers, miners, chauffeurs, lawyers, doctors, engineers, etc.

Interviews

In each camp, children were selected for interviewing by the children's governing council, called the *Druzhina* (councils are elected by the children as their representatives), after instructions from us that they select those who would be the most articulate from each annual age cohort between ten and fifteen years old. Often, it seemed, the council members chose themselves and their friends.

To verify that we could interview any child we wished, so as to control for the possibility that the children who were selected might have been told what to say beforehand in response to our interview questions, we chose children by ourselves as well, without consultation with campers or staff. These choices were based on our own interactions with the children during the three days we spent at each camp. We were allowed to interview every child we picked. Preparation on the part of the camp administration would have been extremely difficult in any case; there would have been less than a day to instruct the children, as the selection process was revealed to the camp directors only the evening before the interviews. At Orlyonok in particular, the logistics would have been almost impossible, as we were given the opportunity to choose any of the five subcamps, each composed of several hundred youngsters. We selected the Star Camp for our interviews. This subcamp included about 540 children from republics throughout the USSR, out of the 2800 in the entire camp. Our choice was made at the last moment, so that any instruction for these hundreds of campers would have had to be given overnight. Moreover, we did not discuss the specific questions we planned to ask at either camp before the interviews to guard further against preparation. Finally, we wandered about both camps asking children of all ages, through our interpreter (a Russian-speaking American), what they had been told about why we were there. This was done in the absence of camp personnel. In every case, the stories matched: the campers had been told that a team of Americans was coming to make a film about Soviet children, but they did not learn the subject of the film until after we had told the council members; that is, on the day before the interviews.

Children were interviewed singly and in groups of three to seven. At Gargarin, four groups of children were selected, ages 10–15, totaling 23 children. In addition, four children were given in-depth individual interviews, and several others were asked about their drawings during an art contest we held, the subject being their greatest hope and their greatest fear for the future. At Orlyonok, five more groups were studied, ages 11–15, totaling 20 children, in addition to three children interviewed singly. Thus 50 young people in all were interviewed.

The interviews were done in the following manner. A psychiatrist (EC, JEM, or JPW) would ask questions in English, which were translated into Russian by our interpreter (CL) for the children. Their Russian answers were then simultaneously translated back into English and whispered into the ear of the interviewer so that he could be prepared for the next question. In a few cases, individual interviews were done only in Russian (by CL) to attempt to overcome the potential barrier of the double translation format. All interviews were performed out of doors, generally in the absence of camp personnel, and were videotaped by a Gosteleradio crew with standard broadcast-quality ¾″ portable equipment. The crew consisted of a director, camera operator, sound technician, and assistant. Tapes were checked for their picture and sound quality on-site, and then were given to us, unedited, to bring back to the United States for final preparation. In the United States, the tapes were transferred from Soviet to American format (Secam to NTSC), after which a voice-over English translation was dubbed for the Russian responses on a second channel, as it was not possible to hear the original whispered English translation.

Generally, all of the questions enumerated below, or their equivalents, were asked of each group (the individual interviews were somewhat more varied). In addition, some questions of a more directly political nature were asked. No question or response was censored at any time, and the interviews proceeded as directed by us without interruption. The questions were: 1) At what age did they learn about the effects of nuclear weapons? 2) What were their sources of information? 3) What did they know about the consequences of nuclear war? 4) Did they believe there would be a nuclear war in their lifetimes? 5) Did they believe they would survive a nuclear war? 6) Did they believe shelters would help them survive? 7) How did thinking about and imagining a nuclear war make them feel? 8) How did these thoughts and feelings affect their plans for the future?

Questionnaire Study

In an effort to acquire some systematic empirical data from Soviet children, which might allow for rough comparison with a large sample of American children, we adapted a questionnaire recently used to survey 913 junior and senior high school students from six schools in the Los Angeles and San Jose areas of California.[14] The questionnaire first asked the students to rate concern about nuclear war in comparison to a variety of other concerns by numbering these concerns from *one* (does not bother me) to *four* (very disturbing), and then to answer questions specifically addressing the issue of nuclear war. The advantage of this format was the burial of the nuclear war issue among other issues, so as not to prejudice, at the outset, the students' responses.

We adapted the California questionnaire in the following ways to suit a Soviet sample: In the first section, where nuclear war was included among other items, we removed "getting hooked on drugs," "getting pregnant or making someone pregnant," and "being the victim of a violent crime," not because these problems do not exist in the Soviet Union, but because we believed they would be unnecessarily provocative to Soviet authorities whose approval we would seek for this project, and unsuitable for the younger age group we expected to survey. We also removed "nuclear power plants leaking," because this is generally not recognized as a serious problem in the Soviet Union, as it is in the USA. Finally, in the first section, we changed the item "not being able to find a job someday" to "not being able to find satisfying work," as there is said to be no unemployment in the Soviet Union. Thus, the list of problems that the Soviet youngsters were asked to rate included, in the following order: *a)* getting cancer; *b)* earthquakes; *c)* people will not like me; *d)*will be unable to find satisfying work; *e)* necessity of moving; *f)* nuclear war; *g)* being considered physically unattractive; *h)* divorce of parents; *i)* environmental pollution; *j)* death of parents; *k)* your own death; *l)* overpopulation of the planet; *m)* sickness or disability or accident; *n)* insufficient family resources (*i.e.,* poverty); *o)* world hunger; *p)* poor grades.

In order to keep the questionnaire to a single page, we selected only four of the 12 questions from the second section of the California study for our Soviet sample. In this section, respondents were asked for ratings from *one* (definitely no) to *five* (definitely yes) for the following questions: (*A*) Do you think that nuclear war between the USSR and the USA will occur within your lifetime? (*B*) Do you think that you and your family could survive a nuclear war? (*C*) Do you think the Soviet Union and the United States could survive a nuclear war? (*D*) Do you think it is possible to prevent a nuclear war between the USSR and the USA?

All these questions were identical to those in the California questionnaire, except that *1)* the Soviet questions (*A*) and (*D*) reversed the order for the USA and the USSR, putting the USSR first, and 2) question (*C*) asked whether both the Soviet Union and the United States could survive a nuclear war, whereas the California survey asked only about United States survival. The Soviet children were asked, therefore, about the probability of an even more devastating event, that is the destruction of both the USA and USSR. These changes in the content of the questions from the California survey limit the comparability of results across samples for those questions.*

The questionnaire study was carried out only at Orlyonok, in contrast to the interviews which were conducted at both camps. Of the five sub-camps at Orlyonok, we selected another, the Sun Camp, for the questionnaires; it was separated physically and administratively from the Star Camp, so that there would be less chance for Sun Camp children to be influenced by the interviews taking place at the Star Camp. All the children at Sun Camp came from the Russian Republic or from one of the autonomous republics in the Russian Federation. Although the deputy director of Orlyonok briefly saw the questionnaire and approved its being administered, he did not keep a copy, so that neither the camp personnel nor the children surveyed saw its contents beforehand. On the day following our selection of the Sun Camp, we passed out our questionnaires among the approximately 400 children (of the total of 700 campers) who were free at the time we chose for the study. As we had only 293 copies, those children who did not get one filed out of the gymnasium. Instructions for filling out the questionnaire were given by the Sun Camp manager. It was explained that we were a group of Americans trying to learn how Soviet children felt about a variety of issues. Nuclear war was not mentioned, and we were assured that the children had not been told the subject of our study. The children were then asked to fill out the questionnaire as best they could, independently, without consulting their neighbors. They were told that there were no right or wrong answers, and that they should not sign their names. Within 20 minutes, they had finished and left the gymnasium.

RESULTS

Interviews

Of the 50 children formally interviewed at the two camps, 29 (58%) were girls. The mean age for the girls was 12.2 years, and for the boys

---

*Copies of the questionnaire used in this study, in its Russian version and the English translation, are available from the authors.

13.2 years, with a mean age for both of 12.7 years. Children at Orlyonok, both boys and girls, tended to be somewhat older than those at Gargarin in our sample. The greater proportion of girls to boys reflected the make-up of the children's councils at both camps. All of the children at Gargarin came from the Moscow area, while those at Orlyonok came from all over the Soviet Union, from Estonia to Yakutsk (near Siberia), from Leningrad, Moldavia and the Ukraine to Kazakhstan, with fewer than one in five being from Moscow. The children interviewed at both camps were likely to be above average in intelligence and achievement when compared to a typical cross-section of Soviet children. At Gargarin, this was probable because we interviewed several children who were friends of council members as well as the council members themselves, a select group of above-average ability, chosen for their leadership skills. This selectivity also existed at Orlyonok, but was further heightened by the preselection process there, which chose students with the highest levels of achievement.

In the interviews, Soviet children uniformly reported that they first learned about nuclear weapons some time between the ages of six and eight:

> Sveta, an 11-year-old girl from a small town in Central Russia, for example, said, "I was seven years old. They told us in school, and I also saw a documentary film."

American children seem, on the average, to be slightly older when they become aware of the nuclear threat. Beardslee and Mack[5] found that about 40% of the children they surveyed between 1978 and 1980 became aware of nuclear war by age 12 (so that a majority were older than 12), and Goldenring and Doctor (personal communication, RD) found that in their California survey[14] less than 25% of their total sample of 913 reported learning about nuclear war before the age of eight, 33% between the ages of 8–10, and approximately 41% between 11–13. Chivian and Snow,[8] on the other hand, found that many six- and seven-year-olds, in a first grade classroom in Brookline, Massachusetts, knew about nuclear weapons, as did a majority of Brookline third graders (8–9 years old). These findings suggest that the age of first exposure to this subject in the Soviet Union is approximately the same for all children, perhaps because of standardized programs in schools, camps, or through the mass media, whereas there is greater variation among American children. This hypothesis requires further study.

The sources of information about nuclear weapons for Soviet children were many—television, radio, documentary and feature films, school curricula, books, newspapers and journals, and their parents. Their main source seemed to be television, followed by school, a finding identical to that for American children:[5]

> Irina, a 13-year-old girl from Moscow, said, "I learned about nuclear war from the television shows 'Vremya'* and 'International Panorama.' A lot is said on these shows about this, almost every day." .
> And Katya, a 14-year-old girl from Moscow, said, "In our third and fourth grade they started telling us what nuclear war is, telling us about Hiroshima and Nagasaki."

As with American children, Soviet children seemed to be inundated by discussion of nuclear weapons and imagery of nuclear war:

> Vovo, a 12-year-old boy from Moldavia, said, "I think about it [nuclear war] almost every day because I watch the television show 'Vremya.' They constantly show how there shouldn't be any nuclear weapons."

Information about nuclear weapons effects was detailed, accurate, and, in some cases, surprisingly advanced among the Soviet children we interviewed. All seemed knowledgeable about Hiroshima and Nagasaki from documentaries they had seen in their schools, and some were able to extrapolate from the comparatively small single weapons used there to what a present-day nuclear war would be like:

> Katya, age 14, from Moscow, said: "I remember seeing a film on Hiroshima of a bridge that was located not far from the epicenter of the explosion, and the only thing that was left of people were their shadows. And an explosion that would happen now, an explosion that would be much more powerful than that one, it is hard to imagine what it would be like. I can't imagine what would become of people."

Even young children knew about such things as radiation sickness, and the lasting effects of radiation:

---

*"Vremya" (which means "time") is the daily news program and reportedly has an audience of over 100 million. Other TV shows mentioned that had programs about nuclear weapons were "International Panorama" and "Today In the World."

> Oksana, age 11, from Moscow, described the aftermath of nuclear war by saying, "Some will live, but become diseased from the radiation and there is very little chance that they could be cured." She added that, "The atomic bombs were dropped a fairly long time ago, but children are still being born with the effects of radiation."

Others were familiar—even before the 1982 joint US-Soviet Scientists' conference on "nuclear winter" was shown on Soviet national television[22] and widely publicized in the Soviet Union—with atmospheric effects following a nuclear war:

> Thirteen-year-old Irina, from Estonia, said that in a nuclear war: "The air would be destroyed; the atmosphere would be destroyed. It would be impossible to live."

These Soviet children imagined nuclear war as a global event after which all living things die. In an art contest we held at Gargarin, they drew the Earth shattered by nuclear weapons or all in flames. And in the interviews they described the world after a nuclear war as devoid of life (one child even said that all micro-organisms would die), with devastation that would be complete. The words "wasteland" and "desert" were used repeatedly:

> Alexei, 14 years old, from a town called Tambovskoye, summed up this theme: "The entire earth will become a wasteland . . . all living things will perish. No grass, no trees, no greenery."

And the effects were seen as extending over time, making impossible the survival of any who were somehow still alive:

> Sergei, a 13-year-old from Moscow, said, "All living things would die . . . and even if people lived, the consequences last for thousands and millions of years and the race won't survive."

In response to the question of whether they thought there would be a nuclear war in their lifetimes, Soviet children in the interviews were in general hopeful and optimistic, having great faith in the USSR's struggle for peace and in the activities of peace-loving people around the world, including the United States:

Sveta, a 13-year-old girl from the Riazan region, said, "War will never happen, because the Soviet Union and America will come to terms."

Oleg, a 15-year-old from the Ukraine, voiced the optimism of many of his fellow Pioneers: "If all humanity gathers together, they can curtail the nuclear war. And that's why I don't think it will happen, not in our lifetime or after our lifetime."

Yet, in the midst of this optimism, there was a nagging anxiety that a nuclear war could start at any time, either by design or by accident:

Valery, a 14-year-old Muscovite, stated, "It seems to me that one person could do it all. Could push the button and that would be it. Rockets would be launched at us and we would launch rockets back." [It was interesting for us to note that Soviet scenarios for the initiation of a nuclear war had the United States firing first, the mirror image of American scenarios.]

Kira, a 14-year-old girl from Minsk, expressed a concern that a computer would start a war: "Nuclear war is very possible. It could start from any simple accident. If an American computer or our computer made a mistake, there would be war, accidentally." [This seemed a common concern. We were told about a Soviet feature film, *Quadrant 38–80*, in which an American ship in the Mediterranean, armed with nuclear missiles, has a computer error which results in its nearly launching its rockets and starting a nuclear war.]

While there was general optimism that there would not be a nuclear war, there was uniform pessimism (or realism) among interviewed Pioneers about surviving a nuclear war. Not one child believed survival was possible, even when specific questions were asked about the use of civil defense shelters. Radioactive fallout was understood to spread over great distances and to last for very long periods of time. And the global nature of nuclear war, they believed, coupled with the death of living things, made long-term survival impossible for any who had lived through the early period following a nuclear war:

Alla, a 14-year-old girl from Minsk, said, "If such an explosion were to happen somewhere, then for tens and hundreds of kilometers around, the atomic particles will be distributed and everything will be destroyed . . . no animals, no plants."

Alexei, a 14-year-old from Tambovskaya, said, "It would be impossible to make a big enough bomb shelter to save the entire world."

Sergei, 13 years old, from Moscow, said, "The nuclear radioactivity remains for a very long time. And even if a person goes underground, no matter how much he wants to live, he wouldn't."

Larissa, a 13-year-old from Serov: "And when you come out of the bomb shelter after that kind of catastrophe, . . . there wouldn't be anything left alive. And how can that be? You'd have to start life all over again."

Eleven-year-old Sveta may have been referring to civil defense instruction that she had received (and that she maintained she did not believe in) when she said: "They told us what we can do to save ourselves, but I think you can try, but you won't be saved from nuclear war."

We did not ask specifically about civil defense instruction during this study in 1983, but did during our visit in October 1984. In brief, we learned that there is some nuclear war civil defense training for 15–17-year-olds in the school. At the same time, however, the media give a contradictory message which is clearly more convincing—that if there were a nuclear war, children, their families, their neighborhoods, their country, in fact, the entire world, would be destroyed. This belief in total devastation was widespread among the Soviet children we interviewed, as our questionnaire results, to be discussed below, suggest.

It was at first difficult for us to elicit affect or descriptions of how the children felt about the subject of nuclear weapons and the possibility of nuclear war. Although the Soviet children seemed as playful, unrestrained, and rambunctious as a comparable group of American children when they were among themselves, the Pioneers from Gargarin and Orlyonok became shy and restrained when with us, showing little nonverbal expression. When we asked them, in open-ended questions, what they were feeling as we were discussing nuclear weapons, there was often silence. The Soviet adults who accompanied us explained that, in contrast to the United States, in the Soviet Union feelings about subjects as profound as nuclear war, or about some of the items covered in the questionnaire such as divorce, are a very personal matter, shared only with family and close friends. Not only were we strangers from another country, but we were asking these children to reveal themselves in front of television cameras. Another difficulty may have been their reluctance to label with words intense emotions they felt could not be named, as we were more successful when we explained that words could not adequately describe feelings, but we wanted them to tell us the best word or words that described how they were feeling inside. Then we heard about their sadness, pain, and despair, their bitterness, and their great anxiety that a nuclear war could happen. These feelings were similar to those expressed by American children, although there was, perhaps, less anger and less outward display of emotion:

> Boris, a 13-year-old from Minsk, said, "We feel great despair. We can't imagine life without our parents, friends, brothers and sisters, relatives."

Others in his group echoed this fear of abandonment in mournful tones. In other groups, a great deal of anxiety was expressed about the possibility of war starting at any moment:

> Sveta, age 11, translated media accounts about nuclear weapons into a personal threat: "When I watch films or listen to the radio, I can imagine how bombs will fall on my village. And sometimes, at night, I cover myself with the blankets, because I'm afraid."

> Oleg, 15, from the Ukraine, eloquently expressed the anxiety that several of the children referred to: "There is a film [*Quadrant 38–80*] that tells how a war broke out between America and the Soviet Union, and after that I didn't sleep for several nights thinking about this, about how war almost broke out and how our existence is hanging on a thread."

While the Soviet Pioneer children did not believe in the possibility of surviving a nuclear war, they were optimistic that children could help prevent one. Their numerous activities in this area, most of which seemed to be officially organized by the state-run schools and by the Pioneer organization, perhaps explained this optimism (discussed further, below). Involvement in these activities seemed to convince Soviet children that something can be done.

As in our interviews with American children, we asked the Soviet children at Gargarin and Orlyonok whether their thoughts about nuclear war had affected their plans for the future. We were unable to analyze their responses, however, because all the children answered this question by projecting themselves into a future post-nuclear-war world which nullified their plans, rather than by responding about the effect on the formulation of future plans in the present:

> A typical response to this question was Sergei's: "Of course it affects them, because we all have plans for the future and if a nuclear war suddenly begins that's the end of our plans."

We attempted to ask this question in other ways to clarify what we wanted to know about the planning process itself, but the confusion persisted and we abandoned this area of inquiry.

Questionnaire Responses

The questionnaire study of Goldenring and Doctor[14] surveyed 913 California junior high school and high school students, having a mean age of approximately 16. The Soviet sample of 293 Pioneers ranged from 9–17 years old, with a mean age of 12.8. Because of this discrepancy, we selected an American subsample of seventh, eighth, and ninth graders from the total, made up of 201 students with a mean age of 13.6 and a somewhat similar age distribution (see TABLE 1). Most of the California subsample came from the Center for Enriched Study in the San Fernando Valley of Los Angeles County, a "magnet school" that accepts good students from a broad socioeconomic range in Los Angeles who desire an enriched curriculum. The American sample, therefore, like the Soviet Pioneer sample with which it is compared, is made up primarily of academic achievers with above average intelligence.

Table 1
Age Distribution of American and Soviet Samples

AGE GROUP	USA	USSR
9-11 years	.5%	10.6%
12-14 years	79.5%	80.5%
15-17 years	17.9%	8.9%
Mean	13.6 yrs	12.7 yrs

The American subsample was 59.7% male and 39.3% female, while the Soviet sample had an inverse sex ratio—43% male and 57% female. Although the authors recognize the sex differences regarding concern for the nuclear war issue among adults in the USA,[23] children in Finland[27] and Sweden,[17] and a sample of teenage Soviet emigrees to the United States (personal communication, Mischa Galperin, 1984), our Soviet sample and American age-matched subsample (hereafter referred to as the "sample") showed few significant differences for any of the 15 items of general concern on the questionnaire (see TABLE 2). There were significant differences ($p < .01$) on only two items: American boys were more disturbed by "earthquakes" than American girls, and Soviet boys were more concerned about "getting cancer" than Soviet girls. On the nuclear war item, the mean scores for boys and girls, among both the Americans and the Soviets, were almost identical.

In the first section of the questionnaire, respondents were asked to rate their degree of disturbance in regard to a variety of concerns, from "being considered physically unattractive" and "poor grades" to "death of parents" and "nuclear war." Ratings were from *one* to *four*, with the higher number indicating greater disturbance. For the American sample, the item of greatest concern was "parent dying" with a mean of 3.30, whereas for the Soviet sample, the item of greatest concern was "nuclear war" with a mean of 3.86 (see TABLE 3). Almost 99% of the Soviet

Table 2

Summary of Means, by Sex, for American and Soviet Ratings of Problem Items

PROBLEM[1]	USA			USSR		
	M	F	*t*	M	F	*t*
Getting cancer	2.27	2.20	0.20	2.46	2.13	8.99**
Earthquakes	2.71	2.30	7.49*	1.87	1.67	3.15
Not being liked	2.27	1.94	4.83	2.83	2.77	0.28
Having to move	1.90	1.77	0.85	1.54	1.54	0.00
Nuclear war	3.00	2.95	0.12	3.89	3.84	0.82
Being considered ugly	2.28	2.07	2.57	1.79	1.80	0.02
Parental divorce	2.16	2.18	0.01	2.60	2.74	1.00
Pollution	2.29	2.25	0.06	3.23	3.39	2.68
Death of parents[2]	3.39	3.19	1.88	3.70	3.63	0.76
Own death	2.79	2.66	0.51	2.74	2.83	0.39
World overpopulation	2.08	2.14	0.17	2.60	2.33	3.95
Becoming sick/crippled	2.79	2.81	0.01	2.89	2.79	0.73
Family poverty	2.66	2.43	1.89	2.30	2.25	0.18
World hunger	2.83	2.54	3.68	3.69	3.50	4.14
Bad grades	2.96	2.86	0.34	2.82	2.91	0.76

[1]Comparative data on the item relating to job satisfaction/unemployment are not presented here due to lack of comparability between samples.
[2]USA questionnaire specified "parent death" (singular), whereas Soviet questionnaire gave plural version, as above.
* $p<.007$; ** $p<.003$; all other M–F (boy-girl) differences=NS ($p>.01$).

Table 3
Summary of Means Comparing American and Soviet Ratings of
Problem Items

PROBLEM[1]	USA	USSR	t
Getting cancer	2.22	2.32	1.18
Earthquakes	2.46	1.79	− 7.25*
Not being liked	2.08	2.80	8.00*
Having to move	1.85	1.54	− 3.86*
Nuclear war	2.99	3.86	11.26*
Being considered ugly	2.15	1.79	− 3.79*
Parental divorce	2.20	2.67	4.12*
Pollution	2.27	3.30	11.92*
Death of Parents[2]	3.30	3.68	4.54*
Own death	2.72	2.79	.62
World overpopulation	2.13	2.49	3.52*
Becoming sick/crippled	2.80	2.86	.60
Family poverty	2.58	2.28	2.86*
World hunger	2.67	3.60	10.83*
Bad grades	2.89	2.86	− .38

[1]Comparative data on the item relating to job satisfaction/unemployment are not presented here due to lack of comparability between samples.
[2]USA questionnaire specified "parent death" (singular), whereas Soviet questionnaire gave plural version, as above.
*$p < .001$.

children regarded the prospect of nuclear war as "disturbing" or "very disturbing," compared with 72% of the American group (see TABLE 4). Only one Soviet child out of the total of 293 did not report being bothered by nuclear war, compared to 12.7% of the American sample. It should be noted that the American questionnaire asked about "parent dying" while the Soviet questionnaire stated "death of parents," and therefore they cannot be compared, although some American children might have interpreted the item as death of both parents because of the ambiguity of the phrase. Yet, the Soviet children, even when presented with the loss of both parents, were still more concerned about nuclear war, perhaps because they saw nuclear war as all inclusive—encompassing not only the death of both parents, but of everything. This was borne out by the interviews with Pioneers at both Gargarin and Orlyonok. For youngsters in both the American and Soviet samples, concern about nuclear war was greater than concern about their own deaths. It is of great interest that the Soviet sample was also significantly more con-

Table 4
Percentages of American and Soviet Ratings of "Nuclear War"
Problem Item

RATING	USA	USSR
1. Does not bother me	12.7%	0.3%
2. Somewhat bothersome	15.2	1.0
3. Disturbing	32.5	9.9
4. Very disturbing	39.5	88.7

cerned about global issues such as world overpopulation, world hunger, and pollution. Some of their worry about nuclear war, then, may relate to their greater association of nuclear war with global destruction when compared to the American sample. Preliminary examination of the interviews, in which Soviet children spoke about nuclear war as a global event in which every living thing would be killed, and of drawings of nuclear war by Soviet children at the Gargarin camp, representing the Earth engulfed in flames or shattered into many pieces, tend to support this view. This is an area that requires further study, in particular the question of how this global outlook among Soviet young people is formed.

The American children were significantly more concerned about some family and personal issues such as "looking ugly," "having to move," and "family poverty." On the other hand, Soviet children were significantly more disturbed than American children about "divorce of their parents" and about "not being liked." For the former, it is of interest that the rate of divorce per 1000 population in the Soviet Union is second in the world (3.48 in 1981)[30] only to the United States (5.10 in 1982).[21] The Soviet rate might be even higher if one excluded the populous Moslem sections of the country, where divorce is rare. For the item "not being liked," the higher levels of concern by Soviet children, compared to the American sample, may be explained by the overriding importance given to interpersonal relationships in the USSR.

For the American sample, the items that caused the most concern were, in order: parent dying, nuclear war, bad grades, being sick or crippled, and their own deaths. Among the Soviet Pioneers, the major worries, ranked as: nuclear war, parents dying, world hunger, pollution, and, tied for fifth, bad grades and being sick or crippled. While there is much agreement between the two groups, with four of five of the

American children's concerns showing up on the Soviet list, there are also major differences. For the Soviets, for example, personal death ranked eighth, whereas it was fifth among the Americans; for the Americans, world hunger ranked sixth, and pollution ninth, as compared to third and fourth, respectively, for the Soviets. Also striking is the higher level of worry among the Soviet sample when all the means are averaged—2.71 for the Soviets, 2.49 for the Americans. Does this indicate generally higher levels of anxiety or social concern among Soviet when compared to American young people? Further studies are needed to answer this question.

The second section of the questionnaire presented specific questions about nuclear war. As shown in TABLE 5, the Soviet Pioneers were significantly more optimistic than the American sample that nuclear war between the USSR and US (Question A) would not occur in their lifetime. The percentage of respondents who said that it would definitely not occur was ten times that of the American sample, while those who thought it would probably or definitely occur was less than one-third the percentage of the Americans (12.6% compared to 38.4%). This statistic for California children, consistent with other studies in the USA and abroad,[5,10,17,18] indicates that almost four in ten believed that a nuclear war is probable or certain in their lifetimes. In both samples, the levels of uncertainty were high. Similarly, with regard to preventing nuclear war (Question D), the Soviets were significantly ($p < .001$) more optimistic. Almost three times as many Soviet Pioneers felt positive about the possibility of prevention than did the American students (75.1% compared to 25.9%), while those Soviet children who were definitely or

Table 5

Responses of American and Soviet Samples to Questions[1] on Prospects for Nuclear War

RESPONSE	QUESTION A		QUESTION B		QUESTION C		QUESTION D	
	USA	USSR	USA	USSR	USA	USSR	USA	USSR
1. Definitely not	2.5%	24.9%	11.9%	45.1%	11.9%	54.3%	4.5%	2.0%
2. Probably not	14.4%	28.3%	29.4%	35.5%	25.9%	22.5%	10.0%	0.7%
3. Uncertain	44.8%	33.8%	40.8%	16.4%	39.8%	15.4%	19.9%	4.8%
4. Probably yes	28.9%	9.2%	11.4%	2.4%	16.9%	3.1%	39.3%	16.7%
5. Definitely yes	9.5%	3.4%	5.0%	0.3%	5.0%	3.8%	25.9%	75.1%
Mean rating	3.30	2.38	2.67	1.77	2.77	1.78	3.73	4.63
t	−10.33*		−10.50*		−10.28*		10.10*	

[1]A=Do you think that nuclear war between the USSR and the USA will occur within your lifetime?
B=Do you think that you and your family could survive a nuclear war?
C=Do you think the Soviet Union and the United States could survive a nuclear war? (American sample asked only about U.S. survival.)
D=Do you think it is possible to prevent a nuclear war between the USSR and USA?
*$p < .001$.

guardedly negative (2.7%) constituted a small fraction of the Americans in the negative categories (14.5%). Both the American and the Soviet samples expressed greater optimism and less uncertainty in regard to preventing nuclear war (Question D) than in regard to its inevitability in their lifetimes. This may reflect the wording of the two questions, one of which asks about the possibility of prevention, suggesting that the respondents may have some control over the outcome (and thus eliciting a more positive response), whereas the other simply asks whether the event will occur, presenting an impersonal actuality or inevitability (and thus a less hopeful response).*

We can only speculate on why the Soviet children in our sample seem to be generally more optimistic about the possibility of averting nuclear war than are the youngsters in the American sample. One possibility was suggested in our interviews with the Pioneers, in which many of the Soviet children referred to their involvement in peace-related activities:

> Julia, a 15-year-old, spoke about Pioneer efforts for peace: "We collect petitions against nuclear war, we go door to door, write postcards and conduct meetings."

> Oleg, a 14-year-old from the Siberian city of Yakutsk, told about the contribution children can make: "We can help them [adults] by struggling against nuclear war—by sending letters, designing banners. These are the things that we can contribute."

> The role of friendship with children in other parts of the world was cited by Larissa, a 13-year-old from the mountain village of Serov: "It's very important for all the children of the world to become friends. We have a club in school [the International Friendship Club] where we correspond with people in other countries. They become friends that way . . . become nearer to each other, understand each other."

---

*In two recent studies of young people from "non-super-power" countries there was even more pessimism than among American youth on the question of preventing nuclear war. Among British respondents[7] 28.7%, and among Swedish youth[17] 32% said "definitely or probably no" when asked to assess the probability of preventing nuclear war between the USA and USSR. Their greater expression of pessimism may derive from a perception of even less personal control over USA-USSR actions and policy than is felt by American or Soviet youngsters.

These activities, coupled with strong messages in the media (*e.g.*, showing antinuclear demonstrations around the world) and the schools (through the Friendship Clubs) that the people of all countries are similar, and are united in their desire for peace, may underlie the Soviet children's optimism. That is, the official sanction by Soviet adults in sponsoring activities for children designed to prevent war carries with it the clear message that these activities will be successful. By contrast, in the United States, antinuclear activities among children are scattered, confined to a minority, and are not in general supported by the government, schools, or other official bodies.

In addition, some of the optimism among the Soviet children we surveyed may be a function of the tone in which world events are presented to the Soviet people. For example, the national news program, "Vremya," presents crises in a calm, reassuring manner, which seems to suggest that although there are complex and potentially dangerous problems in the world, they are manageable and being taken care of. By contrast, after viewing the nightly news on American network television, one is often left with the feeling that there are crises all over the world that are out of control, dangerous, and insoluble. We suspect these disparate messages filter down to both Soviet and American children and are involved in their feelings about the possibility of nuclear war.

On the two questions dealing with survival in nuclear conflict (Questions B and C), our findings indicate a significantly greater degree of pessimism (or, perhaps more accurately, realism) among the Soviet Pioneers, compared to the American sample. On the questions concerned with individual and family survival following a nuclear war, only 2.7% of the Soviet children thought this probable or definite, compared with 16.4% among the Americans, a six-fold difference. But both groups, it appears, hold out little hope for survival. More than four in ten of the American sample thought they would probably or definitely not survive, and a similar percentage was uncertain. Among the Soviet children, eight out of ten thought survival unlikely or impossible, and the percentage of those uncertain was much lower. This finding is of interest in light of the publicity in the USA about extensive Soviet nuclear civil defense efforts involving all parts of the population, including children.[6, 11,13,29,34] The response of our Soviet sample may be a result of the extensive reporting, particularly on Soviet television, that nuclear war would totally destroy the Soviet Union and kill the population.[22,32,35]

The questions of national survival follow a pattern similar to that of personal and family survival. It is not, however, possible to compare the

American and Soviet data on this question, as the American children were asked only about survival of their own country, while the Soviet children were asked about both the USA and USSR. One might expect, considering the more devastating scenario presented to the Soviet children, that the differences between the two groups might be smaller. However, this was not the case; percentages in both groups were almost identical to those for the question on family survival. Although the question is vague, since it is not clear what survival of a country means, this finding tends to indicate that, for Soviet and American children alike, nuclear war is seen as destroying everything, there being no clear boundary between loss of individuals and the loss of nations.

CONCLUSIONS

In summarizing the principal findings of this preliminary exploration of the experience of Soviet children in relation to the threat of nuclear war it is important to acknowledge once again the several limitations of the study. The sample was small—50 children were interviewed and 293 completed questionnaires. All of the children were from two Pioneer camps which our hosts selected for us in advance, although the children themselves, as far as we could ascertain, were not prepared for our arrival or for the questions they would be asked. The interview questions were directed only to the subject in which we were interested, and there was little time to establish a relationship with the children, both of which may have hindered our understanding their answers in a broader psychological and social context. There were added difficulties related to cultural differences, the problems associated with translation, and possibly the desire of the children to please, or to give "correct" answers. With these reservations in mind, we would highlight the following findings of this exploratory study:

1. The Soviet children reported learning about the facts of nuclear war by six to eight years old—earlier than American children who have been studied.

2. Soviet children seem to be exposed consistently to more detailed, accurate information about nuclear weapons and their physical and biological effects than are American children, whose information is likely to be obtained sporadically through the media or in the relatively few schools that offer courses on this subject. The Soviet children learn about nuclear weapons through courses in school, television news and information programs, and discussions in the home. The subject seems to be

less taboo in Soviet families than among families in the United States.[37] Still, television appeared to be the most frequent source of information for Soviet children, as it is with American children.[5]

3. There has been a great deal of attention given to nuclear worries and fears among American children and adolescents in recent years. However, the Soviet children questioned were, virtually without exception, concerned about the nuclear threat, while in American studies varying percentages of our youth professed not to be troubled about it at all.

4. A higher level of worry or concern generally was shown in the Soviet children's responses on the questionnaire items when compared to a partially age-matched American sample, especially on global issues such as pollution, world overpopulation, and world hunger, as well as on nuclear war.

5. The Soviet children were more pessimistic (or realistic) than American children studied about the chance that they, their families, the Soviet Union, or the United States could survive a nuclear war. With very few exceptions they believed survival would not be possible. Those interviewed also had quite vivid, well-informed images of what the world would be like after a nuclear war, seeing it as totally destroyed, devoid of life, a "wasteland." Whatever the Soviet children were taught about civil defense preparations for nuclear war had not convinced them that protection is possible. In fact, all the children with whom we spoke dismissed civil defense measures as useless.

6. Compared to the American sample, the Soviet children were more optimistic that nuclear war between the two countries could be prevented.

7. Virtually all the Soviet children in our sample had taken part in officially organized peace education and activities, such as sending letters to world leaders, designing banners and posters, collecting names for petitions, and taking part in meetings and demonstrations.

On February 9, 1983, Moscow correspondent Don McNeil stated on the CBS Evening News that Soviet children

> . . . are never taught about the possible horrors of a nuclear conflict. The reason: according to Soviet military policy, nuclear missiles are the decisive weapons of the future, not an irrational choice for oblivion, and Soviet children must never be allowed to fear the prospect of war in defense of the motherland. In fact, they are taught the opposite.

The findings of the present study indicate that this statement, which was broadcast with confidence to millions of Americans, is so completely at odds with current reality that we cannot help but wonder how much else that we have been presented with as factual about Soviet society—and in particular about the attitudes and knowledge of the Soviet people with regard to nuclear war—is equally without foundation.

REFERENCES

1. Adams, J. 1963. Adolescent opinion on national problems. Pers. Guid. J. 42(4):397-400.
2. Austill, C., ed. 1983. Decision Making in a Nuclear Age. Halcyon House, Weston, Mass.
3. Allerhand, M. 1965. Children's reactions to societal change: cold war crisis. Amer. J. Orthopsychiat. 35:124-130.
4. Bachman, J. 1983. American high school seniors view the military: 1976-1982. Armed Forces and Society 10(1):86-94.
5. Beardslee, W. and Mack, J. 1982. The impact on children and adolescents of nuclear developments. *In* Psychosocial Aspects of Nuclear Developments. Task Force Report No. 20, American Psychiatric Association, Washington, D.C.
6. Central Intelligence Agency. 1978. Soviet Civil Defense. Central Intelligence Agency, Washington, D.C.
7. Chivian, E. and Tudge, J. British children and the threat of nuclear war: a preliminary study. Paper in preparation.
8. Chivian, E. and Snow, R. 1983. There's a nuclear war going on inside me. Videotape of interviews with 6–16-year-olds, International Physicians for the Prevention of Nuclear War.
9. Darr, J. 1963. The impact of the nuclear threat on children. Amer. J. Orthopsychiat. 33:203-204.
10. De Jong, J. 1981. Teaching About Nuclear Weapons. Institute of Polemology, University of Groningen, Groningen, Netherlands.
11. Douglass, J. and Hoeber, A. 1979. Soviet Strategy for Nuclear War. Hoover Institution Press, Stanford, Calif.
12. Escalona, S. 1965. Children and the threat of nuclear war. *In* Behavioral Science and Human Survival, M. Schwebel, ed. Science and Behavior Books, Palo Alto, Calif.
13. Gillette, R. 1983. Soviet way: militarism at early age. Los Angeles Times (July 21).
14. Goldenring, J. and Doctor, R. 1985. California adolescents' concerns about the threat of nuclear war. *In* Impact of the Threat of Nuclear War on Children and Adolescents: Proceedings of an International Research Symposium, T. Solantaus et al, eds. International Physicians for the Prevention of Nuclear War, Helsinki.
15. Goodman, L. et al. 1983. The threat of nuclear war and the nuclear arms race: adolescent experience and perceptions. Polit. Psychol. 4(3):501-530.
16. Haas, S. 1983. Psychological effects upon adolescents of living under nuclear conflict. Presentation at Beth Israel Hospital, Boston (Jan. 13).
17. Holmborg, P. and Bergstrom, A. 1985. How Swedish teenagers, age 13-15, think and feel concerning the nuclear threat. *In* Impact of the Threat of Nuclear War on Chil-

dren and Adolescents: Proceedings of an International Research Symposium, T. Solantaus et al, eds. International Physicians for the Prevention of Nuclear War, Helsinki.

18. Klavens, J. 1982. Survey of Newton North High School students. Unpublished manuscript, Newton, Mass.

19. Mack, J. 1981. Psychosocial effects of the nuclear arms race. Bull. Atom. Sci. 37(4):18-23.

20. Mikolajczak, O. 1984. Impact of the threat of nuclear war on young adults and adolescents. Presented to the International Physicians for the Prevention of Nuclear War, Helsinki.

21. National Center for Health Statistics. 1982. Monthly Vital Statistics Reports 31(12). U.S. Dept. of Health and Human Services, Washington, D.C.

22. Nuclear war: the incurable disease. 1982. Soviet National Television (June 24).

23. Public Agenda Foundation. 1984. Voter Options on Nuclear Arms Policy. Public Agenda Foundation, New York.

24. Remmers, H. et al. 1947. Youth Looks at War and Peace. Poll No. 16, Purdue Opinion Poll for Young People, Division of Educational Reference, Purdue University, Lafayette, Ind.

25. Richter, H. 1982. Psychological effects of living under the threat of nuclear war. J. Royal Coll. Gen. Practit. (June):377-379.

26. Schwebel, M. 1965. Nuclear cold war: student opinions and professional responsibility. *In* Behavioral Science and Human Survival, M. Schwebel, ed. Science and Behavior Books, Palo Alto, Calif.

27. Solantaus, T., Rimpela, M. and Taipale, V. 1984. The threat of war in the minds of 12-18 year olds in Finland. Lancet 1(8380):784-785.

28. Sommers, F. et al. 1985. The nuclear threat and Canadian children. Canad. J. Pub. Hlth 76:154-156.

29. Temko, N. 1983. Soviets try for "survivability" in war. Christian Science Monitor (July 11):4.

30. United Nations. 1981. Demographic Yearbook. United Nations, New York.

31. Valentine, J. and Gray, B. 1985. Nuclear war: the knowledge and attitudes of New Zealand secondary school children. *In* Impact of the Threat of Nuclear War on Children and Adolescents: Proceedings of an International Research Symposium. T. Solantaus et al, eds. International Physicians for the Prevention of Nuclear War, Helsinki.

32. Voice of physicians of the planet: protect peace, protect life. 1981. Interview with Y. Chazov, M.D. Komsomolskaya Pravda (Apr. 10).

33. Washington Post-ABC News Poll. 1982. Boston Globe (Mar. 24).

34. Wigner, E. 1982. Civil defense: our no. 1 requirement. J. Civ. Defense 15(6):6-9.

35. World after nuclear war: a dialogue between U.S. and Soviet scientists. 1983. Soviet National Television (Nov. 1).

36. Wrightsman, L. 1964. Parental attitudes and behaviors as determinants of children's responses to the threat of nuclear war. Vita Humana 7:178-185.

37. Zeitlin. S. 1984. What do we tell Mom and Dad? Fam. Ther. Networker 8(2).

17

Family Interaction Patterns Among Japanese-American and Caucasian Families in Hawaii

Jing Hsu, Wen-Shing Tseng, Geoffrey Ashton, John F. McDermott, Jr., and Walter Char

John A. Burns School of Medicine
University of Hawaii, Honolulu

The authors compared the family interaction patterns of Japanese-American and Caucasian families in Hawaii by rating videotapes of structured family interactions. There were significant differences between the two groups in many aspects of family interaction, such as power, coalition, closeness, negotiation, clarity of self-disclosure, responsibility, invasiveness, affect, and empathy. The differences in family interaction could be explained by the cultural differences between the two groups and indicate that profiles of healthy families differ between distinct cultures, and there is a need to establish a culturally relevant family interaction profile; otherwise normal interactions in families outside the mainstream could be misinterpreted as pathological.

Reprinted with permission from the *American Journal of Psychiatry*, 1985, Vol. 142, 577–581. Copyright 1985 by the American Psychiatric Association.

Presented at the Japanese Culture and Mental Health Conference, Honolulu, Aug. 15–19, 1983.

The authors thank Joy Ashton for her assistance in this project.

The role of the family in mental illness and health has gained recognition over the past three decades, and studies concerning families have proliferated at a fast pace (1). Most family studies in the past dealt with the clinical population, namely, families with identified patients or problems. However, there have been several large-scale studies of healthy family interactions (2–6). On the basis of these findings, derived from predominantly middle-class Caucasian families, profiles of healthy families have been established and have been used to measure the degree of normality or pathology of families, including those of non-Caucasian heritage. Even though efforts have been made to study black American families (7, 8), relatively few studies have dealt with Asian-American families, especially with regard to what are considered healthy family interaction patterns (9, 10). McGoldrick et al.'s book on ethnicity and family therapy (11) devoted only one chapter to Asian families, while numerous chapters were given to various Caucasian families.

We conducted a study that compared the family interaction patterns in families without identified problems who belonged to four ethnic groups in Hawaii: Caucasians, Chinese-Americans, Japanese-Americans, and Hawaiians. In this paper we present our findings from the comparison of Americans of Japanese ancestry (the Japanese) and Americans of European ancestry (the Caucasians).

METHOD

We asked 407 families in the Hawaii Family Study of Cognition (12) to participate in a questionnaire survey aimed at identifying ethnic differences in family values (13). Twelve families from each ethnic group were then selected to participate in the present family interaction study. We selected only families in which the parents were of the same ethnicity and were living together and at least two of their children (aged 10–30 years) were unmarried and were still living at home.

Through a television monitor the researcher instructed the family to perform three tasks, and the family members' interactions were videotaped through a one-way mirror. The tasks were planning an activity, discussing how the family responds to an upsetting situation, and discussing the family's strengths and weaknesses. The parents were asked to perform two additional tasks: discuss the circumstances of their first meeting and their decision to marry each other and describe how decisions were made at home.

The resulting videotapes were rated by nine raters using the Timberlawn Family Evaluation Scale and the Couple Interaction Scale. The

Family Evaluation Scale (3) assesses the family's functioning on a continuum of competence and the Couple Interaction Scale was developed by the research team to assess how intimacy is expressed in a couple's interaction and how power is distributed between the partners. The raters were, by design, of different ethnic groups: two Chinese-American, four Japanese-American, and three Caucasian.

Analysis of variance revealed highly significant differences between the scores of the individual raters for most of the measures. To correct for this, differences among raters were removed by subtracting from each rater's score that rater's deviation from the mean score for all raters on a particular measure. This procedure assumes that scores are independent of associations between the rater's ethnicity and the subject's ethnicity. In fact, analysis of covariance showed this to be so; no significant interaction between family's ethnicity and rater's ethnicity was detected for any measure.

The scores, corrected for rater variation, were then subjected to one-way analysis of variance to test the significance of differences in mean scores between the Japanese and Caucasian families. The proportion of the variation due to ethnic differences (r^2) was also determined. In most but not all instances this was not significant, indicating that between-family variation generally exceeded variation between ethnic groups.

RESULTS

Family Interaction

All the scores on the Family Evaluation Scale fell within the normal range. This is not surprising, as only "functioning" families were included in the study. However, significant differences between the Caucasian and Japanese families are evident in the subscale scores shown in table 1.

With regard to the distribution of power between the parents, the Japanese couples were rated as interacting with slightly more dominance and submission than were the Caucasian couples. The Caucasian parents were rated as having stronger parental coalitions than the Japanese parents, but there was no evidence for rigid parent-child coalitions in either group.

Mythology refers to the family members' shared belief of how they function as a group. It measures the degree of congruence between the family's belief and the actual behavior observed by the raters. The raters perceived the Japanese families' beliefs about their interactions as being

TABLE 1. Scores[a] on the Timberlawn Family Evaluation Scale and the Couple Interaction Scale of 12 Japanese-American and 12 Caucasian Families

Measure	Japanese-American Families		Caucasian Families		Analysis of Ethnic Differences		Analysis of Variation Explained by Ethnicity	
	Mean	SD	Mean	SD	F (df = 1, 214)	Significance	r^2	Significance
Family Evaluation Scale								
Power	2.02	1.05	1.72	0.97	4.36	p<.05	.022	n.s.
Coalitions	1.87	0.64	1.70	0.52	4.35	p<.05	.020	n.s.
Closeness	2.10	0.74	1.80	0.53	11.78	p<.001	.052	n.s.
Mythology	2.41	0.83	2.04	0.58	14.87	p<.001	.065	p<.01
Negotiation	2.49	0.84	2.35	0.83	1.60	n.s.	.007	n.s.
Clarity	2.31	0.76	1.83	0.59	27.76	p<.001	.115	p<.001
Responsibility	2.34	0.69	2.05	0.70	9.62	p<.01	.043	n.s.
Invasiveness	2.14	0.77	1.88	0.58	8.01	p<.01	.036	n.s.
Permeability	2.21	0.61	2.08	0.74	1.97	n.s.	.009	n.s.
Expressiveness	2.25	0.78	1.62	0.51	49.84	p<.001	.189	p<.001
Mood	1.82	0.62	1.62	0.56	6.34	p<.01	.029	n.s.
Conflict	1.87	0.68	1.78	0.70	1.08	n.s.	.005	n.s.
Empathy	2.13	0.78	1.83	0.56	10.59	p<.001	.047	n.s.
Couple Interaction Scale								
Revelation manner	3.37	1.10	2.58	0.89	33.88	p<.001	.137	p<.001
Comfort	3.21	0.97	1.92	0.68	90.74	p<.001	.376	p<.001
Discussing style	3.13	1.02	2.13	1.12	31.13	p<.001	.127	p<.001
Decision making	2.96	1.07	2.34	1.03	18.87	p<.001	.081	p<.01
Congruence	1.94	0.66	1.78	0.65	3.51	n.s.	.016	n.s.
Satisfaction	1.93	0.62	1.63	0.47	15.72	p<.001	.068	p<.05
Mood	1.89	0.58	1.48	0.39	36.79	p<.001	.147	p<.001
Future relationship	1.95	0.69	1.53	0.47	25.52	p<.001	.114	p<.001

[a]After removal of rater differences. Lower score indicates higher competency or functioning, but all scores fell within the normal range.

less congruent with the observed family interaction than the beliefs of their Caucasian counterparts.

The two groups of families were seen as quite different with regard to variables thought to influence the development of individual autonomy: clarity, responsibility, invasiveness, and permeability. The Caucasians were rated as significantly clearer in self-disclosure than the Japanese, who were seen to be somewhat vague and reticent in expressing individual thoughts and feelings. The difference in clarity also contributes significantly to the total causes of variation between the two groups. The responsibility subscale measures the degree to which family members accept responsibility for their own feelings, thoughts, and actions, and the invasiveness subscale measures the degree to which the members speak for one another or make "mind reading" statements. The Caucasians were seen as able to accept more responsibility and as less invasive in their interactions than the Japanese. No significant difference was found in "permeability," which measures the members' responsiveness to each other.

The Caucasian families were seen as open and direct in expressing their feelings, while the Japanese were seen as more restricted and more uncomfortable. The Japanese were perceived as showing more "restraint, without impressive warmth or affection"; the Caucasians were seen as "usually warm and affectionate."

Global Health-Pathology

After having rated the specific aspects of the families' interactions, the raters were asked to make a global assessment of each family on a 10-point scale, based on their subjective impressions. The raters judged the Caucasian families to be significantly healthier (F = 9.58, df = 1,208, p < .01) than the Japanese families, even though both ratings were within the healthy range.

Couple Interaction

The couples' scores on the Couple Interaction Scale are also given in table 1.

Each couple was asked to discuss the circumstances of their first meeting and their decision to marry, and their subsequent interaction was rated. A significant difference was found in the way the couples described their initial encounters. The Japanese couples described their first encounters in a more narrative manner, with less expressed affection, while the Caucasian couples spoke with more affection and recall of feelings.

The Japanese couples were also rated as being less comfortable (even uncomfortable) in discussing private and personal matters, while the Caucasian couples evidently felt much more at ease. There were significant differences in the way each spouse contributed to the discussion; there were more simultaneous utterances by the Caucasian partners, while the Japanese couples tended to speak in alternation.

Significant differences were also found in the ways the couples made decisions. The Caucasian couples based their decisions more on mutual consent, while the Japanese couples made more unilateral decisions. The Caucasian couples' descriptions of their decision-making patterns were seen as more congruent with the raters' impressions; those couples were also seen as being more satisfied with their own decision-making patterns.

The differences between the two groups in managing affect were akin to those differences observed in family interaction, and these differences became more evident when the spouses were together without the children.

The raters were asked to predict the future relationship of the couples after their children had grown and left home. The Caucasian couples were rated as being more likely to have a satisfactory future relationship than were the Japanese couples.

In summary, in both family and couple interaction, considerable differences in the mean scores were found between the two groups on almost every measure.

DISCUSSION

The differences between the Japanese-American and Caucasian families could be due to many variables, such as socioeconomic status, stage of family development, level of competence, and ethnic-cultural background.

The families included in our study were primarily middle-class and had similar socioeconomic characteristics. They were also in a similar developmental stage; two adolescent children in the same age range were living at home and the parents were in the same age group. All families were from a research pool of families without identified problems. Even though it has been demonstrated that even healthy families can be quite different in their levels of competency (8), there is no evidence that less competent Japanese families volunteered for the family interaction stud-

ies. Therefore, it is reasonable to assume that the differences observed
are primarily related to the ethnocultural background of the families.

The interaction of Japanese-American families, who are subject to the
influences of both the American and Japanese cultures, depends on the
degree of acculturation in these families. Our sample, because of the
selection criteria, may have been somewhat biased toward Japanese-
Americans who have retained more traditional Japanese cultural values.
For example, our criteria required that both parents be Japanese; therefore, Japanese-Americans who married out of their race were excluded.
However, the Japanese as a group have the lowest rate of interracial
marriage in Hawaii. During the period when the majority of the parents
in our sample were married (1956-1960), the interracial marriage rate
for Japanese in Hawaii was 17%, as compared with 49% for the Chinese
and 77% for the Koreans (14). Thus, our sample is still representative
of that particular age group. The rate of interracial marriage for the
Japanese in Hawaii in 1980 was 59% (76% for Chinese and 83% for
Koreans) (15).

Our comments will refer to the cultural roots that clearly relate to the
Japanese family's behavior patterns reflected in this study.

The Japanese families were seen as being "less direct, somewhat vague,
and concealing" in expressing individual thoughts and feelings. Such
phenomena may be related to their concern for maintaining harmonious
social relationships. It is important for a Japanese person to conform to
the group norm and to refrain from expressing disagreement (16). As
clear statements of individual feelings and thoughts may risk disagreement, it is culturally adaptive for one to be more indirect and ambiguous.
The Japanese also value implicit, nonverbal, intuitive communication
over explicit, verbal, and rational exchange of information. Family and
in-group members rely more on nonverbal cues and physical contact for
real communications. One should, they believe, be sensitive to what is
implied rather than what is expressed. Such in-group communication
might be perceived as vague and imperceptible by the outsider.

This attitude toward verbal communication is evident even in their
early child-rearing practice. By studying the behavior of mothers and
infants in Japan and the United States, Caudill and Weinstein (17) noted
that the American mothers had more vocal interaction with their infants
and the Japanese mothers had more bodily contact with their infants.

The Japanese families in our study were also seen as having difficulty
in expressing affection and in revealing private matters and as displaying
incongruence between their stated and observed behaviors. Such manifestations may be related to the Japanese attitude toward expressing

personal feelings in public. Doi (18) stipulated that the Japanese have a twofold structure of psychological functioning, conveyed by two Japanese words, *omote* (front, public) and *ura* (back, private), which the Japanese use to indicate contrasting attitudes in dealing with social situations. Certain behaviors are observed more in one setting than in another, depending on whether the situation is considered intimate and private or ritualistic and public. The expression of intimate feelings and revelation of private matters may not be seen as appropriate in a situation considered *omote* (front), such as in front of a videotape camera. Thus, a lack of expression of affection in public should not be equated with a lack of affection in actuality.

The duality of the Japanese response to a situation is also illustrated by the concepts of *honne* and *tatema*. The Japanese believe that there is a normative way of doing certain things; they value adherence to this normative behavior and believe that is what a person can show or tell the other (*tatema*). *Honne* is how one really feels or what one actually does, something one may confine to only family members or close friends. It is not that *honne* is truth and *tatema* is a lie; both are aspects of the truth for the individual (H. Wagatsuma, unpublished paper). This dual concept may partially explain why, in the observer's eye, there seems less congruence between what the Japanese purport to believe and what they actually do.

One unexpected finding was the ratings of empathy. Social scientists often stress that the Japanese are highly sensitive to other people's feelings in social encounters. Thus, it came as a surprise to us that in this study the Japanese were seen as less empathetic than the Caucasians. A possible explanation of this finding may lie in the manner of communication among the Japanese. As the Japanese were constantly anticipating and meeting each other's needs in subtle and nonverbal ways, the raters, who were watching for more observable empathetic responses, may have failed to notice such communication.

Even though the raters were of different ethnic groups, there was no evidence that the differences were related to the ethnicity of the raters or that the ethnicity of the raters interacted with the family's ethnicity in any particular way. This finding may be due to the influence of two circumstances: 1) the raters as a group had more mainstream (Caucasian) cultural values than the Japanese families as a group; the raters were younger than the parents in the Japanese families in our sample, and studies have shown that the immigrant family becomes acculturated after three or four generations (19), and 2) the raters were trained to use the mainstream profile to view family interaction. Perhaps, because of their mainstream position, the raters considered the Japanese families less competent and less healthy, even though our samples were nonclinical families and the common indicators of potential psychopathology, such as rigid parent-child coalition, unresolved chronic conflict, and "invasiveness," were absent from both groups. This observation emphasizes the need for establishing culturally relevant profiles for different ethnic groups, especially with regard to cultural aspects that may differ from the mainstream family model. Clinical observations interpreted without considering their culture context could be misleading.

The findings from this study do not necessarily represent all Japanese-American families. The study of a larger number of families would obviously be more representative. Further investigation is also necessary to study the behavior of Japanese families in Japan and other Asian-American families to understand which attributes are unique to Japanese-American families.

REFERENCES

1. Gurman, A. S., Kniskern, D. P.: Family outcome research: knowns and unknowns, in Handbook of Family Therapy. Edited by Gurman, A. S., Kniskern, D. P. New York, Brunner/Mazel, 1981.
2. Epstein, N. B., Bishop, D. S., Levin, S.: The McMaster model of family functioning. J Marriage and Family Counseling 4:19-31, 1978.
3. Lewis, J. M., Beavers, W. R., Gossett, J. T, et al.: No Single Thread: Psychological Health in Family Systems. New York, Brunner/Mazel, 1976.
4. Moos, R. H., Moos, B. A.: A typology of family social environments. Fam. Process 15:357-371, 1976.
5. Olson, D. H., McCubbin, H. I.: Families, What Makes them Work? Beverly Hills, Calif., Sage Publications, 1983.
6. Reiss, D.: Varieties of consensual experience, III: contrast between families of normals, delinquents and schizophrenics. J. Nerv. Ment. Dis. 146:384-403, 1968.
7. McAdoo, H. P.: Black Families. Beverly Hills, Calif., Sage Publications, 1981.
8. Lewis, J. M., Looney, J. G.: The Long Struggle: Well-Functioning Working-Class Black Families. New York, Brunner/Mazel, 1983.
9. Sue, S., Morishima, J. K.: Understanding the Asian American family, in The Mental Health of Asian Americans. San Francisco, Jossey-Bass, 1982.
10. Hsu, J.: Chinese family: relations, problems and therapy, in Chinese Culture and Mental Health. Edited by Tseng, W. S., Wu, D. New York, Academic Press (in press).
11. McGoldrick, M., Pearce, J. K., Giordano, J.: Ethnicity and Family Therapy. New York, Guilford Press, 1982.
12. Ashton, G. C., Polovina, J. J., Vandenberg, S. G.: Segregation analysis of family data of 15 tests of cognitive ability. Behav. Genet. 9:329-347, 1979.
13. McDermott, J. F., Jr., Char, W. F., Robillard, A. B., et al.: A study of cultural variations in family attitudes. J. Am. Acad. Child Psychiatry 22:454-458, 1983.

14. Sanborn, K. O.: Intercultural marriage in Hawaii, in Adjustment in Intercultural Marriage. Edited by Tseng, W-S., McDermott, J. F., Jr., Maretzki, T. W., et al. Honolulu, University of Hawaii Press, 1977.

15. Kitano, H. L., Yeung, W. T., Chai, L., et al.: Asian-American interracial marriage. J. Marriage Fam. 46:179-190, 1984.

16. Lebra, T. S.: Japanese Patterns of Behavior. Honolulu, University Press of Hawaii, 1976.

17. Caudill, W., Weinstein, H.: Maternal care and infant behavior in Japan and America, in Japanese Culture and Behavior. Edited by Lebra, T. S., Lebra, W. P. Honolulu, University Press of Hawaii, 1974.

18. Doi, L. T.: Omote and ura: concepts derived from the Japanese 2-fold structure of consciousness. J. Nerv. Ment. Dis. 157:258-261, 1973.

19. Yamamoto, J., Wagatsuma, H.: The Japanese and Japanese-Americans. J. Operational Psychiatry 11:120-135, 1980.

18

Cognitive Performance and Academic Achievement of Japanese, Chinese, and American Children

Harold W. Stevenson, James W. Stigler, Shin-ying Lee, and G. William Lucker
University of Michigan

Seiro Kitamura
Tohoku Fukushi College

Chen-chin Hsu
National Taiwan University

Chinese, Japanese, and American children at grades 1 and 5 were given a battery of 10 cognitive tasks and tests of achievement in reading and mathematics. Samples consisted of 240 children in each grade in each culture. 2 major purposes of the study were to determine possible differences in cognitive abilities of Japanese, Chinese, and American children and to investigate the possible differential relation of scores on cognitive tasks to reading by children of the 3 cultures. Similarity was found among children of the 3 cultures in level, variability, and structure of cognitive abilities. Chinese children surpassed

Reprinted with permission from *Child Development*, 1985, Vol. 56, 718–734. Copyright 1985 by the Society for Research in Child Development, Inc.

This study was supported by grant MH30567 from the National Institute of Mental Health. We want to express our gratitude to the children, teachers, parents, and school officials who made it possible for us to conduct this study; to the examiners who worked so effectively; and to Ai-lan Tsao, our coordinator in Taipei, Elizabeth Clarke, our coordinator in Minneapolis, and Susumu Kimura and Tadahisa Kato, who coordinated the project in Sendai. James Stigler is now at the University of Chicago, and William Lucker at the University of Texas, El Paso.

Japanese and American children in reading scores; both Chinese and Japanese children obtained higher scores in mathematics than the American children. Prediction of achievement scores from the cognitive tasks showed few differential effects among children of the 3 cultures. The results suggest that the high achievement of Chinese and Japanese children cannot be attributed to higher intellectual abilities, but must be related to their experiences at home and at school.

Students in Japan are consistently among the top performers in international studies of achievement in mathematics and science (Comber & Keeves, 1973; Husen, 1967). Scores received by American children, on the other hand, typically lag behind; rarely does the average score of American children fall within the range of averages for the top countries. The high level of academic success of Asian-American children is a well-known feature of American society. Many hypotheses have been advanced to account for the high levels of achievement of children from families with Asian backgrounds, including the possibility that the cognitive abilities of these children exceed those of American children.

Evidence presumed to support such a possibility had recently been published by Lynn (1982), and the research by Lynn has generated a great deal of interest in both scientific journals and in the popular press. Lynn, on the basis of an analysis of cognitive functions tapped in the revised version of the Wechsler Intelligence Scale for Children (WISC-R), claimed that the average IQ of Japanese children significantly exceeds that of American children. "At 111," Lynn wrote, "the mean IQ in Japan is the highest recorded for a national population by a considerable order of magnitude" (p. 223). Several earlier studies by Lynn had yielded similar but less extreme results (Lynn, 1977; Lynn & Dziobon, 1980).

Lynn's claim, if correct, is of great importance. If Japanese and other Asian children are indeed so capable in cognitive functioning, information about this phenomenon would be an important addition to our understanding of cultural differences in achievement; it would also increase our knowledge about the genesis of cognitive processes.

Before Lynn's conclusion is accepted, however, his study must be examined in detail. This has been done by Stevenson and Azuma (1983), who conclude that methodological problems in Lynn's analyses prohibit meaningful generalizations about differences in the cognitive functioning of Japanese and American children. Their discussion is based on the following arguments.

Lynn did not gather data himself, but based his analyses on data available in the descriptions of the standardization of the WISC-R in the United States (Wechsler, 1974) and in Japan (Kodama, Shinagawa, & Moteki, 1978). Lynn sought to compare national averages in intelligence by asking what scores Japanese children would receive if their responses were scored according to American norms. However, the norms were not obtained in a comparable manner in the two countries. The major factor invalidating Lynn's procedure is the failure to control for socio-economic status and location of residence (rural vs. urban) of the children in the Japanese sample. The standardization sample in the United States was chosen to be representative of the nation according to these variables, but both variables were ignored in selecting the standardization sample in Japan. The Japanese sample consisted primarily of children from families in large urban centers. Other factors, such as using only performance items rather than including both performance and verbal items in estimating IQ, increase the need to interpret Lynn's results with great caution.

A more direct approach to answering the question that Lynn sought to investigate is necessary. Rather than relying on tests translated from one language to another and on norms obtained in one country for evaluating children from another country, data in cross-cultural studies should be derived from tasks designed specifically for use in cross-national comparisons. Data for the present study were obtained in such a manner. As part of a large cross-national study of elementary school children's scholastic achievement, 10 cognitive tasks were constructed for use among Japanese, Chinese, and American children. Tasks falling into traditional "verbal" and "performance" categories were developed by a team with members from each of the three cultures. Two criteria were adopted for selecting tasks: first, some tasks frequently included in standard intelligence tasks were chosen because they are presumed to be effective measures of intellectual functioning; second, some tasks were selected because they were hypothesized to assess cognitive components of reading ability. (The major focus of our larger study was on reading.) Items were constructed simultaneously in the three languages and were judged by professionals from each culture to be culturally fair, that is, within the children's expected experience. The tasks were then given to samples of children selected in a comparable manner in each culture. Biases derived from the testing materials and from the selection of the samples characteristic of previous cross-cultural studies involving Asian and Asian-American children were avoided through these procedures. (For a review of the studies of Asian-American children, see Vernon, 1982.)

This report therefore has two purposes. First, we are interested in responding to the question of whether children in the three cultures differ significantly in their scores on cognitive tasks. Second, we seek to determine whether there are differential relationships between the measures of cognitive ability and scholastic achievement of Chinese, Japanese, and American elementary school children. Primary emphasis is placed upon the children's achievement in reading, but analyses of achievement in mathematics also are conducted.

METHOD

Subjects

The study was conducted with first- and fifth-grade children from three cities chosen to represent the three cultures. It was impossible to test children in more than a single city in each culture because of logistical and financial constraints. The Minneapolis metropolitan area was chosen as the American site for the study. Relatively few residents of Minneapolis are from minority groups or from non-English-speaking families; most are from Northern European backgrounds. All but four of the children in our sample were born in the United States, as were all but 10 of the mothers and six of the fathers. Thus, our sample is not representative of all American children, but of children from white, English-speaking, native-born families. These constraints must be kept in mind when we refer to our American sample.

Having chosen the American city, we faced the problem of selecting a comparable site in Japan for our study. After discussions with colleagues in Japan and the United States, it was agreed that the Japanese city most similar to Minneapolis in size and other characteristics was Sendai. Both Minneapolis and Sendai are economically successful cities with relatively traditional cultures. All but two children in our Sendai sample were born in Japan. Seven mothers and 10 fathers were born in Japanese families residing in another Asian country.

Only two large Chinese cities were potential sites for the study: Hong Kong and Taipei. We chose Taipei for several reasons, but primarily because it is a large, modern city, comparable in size to Minneapolis, and with a Chinese-speaking population. Three of the Chinese children were not born in Taiwan; two were born in mainland China and one in another

Asian country. All of the parents were Chinese and all but three who were born in another Asian country were born in Taiwan or mainland China. The sample of Chinese children are representative, therefore, of the populations that have migrated to Taiwan from southern regions of China over the past centuries and of the more recent migrations in the late 1940s of persons from all over China.

A procedure for selecting our subjects was adopted that would insure our obtaining representative samples of children from within each city. Over 99% of all children of elementary school age attend school in all three cities. Promotion from one grade to another is automatic in Taipei and Sendai elementary schools, and retention of a child in a grade is very rare in elementary schools in Minneapolis. Sampling by grade is equivalent, therefore, to sampling by age, for there is a narrow age range within each country in each grade.

Our first step was to select stratified random samples of 10 schools in each city. The selection was based on a demographic analysis of the characteristics of both public and private schools. In consultation with educational authorities, a list of schools stratified by region and socio-economic status of the families was obtained. Schools were then selected at random with the restriction that the 10 schools constitute a representative sample of public and private schools within the cities. Within each school two classrooms were selected at random at each of the two grade levels, yielding a total of 20 first-grade and 20 fifth-grade class-rooms in each city. The only exception to this procedure occurred in Minneapolis. Since there was not a sufficient number of first- and fifth-grade classrooms in the 10 schools initially selected, it was necessary to visit 13 schools to obtain the required 40 classrooms.

In Minneapolis, all children suspected of mental retardation had been examined by a school psychologist during kindergarten or early in the first grade and had been assigned to special classes. It was necessary, therefore, to eliminate mentally retarded children from our sample in Taipei and Sendai. Children in Taipei are automatically given the Raven's Progressive Matrices Test in their school; thus these scores were available for all children. To insure comparability, the Raven's test was given in Sendai when either the teacher or examiner had reason to question the child's level of intelligence. Children were not included in the sample when they had scores comparable to IQs below 70. On this basis, 2.5% of the children in the classrooms visited in Taipei and 0.6% of the children in the Sendai classrooms were eliminated from testing.

Within each culture, 240 first- and 240 fifth-grade children were stud-ied. They were selected in the following manner. Approximately 4 months after the beginning of the school year we had tested all children in each classroom with a test of reading ability. The sample of children tested in each classroom was constituted by randomly selecting two boys and two girls from the upper, middle, and lower thirds of the classroom according to their performance on the reading test. The actual number of children departed slightly in several cases from 240. The *N* for individual cells varied from 237 to 246.

The mean ages of the first graders in Minneapolis, Taipei, and Sendai were, respectively, 6.8, 6.7, and 6.8 years, and of the fifth-graders, 10.9, 10.8, and 10.9 years. The children in Taiwan were, therefore, approximately 1 month younger on the average at the time of testing than the children in Japan and the United States.

Cognitive Tasks

Our primary goal in including cognitive tasks in the major study of which this is a part was to assist us in understanding possible differences among Chinese, Japanese, and American children in their reading ability. If the children's scores in different cultures differ both on cognitive measures and on reading tests, it is appropriate to infer that differences in reading may be one index of more general differences in cognitive functioning. If, on the other hand, the scores of the children in the three cultures differ on the test of reading achievement but not on the other indices of cognitive level, we assume differences in reading achievement are due to other factors, such as differences in the children's experiences at home and school. A secondary purpose in including cognitive tasks in our larger study was to assess the differential effectiveness of several cognitive tasks in predicting reading skills in Chinese, Japanese, and English. These tasks were devised to tap abilities that have been proposed by some writers to be related more strongly to reading one language than the others.

Since no comparative studies of the cognitive abilities of children in these three cultures have been undertaken, it was necessary to develop our own battery of tasks. We attempted to include as wide a range of tasks as possible within the limitations of time and cross-cultural comparability with which we were faced. Some performance tasks already available for use with young children were considered to be appropriate in form, but their content had to be modified. The content of all verbal tasks had to be written especially for this study.

In addition to paying careful attention to the cultural appropriateness of the tasks, we were guided by several other criteria. We wanted to include both verbal and performance tasks, and in an effort to increase reliability, we planned to administer all tasks to individual children. Other criteria included their relevance as measures of intellectual functioning, potential interest to young children, comparability in terms of language, the appropriateness of the tasks for the developmental levels of the children, and the ease with which they could be administered and scored.

Since all tasks were constructed simultaneously in three languages, many of the problems associated with translation from a single language were avoided. Preliminary forms of each task were pretested with children in each city before the final version was developed. The tasks are described briefly in the following paragraphs.

Coding. The coding task was similar to that used in many tests of children's intelligence. The code consisted of nine paired elements; one element was a numeral from 1 to 9, and the second, a simple figure such as ⌐ or ⌐. Nearly all figures required the detection of spatial differences involving up-down or left-right relations, dimensions of difference found to produce problems among young children learning to read English. After the child was guided through seven practice items, 2 min were allowed for the child to complete as many of the test items as possible. Each test item consisted of a symbol, below which the child was to write the associated numeral.

Spatial relations. This task was adapted from the Thurstone Primary Mental Abilities Battery. For each item, the child was asked to choose one of four alternative geometric shapes that, when combined with a target shape, would form a square. Simpler shapes were used for the first graders than for the fifth graders. The first-grade test consisted of two practice items and 12 test items. For the fifth graders there were three practice and 21 test items. The younger children were allowed 3 min, and the older children, 4 min, to complete as many items as possible. This task was included in order to determine whether, especially for the first graders, performance would be more closely related to reading spatially organized Chinese characters than to reading English letters.

Perceptual speed. This task also was adapted from the Thurstone Battery. On each of 18 items, a target was to be matched by one of four alternative choices. First-grade items consisted of line drawings of common objects and of simple shapes; for fifth graders the line drawings were of more complex shapes. First graders were allowed 2 min, and fifth graders, 4 min, to complete as many items as possible. It was assumed that this task would be more closely associated with reading of the characters used in Chinese and Japanese, which often require the perception of small elements of difference, than with reading of English words.

Auditory memory. Many persons have suggested that memory for auditory sequences may be related to reading English. Because of differences among Chinese, Japanese, and American cultures in musical and speech tones, and in experience with auditory material, we constructed a task that involved memory for atonal sequences of different duration. The examiner tapped out a pattern of sounds with a pencil shielded from the child's vision. The child was asked to repeat exactly what the examiner had done. Patterns consisted of long (1.5 sec) and short (.5 sec) intervals between taps. The 13 progressively more difficult patterns varied from simple ones such as short-long-long (S-L-L) to complex patterns such as S-L-S-S-L-S-S-L-S-S. If four successive items were failed, testing was discontinued.

Serial memory for words. Chinese children are required to learn and remember 3,000 characters during the elementary school years, and Japanese children are required to learn 1,000. As part of our effort to assess children's memory ability, two short-term memory tasks were used. The first involved memory for series of words, and the second, memory for series of numbers. The lists of words varied from three to six words for first graders and from four to six words for fifth graders. The length of each successive list increased by one word. Words were chosen that would be equally familiar to children in each of the three locations, that would not contain differential mnemonic cues among the three languages, and that could be pronounced relatively easily. The words for first graders were concrete nouns (e.g., pencil, rabbit, airplane). Two lists of abstract nouns (e.g., experiment, peace, curiosity, satisfaction) were added for the fifth-grade test. Children began with a list of three (first graders) or four (fifth graders) words and continued with successive lists until they were unable to repeat two consecutive lists correctly. The score was the total number of words in each list recalled in the correct order.

Serial memory for numbers. Lists were composed of randomly selected digits. Three constraints were imposed in constructing the list. No digit was repeated in a list, no successive numbers (e.g., 2-3) followed each other, and sequences of numbers that contained mnemonic cues in any language were eliminated (e.g., 1-7 was not allowed because the words in Japanese for these numbers are pronounced ichi-shichi). Lists varied in length from four to seven numbers. Two lists of each length were presented. After practice with a list containing three numbers, testing continued until the child missed both lists of a given length. The score for each list was the total number of successive digits repeated correctly.

Verbal-spatial representation. This task was designed to tap children's ability to identify or draw figures on the basis of verbal directions. The task of 13 items was an adaptation and extension of an earlier task constructed by Y. Ko of National Taiwan University, who recently found that children's ability to draw figures varying in their spatial arrangements on the basis of verbal directions is related to the rate at which children learn Chinese characters. Items were arranged in order of increasing difficulty. An example of a simple item is the following. The child is shown a linear array containing four crosses and a triangle. The examiner asks the child to point to the "one that is different from the others." In one of the more complex items the child was shown a square and was told, "Inside the square draw a cross that divides the square into four parts. In the upper right box draw a small circle and in the lower left box draw a small triangle." The test was discontinued when four successive items were missed.

Verbal memory. Many studies have found that scores on tests of memory for the content of a short text, commonly included in scales of intelligence, are significant predictors of reading ability. Comprehension and memory of what is read to children should logiccally be related to children's understanding and memory of what they read themselves. Two brief stories were written that would be suitable for use in the three cultures. The theme of the story written for each grade involved the visit of a family to the beach and the discovery by one of the children of an object in the sand. The child was forewarned that questions about the story would be asked later. The stories were judged by members of each culture to be culturally fair and linguistically comparable. First graders were asked nine questions, and fifth graders, 11.

Vocabulary. Vocabulary tests are among the most frequently used tests of verbal intelligence. Children were asked to define words. The words were obtained from many different sources: the lexicon of all words contained in the readers used in the elementary schools of the three cities; popular books and magazines for children from each culture; and the Japanese, Chinese, and American versions of the WISC-R. Words were reviewed by native speakers of each language who also were skilled with at least one of the other languages. The final list contained 25 words that were judged to be of equal difficulty in the three languages, were considered to have precisely the same meaning in the three languages, and could be scored reliably. Testing was continued until the child was unable to define four successive words correctly.

General information. Another type of task found in most tests of intelligence is one in which children are asked questions tapping common knowledge. A distinction was made between questions requiring inferential reasoning and those dependent upon factual knowledge. It was decided to minimize the number of the first type since the purpose of the task was to assess the amount of common knowledge the child had acquired through everyday experience. The procedure for developing items was similar to that used in the selection of vocabulary words. After reviewing a large number of possible questions, 26 questions were selected for the final list. Testing was discontinued when four successive items were missed.

Scoring was done in the United States by graduate students from each culture. All tasks were coded independently by two different coders to insure accuracy. When disagreement between the two coders occurred, a final score was obtained by consensus following discussion in a group meeting attended by representatives from each culture. Objective criteria were available for all tasks except vocabulary and general information. Coding systems for these tasks were developed empirically through examination of a large sample of the responses to each question.

Reliability of the Tasks

Reliabilities were calculated when possible by means of Cronbach's alpha statistic. Values obtained for coding, spatial relations, perceptual speed, auditory memory, vocabulary, and general information were uniformly high, as can be seen in Table 1. Values obtained for each grade level and culture ranged from .73 to .98, with a median value of .86.

TABLE 1

RELIABILITIES OF THE TASKS (Cronbach alpha)

TASK	JAPAN		TAIWAN		UNITED STATES	
	Grade 1	Grade 5	Grade 1	Grade 5	Grade 1	Grade 5
Coding	.94	.95	.98	.95	.94	.95
Spatial relations	.80	.81	.84	.83	.83	.87
Perceptual speed	.87	.85	.85	.92	.87	.79
Auditory memory ...:	.74	.73	.76	.69	.82	.80
Verbal-spatial	.78	.45	.77	.47	.77	.81
Verbal memory	.57	.72	.55	.48	.63	.70
Vocabulary	.82	.87	.71	.86	.88	.87
General information .	.91	.86	.88	.79	.90	.86
Mathematics	.92	.94	.93	.95	.93	.94

Two tasks, verbal memory and verbal-spatial representation, were less reliable. For the former, the range of values was from .48 to .72, and for the latter, .45–.81. The small number of items in serial memory for words and serial memory for numbers precluded computation of the reliability statistic.

Tests of School Achievement

In addition to a test of reading ability, children were also given a mathematics test. We included the mathematics test in order to provide information about achievement in more than a single subject. Mathematics was chosen because of its importance in the elementary school curriculum. The construction of the reading and mathematics tests is described in the following paragraphs.

Reading test. Although there are many individual reading tests in the United States, and there are group reading tests in Japan, surprisingly, no reading tests exist in Chinese. We did not consider translating American or Japanese reading tests into the other two languages, for we sought to develop an individually administered test, and we were especially concerned that the test reflect what was actually being taught to the children in the three cultures. Details of the construction of the test are described elsewhere (Stevenson, Stigler, Lucker, Lee, Hsu, & Kitamura, 1982).

The reading test was constructed to yield three scores: sight reading of vocabulary, reading of meaningful textual material, and comprehension of the text. We began our work by compiling lists of each vocabulary word introduced in elementary school textbooks from each country. Preparation also included a search through the textbooks for the grades at which various grammatical structures were introduced. All of the stories included in the text were summarized. This information made it possible for us to construct three versions of the test (Chinese, Japanese, English) that were of comparable difficulty in terms of vocabulary and grammatical complexity and that were of comparable familiarity to children of all three cultures. Items in all three languages were identical through grade 3. However, because of divergent vocabularies, it was necessary to use different words in the three languages for items after grade 3. Words were chosen for the items after grade 3 that were comparable in terms of the grade at which they were first introduced and their frequency of usage in printed materials in each culture. The three portions of the test were highly intercorrelated, and the correlations were similar for the Chinese, Japanese, and American samples (see Table 2). It is apparent that the test is highly reliable.

TABLE 2

INTERCORRELATIONS OF THE SUBTESTS OF THE READING TEST

	JAPAN		TAIWAN		UNITED STATES	
	Grade 1	Grade 5	Grade 1	Grade 5	Grade 1	Grade 5
Vocabulary, reading text	.91	.92	.96	.90	.96	.94
Vocabulary, comprehension	.89	.88	.92	.87	.94	.86
Reading text, comprehension	.94	.78	.95	.76	.97	.87

Mathematics test. Our first step in constructing the mathematics test was to analyze the content of elementary school textbook series used in each culture. A list was compiled of each concept and skill introduced, and the grade and semester in which it first appeared. The task was greatly simplified by the fact that Arabic numerals and a common international system of mathematical notation were used in all mathematics texts. Items were constructed to tap concepts and skills introduced at comparable grade levels in each culture. Both computational and word problems were included. The items were identical for each culture.

The test was individually administered, and all word problems were read to the child to avoid the possibility that failure to solve the problems was due to poor reading ability. Reliability of the test was assessed by computing Cronbach's alpha separately for each grade and country. As can be seen in Table 1, the test has very high degrees of reliability. A complete description of the construction of the test can be found in an article by Stigler, Lee, Lucker, and Stevenson (1982).

Procedure

All examiners were residents of the cities in which the children lived. They had professional experience with children or were preparing for careers in psychology, education, or social work. Examiners were carefully trained in the administration of the tasks. During this training period a project coordinator demonstrated the tasks, supervised practice sessions, and observed the examiners administer the tasks to children before scheduling the actual testing sessions.

Testing was conducted for the reading test 4–5 months after the school year began, and for the remaining tasks, 2–3 months later. Children were taken individually from their classrooms to a room made available in each school. Motivation was very high and testing was completed for all children for whom testing was begun. Tasks were presented in one of four random orders.

RESULTS

Analyses of the data took several forms. An overview of these analyses will be of assistance in following the presentation of the results. We first will describe the analyses of variance of the cognitive variables undertaken to assess the significance of differences among cultures. The structure of cognitive ability as represented by these cognitive tasks is then compared by reviewing factor analyses of the tasks. Children's performance on the achievement tests is then evaluated, and finally, the relation between the cognitive tasks and achievement in the three cultures is discussed in terms of regression analyses conducted separately by grade and culture.

Cultural Differences

The average scores and standard deviations obtained by the first and fifth graders in each culture on each of the cognitive tasks are presented in Table 3. Scores on these tasks were subjected to analyses of variance

TABLE 3

PERFORMANCE OF THE CHILDREN ON THE COGNITIVE TASKS

GRADE AND TASK	JAPAN		TAIWAN		UNITED STATES	
	$\bar{X}$	SD	$\bar{X}$	SD	$\bar{X}$	SD
Grade 1:						
Coding	23.61	7.64	25.53	7.28	24.71	8.00
Spatial relations	10.68	1.53	9.92	1.93	10.19	1.49
Perceptual speed	13.22	3.16	13.73	2.99	15.05	2.68
Auditory memory	6.19	2.29	4.42	2.64	5.56	2.26
Verbal-spatial	12.02	3.97	10.33	5.87	11.51	3.95
Serial memory (words)	7.90	3.07	9.45	3.03	9.58	3.06
Serial memory (numbers)	14.85	8.55	36.30	8.71	21.13	9.89
Verbal memory	5.13	1.80	5.17	1.91	5.87	1.88
Vocabulary	11.93	4.11	10.07	5.18	14.88	3.81
General information	12.05	5.52	10.41	6.07	14.46	4.40
Grade 5:						
Coding	48.96	8.95	50.95	8.61	50.69	8.34
Spatial relations	16.28	2.64	14.54	2.73	15.00	2.71
Perceptual speed	17.58	1.05	17.00	1.67	17.34	1.31
Auditory memory	8.73	2.36	6.69	3.18	7.70	2.15
Verbal-spatial	18.03	2.94	16.99	4.14	17.65	3.25
Serial memory (words)	9.80	4.96	11.62	5.66	11.03	4.94
Serial memory (numbers)	26.41	9.30	41.77	3.95	29.92	10.29
Verbal memory	8.05	2.57	9.95	2.21	10.37	1.65
Vocabulary	27.14	5.61	27.50	6.83	27.72	4.96
General information	32.92	8.32	32.35	7.47	31.51	7.33

in which the indepedent variable was culture. These analyses are summarized in Table 4.

The question of primary interest is whether the scores of Japanese, Chinese, and American children differed significantly. The answer is yes. Before making statements about general cultural differences, however, we must determine whether the rank order of the children's average scores in the three cultures was consistent across the various tasks. Scheffé contrasts comparing the children's performance on each task according to culture were computed separately for each grade (see Table 4). Each column of the table reports the results for the comparison between the children of two cultures.

For first graders, the most outstanding features of the Scheffé contrasts are (*a*) the large number of tasks on which the scores of the American children exceeded those of both the Chinese and Japanese children, and (*b*) the high frequency with which the scores of the Japanese children exceeded those of the Chinese children.

There was less consistency at fifth grade. The advantage of the American children had disappeared. The characteristic finding in comparisons

TABLE 4

ANOVA RESULTS AND THE ASSOCIATED PAIRED COMPARISONS OF AVERAGE PERFORMANCE OF THE JAPANESE, CHINESE, AND AMERICAN CHILDREN

				SCHEFFÉ CONTRASTS		
GRADE AND TASK	F	df	η^2	J vs. C	J vs. A	C vs. A
Grade 1:						
Coding	3.87	2,642[a]	.01	J < C*	N.S.	N.S.
Spatial relations	12.95	2,715	.04	J > C**	J > A**	N.S.
Perceptual speed	24.32	2,714	.06	N.S.	J < A**	C < A**
Auditory memory	33.45	2,715	.09	J > C**	J > A*	C < A**
Memory (words)	22.43	2,714	.06	J < C**	J < A**	N.S.
Memory (numbers)	356.28	2,715	.50	J < C**	J < A**	C > A**
Verbal-spatial	8.21	2,713	.02	J > C**	N.S.	C < A*
Verbal memory	11.72	2,715	.03	N.S.	J < A**	C < A**
Vocabulary	72.09	2,715	.17	J > C**	J < A**	C < A**
General information	34.28	2,715	.09	J > C**	J < A**	C < A**
Grade 5:						
Coding	3.78	2,722	.01	J < C*	N.S.	N.S.
Spatial relations	26.97	2,723	.07	J > C**	J > A**	N.S.
Perceptual speed	10.66	2,723	.03	J > C**	N.S.	C < A*
Auditory memory	36.91	2,723	.09	J > C**	J > A**	C < A**
Memory (words)	7.72	2,723	.02	J < C**	J < A**	N.S.
Memory (numbers)	224.40	2,723	.38	J < C**	J < A**	C > A**
Verbal-spatial	5.54	2,722	.02	J > C**	N.S.	N.S.
Verbal memory	78.56	2,723	.18	J < C**	J < A**	N.S.
Vocabulary	.62	2,723	.00	N.S.	N.S.	N.S.
General information	2.06	2,723	.01	N.S.	N.S.	N.S.

[a] Data for 76 children from the American sample were invalidated by a change in testing procedure introduced for this task.

* $p < .05$.

** $p < .01$.

made between American and Chinese or Japanese children was a lack of significant differences. When there were differences between Chinese and Japanese fifth graders, scores of the Chinese children exceeded those of the Japanese children as often as the reverse occurred.

Performance on several tasks merits special comment. The largest cultural difference occurred for serial memory for numbers, where Chinese children at both first and fifth grades displayed remarkable superiority. Over one-third of the first-grade and 68% of the fifth-grade Chinese children received perfect scores. These children were able to recall perfectly each of two lists of four, five, six, and seven digits. Among the Japanese and American children, fewer than 5% of the first graders and 17% of the fifth graders were able to do this. The superior serial memory of the Chinese children did not extend to words; for example, only one Chinese first grader and 10 Chinese fifth graders received perfect scores on the word-memory task. Nevertheless, the correlations between the scores for the two serial memory tasks were significant for the Chinese children at both first, $r = .56$, and fifth, $r = .33$, grades. (The correlations were also significant for the American and Japanese children, r's $= .48–.53$.) We have no hypothesis to account for the superiority of the Chinese children in this task.

The consistently low scores of the Japanese children on memory tasks involving verbal materials also merit comment. Japanese children received significantly lower scores than Chinese and American children on verbal memory at the fifth grade and on serial memory for words and for numbers at both grades. At the same time, the Japanese children at both grades received the highest scores on auditory memory, a nonverbal memory task. Again, the basis of these findings is not clear.

A detailed picture of the children's performance can be seen in Figure 1. With few exceptions, the forms of the distributions obtained for the Japanese, Chinese, and American children are remarkably similar. Moreover, variability of scores did not differ greatly among the three groups of children at either grade. Despite our pretesting, ceiling effects were found for one task at first grade (spatial relations), and two at fifth grade (coding and perceptual speed). As will be apparent, the skewness found in these three instances appeared to have no systematic influence on the outcomes of other analyses presented here.

A second feature of the distributions of scores should be mentioned. Although the differences between the means for the children of each culture are frequently significant statistically, the variability of scores within each culture is much greater than the variability among the three cultures (see Table 4). This is reflected in the small values of eta-squared,

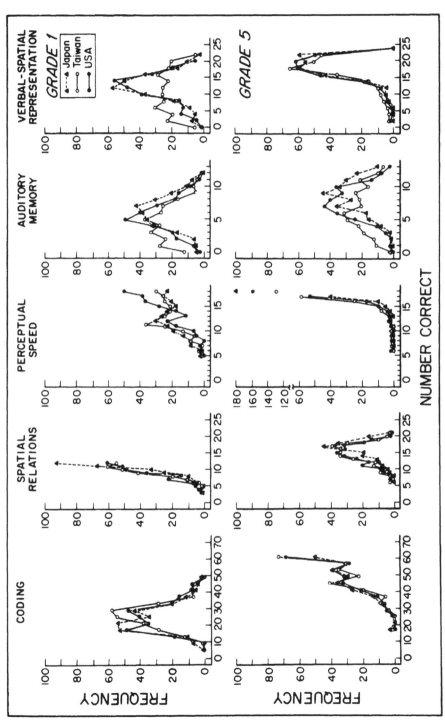

FIG. 1.—Children's performance on the 10 cognitive tasks

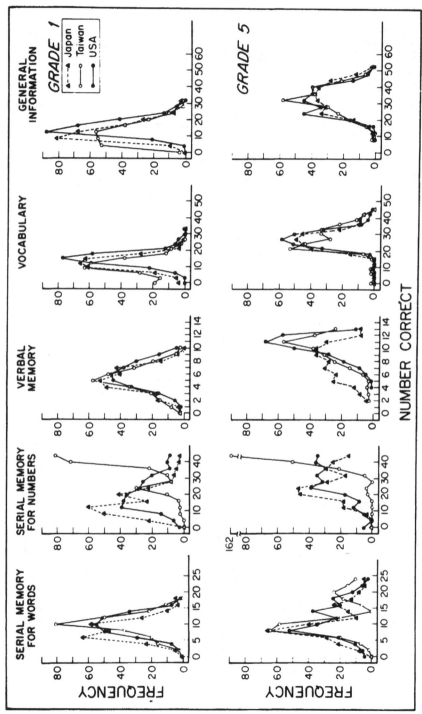

Fig. 1.—*Continued*

which represent the relation of between-culture variability to within-culture variability. The values ranged from .00 to .18 for all tasks except for serial memory for numbers, where the value was .50 for first graders and .38 for fifth graders.

Sex Differences

Among the 60 comparisons (10 tasks × two grades × three cultures), few significant sex differences in performance were found. Some systematic effects were found on two tasks. On coding, girls received higher scores than boys at first grade in Taipei and Sendai and at fifth grade in Minneapolis, F's$(1,238-243 = 5.77-8.52, p$'s $< .05$. On general information, boys received higher scores than girls in first grade in Sendai and in fifth grade in Minneapolis and Taipei, F's$(1,237, 239) > 4.65, p$'s $< .05$. In addition, auditory memory was higher for girls than boys in first grade in Minneapolis and in fifth grade in Sendai, verbal memory for words was higher for first-grade American girls, and spatial relations were higher for boys and verbal memory was higher for girls among Japanese fifth graders, F's$(1,235-243) > 5.08, p$'s $< .05$.

Item Analyses

A problem commonly encountered in cross-cultural research is the possibility that the children were tested with culturally biased items. This is especially true when the items involve verbal material. To ascertain whether this problem was successfully avoided in the present study, we conducted item analyses for the three tasks that required complex verbal responses: general information, vocabulary, and verbal memory.

General information. Little evidence of cultural bias appeared in the questions asked of first graders. Large differences in the percentage of children failing an item (which would indicate the possible presence of bias) occurred only when the children were asked the name of their thumb, how many pencils are in a dozen, and the name of an animal that hibernates in winter. Chinese children called their thumb "number one," reflecting the custom of raising their thumb to indicate being first or the best. Japanese first graders were less familiar than we expected with the unit of a dozen, and many Chinese children had apparently not heard of animals that hibernate. At the fifth grade, large differences were found only on the question, "What color do you get when you mix yellow and blue paint?" More Chinese and Japanese than American children missed this item.

Vocabulary. Chinese children had more difficulty in defining words than did Japanese and American children. For example, more Chinese than Japanese and American first graders were unable to define 13 of the first 15 words. While Chinese children experienced this overall difficulty, there was little evidence that this was due to biased content in any particular items. By the fifth grade these differences had disappeared.

Verbal memory. The major question is why the Japanese children performed so poorly on this task at the fifth grade. Their low scores were derived from failure to answer questions both of central importance and questions of incidental significance. It is difficult to attribute the low scores among the Japanese children to bias in certain types of questions. For example, whereas only 2% of the American children and 11.2% of the Chinese children failed to answer a central question in the story, such as who owned an item that was lost, 39.3% of the Japanese children were unable to do so. Similarly, 89.3% of the Japanese children were unable to describe three of the incidental characters in the story, while only 28.5% of the American and 29.0% of the Chinese children could not.

Factor Analyses

To explore the structure of abilities represented in the cognitive tasks, factor analyses using a principal component solution were conducted separately for each grade in each culture. The results are summarized in Table 5. In all cases, the greatest percentage of variance is accounted for by a general cognitive factor in which all tasks are included. Two of the tasks tended to be common to a second factor: serial memory for words and serial memory for numbers. In several instances a third factor appeared, but its interpretation is obscure. We conclude, both from the factor structure and from the percentage of variance accounted for by the factors, that the organization of cognitive abilities tapped in these tasks was very similar among the children in the three cultures and was represented primarily by general cognitive and serial memory factors.

Classroom Analyses

Significant relationships are often reported between socioeconomic variables and children's cognitive abilities (e.g., Lesser, Fifer, & Clark, 1965). Since our samples included children from regions of each city selected to represent neighborhoods of different socioeconomic levels,

TABLE 5

GRADE, COUNTRY, AND VARIABLE	FACTOR LOADING		
	1	2	3
Grade 1, Japan:			
Coding	.582	...	
Spatial relations	.472	...	
Perceptual speed	.568	...	
Auditory memory	.505	−.322	
Verbal-spatial	.743	...	
Serial memory (words)	.554	−.561	
Serial memory (numbers)	.524	−.612	
Verbal memory	.672	...	
Vocabulary	.564	.460	
General information	.690	...	
Variance accounted for	35.2	47.9	
Grade 5, Japan:			
Coding	.627	...	−.367
Spatial relations	.539	...	−.523
Perceptual speed	.392	...	−.404
Auditory memory	.548	...	...
Verbal-spatial	.649	...	...
Serial memory (words)	.511	−.507	.466
Serial memory (numbers)	.457	−.659	...
Verbal memory	.562	.465	...
Vocabulary	.664	.358	...
General information	.735	.355	...
Variance accounted for	33.3	46.6	56.9
Grade 1, Taiwan:			
Coding	.499	−.560	
Spatial relations	.523	...	
Perceptual speed	.349	−.588	
Auditory memory	.514	...	
Verbal-spatial	.699	...	
Serial memory (words)	.512	.569	
Serial memory (numbers)	.555	.484	
Verbal memory	.772	...	
Vocabulary	.762	...	
General information	.778	...	
Variance accounted for	37.5	50.4	
Grade 5, Taiwan:			
Coding	.463	...	
Spatial relations	.580	−.667	
Perceptual speed	.461	−.400	
Auditory memory	.489	−.464	
Verbal-spatial	.646	...	
Serial memory (words)	.449	...	
Serial memory (numbers)	.485	.398	
Verbal memory	.686	.357	
Vocabulary	.744	...	

(continued)

TABLE 5 (Continued)

GRADE, COUNTRY, AND VARIABLE	FACTOR LOADING		
	1	2	3
General information	.760	...	
Variance accounted for	34.6	46.5	
Grade 1, United States:			
Coding	.517	...	−.614
Spatial relations	.416	...	...
Perceptual speed	.359	...	−.774
Auditory memory	.469	−.507	...
Verbal-spatial	.760	...	...
Serial memory (words)	.356	−.656	...
Serial memory (numbers)	.470	−.667	...
Verbal memory	.662	...	.307
Vocabulary	.621	.329	...
General information	.705	.353	
Variance accounted for	34.4	45.4	57.1
Grade 5, United States:			
Coding	.410	...	.360
Spatial relations	.532	...	.319
Perceptual speed	.356	...	.615
Auditory memory	.513	−.317	...
Verbal-spatial	.703	...	...
Serial memory (words)	.537	−.607	...
Serial memory (numbers)	.439	−.708	...
Verbal memory	.403	...	−.531
Vocabulary	.624	.497	...
General information	.689	.353	−.304
Variance accounted for	28.4	43.3	54.9

NOTE.—Factor loadings below .30 are omitted.

we would expect different levels of performance among the classrooms in which the children were enrolled. To assess these differences, one-way analyses of variance were conducted with classroom as the independent variable. The results were straightforward: there was moderate diversity among the means for the American classrooms, high diversity among the Chinese classrooms, and remarkable homogeneity among the means for the Japanese classrooms.

Differences among the American first-grade classrooms were significant, F's$(19,217) = 1.66$–3.39, $p < .05$, for all but three tasks (spatial relations, serial memory for numbers, and verbal memory). Among the Chinese classrooms, all but two of the differences (serial memory for numbers and coding) were significant, F's$(19,221) = 2.36$–6.35, $p < .01$. In contrast, the only task for which the means among Japanese first-grade classrooms did differ significantly was serial memory for words, $F(19,219) = 2.13$, $p < .01$.

Similar results were found at the fifth grade. Again, the greatest diversity occurred among Chinese classrooms. Differences among the means for the Chinese classrooms were significant, F's$(19,221)$ = 1.69–7.00, $p < .05$, for all but two tasks (serial memory for words and verbal memory). The only tasks for which there were significant differences among the classroom means for the Japanese children were serial memory for words, vocabulary, and general information, F's$(19,220)$ = 1.67–3.85, $p < .05$, and for the American children, auditory memory, serial memory for words, vocabulary, and general information, F's$(20,225)$ > 1.64, $p < .05$.

Neighborhoods in Sendai appear to be more similar to each other than is the case in Taipei or Minneapolis. This is supported by one's general impressions and from certain statistics. For example, the diversity in the average levels of parental education paralleled the degree of diversity of the classroom means for the cognitive tasks. That is, there was greater homogeneity in the level of education attained by the parents of the children in the 20 classrooms at each grade in Sendai than in Taipei or Minneapolis.

School Achievement

Children's scores on the tests of achievement in reading and mathematics are presented in Table 6. For reading, three scores were available: the number of words read correctly in the vocabulary portion of the test, the percentage of words of meaningful text read correctly, and the

TABLE 6

PERFORMANCE OF THE CHILDREN ON THE TESTS OF READING AND MATHEMATICS ACHIEVEMENT

	JAPAN		TAIWAN		UNITED STATES	
GRADE AND SCORE	$\bar{X}$	SD	$\bar{X}$	SD	$\bar{X}$	SD
Grade 1:						
Vocabulary	7.16	6.21	10.78	9.11	9.95	9.63
Comprehension	22.76	13.17	25.65	18.68	21.27	18.23
Reading text (% correct)	.15	.13	.20	.21	.16	.18
Mathematics	20.07	5.17	21.17	5.46	17.11	5.34
Grade 5:						
Vocabulary	46.98	8.99	49.79	7.13	48.43	9.13
Comprehension	82.53	8.53	84.58	7.16	82.65	10.49
Reading text (% correct)	.85	.09	.85	.11	.85	.12
Mathematics	53.27	7.51	50.76	5.73	44.39	6.24

number of correct answers to questions related to comprehension of the text. For mathematics, the value is the average number of items passed.

Differences among the scores on the reading test made by the children in the three cultures were significant at each grade for each of the measures, F's$(2,715 - 725)$ = 4.09–12.09, $p < .05$, except for reading of text at fifth grade, $p > .05$. The Chinese children tended to receive the highest scores. Scheffé contrasts indicated superiority of the Chinese children over the American children on comprehension and reading of text at the first grade and on comprehension at fifth grade, $p < .05$. Chinese children received significantly higher scores than the Japanese children in reading vocabulary at both grades, in comprehension at grade 5, and in reading of text at grade 1, $p < .05$. Scores of the Minneapolis children exceeded those of the Sendai children on vocabulary at the first grade, $p < .001$.

Cultural differences among the scores on the mathematics test were large and significant at both the first grade, $F(2,715)$ = 37.12, $p < .001$, and fifth grade, $F(2,715)$ = 116.95, $p < .001$. At both grade levels, American children received significantly lower scores than the Chinese and Japanese children (Scheffé contrasts, $p < .01$). Scores for boys and girls did not differ significantly from each other in any country at either first or fifth grade, all t's < 1.84, p's $> .05$.

Regression Analyses

As we indicated earlier, the cognitive tasks were selected for several purposes, one of which was to assess their possible differential relation to reading ability in the three writing systems. Cues about possible bases of difference in the children's performance on the reading task may be found in these relationships. For this purpose, regression analyses were conducted in which the scores on the 10 cognitive tasks were used to predict a summary score combining the three components of the reading test.

The analyses (see Table 7) indicate a great similarity in the prediction of reading scores of first-grade Chinese, Japanese, and American children. Two tasks entered significantly into all three regression equations: general information and verbal-spatial representation. At fifth grade, general information was the only task common to all three regression equations. Auditory memory, as predicted, proved to be significant only for the American first and fifth graders. Little other evidence was found for the predicted differential contributions of the cognitive tasks to reading skill among the children in the three cultures. Prediction was least

TABLE 7

REGRESSION ANALYSIS PREDICTING READING ACHIEVEMENT FROM THE COGNITIVE TASKS

	JAPAN		TAIWAN		UNITED STATES	
GRADE AND TASK	β	t	β	t	β	t
Grade 1:						
Coding	.21	3.61***	.09	1.53	.14	1.94
Spatial relations	.10	1.78	.11	1.82	.14	2.04*
Perceptual speed	−.02	−.32	−.04	−.65	.08	1.14
Auditory memory	.08	1.54	.00	.03	.22	3.07**
Verbal spatial representation	.20	3.09**	.13	2.01*	.19	2.33*
Memory for words	.18	3.01**	−.07	−1.17	−.03	−.40
Memory for numbers	−.03	−.48	.17	2.69**	−.05	−.63
Verbal memory	.01	.12	.17	2.33*	.12	1.56
Vocabulary	.03	.54	.01	.13	.03	.38
General information	.26	4.08***	.25	3.29**	.18	2.23*
F	18.72***		13.23***		10.29***	
N	238		240		164	
R²	.45		.37		.40	
Grade 5:						
Coding	.02	.45	.01	.09	.14	2.66**
Spatial relations	.13	2.51*	.07	1.20	.02	.35
Perceptual speed	.01	.28	.04	.72	.14	2.61**
Auditory memory	−.08	−1.56	−.10	−1.74	.12	2.23*
Verbal spatial representation	.15	2.92**	.06	.93	.04	.73
Memory for words	−.03	−.58	.05	.88	.12	1.97
Memory for numbers	.13	2.47*	.04	.67	.03	.55
Verbal memory	.25	4.73***	.26	3.91***	.01	.26
Vocabulary	.20	3.46***	.07	1.03	.16	2.46*
General information	.29	4.75***	.27	3.68***	.35	5.36***
F	28.52***		11.74***		19.03***	
N	239		240		245	
R²	.56		.34		.45	

* Significant at the .05 level.
** Significant at the .01 level.
*** Significant at the .001 level.

successful for Chinese children, and most successful for the Japanese children. Perhaps the most unexpected result was the greater contribution of the verbal tasks to the prediction of the fifth-grade reading scores for the Japanese than for the American or Chinese children.

For exploratory purposes, regression analyses involving the prediction of performance in mathematics were also conducted. These are summarized in Table 8. The cognitive tasks were no more effective in predicting mathematics scores of Japanese and Chinese children than of American children. Despite the fact that some of the tasks were selected because of their presumed relation to reading, the tasks tended to be more effective in predicting mathematics than reading scores. Five tasks appeared frequently in the regression equations for mathematics: general information, coding, spatial relations, verbal-spatial representation, and verbal memory. From these analyses it appears that general cognitive abilities were more strongly involved in mathematics than in reading.

TABLE 8

REGRESSION ANALYSIS PREDICTING MATHEMATICS ACHIEVEMENT FROM THE COGNITIVE TASKS

GRADE AND TASK	JAPAN β	JAPAN t	TAIWAN β	TAIWAN t	UNITED STATES β	UNITED STATES t
Grade 1:						
Coding	.14	2.39*	.07	1.21	.14	2.09*
Spatial relations	.19	3.60***	.18	3.48***	.17	2.83**
Perceptual speed	−.05	−.88	−.02	−.45	.03	.53
Auditory memory	.05	.96	−.03	−.51	.08	1.17
Verbal spatial representation	.31	4.90***	.12	1.96	.13	1.66
Memory for words	.08	1.50	−.02	−.38	−.03	−.39
Memory for numbers	.07	1.15	.03	.54	.13	1.89
Verbal memory	−.04	−.65	.28	4.41***	.17	2.39*
Vocabulary	.43	.76	.18	2.60*	.09	1.34
General information	.23	3.79***	.16	2.31*	.24	3.19**
F		21.12***		22.91***		14.73***
N		238		240		164
R²		.48		.50		.49
Grade 5:						
Coding	.20	3.52***	.14	2.52*	.06	1.24
Spatial relations	.14	2.60*	−.02	−.33	.18	3.42***
Perceptual speed	−.02	−.36	.00	.08	.18	3.61***
Auditory memory	−.04	−.82	.01	.17	.16	3.02**
Verbal spatial representation	.23	4.07***	.14	2.37*	.13	2.27*
Memory for words	.05	.84	.02	.37	.06	1.07
Memory for numbers	.11	1.90	.15	2.74**	.07	1.16
Verbal memory	.13	2.26*	.24	3.97***	.03	.62
Vocabulary	.02	.31	.00	.02	.05	.75
General information	.21	3.19**	.31	4.65***	.32	5.12***
F		20.00***		19.16***		23.36***
N		239		240		237
R²		.47		.46		.51

* Significant at the .05 level.
** Significant at the .01 level.
*** Significant at the .001 level.

DISCUSSION

This study offers no support for the argument that there are differences in the general cognitive functioning of Chinese, Japanese, and American children, nor for the contention (Lynn, 1982) that the superiority of Japanese children in mathematics and science is due to a generally higher level of cognitive functioning than is found in American children. Positing general differences in cognitive functioning of Japanese and Chinese children is an appealing hypothesis for those who seek to explain the superiority of Japanese and Chinese children's scholastic achievement, but it appears from the present data that it will be necessary to seek other explanations for their success. Children in each culture have strengths and weaknesses, but by the time they are enrolled in the fifth grade of elementary school, the most notable feature of their performance is the similarity in level, variability, and structure of their scores on the cognitive tasks. Two factors emerged at both grades in all three cultures, one representing a general cognitive ability, and a second, serial memory ability.

The tendency of the Chinese first graders to receive low scores on a number of the verbal tasks was due, we believe, to their lack of experience in responding to adult questions. In Chinese culture, a good child is considered to be thoughtful but not talkative. By the fifth grade, however, the Chinese children had experienced frequent opportunities in school for verbal interactions with adults, and they encountered little difficulty in responding to the questions posed by the unfamiliar adult examiner.

The initial superiority of the American children on a number of the tasks may be related to their more frequent exposure to events outside the home and neighborhood. For example, in our interviews with the children's mothers, we found that among the American families, 91% indicated that they had taken their children on an outing to such places as a museum, movie, sporting event, zoo, or theater during the preceding month. This occurred less frequently among the Chinese (61%) and the Japanese (30%) families. However, school provides exposure to many new experiences, including those encountered on school outings. Differences in environmental experiences of the children will be discussed more thoroughly in a subsequent report.

Claims for the cognitive superiority of children of one culture over those from other cultures are often made without considering the pervasive and subtle problems that must be overcome before the claims have validity. Translating tests from one culture to another, employing normative data collected in one culture as a basis for describing children in another culture, and failing to obtain random samples of children are some of the most serious obstacles that must be overcome. Such problems were taken into account in planning the present study, and we believe they were minimized or avoided.

We conclude, therefore, that the data do not support an explanation of cultural differences in achievement in school in terms of more general differences in level of cognitive functioning among children in these three cultures. Striking differences appeared in mathematics and some differences appeared in reading scores, but similarities rather than differences characterized the cognitive functions among the children of these cultures. Although we expected that some of our tasks would be more strongly related to reading one language rather than another, the results failed to conform to these expectations. Instead, the relations between cognitive performance and reading were uniformly similar for these children living in diverse cultures, speaking unrelated languages, and reading different orthographies. These relations merit further scrutiny.

REFERENCES

Comber, L. C., & Keeves, J. (1973). *Science achievement in nineteen countries.* New York: Wiley.

Husen, T. (1967). *International study of achievement in mathematics: A comparison of twelve countries.* New York: Wiley.

Kodama, H., Shinagawa, F., & Moteki, M. (1978). *Wechsler Intelligence Scale for Children—Revised.* Tokyo: Nihon Bunka Kagakusha.

Lesser, G. S., Fifer, G., & Clark, D. H. (1965). Mental abilities of children from different social-class and cultural groups. *Monographs of the Society for Research in Child Development,* **30**(4, Serial No. 181).

Lynn, R. (1977). The intelligence of the Japanese. *Bulletin of the British Psychological Society,* **30**, 69-72.

Lynn, R. (1982). IQ in Japan and the United States shows a growing disparity. *Nature,* **297**, 222-223.

Lynn, R., & Dziobon, J. (1980). On the intelligence of Japanese and other Mongoloid peoples. *Personality and Individual Differences,* **1**, 95-96.

Stevenson, H. W., & Azuma, H. (1983). IQ in Japan and the United States: Methodological problems in Lynn's analysis. *Nature,* **306**, 291-292.

Stevenson, H. W., Stigler, J. W., Lucker, G. W., Lee, S. Y., Hsu, C. C., & Kitamura, S. (1982). Reading disabilities: The case of Chinese, Japanese, and English. *Child Development,* **33**, 1164-1181.

Stigler, J. W., Lee, S. Y., Lucker, G. W., & Stevenson, H. W. (1982). Curriculum and achievement in mathematics: A study of elementary school children in Japan, Taiwan, and the United States. *Journal of Educational Psychology,* **74**, 315-322.

Vernon, P. E. (1982). *The abilities and achievements of Orientals in North America.* New York: Academic Press.

Wechsler, D. (1974). *Wechsler Intelligence Scale for Children—Revised.* New York: Psychological Corp.

Part V
TEMPERAMENT STUDIES

Temperament studies continue to constitute one major focus of childhood developmental research activity. This attention undoubtedly reflects, at least in part, an increasing awareness of the significance of temperament for both normal and deviant development.

One of the challenging problems in temperament research concerns the issue of developing a reliable measure of temperament in the neonate. The behavioral state of the neonate is influenced by so many adventitious factors, such as the residual effects of the delivery process, the radical adjustment from the intra- to the extra-uterine environment, and the influence of maternal hormones still circulating in the neonate's blood, that the task of teasing out those behaviors that can constitute reliable measures becomes a formidable undertaking. It was for this reason that we ourselves, with our limited initial resources, decided to start our data gathering at the 2 to 3 month age-period rather than at birth.

Given the problems of rating temperament in the neonate, the report by Matheny and his coworkers from the highly productive Louisville Twin Study Project is indeed a welcome one. Using a substantial sample of 55 twin-pairs, extensive and detailed behavioral data were obtained that permitted reliable ratings of irritability, resistance to soothing, reactivity, level of activity, reinforcement value, and response to manipulation. Factor analysis identified two basic types of infants: those who were more difficult to soothe, fussy when handled, and negatively reinforcing to the examiner. The other type showed the opposite characteristics (less irritability, etc.). A crucial aspect of the study was the correlation of these neonatal characteristics with temperament ratings made on the same twins at 9 months. In other words, did the neonatal ratings reflect evanescent characteristics, or were they predictive of temperament in later infancy. Significant correlations were found especially in the category of emotional activity, which is a significant component, however it may be labeled, of the temperamental typologies formulated by various other

351

researchers including ourselves. This finding of the Matheny group bears significantly on the debate over whether temperament begins as an inborn characteristic of the child, or whether it is shaped primarily by the influences of the early postnatal environment. It should be pointed out that other aspects of temperament that can be rated in older infants, such as distractibility, persistence, and adaptability, and that have functional significance for the child's developmental course, may be very difficult if not impossible to measure in the neonatal period. Thus, the authors' conclusion that "emotional activity appeared to be the core dimension stretching over ages" is justified for the neonatal to 9-month period from their study, but may require modification for later age-periods.

Stevenson and Fielding report a British study of a very large sample of twins of different ages, in which temperament ratings were obtained from the parents not only on the children, but also on themselves and on their spouses. The wide scope of these data enabled the authors to make a number of useful analyses. They confirmed the findings of Lyon and Plomin that parental projection does not take place in rating each other, and only the mothers' rating of emotionality showed any indications of projection in the ratings of the children. These findings are highly relevant as negative evidence for the assertion of some investigators that the mother's rating of the child's temperament reflects primarily a projection of her own biases and attitudes, rather than reliable evidence of the child's own characteristics. The importance of the findings of Stevenson and Fielding is enhanced by the large size of their sample (576 pairs of twins), and the fact that temperament data were gathered on the parents as well as the children. The authors also report the interesting finding that correlations of the mothers' and fathers' temperament were extremely small and negative. Perhaps "likes" do not marry "likes" as a rule. Variable genetic influences were found, using the comparison of intrapair MZ and DZ twins model. This casts doubt on the use of a genetic origin for temperament as a basic factor in the conceptualization of temperament. Differences in the findings for males and females lead the authors to reaffirm the principle that the origin of individual differences needs to be studied separately in boys and girls.

Oberklaid and his coworkers report an Australian study of premature infants who were rated at 4 to 8 months with the Carey Infant Temperament Questionnaire, which had been revised and revalidated for an Australian population. When compared to a control group of infants born at term, there were no significant differences between the two groups. This confirms the finding of Hertzig on a New York sample, rated by maternal interviews rather than questionnaire, that infants born prematurely did not differ from a sample of infants born at term with regard to the rating of difficult versus easy temperament. Again, these findings bear on the contention of some that maternal ratings of difficult temperament reflects maternal characteristics such as anxiety rather than the child's attributes. If this contention were valid, we would expect that mothers of premature infants who, as a group, are more anxious about their infant's well-being and development would report a higher percentage of difficult temperament in their children than mothers of full-term infants.

The final paper by Maziade and his coworkers reports a Quebec study showing that children rated as having difficult temperament at 7 years of age were at higher risk for behavior disorder development when reevaluated 5 years later. This study confirms previous reports, but is valuable because of the large sample from which the target study subjects were selected and the different cultural milieu as compared to other reports. The authors also obtained a measure of family functioning and found that in dysfunctional families, in terms of behavior control, the risk of behavior disorder development in the children with difficult temperament was increased. This lends additional specific evidence to the thesis that it is not temperament alone that creates behavior disorders, but rather the interaction between the child's temperament and the family's functioning.

It is of interest that these four fruitful studies of temperament come from such different parts of the globe—the United States, Great Britain, Australia, and Canada. Added to the studies from other parts of the world, such as the Scandinavian countries, Israel, and Kenya, the ubiquity of temperament as a functional behavioral characteristic of children is evident. Specific temperamental attributes may be expressed differently and their functional significance may be different in different cultures, but they are not produced by the culture itself.

PART V: TEMPERAMENT STUDIES

19

Rudiments of Infant Temperament: Newborn to 9 Months

Adam P. Matheny, Jr., Marilyn L. Riese, and Ronald S. Wilson

School of Medicine, University of Louisville

Temperament was assessed for newborn twins, using a comprehensive neonatal exam that focused on irritability, resistance to soothing, activity, and reinforcement value. The same infants were later assessed at 9 months in a structured laboratory setting, where measures of emotional tone were obtained under a wide variety of instigating conditions. Summary ratings of emotional activity were compiled for each infant, representing the preponderant reaction of the infant in both settings. Individual differences were markedly evident, ranging from wailing distress to smiling and contentment. The neonatal variables correlated significantly with emotional tone at 9 months (rs in mid–0.20 s, p < .05), and a further analysis revealed a generalized multiple correlation of R = 0.32 between the neonatal variables and the 9-month measures of temperament. When extreme groups on emotional tone were selected at 9 months (crying and distress vs.

Reprinted with permission from *Developmental Psychology*, 1985, Vol. 21, 486–494. Copyright 1985 by the American Psychological Association, Inc.

This research was supported in part by research grant OCD 90-C-922 from the Office of Child Development and by a research grant from the John D. and Catherine T. MacArthur Foundation.

We are indebted to the administrators and nurses in the participating hospitals where the neonatal assessments were carried out; and to the many co-workers who participated in the lab assessments, including Sharon Nuss, Patricia Gefert, Ruth Arbegust, Jane Lechleiter and Deborah Sanders.

smiling and contentment), the groups were significantly discriminated by their neonatal scores, with 70% of the infants being correctly assigned to the appropriate extreme group. Overall, the irritable, difficult-to-soothe neonate was likely to be fussier and more distressed in the lab assessment than the more tractable neonate. The results affirmed a significant predictive linkage between neonatal behaviors and later measures of temperament and thus gave credence to the premise of some stability in infant temperament. Emotional activity appeared to be the core dimension stretching over ages, and it is discussed in relation to other formulations of infant temperament. The results demonstrated the utility of a comprehensive neonatal assessment specifically designed to measure temperament, which could be coordinated with laboratory measures of temperament at later ages.

Research in infant temperament has become particularly active in the past few years, with a notable increase in observational studies to supplement the earlier questionnaire studies. Two recent reviews have drawn attention to some of the limitations in questionnaire studies and urged that controlled laboratory studies be performed (Goldsmith & Campos, 1982; Hubert, Wachs, Peters-Martin, & Gandour, 1982).

The problem of measurement has been particularly troublesome in looking for relations between neonatal behavior and later measures of temperament. Most such studies have employed Brazelton's (1973) Neonatal Behavioral Assessment Scale (NBAS), with the follow-up measures typically being obtained from parental questionnaires. The results have generally been low-order and disappointing (Goldsmith & Campos, 1982; Hubert et al., 1982; Sameroff, 1978). If there are reliable individual differences in temperament that appear at birth and remain reasonably stable during infancy, they have not been adequately detected in the studies to date.

As the above reviews point out, however, Brazelton's NBAS was not designed as a measure of temperament but rather as a means of illustrating the complex social/emotional responses that the neonate might display. It has been pressed into service because its dimensions seemed closer to temperament-like variables than other neurologically oriented scales. The weak predictive relationships may therefore reflect an application of the NBAS for which it was not designed.

Assessment of neonatal behavior has remained a ranking interest because it captures the infant's behavior before the extended socializing contacts with the parents have begun. Most conceptions of temperament propose a constitutional basis reflecting genetic and prenatal effects, and most call for some stability in the expression of temperament over time (Buss & Plomin, 1984; Rothbart & Derryberry, 1981). Rothbart has put these characteristics at the center of her formulation, and she has employed longitudinal observations at home plus parental questionnaires to assess the stability of each infant's temperament. Although there was no neonatal assessment, temperament stability increased from 3 to 9 months, and there was greater convergence between the home observations and the parents' reports (Rothbart, in press).

Rothbart also noted that, whereas home observations have the advantage of a natural setting, they inevitably confound the characteristics of the home setting with the features of the infant's temperament. What one observes is the product of the infant's temperament plus the modifying effects of a particular family environment. Home settings are widely diverse, and they introduce a large element of uncontrolled variance when comparing individual differences in temperament.

RELATED BACKGROUND STUDIES

In a prior longitudinal study of infant twins, a battery of standardized laboratory procedures was developed to serve as probes for temperament (Matheny, Wilson, & Nuss, 1984; Wilson & Matheny, 1983). The infant was presented with some age-appropriate challenges, the most notable being separation from the mother, and then a structured series of play activities and soothing techniques were employed to alleviate distress and upset. The infant's behavior was rated from videotapes by trained observers to yield a composite measure of each infant's temperament profile.

In addition, a detailed neonatal assessment has been developed (Riese, 1983), which focused on behaviors expressive of temperament (e.g., irritability, resistance to soothing, activity, and reactivity). The procedure searched for the predominant characteristics of each neonate as displayed during a 3-hour appraisal of feeding, sleeping, orienting behaviors, and responsiveness to noxious and soothing stimuli. If the rudiments of temperament have a constitutional basis and are evident shortly after birth, they should be detected by this assessment. And if these rudiments continue to shape the infant's behavior, then there should be some stability between neonatal reactions and later temperament. As Rothbart and Derryberry (1981) noted, although maturation may promote transformations in temperament over age, nevertheless, some degree of consistency is expected.

The purpose of this study was to obtain a detailed behavioral assessment of the neonate, and to follow up with a laboratory assessment of temperament at 9 months. The focus was on standardized laboratory procedures and objective ratings as the means of quantifying each infant's temperament. Although several dimensions would be measured, the primary interest was in emotional activity, as expressed by such terms as *negative mood, irritability,* and *distress* versus *smiling* and *contentment, cuddliness,* and *positive mood.* Infants differ widely in these characteristics, and if the characteristics have a constitutional basis, they should be expressed with some consistency during early infancy.

METHOD

Subjects

The newborn infants were recruited as part of an ongoing longitudinal study of twins. The recruiting procedures have been described in more detail elsewhere (Wilson, 1978), but briefly, the recruits were drawn from the entire twin-birth registry in the metropolitan area of Louisville, Kentucky. Special efforts were made to recruit and retain families of low socioeconomic status (SES), so that the full range of social class would be represented in the sample. According to the SES scale as described in Reiss (1961), 27% of the families were classified in the lowest two deciles, and the remaining families were distributed in somewhat equal proportions throughout the other eight deciles (exception: 4% in highest decile).

Recruited twins made quarterly visits to the research center during the first year, but for purposes of the study, the visit at 9 months was chosen as the criterion age for the follow-up assessment. This selection was based on several factors: (a) prematurity effects have substantially waned by 9 months; (b) the infants are more competent in motor skills, and a broader range of activities can be employed; (c) separation from the mother is a more potent challenge; and (d) prior studies have shown a clearer consolidation of temperament variables at this age (e.g., Rothbart, in press).

Complete data were available for 110 infants at both the newborn period and 9 months. The 110 infants were drawn from 23 male-male twin pairs, 21 female-female pairs, and 11 opposite-sex pairs. For technical and psychological reasons, the twins are not bloodtyped until they are 3 years old; therefore, twin analyses were deferred until zygosity could be verified by bloodtyping.

Neonatal Assessment

Procedure. The detailed procedures for the neonatal assessment have been described elsewhere (Riese, 1982, 1983). By way of brief overview, neonates were generally examined between Days 1 and 4 of life. If medical complications occurred, the infant was tested shortly before discharge from the hospital.

The examination sequence took place during an entire metabolic cycle; that is, from one feeding to the next (about 3 hr). The following assessments were made.

1. Ratings of behavioral state, irritability, and activity were noted before, during, and after feeding.

2. State organization and state changes were recorded after feeding, as well as spontaneous behaviors and activity during sleep.

3. At the midpoint between feeding, the infant was awakened so that maturational level, sensorimotor status, and orienting behaviors believed to involve cortical processing could be assessed, using a series of items adapted from the Einstein Neonatal Neurobehavioral Assessment Scale (Kurtzberg et al., 1979). Also included was a rating of the infant's reinforcement value to the examiner, as adapted from Lancioni, Horowitz, and Sullivan (1980).

4. Reactivity to a stressor was studied by placing a cold disc on the infant's thigh and recording behavioral responsivity, irritability, and soothability (adapted from Birns, 1965).

5. Throughout the assessment period, an evaluation was made of spontaneous irritability and consolability. Various types of soothing techniques were applied, including acceptance of a pacifier, vocal stimulation, manual stimulation, placement in the prone position, lifting to shoulder, cradling in arm, and swaddling in blanket. Individual responsivity to the various types of soothing and degree of intervention necessary for soothing were assessed.

Observations and scoring. The neonatal observations were rated on 5-point scales, with a higher score indicating a higher level of the attribute being measured. From the entire assessment, those items considered of interest for the study of neonatal temperament were combined or aggregated within six categories of behavior, as described below. Interrater reliabilities,[1] as determined by intraclass correlations, are presented in parentheses following the behavioral headings.

Irritability ($r = .94$). The sum of ratings of irritability from the various situations in the assessment (i.e., irritability before feeding, and irritability in response to visual stimuli, auditory stimuli, and aversive stimuli).

Resistance to soothing ($r = .99$). The sum of ratings of the neonate's response to soothing procedures during various parts of the assessment (i.e., console latency after withdrawal reflex to pinprick, soothability after the cold disc, and soothability after spontaneous irritability).

Reactivity ($r = .94$). The sum of ratings of the neonate's responsivity and degree of orienting (i.e., visual following of bull's-eye; auditory orienting to rattle, bell, and voice; and alertness during presentation of orienting items).

Activity awake ($r = .79$). A rating summarizing the level of activity while the neonate was awake and stimuli were being presented.

Reinforcement value ($r = .90$). A rating summarizing the effect of the infant's behavior on the attitude of the examiner toward the infant.

Response to manipulation ($r = .83$). A rating summarizing the degree of fussiness or irritability during manipulation (e.g., undressing after feeding, diaper changes, or repositioning).

These six summary scores furnished a condensed behavioral profile for each neonate, based on most of the responses elicited during the neonatal exam.

Laboratory Assessment of Infant Temperament

Procedures. The standardized procedures, including the sequence of play activities and toys used, may be found in Matheny and Wilson (1981). The basic outline for the lab visit consisted of the following: (a) a brief warm-up episode, after which the mother left both twins alone with the staff while she was being interviewed; (b) subsequently, a solo episode with the staff with each twin, while the alternate twin, accompanied by the mother, was taken for mental testing.

During these episodes with the mother absent, the staff engaged each twin in a prescribed set of activities, or vignettes, for a fixed period of

---

[1]Interrater reliabilities were obtained for 13 infants observed by two independent raters throughout the entire assessment procedure. For all other assessments, one examiner (MLR) conducted the procedures and rated the infants.

time. Some vignettes were designed to promote happy, enthusiastic play by the infants, while others probed for frustration tolerance, reactions to novelty, and responses to goal blocking. The sequence of vignettes was carefully organized to yield 1 hr of videotaping for each pair, and in a format that was standardized for all twins.

For illustration, two of the vignettes presented at 9 months are briefly described below.

1. Imitative game (2 min). *E* instigates a game (pat-a-cake, waving bye-bye, peak-a-boo), combining gestures with animated expressions and vocalizations. The cadence of activities is repeated so that the infant can spontaneously continue the game with enthusiasm.

2. Visible barrier (2 min). The infant is seated and given an attractive small toy. When the infant holds the toy and proceeds to play with it, the toy is taken away, but placed within reach. As the infant reaches for the toy, a transparent Plexiglas screen is placed upright between the infant and the toy.

Observations and scoring. After the visit was completed, independent raters worked from the videotape and rated the infant's behavior for each successive 2-min period. The ratings were made on 9-point scales drawn initially from Bayley's (1969) Infant Behavior Record, then refined by extensive pretesting (see Matheny & Wilson, 1981). The scales are outlined below.

Emotional tone. Refers to the principal emotional state during the rating period: (1) *Extremely upset, crying vigorously;* (3) *upset, but can be soothed;* (5) *bland, no apparent reaction;* (7) *contented, happy;* (9) *excited or animated.*

Attentiveness. Refers to the degree to which an infant is alert to and maintains attention on objects and events: (1) *Unoccupied, nonfocused vacant staring;* (3) *minimal or fleeting attention, easily distractible;* (5) *moderate attention, generally attentive but may shift;* (7) *focused and sustained attention;* (9) *continued and persistent attention to the point of being "glued" to object or event.*

Activity. Refers to body motion with or without locomotion; may involve whole or part body movements: (1) *Stays quietly in one place, with practically no self-initiated movement;* (3) *usually quiet and inactive but responds appropriately in situations calling for some activity;* (5) *moderate activity;* (7) *in action for much of period;* (9) *hyperactive; cannot be quieted for sedentary tests.*

Social orientation: Staff. (1) *actively negativistic, struggling, strongly avoidant;* (3) *wary, hesitant, passively resistant;* (5) *indifferent or ignoring;* (7) *positive, friendly, approachful;* (9) *very strongly oriented, demanding, possessive of interaction.*

When the ratings were completed,[2] they were summed across all 2-min periods to yield an aggregate score for each rating scale. The four scores thus represented a composite index of the infant's temperament as revealed during the laboratory assessment.

After the lab session was completed, the infant was undressed and measured for head circumference, weight, and recumbent length. Some infants became distressed at the restraint involved, and ratings of emotional tone were made during the physical measurements. This summary score was added to the lab scores, as a measure of temperament under a very different type of challenge. The five scores collectively represented the preponderant reactions of the infant throughout the visit, and they furnished the predictive criteria for the neonatal scores.

RESULTS

Neonatal Assessment

The scores derived from the neonatal assessment were intercorrelated and factor analyzed, and the results are shown in Table 1.

It is apparent that all of the six variables were moderately intercorrelated, with irritability, resistance to soothing, reinforcement value, and response to manipulation forming the core of the temperament relation (also see Riese, 1983). At one extreme, the core represented the neonates who were more irritable, difficult to soothe, fussy when handled, and negatively reinforcing to the examiner. At the other extreme, the core

Table 1
Correlations Between Neonatal Assessment Scores

Variable	1	2	3	4	5	6	First factor loadings
1. Irritability	—	.63**	.35**	−.38**	−.47**	.50**	.80
2. Resistance to soothing		—	.51**	−.18	−.43**	.42**	.75
3. Activity awake			—	−.06	−.32**	.27**	.56
4. Reactivity				—	.50**	−.35**	−.57
5. Reinforcement value					—	−.62**	−.80
6. Response to manipulation						—	.71

Note. N = 110.
* p < .05, ** p < .01.

---

[2]Interrater reliabilities were computed for 22 infants whose videotapes were completely rescored by separate examiners. The percentage of agreement (within one point) averaged 97.2% for emotional tone, 95.7% for attentiveness, 96.2% for activity, and 96.7% for orientation to staff.

represented those neonates who were less irritable, easier to soothe, more adaptable to handling, and more positively reinforcing.

The fussy, irritable neonates also tended to be more active but less responsive to auditory and visual stimuli. These relations, however, were somewhat weaker than the interlocks among the four core variables, and it seemed appropriate to designate the core variables as the basic constituents of neonatal temperament. Although reinforcement value technically measured a qualitative judgment of the examiner rather than a behavioral rating, it clearly depended on behavior that was engaging and socially evocative by the neonate, a point that has been illustrated many times by Brazelton.

Laboratory Assessment

The summary scores from the 9-month laboratory visit were intercorrelated and factor analyzed, and the results are shown in Table 2.

The results revealed that emotional tone was the central variable of the temperament cluster, as refelcted by its moderate-to-high correlations with other variables. Infants who were emotionally positive during the lab vignettes were also likely to be attentive, active, socially oriented to the staff, and not upset by the restraints of physical measurements. By contrast, infants who were distressed and difficult to soothe tended to be inattentive, low in activity (generally sitting and crying), unresponsive or negative to the staff, and provoked by physical measurements.

Aside from emotional tone, the intercorrelations among the other variables were lower, especially for physical measurements. Although the correlations were all positive, there was no strong nucleus of separate relationships, and these variables were all given meaning through their relation to the central variable of emotional tone. As in the neonatal data, there seemed to be a primary dimension of tractability versus distress along which these infants were arrayed.

Table 2
Correlations Between the 9-Month Infant Lab Assessment Scores

Variable	1	2	3	4	5	First factor loadings
1. Emotional tone	—	.52**	.76**	.41**	.45**	.86
2. Activity		—	.33**	.32**	.01	.73
3. Attentiveness			—	.28**	.36**	.74
4. Social orientation: Staff				—	.07	.54
5. Emotional tone: Physical measures					—	<.30

Note. $N = 110$.
* $p < .05$. ** $p < .01$.

Predictive Relations

If emotional activity was the core dimension at both ages, to what extent were individual differences maintained with some consistency from birth to 9 months? Initially, the correlations between all neonatal variables and 9-month lab variables were computed, and the results are shown in Table 3.

The correlations revealed significant although modest relationships between birth and 9 months, especially for the marker variable of emotional tone. Note that low scores on emotional tone in the lab were indicative of distress and upset, so the negative correlations with the neonatal variables actually signified that irritable, difficult-to-soothe neonates were more upset and distressed at 9 months. By contrast, the infants who were more reinforcing as neonates were more positive and good-humored at 9 months. On the core dimension of emotional activity, some consistency of individual differences was being maintained from birth onward.

Multivariate Analysis

Although the correlations illustrated the main connective links between birth and 9 months, they did not capitalize on the patterning of variables at each age and the multivariate linkage between the two sets of variables. For this purpose, a canonical correlation analysis (Cooley & Lohnes, 1971) was performed to examine the joint relation between the neonatal scores and the 9-month scores. The analysis searched for the linear combinations of variables in each set that would maximize the relation between sets; and after all such combinations had been extracted, it yielded a measure of variance accounted for in the 9-month

Table 3
Predictive Correlations Between Neonatal and 9-Month Assessments

	9-month variable				
Neonatal variable	1: Emo.	2: Act.	3: Atn.	4: Soc.	5: Em: P.
1. Irritability	−.24*	−.10	−.12	−.18	−.23*
2. Resistance to soothing	−.21*	−.17	−.08	−.06	−.20*
3. Activity awake	−.22*	−.13	−.05	−.16	−.06
4. Reactivity	.09	−.11	.06	−.04	.06
5. Reinforcement value	.28**	.24*	.22*	.07	.05
6. Response to manipulation	−.27**	−.26**	−.15	−.25**	−.04

Note. N = 110. For 9-month variables, Emo. = emotional tone, Act. = activity, Atn. = attentiveness, Soc. = social orientation to staff, Em: P. = emotional tone in physical measurements.
* *p* < .05. ** *p* < .01.

set by prediction from the neonatal set. The results of the canonical analysis are summarized in Table 4.

The first canonical variate yielded $R = .42$ ($p < .02$), and the three primary linking variables in each set are shown in Table 4, with their respective canonical weights. Each linking variable was also significantly associated with all variables of the opposing set, via multiple correlation. Collectively, 10.6% of the variance in the 9-month scores was predicted from the neonatal scores, and this composite predictive relation between the two data sets could be expressed as $R_{mult} = .32$.

The individual differences in temperament detected in the neonatal exam thus remained with some consistency over 9 months and were significantly expressed in the lab setting. Given the time span involved, plus the powerful complications of rapid growth and maturation during this period, it was gratifying to find a significant relation between these two observational measures of temperament.

Discriminant Function

Among the characteristics assessed in the laboratory, emotional tone clearly stood out as the central variable in the temperament cluster. In qualitative terms, the predominant emotional tone of the infant—whether positive or negative—had a major influence on all other activities in the lab; and in this sense, emotional tone served as the principal marker variable of infant temperament.

With this in mind, the next analysis was designed to test whether the extreme groups on emotional tone in the lab were accurately predicted by their neonatal scores. Did the distraught 9-month infant have a different profile as a newborn than the positive, tractable infant?

Table 4
Summary of Canonical Analysis for Newborn and 9-Month Temperament Scores

Primary variables	First canonical loading	First canonical R	Total predictive variance	Predictive multiple R
Neonate				
Irritability	−.46	.42*	10.6%	
Reinforcement value	.59			
Response to manipulation	−.79			
9 months				.32**
Emotional tone	.72			
Activity	.86			
Social orientation	.68			

Note. N = 110.
* $p < .02$. ** $p < .01$.

The upper and lower quartiles on emotional tone were designated as the extreme groups, then a discriminant-function analysis was performed to identify the combination of neonatal variables that would produce maximum separation of the groups. The three primary neonatal variables from the canonical analysis were initially selected as the set of predictors for separating the extremes on emotional tone.

These three variables (irritability, reinforcement value, and response to manipulation) produced a highly significant discrimination (Wilks's lambda = 0.0523; approximate F = 320.4), and each variable contributed significantly to the overall discriminant function. In terms of classification, 70.2% of the cases were correctly assigned to the appropriate extreme group, based on their neonatal scores, $\chi^2(1, N = 57) = 9.52$, $p < .01$. Distressed infants in the lab had initially been more irritable, nonreinforcing, and fussy when handled as neonates, and the opposite was true for happy, outgoing infants.

The use of extremes helped clarify the relationship, a feature that was also noted by Garcia-Coll (1982) in studies of inhibition. At this early stage, midrange scores on emotional tone were uninformative about prior status, but the extremes did relate in a coherent way to the irritability/fussiness index of the newborn. By the same token, not all irritable newborns remained that way for 9 months, nor did all placid neonates turn out to be easygoing in the lab. But if an infant was distraught in the lab assessment, the chances were 2-to-1 of that infant being correctly classified from the neonatal scores.

DISCUSSION

As Rothbart (in press) has observed, developing adequate techniques for assessing temperament in the early months of life has become a major challenge for students of development. In the present study, the emphasis was placed on detailed behavioral observations in a structured laboratory setting —or in the case of the neonates, an equivalently structured hospital assessment. Each assessment was constructed to pose a wide range of challenges and opportunities to the infant for expression of temperament, and each assessment compiled many ratings of the infant's behavior into summary scores on the primary temperament variables.

By aggregating across a variety of challenges, and by compiling multiple ratings into summary scores, the preponderant reaction of each infant was more dependably detected (cf. also Goldsmith & Campos, 1982). This in turn yielded a more reliable spectrum of individual differences and a better prospect for demonstrating stability over age. During an age period when so many extraneous factors can confound the appraisal of temperament, a protocol for extracting the infant's preponderant reaction from the background noise becomes vitally important.

Emotional tone—and more broadly, emotional activity—emerged as the core variable in these data. It is consonant with the prominent weighting of emotional tone in the temperament cluster at later ages (Matheny, Wilson, & Nuss, 1984; Wilson & Matheny, 1983), and it comports with the central position given to emotional activity in the formulations of Rothbart and Derryberry (1981), Buss and Plomin (1984), and Goldsmith and Campos (1982). The primary marker variable on which infants arrayed themselves was emotional tone, as graded from wailing distress to animated laughter.

Because emotional tone played the central role, and because it was rated as a bipolar variable, it may be compared with the four categories in Rothbart's (in press) protocol that measured emotional activity: fear, smiling and laughter, distress to limitations, and soothability. Both the fear and distress categories were operationalized as crying and fussiness, with the category distinction being based on what had evoked the crying. Soothability was operationalized as a reduction in crying and fussiness after the mother commenced soothing procedures. Smiling and laughter were scored as a frequency count of these positive reactions over a variety of situations.

At the level of actual behavior, therefore, Rothbart's categories ultimately reduced to a bipolar measurement of emotional tone. In terms of instigating conditions, Rothbart depended on spontaneous home situations to create the occasions for fear or distress to limitations, whereas in the present study the lab vignettes incorporated standardized probes along these dimensions.

Given the general parallel between the two studies, it was gratifying to find the results in basic agreement. Rothbart (in press) reported increasing convergence among the emotional activity measures at 9 months, both as rated by observers and as reported by parents. Age-to-age stability was also apparent for smiling and laughter, and to a lesser degree for fear and distress to limitations. Collectively, both data sets pointed to a more dependable assessment of temperament at 9 months, and the prominent role played by emotional activity.

Turning to the neonatal assessment, the four primary variables of irritability, resistance to soothing, reinforcement value, and response to manipulation all funneled into a basic dimension of emotional activity. The bipolar character of the dimension was less sharply drawn—neonates did not display the smiling and animated laughter of the 9-month in-

Annual Progress in Child Psychiatry and Development

fant—but a positive quality was still picked up by the category of reinforcement value.

The fact of finding some stability in this basic dimension over 9 months may be attributed to the use of a neonatal examination that was specifically designed to measure temperament. Replication of the results is necessary, but it opens up the prospect of demonstrating greater stability and predictive potential for neonatal temperament than has heretofore been shown. Goldsmith and Campos (1982) have carefully reviewed some methodological problems in earlier studies with the NBAS, and the present results may offer a more optimistic view for detecting links between neonatal behavior and later temperament.

From this perspective, the basic rudiment of early infant temperament would appear to be emotional activity. As noted previously, it appears to have a constitutional basis, it is progressively elaborated through maturation and learning, it has a powerful impact on the parent-infant relationship, and it is the nuclear characteristic around which the other variables are clustered. A distraught infant who is active and inattentive poses a challenge that is very different from a smiling, good-humored infant with the same characteristics. If temperament is defined as individual differences in reactivity and self-regulation (Rothbart & Derryberry, 1981), then emotional activity represents the primary behavioral variable on which such differences are expressed.

Finally, there still remains a major source of variance in the temperament data that must be attributed to change, or transformations in temperament. Even after all errors of measurement and extraneous influences have been set aside, it is apparent that some infants markedly change in predominant emotional tone over age. The theme of transformations in temperament was the focus of a recent conference (Plomin, 1984), and both maturational changes plus the family environment were discussed in detail as potentiating agents. One might speculate that there is an ebb and flow in temperament development, analogous to the spurts and lags in mental development (Wilson, 1978). If so, the pattern of transformations may depend in part on intrinsic programming, and thus may follow parallel paths for identical twins. Longitudinal data are presently being collected to address this point.

REFERENCES

Bayley, N. (1969). *Bayley scales of infant development.* New York: Psychological Corporation.
Birns, B. (1965). Individual differences in human neonate's responses to stimulation. *Child Development, 36,* 249-256.

Brazelton, T. B. (1973). *Neonatal Behavioral Assessment Scale*. Philadelphia: Lippincott.

Buss, A. H., & Plomin, R. (1984). *Temperament: Early developing personality traits*. Hillsdale, NJ: Erlbaum.

Cooley, W. W., & Lohnes, P. R. (1971). *Multivariate data analysis* (2nd ed.). New York: Wiley.

Garcia-Coll, C. T. (1982, October). *A temperament dimension of behavioral inhibition in infants*. Paper presented at Fourth Occasional Temperament Conference, Salem, MA.

Goldsmith, H. H., & Campos, J. J. (1982). Toward a theory of infant temperament. In R. N. Emde & R. J. Harmon (Eds.), *The development of attachment and affiliative systems*. New York: Plenum.

Hubert, N. C., Wachs, T. D., Peters-Martin, P., & Gandour, M. J. (1982). The study of early temperament: Measurement and conceptual issues. *Child Development, 53*, 571-600.

Kurtzberg, D., Vaughan, Jr., H. G., Daum, C., Grellong, B. A., Albin, S., & Rotkin, L. (1979). Neurobehavioral performance of low-birthweight infants at 40 weeks conceptional age: Comparison with normal full term infants. *Developmental Medicine and Child Neurology, 21*, 590-607.

Lancioni, G. E., Horowitz, F. D., & Sullivan, J. W. (1980). The NBAS-K; I. A study of its stability and structure over the first month of life. *Infant Behavior and Development, 3*, 341-359.

Matheny, A. P., & Wilson, R. S. (1981). Developmental tasks and rating scales for the laboratory assessment of infant temperament. *JSAS Catalog of Selected Documents in Psychology, 11*, 81-82 (Ms. No. 2367).

Matheny, Jr., A. P., Wilson, R. S., & Nuss, S. N. (1984). Toddler temperament: Stability across settings and over ages. *Child Development, 55*, 1200-1211.

Plomin, R. (1984, March). Proceedings of the Fifth Occasional Temperament Conference. Keystone, CO.

Reiss, A. J. (1961). *Occupations and social status*. New York: Free Press of Glencoe.

Riese, M. L. (1982). Procedures and norms for assessing behavioral patterns in full-term and stable pre-term neonates. *JSAS Catalog of Selected Documents in Psychology, 12*(6) (Ms. No. 2415).

Riese, M. L. (1983). Behavioral patterns in full-term and preterm twins. *Acta Genet. Med. Gemellol., 32*, 209-220.

Rothbart, M. K. (in press). Longitudinal observation of infant temperament. *Developmental Psychology*.

Rothbart, M. K., & Derryberry, D. (1981). Development of individual differences in temperament. In M. Lamb & A. Brown (Eds.), *Advances in developmental psychology* (Vol. 1, pp. 37-86), Hillsdale, NJ: Erlbaum.

Sameroff, A. J. (Ed.) (1978). Organization and stability of newborn behavior: A commentary on the Brazelton neonatal behavioral assessment scale. *Monographs of the Society for Research in Child Development, 43*, (5-6, Serial No. 177).

Wilson, R. S. (1978). Synchronies in mental development: An epigenetic perspective. *Science, 202*, 939-948.

Wilson, R. S., & Matheny, A. P., Jr. (1983). Assessment of temperament in infant twins. *Developmental Psychology, 19*, 172-183.

20

Ratings of Temperament in Families of Young Twins

Jim Stevenson and Jane Fielding

The University of Surrey
Surrey, Guildford, United Kingdon

We studied a sample of 576 pairs of twins in three age groups (0-2, 2-5, 5 + years), and obtained for each family a set of temperament ratings which provided isomorphic dimensions for parents and children (EASI Temperament Survey). Both parents were asked to rate independently themselves, their spouse and each of the twin children. The results confirm the findings of Lyon & Plomin (1981) that parental projection does not take place in the rating of each other. Only the mothers' rating of Emotionality shows any indications of projection in the rating of children, and parental agreement on children's temperament shows modest levels of reliability (r = 0.53). There is no evidence of assortative mating for temperament characteristics. The intra-class correlations for monozygotic and dizygotic twins are consistent with Emotionality and Sociability being under some genetic control only in girls, Activity shows increasing genetic influences with age in both boys and girls, and Impulsivity indicates a lower level of genetically determined variance at all ages in both sexes. We concluded that, in common with recent studies on environment associations with temperament, the origin of individual differ-

Reprinted with permission from the *British Journal of Developmental Psychology*, 1985, Vol. 3, 143–152. Copyright 1985 by The British Psychological Society.

The research reported in this paper was funded by an award from the University of Surrey Research Committee. We would like to thank Dr. D. Fulker and the Department of Psychology, Institute of Psychiatry for the assistance with obtaining the sample of twins.

*ences needs to be studied separately in boys and girls. A more general
case is made for the utility of twin studies that include data on other
family members.*

The status of the concept of temperament has become less clear over
the past five years (Rutter, 1982). The notion of behavioural style originally proposed by Thomas *et al.* (1963) has been shown to be significantly
related to children's responses to specific life events (e.g. Dunn *et al.*,
1981) and to be a significant predictor of later behaviour disturbance
(Thomas *et al.*, 1968; Graham *et al.*, 1973). Temperament has been put
forward as a major influence on children's vulnerability to a broad range
of stresses and therefore of central importance in understanding the
development of psychopathology (Rutter, 1981). It has also been placed
as a central construct in a theory of abnormal development based on the
match (goodness of fit) between the child and his physical and social
environment (Thomas & Chess, 1977, 1980). On the other hand major
criticisms have been made both in terms of how temperament is conceptualized and in how it is measured. Bates (1980) has suggested that
the concept of difficult temperament, which was utilized in many of the
predictions of later behaviour problems, was not primarily a characteristic of the child but rather a reflection of the parents' perception of the
child's behaviour. The response to this critique has been made in a
number of papers (Kagan, 1982; Plomin, 1982*a*; Rothbart, 1982) discussing the conflicting propositions that (*a*) temperament represents a
constitutionally based but environmentally modified characteristic of the
child (Thomas *et al.*, 1982), (*b*) that temperament is closely linked to
social relationships of the child especially that with the mother (Dunn
& Kendrick, 1982; Hinde *et al.*, 1982; Stevenson-Hinde & Simpson,
1982) and (*c*) that temperament (especially difficult temperament) has
to be seen as inextricably linked to parental perceptions of the child
(Bates, 1980). It is of course not possible to obtain data on temperament
from parents' reports without such information being influenced by
parental perceptions and, as Plomin (1982*b*) has argued, recourse to
studies of concurrent validity will not resolve the issue, since there is no
agreement on what constitutes an acceptable criterion against which
ratings can be compared. However, the evidence that parental ratings
of temperament do correlate with some independent measures of behaviour (Dunn & Kendrick, 1980; Wilson & Mathney, 1983) is sufficient
to counter the strong form of Bates' argument. The more intractable
problem of the status of difficult temperament and the relationship

between this concept and that of problem behaviour remains to be resolved (Stevenson & Graham, 1982; Wolkind & DeSalis, 1982). To what extent can behavioural style be distinguished from behavioural content, when the latter is the basis for judgements of disturbance?

The possibility of biases in parental ratings of their children's temperament has been directly studied by Lyon & Plomin (1981). They obtained ratings on the EASI Temperament Survey (Buss & Plomin, 1975) for both members of a twin pair by each of their parents and the rating by the parents of their own and their spouse's temperament. They tested specifically whether parents tended to project their perception of their own temperament into their report of their children's temperament. They found no evidence of such projection in the rating of the temperament of others. However, Lyon & Plomin (1981) did not have a large enough sample of twins to establish whether such projection is more or less likely with children at different ages. It is possible that such biases in rating are more likely with younger children when behaviour is more open to distorted reporting or possibly a type of identification takes place for parents as their children become older. The present study was undertaken to extend the Lyon & Plomin procedure to a sample of twins from a wider age range. Results are also reported on the issue of inter-rater reliability and the comparison of monozygotic and dizygotic twin similarity is made to indicate possible age differences in genetic influences on temperament.

METHODS

Sample of Twins

A register of child twins at the Department of Psychology, University of Surrey, provided a sampling frame for this study. It was assembled from two sources: 624 twin pairs from the general population had been collected at various times from volunteer sources by the Institute of Psychiatry, London, and a further 315 twin pairs had been recruited via the Twins Clubs Association. The 939 twin pairs were all under the age of 12 years with a large majority under 5 years of age. They cannot necessarily be considered representative of the total population of twin pairs since they were all volunteered for participation by their parents. However, they were not selected because of the presence or absence of any specific characteristic in the twins or their families.

Questionnaires were sent to 939 twin pairs asking for both the parents to complete ratings of their own, their spouse's and twins' temperament.

Despite requesting cooperation from both parents nearly two-thirds (*n* = 576) of those families contacted returned complete data (61 per cent response rate).

Zygosity

All parents were asked to complete a questionnaire concerning certain general and specific physical and other similarities between the twins (Nichols & Bilbro, 1966). The accuracy of this Twin Similarity Questionnaire (TSQ) when compared to blood typing for zygosity designation has been estimated as between 90 and 95 per cent (Loehlin & Nichols, 1976). A previous study has demonstrated that a similar degree of accuracy can be obtained with older British twins (Graham *et al.*, 1985). The criterion used for designating a pair as monozygotic was that they should obtain 85 per cent or more of the maximum total possible score on the TSQ. Of the 576 pairs on which information was available 35 could not be assigned a zygosity (6·1 per cent).

The remaining twins comprised 106 monozygotic male (MZM), 113 monozygotic female (MZF), 129 dizygotic male (DZM), 85 dizygotic female (DZF) and 108 dizygotic opposite sex pairs (DZO).

Age Ranges

The sample of twins was divided into three age ranges for purposes of data analysis: 0–2 years, 2–5 years and over 5 years of age. The final number of twin pairs in each zygosity group in each age range is given in Table 1.

Temperament Measures

A number of questionnaires are available for the measurement of temperament (McNeil & Persson-Blennow, 1982). In part the present

Table 1. Breakdown of sample of twin pairs by age group and zygosity

Age range (years)	Zygosity				
	MZM	MZF	DZM	DZF	DZO
0–2	22	19	28	17	32
2–5	59	74	78	55	68
5+	25	20	23	13	8

study was designed to replicate and extend the earlier investigation by Lyon & Plomin (1981) and it was therefore necessary to use similar measures. A central concern in these studies is the relationships between child and adult temperament ratings. At the time of the Lyon & Plomin work they concluded that the EASI Temperament Survey (Buss & Plomin, 1975) was the only instrument that provided comparable scales for adults and children and since that time no equivalent scales have been published.

Each parent was asked to complete the 20-item version of the EASI for each of their twins. This version of the EASI includes five items on each of the temperament dimensions Emotionality, Activity, Sociability and Impulsivity. Each item was rated on a five-point scale from 'strongly disagree' to 'strongly agree' in terms of whether the item described the behaviour of the child. These items were scored from 1 to 5 with appropriate reversal of scoring for certain items. The parents were asked to complete separate EASI questionnaires on their own and their spouse's temperament. These were 25 item versions of the EASI which included additional Emotionality items. However, for ease of comparison with the child questionnaires the ratings of adults were only summated to obtain total scores on the four original scales. The following are examples of typical items from the EASI:

He/she is easy going or happy-go-lucky with others.
He/she fidgets at meals and similar occasions.
He/she prefers to play by him/herself rather than with others.
He/she gets bored easily.

The parents were specifically asked not to compare answers with each other until each had completed all the questionnaires. Inspection of the completed questionnaires showed there to be few alterations to the ratings and of course these need not necessarily have been made in response to knowledge of the spouse's rating.

Statistical Analysis

The data were analysed using the SPSS programmes. To obtain intra-class correlations a data file was constructed that contained double entries. That is each twin's data were entered twice under each of two separate variables. Intra-class correlations are equivalent to Pearson product moment correlations between these double entry variables. The factor analyses reported were principal factor solutions orthogonally rotated using the varimax criteria.

Factor Analyses of the Child EASI Terms

The factorial structure of the EASI has been extensively studied (e.g. Rowe & Plomin, 1977). Indeed successive versions of the scales have been developed in part to improve its factorial clarity. However, no previous studies have employed the scale with British children. It might be expected that a different factor structure could be obtained with this population of children. This may particularly be expected for the items concerned with Activity and Impulsivity since consistent cross-national differences in the rates of hyperactivity and attentional deficit have been reported (Rutter, 1984).

Separate factor analyses were conducted for mothers' and fathers' ratings of the first-born and second-born twins. These four analyses each recovered similar factor structures with five factors having eigenvalues greater than 1. One of the factor analyses of the fathers' ratings produced a sixth such factor. This factor structure obtained from parental ratings is similar to that found with American children. That is that the dimensions of Sociability and Emotionality emerge quite distinctly; however, Activity and Impulsivity are less clearly demarcated.

In order to maintain comparability with earlier reports based on the initial structure of the EASI Temperament Survey, the results in this paper will be summarized in terms of the Emotionality, Activity, Sociability and Impulsivity scores using a simple summation procedure for the items as originally devised for the American sample.

RESULTS

Mean Differences Between Groups

The main hypotheses in this study are to be tested using correlations and the differences between correlations. Before presenting these correlations it is of interest to establish whether there are any mean differences between groups that might influence the interpretation of the correlational analyses. In Table 2 the mean scores on each of the four EASI Temperament Scales are compared across zygosity groups. In only one case, father rating of activity, is there a significant difference. The Activity score of the DZ opposite sex twins is lower than that of the MZ and DZ same sex twins. As is usual in twin studies the DZ opposite sex twins will be excluded from MZ and DZ twin comparisons and this isolated mean difference will therefore not affect such comparisons.

Table 3 summarizes comparisons of the mean temperament scores of

Table 2. Mean differences in temperament scores by zygosity of twin pairs

	Total (n = 1082)		Monozygotic (n = 438)	Dizygotic		
	Mean	SD	Mean	Same sex n = 428 Mean	Opposite sex n = 216 Mean	One-way ANOVA F P
Mother rating						
Emotionality	15·27	3·77	15·13	15·48	14·91	1·86 n.s.
Activity	18·13	3·90	18·30	18·18	17·65	2·03 n.s.
Sociability	16·86	3·24	17·12	16·80	16·59	2·11 n.s.
Impulsivity	16·01	3·66	15·93	16·08	16·27	0·60 n.s.
Father rating						
Emotionality	15·19	3·37	15·08	15·13	15·39	0·66 n.s.
Activity	18·22	3·51	18·58	18·22	17·73	4·20 P < 0·05
Sociability	16·49	3·12	16·31	16·75	16·31	2·41 n.s.
Impulsivity	16·06	3·40	15·87	16·26	16·00	1·33 n.s.

Table 3. Mean differences between boys and girls by age group and mother and father ratings

	Emotionality		Activity		Sociability		Impulsivity	
	Mother	Father	Mother	Father	Mother	Father	Mother	Father
Total	n.s.	n.s.	B > G**	B > G**	B > G*	n.s.	B > G**	B > G*
0–2 years	n.s.	n.s.	n.s.	n.s.	n.s.	n.s.	n.s.	n.s.
2–5 years	n.s.	n.s.	n.s.	n.s.	n.s.	n.s.	B > G**	n.s.
5+ years	n.s.	n.s.	B > G**	B > G**	n.s.	n.s.	n.s.	B > G*

n.s. $P > 0.05$; *$P < 0.05$; **$P < 0.01$.
Note. B > G — Boys show significantly higher mean than girls.

boys and girls at different ages. The most consistent results are that boys are rated as more active than girls by both parents and this becomes significant as they get older. A similar pattern is seen for Impulsivity. The only other significant difference was obtained with mothers' rating of Sociability for all age groups combined (boys = 17·11, girls = 16·61).

Inter-rater Reliability

The complete set of ratings obtained from the families of twins provides the opportunity of establishing in a variety of ways the reliability of ratings of temperament. The results of inter-rater correlations based on a number of comparisons are presented in Table 4. These show that inter-rater reliability is consistently in the region of 0·5 both for child and adult subjects and regardless of the temperament dimension. These correlations vary very little when computed separately for boys and girls, for different age groups and for MZ and DZ twins.

Assortative Mating and Projective Rating

An indication of whether assortative mating is taking place can be obtained from the phenotypic correlations between marriage partners. In Table 5 these are shown by the correlation between mother's rating of herself and father's rating of himself and also by the correlation of mother's rating of her husband with the father's rating of his wife. In all cases these correlations are extremely small and negative. The differences between the dimensions of temperament are negligible though consistently Activity shows the highest negative marital correlation.

The results in Table 5 include further correlations which are relevant to the issue of whether projection takes place in rating of spouse. If the correlations between the mother's rating of self and the mother's rating of her husband exceed the other marital correlations above then this

Table 4. Inter-rater reliabilities for the total sample

Correlation	Emotionality	Activity	Sociability	Impulsivity
Mother/self with father rating wife	0·57	0·54	0·58	0·40
Father/self with mother rating husband	0·61	0·53	0·56	0·50
Mother and father rating child	0·51	0·56	0·52	0·52

Table 5. Correlation to test for assortative mating and projective rating (all age groups combined)

Correlation	Emotionality	Activity	Sociability	Impulsivity
Mother/self with father/self	−0·06	−0·11	−0·02	−0·08
Mother/husband with father/wife	−0·10	−0·14	−0·01	−0·13
Mother/self with mother/husband	−0·00	−0·07	0·06	−0·04
Father/self with father/wife	−0·00	−0·08	0·06	−0·12

indicates projection. That is a tendency to rate the spouse in ways that are similar to the person's views of their own temperament. The same reasoning applied to the father's self-rating correlation with father's rating of wife. The results in Table 5 show no evidence that projection takes place in the rating of spouse; indeed if anything the self and spouse ratings are lower than the ratings potentially contaminated by projection.

The presence of projection in ratings can also be explored in the ratings by parents of their children. In this case the comparison can be made between the correlations of a parent's rating of the child and the parents' temperament rated by themselves and by their spouse. If a parent's rating of the child correlates higher with their self-rating than with their temperament as rated by their spouse, then projection can be postulated as having taken place. In the case of parent projection into ratings of their children it is important to analyse the results separately for same sex and different sex parent/child pairs. Such effects may be restricted to one or other of these pairings and may in fact act in opposite directions depending on the parent/child sex match.

The results presented in Table 6 are restricted to all age groups combined. There were no discernible trends in the separate analyses for projection to be increasing or decreasing with age. It can be seen in Table 6 that for fathers no projection is detectable on any of the temperament dimensions for either boys or girls. There is some indication however that in mothers projection is taking place in their ratings of

Table 6. Comparison of correlations between parents' rating of boys and girls temperament and their own and their spouses' rating of their own temperament (all age groups combined)

Mother's rating of child	Boys		Girls	
	Mother rated by		Mother rated by	
	self	husband	self	husband
Emotionality	0·21	0·09	0·31	0·11
Activity	0·08	0·13	0·07	0·11
Sociability	0·19	0·10	0·14	0·05
Impulsivity	0·10	0·03	0·12	0·05

Father's rating of child	Father rated by		Father rated by	
	self	wife	self	wife
Emotionality	0·16	0·16	0·09	0·25
Activity	0·08	0·05	0·06	0·13
Sociability	0·05	0·09	0·06	0·14
Impulsivity	0·12	0·01	0·00	0·13

Emotionality in both their sons and daughters. Of these correlations for boys (0·21 and 0·09) and girls (0·31 and 0·11) only the latter are significantly different ($P < 0.05$).

Origins of Individual Differences in Temperament

By obtaining independent ratings of the twins' temperament from mothers and fathers it is possible to derive three separate estimates of within-pair twin similarity. Intra-class correlations for mothers' ratings and for fathers' ratings can be calculated. In addition the correlation can be derived between mother's rating of one twin and the father's rating of the co-twin. These latter correlations are reported in Table 7 separately for MZ and DZ same sex twins in each of the three age groups.

The advantage of the twin similarity correlation obtained from different parents rating the two twins is that it overcomes an often-made criticism of the twin method, i.e. that greater similarities are obtained for MZ twins through biases in parental ratings. It has been shown earlier that parental bias resulting from projection is minimal. This however does not mean that MZ twins may not be spuriously rated as more similar than DZ twins. However, since the earlier results show a less than perfect correlation between parental ratings of the same twin, the use of the mother and father as relatively independent raters of the twins reduces substantially the possibilities for contamination of the ratings by spurious contrast effects and other biases.

The previously reported finding that the inter-rater reliabilities did not differ for MZ and DZ pairs means that even if such biases are present they are not affecting the ratings of twins of different zygosity in dissimilar ways. This is crucial for the validity of the twin method in identifying genetic influences on individual differences.

In trying to obtain indications of genetic influences on temperament at different ages the differences between the MZ and DZ same sex correlations have been calculated. However, the estimation of broad heritability has not been reported and neither has the fitting of more complex biometrical models been attempted. In common with previous twin studies based upon parental reports the obtained correlations do not necessarily conform to the full set of assumptions underlying the twin method (Plomin, 1981). Some of the DZ correlations are negative and on occasion the heritabilities that would be obtained exceed the theoretical maximum of one.

For Emotionality there are no indications of genetic influences on individual influences in boys. However, for girls there are consistent indications of strong genetic influences at all ages (Table 7). The unweighted average difference in MZ and DZ correlations based on independent mother and father ratings is 0·67.

The results for Activity in Table 7 are somewhat different. Here the influence of genetic factors is seen for both boys and girls. Again in both sexes the size of this effect is greater with the older age ranges of twins.

With Sociability a similar pattern of genetic influences is found to that obtained for Emotionality. However, for Sociability there is a slightly stronger indication that individual differences in boys may be under some genetic control. Impulsivity demonstrates a more modest role of

Table 7. Intra-class correlations for MZ and DZ twin pairs by sex and age based on mother's and father's separate ratings of each twin

	MZ	DZ	(MZ–DZ)
Boys			
Emotionality			
0–2 years	−0·05	0·09	−0·14
2–5 years	0·27	0·05	0·22
5+ years	−0·14	−0·04	−0·10
Activity			
0–2 years	0·21	0·04	0·17
2–5 years	0·31	−0·17	0·48
5+ years	0·30	−0·28	0·58
Sociability			
0–2 years	0·22	0·18	0·04
2–5 years	0·38	−0·18	0·56
5+ years	−0·06	−0·23	0·17
Impulsivity			
0–2 years	−0·19	0·34	−0·53
2–5 years	0·22	−0·11	0·33
5+ years	0·14	−0·31	0·45
Girls			
Emotionality			
0–2 years	0·61	−0·15	0·76
2–5 years	0·40	−0·01	0·41
5+ years	0·48	−0·35	0·83
Activity			
0–2 years	−0·06	−0·41	0·35
2–5 years	0·37	0·00	0·37
5+ years	0·26	−0·42	0·68
Sociability			
0–2 years	0·36	−0·25	0·51
2–5 years	0·44	−0·06	0·50
5+ years	0·59	−0·39	0·98
Impulsivity			
0–2 years	0·16	−0·19	0·35
2–5 years	0·37	−0·02	0·39
5+ years	−0·04	−0·25	0·21

genetic factors but one that is present for both boys and girls. It is seen at all ages, except for the youngest group of boys.

DISCUSSION

The main findings from the study are that there are a few sex differences in the ratings of temperament with older boys being rated as both more active and impulsive than girls and an overall tendency for mothers to see their boys as more sociable than their girls. The factor structure for British children's rating on the EASI was very similar to that obtained with American children. The findings on inter-rater reliability were that with both child and adult subjects reliabilities were only modest (unweighted average 0·53). There was no evidence for assortative mating with respect to phenotypic measures of temperament. In rating their spouses there was no evidence of projection by either parent. However, there was a tendency for mothers to rate their children's Emotionality to be slightly more like their own Emotionality; this was the only indication of projection by either parent in their rating of their children's temperament. Finally, there was some evidence of differential heritability for temperament dimensions that showed some distinct sex differences.

The findings are in agreement with Lyon & Plomin (1981) in the absence of parental projection in the ratings of temperament and on the modest inter-rater reliability of parents' ratings of their children. It should be noted that the present study extends the age range to both younger (less than 2 years old) and older (over 6 years old) children than those studied by Lyon & Plomin.

Before considering any possible conclusions about the origin of individual differences in temperament, it is necessary to establish whether the assumptions underlying the twin method have been met. The first of these concerns whether twins are subject to influences on individual differences that are different from those of the general population. This study was not designed to test this assumption; however, the validity of generalizations from twin data on temperament has been established (Buss & Plomin, 1975).

The second major assumption is that members of MZ and DZ twin pairs share a common environment to the same extent and the findings of the present study were consistent with this. Of particular relevance were the inter-rater reliabilities for MZ and DZ twins. If biases were present making parents respond more similarly to the twins in MZ than DZ pairs, then such a shared set would result in higher parental agreement on the rating of an MZ twin. The findings were that inter-rater reliabilities were the same for twins of different zygosity.

There are aspects of the data that indicate that caution is necessary in the interpretation of the findings. The occasional negative DZ correlation is not consistent with a simple model of influences on individual differences. It is necessary to invoke competitive or compensatory within-pair effects to account for these negative correlations. For these reasons we have been cautious in the genetic interpretation of our data. Heritabilities have not been calculated nor common or specific environmental contributions estimated. Rather differences in MZ and DZ intra-pair similarities have been taken as ordinally related to possible genetic effects. It is with this caution that we now go on to discuss the zygosity differences in similarity.

The findings from the present study are not unusual in suggesting differential genetic influences for temperament dimensions (e.g. Cohen *et al.*, 1977; Torgersen & Kringlen, 1978; Goldsmith & Gottesman, 1981; Wilson, 1982). However, as Plomin (1982*b*) has cautioned, it is necessary to undertake a synthesis of findings from a number of similar studies before conclusions of differential heritability can be reached. However, in one respect the data in the present study do suggest a relatively unexplored possibility. That is that the sex differences in heritability show different changes over time. For example, the pattern of intraclass correlations for Emotionality indicate a strong genetic influence on girls at all ages, but not at any age for boys. In contrast Activity shows increasing genetic influences in both sexes as the children move from infancy to middle childhood. Relatively few of the published twin studies on temperament have been large enough to be sensibly analysed for separate genetic influences on boys and girls. Goldsmith & Gottesman (1981) do present such findings on changes in correlations over time in boys and girls MZ and DZ pairs. However, their measures of temperament were not sufficiently similar to the EASI scales for direct comparisons to be made.

The importance of continuing to investigate influences on temperament separately for the sexes has been made on other grounds by Hinde *et al.* (1982). They found no sex differences in terms of mean temperament scores but found consistent differences in terms of correlations with mother–child interaction. Often these correlations were such that they would cancel one another out if the data from the two sexes were merged.

It is not just twin studies and family studies that have demonstrated the importance of considering the sexes separately when trying to identify influences on temperament. For example, Harburg *et al.* (1982) have shown certain temperamental traits in adult males (Anger and Impulsivity) to be linked to blood markers whereas other traits in females (Sensation seeking) show these links.

We consider that the results presented in this paper indicate the potential value in extending the usual twin study to include data on other family members, in this case parents. As well as providing the opportunity to investigate certain measurement artifacts (such as projection) the data from the two parents provide independent ratings from which heritabilities can be calculated. The data set can of course be extended to include non-twin siblings which would allow the investigation of the influences of the twin situation on temperamental similarity.

The more extensive use of data from families with twins provides the opportunity to explore a range of influences on temperament. The possibility that there is sex limitation in the effects of genetic influences on temperament certainly provides a suitable subject for such studies.

REFERENCES

Bates, J. E. (1980). The concept of difficult temperament. *Merrill-Palmer Quarterly*, **26**, 299-319.

Buss, A. H. & Plomin, R. (1975). *A Temperament Theory of Personality Development*. New York: Wiley-Interscience.

Cohen, D. J., Dibble, E. & Grawe, J. M. (1977). Parental style. Mother's and father's perceptions of their relations with twin children. *Archives of General Psychiatry*, **34**, 445-451.

Dunn, J. & Kendrick, C. (1980). Studying temperament and parent–child interaction: Comparison of interview and direct observation. *Developmental Medicine and Child Neurology*, **22**, 484-496.

Dunn, J. & Kendrick, C. (1982). Temperamental differences, family relationships and young children's responses to change within the family. In M. Rutter (ed.), *Temperamental Differences in Infants and Young Children*; CIBA Foundation Symposium No. 89, pp. 87-101. London: Pitman.

Dunn, J., Kendrick, C. & MacNamee, R. (1981). The reactions of first born children to the birth of a sibling: Mothers' reports. *Journal of Child Psychology and Psychiatry*, **22**, 1-18.

Goldsmith, H. H. & Gottesman, I. I. (1981). Origins of variation in behavioural style: A longitudinal study of temperament in young twins. *Child Development*, **52**, 91-103.

Graham, P., Rutter, M. & George, S. (1973). Temperamental characteristics as predictors of behavioural disorders in children. *American Journal of Orthopsychiatry*, **43**, 328-339.

Graham, P., Stevenson, J., Fredman, G. & McLoughlin, V. (1985). A twin study of genetic influence on behavioural deviance. *Journal of the American Academy of Child Psychiatry* (in press).

Harburg, E., Gleibermann, L., Gershowitz, H., Ozgoren, F. & Kulik, C. L. (1982). Twelve blood markers and measures of temperament. *British Journal of Psychiatry,* **140**, 401-409.

Hinde, R. A., Easton, D. F., Meller, R. E. & Tamplin, A. M. (1982). Temperamental characteristics of 3–4-year-olds and mother–infant interaction. In M. Rutter (ed.), *Temperamental Differences in Infants and Young Children*; CIBA Foundation Symposium No. 89, pp. 66-80. London: Pitman.

Kagan, J. (1982). The construct of difficult temperament: A reply to Thomas, Chess & Korn. *Merrill-Palmer Quarterly,* **28**, 21-24.

Loehlin, J. C. & Nichols, R. C. (1976). *Heredity, Environment and Personality: A Study of 850 Sets of Twins.* Austin: University of Texas Press.

Lyon, M. E. & Plomin, R. (1981). The measurement of temperament using parental ratings. *Journal of Child Psychology and Psychiatry,* **22**, 47-53.

McNeil, T. F. & Persson-Blennow, I. (1982). Temperament questionnaires in clinical research. In M. Rutter (ed.), *Temperamental Differences in Infants and Young Children*; CIBA Foundation Symposium No. 89, pp. 20-31. London: Pitman.

Nichols, R. C. & Bilbro, W. C. (1966). The diagnosis of twin zygosity. *Acta Genetica et Statistica Medica,* **16**, 265-275.

Plomin, R. (1981). Heredity and temperament: A comparison of twin data for self-report questionnaires, parental ratings and objectively assessed behaviour. In L. Gedda, P. Parisi & W. E. Nance (eds.), *Progress in Clinical and Biological Research,* vol. 69**B**. *Twin Research 3,* part B: *Intelligence, Personality and Development.* New York: Alan R. Liss.

Plomin, R. (1982*a*). The difficult concept of temperament: A response to Thomas, Chess & Korn. *Merrill-Palmer Quarterly,* **28**, 25-33.

Plomin, R. (1982*b*). Childhood temperament. In E. Lakey & A. Kazdin (eds.), *Advances in Clinical Child Psychology,* vol. 6. New York: Plenum.

Rothbart, M. K. (1982). The concept of difficult temperament. A critical analysis of Thomas, Chess & Korn. *Merrill-Palmer Quarterly,* **28**, 35-40.

Rowe, D. C. & Plomin, R. (1977). Temperament in early childhood. *Journal of Personality Assessment,* **41**, 150-156.

Rutter, M. (1981). Stress, coping and development, some issues and some questions. *Journal of Child Psychology and Psychiatry,* **22**, 323-356.

Rutter, M. (1982). Temperament concepts, issues and problems. In M. Rutter (ed.), *Temperamental Differences in Infants and Young Children*; CIBA Foundation Symposium No. 89, pp. 1-16. London: Pitman.

Rutter, M. (1984). Beahvioural studies: Questions and findings on the concept of a distinctive syndrome. In M. Rutter (ed.), *Developmental Neuropsychiatry,* pp. 259-279. Edinburgh: Churchill Livingstone.

Stevenson, J. & Graham, P. (1982). Temperament: A consideration of concepts and methods. In M. Rutter (ed.), *Temperamental Differences in Infants and Young Children*; CIBA Foundation Symposium No. 89, pp. 36-46. London: Pitman.

Stevenson-Hinde, J. & Simpson, A. E. (1982). Temperament and relationships. In M. Rutter (ed.), *Temperamental Differences in Infants and Young Children*; CIBA Foundation Symposium No. 89, pp. 51-62. London: Pitman.

Thomas, A. & Chess, S. (1977). *Temperament and Development.* New York: Brunner/Mazel.

Thomas, A. & Chess, S. (1980). *The Dynamics of Psychological Development.* New York: Brunner/Mazel.

Thomas, A., Chess, S. & Birch, H. (1968). *Temperament and Behavior Disorders in Children.* New York: New York University Press.

Thomas, A., Chess, S. Birch, H., Hertzig, M. E. & Korn, S. (1963). *Behavioral Individuality in Early Childhood*. New York: New York University Press.

Thomas, A., Chess, S. & Korn, S. (1982). The reality of difficult temperament. *Merrill-Palmer Quarterly*, **28**, 1-20.

Torgersen, A. M. & Kringlen, E. (1978). Genetic aspects of temperamental differences in twins. *Journal of the American Academy of Child Psychiatry*, **17**, 433-444.

Wilson, R. S. (1982). Intrinsic determinants of temperament. In M. Rutter (ed.), *Temperamental Differences in Infants and Young Children*; CIBA Foundation Symposium No. 89, pp. 121-140. London: Pitman.

Wilson, R. S. & Matheny, A. P. (1983). Assessment of temperament in infant twins. *Developmental Psychology*, **19**, 172-183.

Wolkind, S. & DeSalis, W. (1982). Infant temperament, maternal mental state and child behavioural problems. In M. Rutter (ed.), *Temperamental Differences in Infants and Young Children*; CIBA Foundation Symposium No. 89, pp. 221-234. London: Pitman.

21

Temperament in Infants Born Prematurely

Frank Oberklaid
Royal Children's Hospital, Melbourne, Australia
Margot Prior
Latrobe University, Bundoora, Victoria, Australia
Terrence Nolan
Royal Children's Hospital, Melbourne, Australia
Patricia Smith and Hilary Flavell
Latrobe University, Bundoora, Victoria, Australia

The temperament of infants born prematurely was studied to examine further the notion that prematurity may be a risk factor for an infant's subsequent social interaction. The Infant Temperament Questionnaire of Carey and McDevitt was revised and revalidated for an Australian population and sent to mothers of infants who had been born prematurely (36 weeks or less) and who were aged 4 to 8 months (corrected for prematurity). Two hundred and twenty-six questionnaires were distributed and 110 (49%) returned. There were no differences between respondents and nonrespondents with respect to gestational age, birth weight, method of delivery, Apgar scores, or perinatal complications.

When compared to a control group (N = 240) of infants born at

---

Reprinted with permission from *Developmental and Behavioral Pediatrics*, 1985, Vol. 6, 57–61. Copyright 1985 by Williams & Wilkins Co.
Supported by a grant from the Royal Children's Hospital Research Foundation.
Presented in part at the Society for Behavioural Pediatrics Annual Meeting, San Francisco, April 1984.

term and who came from families with similar demographic charac-
teristics, infants born prematurely did not differ significantly on any
of the nine temperament dimensions. Both groups had similar pro-
portions of "easy," "difficult," and "slow to warm up" infants, and
there were no significant differences in maternal global ratings of
temperament between the two groups. Comparisons of infants of less
than 33 weeks gestation gave results similar to those reported above.
These data indicate that infants born prematurely have temperament
profiles at 4 to 8 months similar to infants born at term.

There is a considerable literature indicating that premature infants
are an "at risk" group in social interactions as well as in physical and
cognitive development,[1-3] and they are overrepresented in child abuse
and failure to thrive populations.[4] While it is increasingly recognized
that the quality of the interaction between infant and care giver is critical
in determining outcomes for infants, [5,6] it has been suggested that premature infants are "behaviorally more difficult social partners."[2] This
is particularly the case where prematurity is associated with neonatal
medical problems.[7] The development of preterm infants can be facilitated provided that the care giver and infant negotiate an optimal interactional style.[8,9] However, this is made more difficult by the reported
behavior of premature infants. It has been stated that premature infants
are often deficient in their capacity to elicit and sustain social interaction,[10] while Field has observed that premature infants are more passive
and less responsive to the social world than full-term infants, and that
their mothers are in turn more stimulating, intrusive, and controlling
than mothers of full terms.[11]

Other workers also have reported that mothers of premature babies
behave differently towards their babies when compared to full-term
infants.[12] However, it is suggested that such differences dissipate with
age and that older premature infants become more similar to their full-
term peers.[13]

The transactional model of development[14] emphasizes the multiple
and complex influences that determine the patterns of the interaction
and underlie the adaptation and adjustment between premature infants
and their care givers. This point is also emphasized in temperament
research,[15,16] where it has been argued that the inborn characteristics of
the infant, in particular the individually typical ways of relating to the
environment, exert a strong influence on the social interactions of the
child and the ways in which his behavior is reciprocated by care givers.

Field and coworkers[7] reported that preterm infants (all of whom had respiratory distress syndrome) were rated by their mothers as more difficult in temperament at both 4 and 8 months of age. The fact that the infants in this study had medical problems may have been a major influence on their being perceived as difficult. However, if these data are considered together with Goldberg's data[2,17] relating to the qualitative differences in interaction patterns of preterm dyads, some relationship between prematurity and difficult temperament may be hypothesized. If it were the case that these infants were rated as difficult by their mothers, it could be suggested that this would be an added dimension of risk in their development. Studies of various groups of children rated as having a difficult temperament have indicated that such children are more likely than those rated as easy to develop behavior and adjustment problems.[15,18,19]

In this study we report the results of the assessment of temperament on a cohort of 110 infants born prematurely.

METHOD

The Infant Temperament Questionnaire (ITQ)[20] of Carey and McDevitt is a 95-item questionnaire for infants aged 4 to 8 months which uses a 6-point rating scale and is completed by the care giver. The items contain precise descriptions of behavior in a variety of daily occurring situations, and the care giver is instructed to rate on the basis of current infant behavior. Scores on nine dimensions of temperament are derived for each infant (activity, adaptability, intensity, approach/withdrawal, mood, rhythmicity, threshold of responsiveness, persistence, and distractibility). An algorithm developed by Carey permits categorization of infants into easy, difficult, slow to warm up, and intermediate groups.

The ITQ was adapted for use with Australian populations. A number of items were altered to conform to Australian language usage, and the instrument was revalidated on a sample of 240 Australian infants.[21] The revised ITQ was mailed to parents along with a face sheet requesting demographic information. Mothers were asked whether their infant had colic, sleep problems, and excessive crying and rated each behavior on a 4-point scale ranging from none to severe. They also rated the temperament of their infant on a 5-point scale, ranging from much easier than average to much more difficult than average.

Names and addresses of infants born prematurely (gestation 36 weeks or less) and who were aged 4 to 8 months (corrected for prematurity) at the time of the study were obtained from three Melbourne metropolitan hospitals. All of these infants were included, and a total of 226 questionnaires was dispatched together with a cover letter inviting parents to participate in the study. Parents were asked to complete the ITQ and face sheet and return them in a stamped, addressed envelope provided.

Details of the births of the infants were obtained by perusing hospital records. Gestational age, weight, type of delivery, and Apgar scores were transcribed directly from the medical record. Because the intensity of resuscitation and extent of any complications were not objectively recorded in the medical history, a 5-point rating scale was derived for both these variables. For resuscitation the scale ranged from 1 (no resuscitation required) to 5 (required intubation and initial manual ventilation). The complications scale ranged from 1 (no complications) to 5 (severe/extensive complications). All ratings were made according to very specific predetermined guidelines by one trained nurse who was otherwise not involved in the study and therefore blind as to temperament ratings of the infants.

Results from this cohort of infants born prematurely were compared with data from a study of 240 infants drawn from a similar (Melbourne) population and which had formed the study cohort for revalidation of the ITQ for Australian populations.[21]

RESULTS

Of the total of 226 questionnaires dispatched, 110 (49%) were returned in time for analysis. There were no differences between respondents and nonrespondents in gestational age, weight, sex, type of delivery, Apgar scores, amount of resuscitation required, and the level of complications (Table 1). Sixty-three percent of the infants were male, and 37% were female. Fifty-five percent were first born, 30% second born, and 15% later born. Mean maternal age at the time of birth was 28.5 years, and 99% of mothers were married. Parental education was normally distributed and ranged from Year 8 of secondary school through to tertiary graduate.

Data from this cohort of premature infants were compared with data from the sample of infants born at term. The two samples did not differ on the demographic characteristics sampled—maternal education, maternal age, infant's birth order, or sex (Table 2).

The means and standard deviations were then computed for each of

TABLE 1. Respondents and Nonrespondents—Comparisons of Infant Variables

	Respondents (N = 113)	Nonrespondents (N = 133)		
Gestational age (mean)	34.08 wk (SD 2.71)	34.80 wk (SD 2.60)	$t = 0.238$	NS
Weight (mean)	2311 g (SD 634)	2250 g (SD 650)	$t = 0.649$	NS
Sex				
Male	71 (63%)	80 (60.2%)	$\chi^2 = 0.19$	NS
Female	42 (37%)	53 (39.8%)		
Delivery				
Normal	42 (37%)	53 (40%)	$\chi^2 = 0.163$	NS
Forceps	25 (22%)	28 (21%)		
Cesarian	46 (41%)	52 (39%)		
Apgar (1 min)	6.8	6.8	$t = 1.49$	NS
(mean, 5 min)	9.7	9.6	$t = 0.475$	NS
Resuscitation				
1	7 (6.2%)	4 (3%)		
2	42 (37.2%)	52 (39%)		
3	35 (31%)	39 (29%)	$\chi^2 = 1.45$	NS
4	5 (4.4%)	8 (6%)		
5	2 (1.8%)	5 (4%)		
Not known	22 (19.4%)	25 (18.5%)		
Complications				
1	49 (44%)	41 (30.8%)		
2	27 (24%)	45 (33.8%)		
3	23 (21%)	28 (21%)	$\chi^2 = 1.81$	NS
4	6 (5.4%)	16 (12%)		
5	6 (5.4%)	2 (1.5%)		

TABLE 2. Comparison of Maternal Education, Maternal Age, Infant's Birth Order, and Sex between Premature and Control Groups

	Premature		Control		Student's t-Test
	Mean	(SD)	Mean	(SD)	
Maternal education	3.61	(1.21)	3.81	(1.19)	1.44 (NS)
Maternal age	28.53	(4.89)	28.07	(4.65)	0.84 (NS)
Infant's birth order	1.66	(0.91)	1.87	(1.07)	1.83 (NS)

	Premature		Control		Chi-Square
	No.	%	No.	%	
Sex					
Male	69	(63%)	125	(52%)	3.46 (NS)
Female	41	(37%)	115	(48%)	

the nine temperament dimensions; these are shown in Table 3. The means from the premature sample did not differ from those obtained from the full-term sample on any dimension, thus indicating that mothers of premature infants did not rate their infants' behavior differently from mothers of full-term infants. The infants were then categorized into subgroups of "easy," "difficult," and "slow to warm up" according to Carey's formula[20] and again comparisons were made between the two samples (Table 4). The proportions of these subgroups were the same for the two samples. Contrary to prediction, premature infants were not rated as being more difficult than average.

We also examined the concordance between actual classification as difficult on the ITQ and mother's global opinion of the infant's temperament on the 5-point rating scale. Seven mothers (6.4%) rated their infants as more difficult than average; two of these infants were actually classified as difficult on the ITQ, while four were intermediate. By contrast 52% of mothers described their infants as easier than average, and 74% of these were classified as easy on the ITQ. The remainder described their infants as average on the 5-point global rating scale. Of the 10 infants classified as difficult on the Carey algorithm 8 were male and 2 female, 6 were first born, 3 were 7 months old, and 7 were 8 months old.

There were no differences between the easy, difficult, and slow to warm up groups in sex ($\chi^2 = 2.01$, NS), age ($\chi^2 = 6.88$, NS), birth order ($\chi^2 = 4.25$, NS), presence/absence of sleep problems ($\chi^2 = 6.64$, NS), or

TABLE 3. Temperament Ratings for Premature and Control Groups

Temperament Dimension	Premature Group		Control Group		Student's t-test
	Mean	SD	Mean	SD	
Activity	3.9393	1.1711	4.1159	1.0527	0.42	NS
Rhythmicity	2.5084	0.6960	2.7513	0.6717	0.91	NS
Approach/withdrawal	2.2748	0.5401	2.4036	0.5006	0.61	NS
Adaptability	2.0929	0.4656	2.1872	0.5324	0.46	NS
Intensity	3.3736	0.7874	3.1809	0.6416	0.63	NS
Mood	2.8597	0.7305	2.7973	0.5248	0.23	NS
Persistence	3.0272	0.3994	3.1408	0.5141	0.52	NS
Distractibility	2.3239	0.4364	2.3402	0.4623	0.09	NS
Threshold	3.6285	0.5267	3.6869	0.4541	0.28	NS

TABLE 4. Percentage of Easy, Difficult, and Slow to Warm Up Infants in Both Groups

Category	Premature (%)	Control (%)
Easy	43	37
Difficult	9	12
Slow to warm up	6.4	7

distribution of maternal educational level ($\chi^2 = 4.91$, NS). However, the groups were significantly different in the reported incidence of:

1. Colic—7 of 46 easy compared to 7 of 10 difficult infants were reported as having colic ($\chi^2 = 17.67$, $p < 0.005$)
2. Excessive crying—2 of 46 easy compared to 4 of 10 difficult infants were reported by their mothers as crying excessively ($\chi^2 = 10.84$, $p < 0.01$)
3. Mother's overall perception—babies classified as easy on the ITQ were more often perceived as easier than average ($\chi^2 = 27.97$, $p < 0.0001$).

We examined specifically the characteristics of the 17 infants of less than 33 weeks gestation. These infants did not differ from the rest of the group in terms of birth order, maternal age or education, presence of colic, excessive crying, or sleep problems. However, results for this latter group should be interpreted with caution because of the lower response rate. Of the 56 (one quarter of total) questionnaires sent to mothers with infants of less than 33 weeks gestation, only 17 (30%) were returned. This difference in return rate is significant ($\chi^2 = 10.01$, $p < 0.005$).

DISCUSSION

The group of premature infants included in this study appeared very similar to the full-term group with whom they were compared and were not rated as more difficult either via the ITQ or in their mothers' stated perception of their temperament. A number of studies have suggested that premature infants are an at risk group in the area of social interaction.[2,7,17] This is believed to be primarily a function of the fact that premature infants' behavior is less responsive to their care giver[10,11] and thus sets up a less than optimal reciprocal interaction. However, in this study preterm infants were not perceived by their mothers as difficult, at least during the 4 to 8 month period. There was a tendency for the opposite to occur, with more than half of the infants found to be "easy," a proportion somewhat greater than usually reported in temperament studies.

There may be a number of explanations for these findings. There is some evidence that early difficulties with premature infants in social/maternal interaction may dissipate with development and be little in evidence after 6 months of age.[2] Most studies of the behavior of premature infants have been during the hospitalization period—these infants were between 4 and 8 months (corrected for prematurity) and assessed on the basis of recent and current behavior; thus they may be outside the age group where such problems are apparent. It may be that the greatly increased sensitivity to problems of prematurity and the improved care and access facilities now available in maternity hospitals may have obviated some of the problems found by earlier researchers.

Sameroff[22] has argued that the notion of "high risk" should be placed into the context of the transactional model where both the child and the environment are seen as actively engaged with each other, changing and being changed by their interactions. This then emphasizes the importance of parental and other environmental attributes (e.g., socioeconomic status) in determining outcome. In our sample the mothers were older (mean age 28.5 years) than those reported in other studies of premature infants. They represented a cross section of educational achievement, and 99% were married and therefore presumably had some supports in their care giving. These mothers may bring to the child rearing situation greater maturity and capability. Thus the mothers were a low risk sample who were managing well and rating their babies positively. The majority of mothers in the sample reported an overall perception of the infants as "easier than average," suggesting minimization of any difficulties. It is of course possible that these mothers were sensitive to the "specialness" of prematurity and were biased towards understatement of problems. On the other hand, researchers have found mothers' assessment of their infants to be reasonably objective.[3]

From the point of view of the infant the only criterion for being included in the study was prematurity—gestation of 36 weeks or less. The infants were not as a group particularly at risk, that is, they were not extremely premature (mean age 34 weeks), and only a minority had experienced severe perinatal stress. Other reports have been of very sick prematures of lower gestational age. The study of Field et al, for example, was of infants with a mean gestational age of 32 weeks who had averaged 3 days on a ventilator.

There are two further issues that may be responsible for our results being at variance with predictions. Firstly there may have been a sampling bias, with a 49% compliance rate for return of questionnaires. It could be argued, for example, that mothers who are more irritated with their infants and are more high risk themselves are less likely to respond to a mail questionnaire. However, it would be just as feasible to argue that the opposite could be true—that mothers having more difficulties with their infants might see the completion of the questionnaires as an opportunity to focus some of their difficulties. The fact that no differences were found between respondents and nonrespondents on the birth history variables cited in Table 1 make it less likely that there was a systematic bias in response and that this affected the results in a predictable manner.

Finally there have been arguments questioning the validity of such measurements of infant temperament, and in particular the difficulties in distinguishing between characteristics of the mothers and the actual behavior of the infant.[23,24] Carey has strongly defended the concept of temperament and its measurement,[16] and the clinical validity of temperament has been well supported in an ever increasing number of studies.

Further studies are under way to attempt to tease out the various biological, behavioral, and environmental strands which influence the transaction between infant and caregiver and affect the outcome of high risk infants. Meanwhile, despite the reservations outlined above, we conclude that prematurity per se does not appear to affect observed temperament—that at least in the period of 4 to 8 months (corrected age) mothers of premature infants do not rate them as being any more difficult than those born at term.

REFERENCES

1. Siegal, L. S.: Reproductive, perinatal and environmental factors as predictors of the cognitive and language development of preterm and full term infants. Child Dev 54:1254-1268, 1983.
2. Goldberg, S.: Prematurity: Effects on parent-infant interaction. J Pediatr Psychol 3:137-144, 1978.
3. Field, T., Dempsey, J., Hallock, N., et al: The mother's assessment of the behaviour of her infant. Infant Behav Dev 1:156-167, 1978.
4. Thoman, E. B.: Infant development viewed within the mother-infant relationship, in Quilligan, E. Kretschmer, N. (eds): Perinatal Medicine. New York, Wiley, 1980.
5. Beckwith, L., Cohen, S. E.: Preterm birth: Hazardous obstetrical and postnatal events as related to caregiver-infant behaviour. Infant Behav Dev 1:403-411, 1978.
6. Cohen, S. E., Beckwith, L.: Preterm infant interaction with the caregiver in the first

year of life and competence at age two. Child Dev 50:767-776, 1979.

7. Field, T., Hallock, N., Ting, G., et al: A first year follow-up of high risk infants: Formulating a cumulative risk index. Child Dev 49:119-131, 1978.

8. Als, H.: The unfolding of behavioural organization in the face of biological violation, in Tronick, E. (ed): Social Interchange in Infancy: Affect, Cognition and Communication. Baltimore, University Park Press, 1982.

9. Thoman, E. B., Acebo, C., Dreyer, C., et al: Individuality in the interactive process, in Thomas, E. (ed): Origins of the Infant's Social Responsiveness. Hillsdale, NJ, Erlbaum, 1979.

10. Brazelton, T. B.: Behavioural competence of the newborn infant. Semin Perinatal 1:35-44, 1979.

11. Field, T. M.: Interaction of high risk infants: Quantitative and qualitative differences, in Sawin, D. B., Hawkins, R. C., Walker, L. D., et al (eds): The Exceptional Infant, vol 4. New York, Brunner/Mazel, 1980.

12. Di Vitto, B., Goldberg, S.: The development of early parent-infant interaction as a function of newborn medical status, in Field, T., Sostek, A., Goldberg, S., et al (eds): Infants Born at Risk. Holliswood, NY, Spectrum, 1980.

13. Brachfield, S., Goldberg, S.: Parent-infant interaction: Effects of newborn medical status on free play at 8 and 12 months. Presented at the South Eastern Conference on Human Development, Atlanta, 1978.

14. Sameroff, A. J., Chandler, M. J.: Reproductive risk and the continuum of caretaking casualty, in Horowitz, F. D., Hetherington, M., Scarr-Salapateks, L., et al (eds): Review of Child Development Research, vol. 4. Chicago, University of Chicago Press, 1975.

15. Thomas, A., Chess, S.: Temperament and Development. New York, Brunner/Mazel, 1977.

16. Carey, W. B.: The importance of temperament-environment interaction for child health and development, in Lewis, M., Rosenblum, L. (eds): The Uncommon Child, New York, Plenum Press, 1981.

17. Goldberg, S.: Premature birth: Consequences for the parent-infant relationship. Am Sci 67:214-220, 1979.

18. Graham, P., Rutter, M., George, S.: Temperamental characteristics as predictors of behaviour disorders in children. Am J Orthopsychiatry 43:328-339, 1973.

19. Earls, F.: Temperament characteristics and behaviour problems in three year old children. J Nerv Ment Dis 169:367-373, 1981.

20. Carey, W. B., McDevitt, S. C.: Revision of the Infant Temperament Questionnaire. Pediatrics 61:735-739, 1978.

21. Oberklaid, F., Prior, M., Golvan, D., et al: Temperament in Australian Infants. Aust Pediatr J 20:181-184, 1984.

22. Sameroff, A. J., Seifer, R.: Familial risk and child competence. Child Dev 54:1254-1268, 1983.

23. Vaughn, B., Taraldson, B., Crichton, L., et al: The assessment of infant temperament: A critique of the Carey Infant Temperament Questionnaire. Infant Behav Dev 4:1-17, 1981.

24. Vaughn, B., Deinard, A., Egeland, B.: Measuring temperament in pediatric practice. Pediatrics 96:510-514, 1980.

PART V: TEMPERAMENT STUDIES

22

Value of Difficult Temperament Among 7-Year-Olds in the General Population for Predicting Psychiatric Diagnosis at Age 12

Michel Maziade, Philippe Capéraà, Bruno Laplante, Maurice Boudreault, Jacques Thivierge, Robert Côté, and Pierrette Boutin

Laval University, Sainte Foy, Québec

The authors assessed the predictive value of "difficult" temperament, as defined in the New York Longitudinal Study, in 12-year-old children from the general population of Quebec City whose temperaments had been determined to be difficult or easy at age 7. The difficult and easy temperament groups were balanced for age, sex, and socioeconomic status. The authors used many convergent measuring devices and were blind to the temperament scores of the children at age 7. Temperamentally difficult children had more clinical disorders at age 12 that qualified for a DSM-III diagnosis. An association with family dysfunction in terms of behavior control seemed to increase this risk: there was a lower rate of clinical disorders among children in superior functioning families than among those in dysfunctional families.

Reprinted with permission from the *American Journal of Psychiatry*, 1985, Vol. 142, 943–946. Copyright 1985 by the American Psychiatric Association.

Presented at the 138th annual meeting of the American Psychiatric Association, Dallas, May 18-24, 1985.

Supported by grants from Santé et Bien-être Social Canada and Le Fonds Richelieu C.S.S. de Québec.

The authors thank the parents and teachers of the children and Chantal Mérette and Germaine Larose for their help.

Although we have some knowledge about factors that contribute to children's vulnerability to psychopathology, little is known about the interaction between risk factors and the way to manipulate them in primary prevention (1, 2). Some risk factors are scientifically well documented: parental discord (3), school effect (4), parental psychopathology (5, 6), and other indexes of adversity (3, 7). The New York Longitudinal Study (8) and other studies (9, 10) have suggested that "difficult" temperament predisposes a child to behavior disorders. Moreover, a typology very similar to the New York study's "difficult" typology has been replicated in diverse cultures and at different age levels (8, 11, 12). The fact that boys in the general population are overrepresented in the temperamentally difficult group of 7-year-olds (13) suggests that temperament may be a contributing factor to the well-documented greater vulnerability of boys to psychosocial stress and their overrepresentation in child guidance clinic attendance.

We undertook this study 1) to verify the hypothesis that difficult temperament increases the probability of psychiatric and behavior disorders in children between the ages of 7 and 12 years; 2) to evaluate the interaction between temperament and family functioning; and 3) to take into account the possible confounding effect of stressful life events and five factors on Rutter's adversity index (7). No one to our knowledge has undertaken a study of the predictive value of the New York study on difficult temperament in a French-speaking nonclinical sample representative of every social class; Thomas and Chess (8) and Cameron (10) studied a middle and upper-middle class, predominantly Jewish sample and Graham et al. (9) studied a sample of children who had parents suffering some form of psychopathology.

We decided to assess the behavior control dimension of family functioning (14) because our clinical experience in family psychiatry suggests that the children who have outwardly directed symptoms (opposition, overactivity, conduct problems, and so on) often live in dysfunctional families in terms of behavior control: the less consensus there is between parents, the fuzzier the rules are, and the more inconsistent their application is, the more likely we are to observe outwardly directed symptoms in children.

METHOD

In 1979, we studied a random sample of 980 7-year-old children from the general population of Quebec City (13), using a French translation of the Thomas, Chess, and Korn Parent Temperament Questionnaire

(8). From this sample, we derived a bipolar factor I very similar to the New York study easy-difficult typology (13). The "difficult" pole of our factor is defined by five main temperamental categories: low adaptability, withdrawal from new stimuli, intensity in emotional reactions, negative mood, and low distractibility.

From this sample, we selected 26 of the most temperamentally difficult subjects. This method of selecting the extreme risk subjects has already been used by others for longitudinal studies (15). In 1979, these 26 subjects scored on two occasions (test-retest) higher than the 70th percentile for at least four of the difficult temperament categories. As a comparison group, we selected 16 children on the "easy" pole of factor I who scored lower than the 30th percentile on two occasions for at least three categories. The selection was made by a research assistant who used only research codes, which allowed the investigators, parents, and teachers to be blind to the 1979 temperament scores. The two groups were balanced for age, sex, and socioeconomic status. In all, 39 families (93%) agreed to participate.

The study group with difficult temperament consisted of 20 boys and four girls (mean age, 12.2 years; range, 11.9–13.1 years). The comparison group consisted of 12 boys and three girls (mean age, 12 years; range, 11.9–13.2 years). The composition of the study group according to the Hollingshead index was as follows: class I, 8%; class II, 12%; class III, 25%; class IV, 38%; and class V, 17%. For the comparison group the distribution was as follows: class I, 13%; class II, 13%; class III, 27%; class IV, 27%; and class V, 20%. The social class distribution of the 1979 sample was very similar (13).

Data gathering was carried out at home and at school. In our first home visit, we explained the study to the family and obtained an informed and signed consent form. In a second visit, a semistructured interview with the child and the parents was performed by a psychiatrist (M.M.) to assess the child's clinical status according to *DSM-III* criteria. This was repeated 2 weeks later by another psychiatrist (B.L.). Medical history, developmental data, and any history of stressful events were obtained by a psychiatrist (B.L.) through a standardized interview resembling the Personal Data Inventory of the ECDEU (16). The parents filled out the Conners Parent Questionnaire (16) and the Children's Behavior Inventory (16) two times. The teacher filled out the Rutter Behavior Questionnaire (17) two times. In a third visit, we assessed the whole family through a semi-standardized interview in terms of behavior control according to the McMaster model of family functioning (14). Behavior control taps the clarity of the family rules, the consensus between parents, and their consistency, firmness, and flexibility when the rules are violated by the children. A psychiatrist (M.M.) audiotaped the interview and rated the McMaster model. Two other family psychiatrists trained with the model (J.T., M.B.) independently reviewed the tapes and also rated the families according to the McMaster 7-point scale, where 4 is normal functioning, less than 4 indicates the degree of dysfunction, and greater than 4 is superior functioning. Each characteristic (rules, consensus, consistency) was rated, and a global rating was also estimated.

RESULTS

Two psychiatrists (M.M., B.L.), blind to temperament scores, separately analyzed their data and decided if the child qualified for a *DSM-III* diagnosis. The percentage of immediate agreement was 79%; in 13% of the cases, the disagreement was slight. The disagreements were more divergent for three cases (8%), which were resolved when all the investigators met and reached consensus by using all the clinical information except the teacher scale. The interrater (M.M., J.T., M.B.) reliability for the family assessment was satisfactory (Kendall's coefficient of concordance, .80). The test-retest reliability (Spearman correlation) on the global scores gave .83 for the Rutter Behavior Questionnaire, .81 for the Children's Behavior Inventory, and .84 for the Conners Parent Questionnaire.

According to Rutter and Graham (18), a score of greater than 9 on the Rutter questionnaire predicted 90% of the children with clinical diagnoses attending clinics and was concordant with 43% of the clinical cases as diagnosed by the clinicians. For our part, 58% of the children with clinical diagnoses had a score of greater than 9 on the Rutter questionnaire and 66% had a score of greater than 6. Among the cases without clinical diagnosis, only 20% had a score of greater than 6.

Among the 24 temperamentally difficult 7-year-old children, 12 qualified for a *DSM-III* diagnosis at age 12 compared with one of the 15 easy subjects (Fisher exact test, $p < .001$). Nine subjects had an oppositional disorder and three had an attention deficit disorder associated with an oppositional disorder; none had a conduct disorder. We identified a child as "clinical" only if he was judged as moderate or severe on the Clinical Global Impressions scale of the ECDEU Assessment Manual (16); we based our judgment on the "clinical-diagnostic" definition of psychiatric disorders as stated by Rutter (19).

We also used a multivariate analysis (log-linear model) (20) in which the variables were temperament, family functioning, and clinical disorders. We found no association between temperament and family functioning (p = .26) or between family functioning and clinical disorders (p = .12), but the association between temperament and clinical disorders remained significant (p = .01).

When we examined this last result in greater detail, we observed a trend suggesting that the significance of the association between temperament and clinical disorders was mainly found in the dysfunctional families: no clinical case among the three easy children living in dysfunctional families (McMaster model rating of less than 4) and seven clinical cases among the 10 difficult children living in dysfunctional families (Fisher exact test, p = .07). In functional families (McMaster model rating greater than or equal to 4), we found one clinical case in the 12 easy children living in functional families and five clinical cases in the 14 difficult children living in functional families (p = .12). Furthermore, when we retained only the difficult children for analysis and looked at only the dysfunctional families and the superior functioning families (McMaster rating greater than or equal to 5), we observed a significant association between family functioning and clinical disorders; although seven of the 10 difficult children living in dysfunctional families had a clinical disorder, only one of the nine difficult children living in superior families had a clinical disorder (Fisher exact test, p < .02).

We could to some extent eliminate the confounding effect of other known risk factors: 1) only three difficult children (one with a clinical disorder) and three easy children (one with a clinical disorder) had manifested in the previous year one of the 12 first stress items of the Holmes and Rahe scale (21); 2) only one difficult subject (with a clinical disorder) and one easy subject (without a clinical disorder) had manifested two of the five stress factors of Rutter's adversity index (7): father's semiskilled job, overcrowding, marital discord, child "ever having been in care," father's offense against the law. We omitted Rutter's sixth stress factor, maternal depression, because we were unable to obtain data assessed in a standard manner.

Finally, our difficult children with clinical disorders had a preponderance of outwardly directed symptoms at home, particularly opposition to authority figures and norms. Paradoxically, at school, even if they displayed some outwardly directed symptoms, these same difficult children with clinical disorders surprisingly showed a preponderance of inwardly directed symptoms: they were described by their teachers as worried, unhappy, tearful or distressed, fearful and afraid of new things, and solitary. The symptoms, therefore, appear specific to the environment, so that our 12-year-old difficult children with clinical disorders often give a more neurotic and internalizing picture in school, while their attitude at home is predominantly externalizing or actively oppositional.

DISCUSSION

Our data, which indicate that the children with a difficult temperament according to the New York Longitudinal Study criteria are at increased psychiatric risk in the French-speaking population of Quebec City, provide a transcultural replication of the New York findings. With the cutoff points presently used on the temperament scores of those children who at 7 years old were temperamentally difficult, one of two displays at age 12 a clinical disorder requiring some form of intervention, a finding that is to some extent applicable to approximately 9% of our general population characterized by such cutoff points. Temperament assessed more than 4 years earlier appears to be as powerful a predictor as an actual dysfunction of parental behavior control. Moreover, there is a trend in our data suggesting that the risk for temperamentally difficult children increases if parents show little consensus and if family rules and demands are not clear or lack firmness and consistency. Conversely, almost no family with superior functioning in terms of behavior control was associated with psychiatric disorder in difficult children. This suggests that a higher than average quality of parental behavior control may be a protective factor against the risk associated with difficult temperament. Methodologically, a possibility exists that in some analyses the statistics did not reach significance because of the small number of subjects; therefore, a replication with a larger sample should be done.

Our findings have implications for the design of future research on child temperament and family interaction and especially for prevention studies on interventions directed toward child-rearing attitudes that best fit the temperamentally difficult children. Our results allow us to formulate a new hypothesis, namely, that a positive change in behavior control in dysfunctional families of difficult children may improve the psychosocial prognosis of the children. This hypothesis must be tested in future studies, and the cost efficiency of such interventions must also be evaluated.

REFERENCES

1. Tarter, R. E.: Vulnerability and risk: assessment and prediction of outcome, in The Child at Psychiatric Risk. Edited by Tarter, R. E. New York, Oxford University Press, 1983.

2. Rutter, M.: Prevention of children's psychosocial disorders: myth and substance. Pediatrics 70:883-894, 1982.
3. Richman, N.: Behaviour problems in pre-school children: family and social factors. Br J Psychiatry 131:523-527, 1977.
4. Rutter, M.: School influence on children's behavior and development: the 1979 Kenneth Blackfan Lecture, Children's Hospital Medical Center, Boston. Pediatrics 65:208-220, 1980.
5. Beardslee, W. R., Bemporad, J., Keller, M. B., et al: Children of parents with major affective disorder: a review. Am J Psychiatry 140:825-832, 1983.
6. Asarnow, R.: Schizophrenia, in The Child at Psychiatric Risk. Edited by Tarter, R. E. New York, Oxford University Press, 1983.
7. Rutter, M., Quinton, D.: Psychiatric disorder—ecological factors and concepts of causation, in Ecological Factors in Human Development. Edited by Gurk, H. M. New York, North Holland, 1977.
8. Thomas, A., Chess, S. (eds): Temperament and Development. New York, Brunner/Mazel, 1977.
9. Graham, P., Rutter, M., George, S.: Temperamental characteristics as predictors of behavior disorders in children. Am J Orthopsychiatry 43:328-339, 1973.
10. Cameron, J. R.: Parental treatment, children's temperament, and the risk of childhood behavioral problems, 2: initial temperament, parental attitudes, and the incidence and form of behavioral problems. Am J Orthopsychiatry 48:140-147, 1978.
11. Persson-Blennow, I., McNeil, T. F.: Factor analysis of temperament characteristics in children at 6 months, 1 year and 2 years of age. Br J Educ Psychol 52:51-57, 1982.
12. Maziade, M., Boudreault, M., Thivierge, J., et al: Infant temperament: SES and gender differences and reliability of measurement in a large Quebec sample. Merrill-Palmer Quarterly 30(2):213-226, 1984.
13. Maziade, M., Côté, R., Boudreault, M., et al: The NYLS model of temperament: gender differences and demographic correlates in a French speaking population. J Am Acad Child Psychiatry 23:582-587, 1984.
14. Epstein, N. B., Bishop, D. S., Levin, S.: The McMaster model of family functioning. J Marriage and Family Counseling 4:19-31, 1978.
15. Moffitt, T. E., Mednick, S. A., Cudeck, R.: Methodology of high risk research: longitudinal approaches, in The Child at Psychiatric Risk. Edited by Tarter, R. E. New York, Oxford University Press, 1983.
16. ECDEU Assessment Manual for Psychopharmacology. Washington, DC, Public Health Service, US Department of Health, Education and Welfare, 1976.
17. Rutter, M.: A children's behaviour questionnaire for completion by teachers: preliminary findings. J Child Psychol Psychiatry 8:1-11, 1967.
18. Rutter, M., Graham, P.: Psychiatric disorder in 10- and 11-year-old children. Proc R Soc Med 59:382-387, 1966.
19. Rutter, M. (ed): Education, Health and Behaviour. London, Longman Group, 1970.
20. Haberman, S. J. (ed): Analysis of Qualitative Data, vol 1. New York, Academic Press, 1978.
21. Holmes, T. H., Rahe, R. H.: The social readjustment scale. J Psychosom Res 11:213-218, 1967.

Part VI

CHILDREN OF DIVORCE

This section comprises two papers by the two leading students, and their coworkers, of the effects of parental divorce on children in this country—Mavis Hetherington and Judith Wallerstein. In the present reports, both workers are concerned with the long-term effects of divorce, and Hetherington also considers the effect of remarriage. This latter consideration is important because 80% of the fathers and 75% of the mothers will remarry. Both articles are rich in valuable information for any mental health professional dealing with divorced parents, whether remarried or not, and their children. Both studies were comprised of populations that were white and middle-class, so caution must be exercised in generalizing to other socioeconomic or racial groups.

Hetherington and her coworkers present their findings of a 6-year follow-up subsequent to the divorce. There were a number of differences between the boys and the girls. For example, the divorce was more disturbing for the boys, while remarriage was more disruptive for girls. Wise advice is offered to stepparents toward making a positive relationship with their stepchildren. Overall, the children did adjust to their parents' marital rearrangements, a conclusion similar to our finding in the New York Longitudinal Study population.

Wallerstein reports a 10-year follow-up, when the children were young adults. She gives a vivid and sensitive account of the long-term effects of the parental divorce on these young adults. Even if they were functioning well, a number were still hindered by vivid memories of their parents' breakup, feelings of sadness and resentment, and a sense of deprivation. They were apprehensive about repeating their parents' unhappy marriages, but, at the same time, determined that this should not happen. Of special interest was the importance of a strong mutually supportive bond between brothers and sisters in helping each other to cope with the trauma of their parent's divorce.

Part VI
CHILDREN OF DIVORCE

23

Long-Term Effects of Divorce and Remarriage on the Adjustment of Children

E. Mavis Hetherington
University of Virginia, Charlottesville
Martha Cox
Timberlawn Foundation, Dallas
Roger Cox
University of Texas Health Science Center, Dallas

This paper presents the results of a 6-year follow-up of a longitudinal study of the effects of divorce on parents and children. It was found that, whereas divorce had more adverse effects for boys, remarriage was more disruptive for girls. The stability of the long-term adjustment of boys and girls differed, with externalizing being more stable in boys and internalizing more stable in girls. Children in divorced families encountered more negative life changes than children in nondivorced families, and these negative life changes were associated with behavior problems 6 years following divorce.

A substantial body of both clinical and research literature has accumulated which shows that most children experience their parents' divorce as a stressful life event and exhibit short-term developmental disruptions, emotional distress, and behavior disorders (see Hethering-

Reprinted with permission from the *Journal of the American Academy of Child Psychiatry,* 1985, Vol. 24, 518–530. Copyright 1985 by the American Academy of Child Psychiatry.

ton (1981), Hetherington and Camara (1984), and Kurdek (1983) for reviews of this literature). The findings of clinical studies (Wallerstein and Kelly, 1980) and intensive multimethod research studies using nonrepresentative samples of convenience (e.g., Hetherington et al. (1982) and Santrock et al., (1982) have been substantiated by large scale surveys studies (Guidubaldi et al., 1983, 1984) and national surveys using representative samples (Peterson and Zill, 1983; Zill and Peterson, unpublished manuscript). In the first few years following divorce, children in divorced families in comparison to children in nondivorced families show more antisocial, impulsive acting out disorders, more aggression and noncompliance, more dependency, anxiety, and depression, more difficulties in social relationships, and more problem behavior in school. The differences in externalizing, impulsive antisocial behavior are more consistently reported than those for internalizing disorders, such as withdrawal, depression, and anxiety. These effects are more severe and enduring for boys than for girls (Guidubaldi et al., 1983, 1984; Hetherington et al., 1982), although problems in heterosexual relationships have been reported for adolescent and young adult girls (Hetherington, 1972; Wallerstein, 1982). Since most of the studies comparing the responses of sons and daughters to divorce have involved preadolescents, it may be that sex differences are more marked in younger than in older children. Although differences in academic achievement and cognitive development, especially in the area of problem solving and quantitative skills, are sometimes reported, they are not as consistently found and are greatly attenuated when the effects of social class are controlled (Guidubaldi, et al., 1983; Hetherington et al., 1983).

There have been many studies of the differences between children of divorced and nondivorced parents; however, few investigators have addressed the possible variations in the sequence of family relationships and life experiences that may occur following divorce. For most children, divorce is only one in a series of family transitions and reorganizations that follow separation and marital dissolution. Following divorce, most children spend a period of time in a one-parent household, usually a mother-headed household. There is some evidence that children show fewer problems if they are in the custody of a parent of the same sex than a parent of the opposite sex (Peterson and Zill, 1983; Santrock et al., 1982; Warshak and Santrock, 1983; Zill and Peterson, unpublished manuscript). For most children, life in a single-parent household is a temporary condition, for 80% of men and 75% of women will remarry, and 25% of children will spend time in a stepparent family before they are young adults. Although good research on stepchildren is meager, there is some suggestion in the literature that whereas divorce has the most adverse effects for boys, perhaps because most of them are in mother-custody homes, remarriage may enhance the development of boys from divorced families. In contrast, the presence of a stepfather may show no effects or have deleterious effects on the development of girls (see Hetherington et al. (1985) for a review of this topic). As was found in the research on divorce, the adverse effects of remarriage tend to decline over time as children adapt to their new family situation. However, since the divorce rate is higher in remarriage than in first marriages, some children encounter a chain of remarriages and divorces, and little is known about the consequences of such a series of family reorganizations for the adjustment of children.

Some of the factors that mediate the long-term outcomes of divorce for children and parents appear to be the multiple life changes encountered following divorce. These include changes in economic status, residence, occupation, child care arrangements, social relationships, support networks, family relationships, and physical and mental health. Such changes have been related to the adjustment and psychological well-being of children and parents (Bloom et al., 1978; Hetherington et al., 1982; Stolberg and Anker, 1983).

This paper presents part of the findings of a 6-year follow-up of a longitudinal study of divorce (see Hetherington et al. (1982) for a summary of this study) and of an expanded cross-sectional cohort involving divorced, remarried, and nondivorced families.

In this article, the topics to be addressed will be:

1. The continuity between children's behavior problems and social competence in the first 2 years following divorce, and a long-term follow-up 6 years after divorce.
2. The relation between behavior problems and socially competent behavior in the family and in the school.
3. The correlations among observational measures, standardized test scores, and reports of behavior problems and socially competent behavior in children.
4. The adjustment of children in nondivorced, divorced mother custody, and remarried stepfather households.
5. Sex differences in the patterns and stability of behavior disorders and socially competent behavior of children in nondivorced, divorced mother custody, and remarried stepfather households.
6. The role of change and stressful life events on the development of behavior problems and socially competent behavior in children.

METHOD

Subjects

The original sample was composed of 144 middle-class white children and their parents. Half of the children were from divorced, mother-custody families, and the other half were from nondivorced families. Within each group, half were boys and half were girls. In the original study, the families were studied at 2 months, 1 year, and 2 years after divorce. The follow-up to be discussed in this paper occurred 6 years after the divorce when the children were an average of 10.1 years of age. As might be expected, by this time many rearrangements in marital relations had occurred; these are summarized in the procedures section.

The subjects were residential parents and children in 124 of an original 144 families who were available and willing to participate in 6-year follow-up study. Sixty of the original divorced families and 64 of the original nondivorced families agreed to participate, although there had been many shifts in marital status in the 6 years since the study began. In the 60 available original divorced families, only 18 of the custodial mothers had remained single (10 with a target daughter and 8 with a target son), and 42 had remarried (20 with a target daughter and 22 with a target son). Two of the parents had redivorced, and there had been 6 changes in custody or residence from the mother to the father (5 sons, 1 daughter). Of the 64 originally nondivorced families, 53 were still married (30 sons, 23 daughters), 11 were divorced (7 daughters, 4 sons). In the newly divorced families, only one of the children, a son, was in the custody of the father.

This was a well-educated, middle-class, white sample. All parents had at least a high school education. Eighty percent of the parents had some education or advanced training beyond high school. At 6 years following divorce, the household income of the nonremarried divorced mothers was significantly lower than that of the nondivorced or remarried families. The average household income of the divorced nonremarried mothers was $16,010, of remarried mothers was $35,162, and of nondivorced families was $36,900.

A new cohort of families was added to the group of participating original families on whom there was complete data (except for noncustodial father measures) in order to expand the size of the groups to 30 sons and 30 daughters in each of three groups—a remarried mother/stepfather group, a mother-custody, nonremarried group, and a nondivorced group—for a total of 180 families. For some analyses, the remarried group was broken down into those remarried less than 2 years and those remarried longer than 2 years. The additional subjects were matched with the original subjects on family size, age, education, income, length of marriage, and, when appropriate, length of time since divorce and time of remarriage.

All longitudinal analyses involve only the original sample; however, cross-sectional analyses of child adjustment and of the relationship between child adjustment and life change 6 years following divorce utilize the expanded sample.

Procedure

Partial data were available in the follow-up study on 124 families. In all cases, this included interviews, tests, and home observations of the residential parents and child. In 18 of these families, complete school data, which included a peer nomination measure, were not available because of lack of willingness of the schools to participate in the study, although with 10 of these families, measures were available from teachers who were contacted directly and who agreed to participate. In addition, telephone interviews and/or take home questionnaire and test material could not be obtained for six of the noncustodial fathers. As was true in the three waves of data collection in the original study, multiple measures of family relations, stresses, and support systems, and parent and child characteristics and behavior were obtained from the child and residential parent, and when possible from the nonresidential parent. These involved standardized tests, interviews, and observations. In addition, teacher and peer evaluations of behavior, observations in school, and information from school records were obtained when possible. Only the measures used in the analyses presented in this article will be described.

Measures of child adjustment were obtained from parents, teachers, peers, and the child. All of these measures were selected or constructed to measure internalizing, externalizing, and socially competent behavior. Although the same types of measures were used in the first three time periods and the 6-year follow-up, they were not identical. Instruments were modified or new ones adopted to make the measures more appropriate for older children and to more directly assess internalizing, externalizing, and socially competent behavior. Many of the older measures were rescored or refactored, or selected items were used to develop measures to assess the three outcome variables of interest in this paper. More detailed information on the earlier sets of measures are available in Hetherington et al. (1978, 1979a, b). The measures listed below are grouped according to type of measure. Thus, although the same parent rating scales were not used in the earlier time periods and the follow-up study, the same method was used, i.e., that of rating.

Parent Rating Scales. In the early assessments, parents rated 49 items on 5-point rating scales, which comprised 7 scales of behavior. These early ratings were factor analyzed to yield three scales containing a total of 40 items. The scales were externalizing, internalizing, and social competence. Test-retest reliabilities administered to a group of 100 parents 1 month apart were 0.81 externalizing, 0.72 internalizing, and 0.75 social competence.

In the 6-year follow-up, the Child Behavior Checklist (Achenbach and Edelbrock, 1983) was used. This is a standardized test using parent ratings, which yields two overall psychopathology factors (internalizing and externalizing) and three social competence scales (activities, social, and school) which can be combined into a single competence scale. Sex differences were dealt with by converting raw scores to t scores. Ratings were made by nonresidential parents and residential parents, including stepfathers.

Teacher rating scales. The items in the teacher rating scales used in the original study were reanalyzed to produce a 3-factor solution involving externalizing, internalizing, and social competence. The same scales were used in the analyses in this paper for the earlier and later measurement periods. Interteacher reliabilities were 0.79 externalizing, 0.69 internalizing, and 0.74 social competence. Test-retest reliabilities for the same teachers 1 month apart were $r = 0.81$ externalizing, 0.72 internalizing, and 0.76 social competence.

Peer nominations. In the three early assessments, peer nominations involved a "guess who" format to assess peers on 30 attributes. Each child received a different set of seven photographs including a subject and a random set of three boys and three girls, since they were too young to be able to cope with the full array of class peers. The child was then asked to " 'Guess who' always does what the teacher asks," " 'guess who' got angry and called another child a bad name," "helped a child who was crying," and so on. The number of peer nominations relative to class size was recorded on internalizing, externalizing, and social competence scales. Test-retest reliabilities 1 month apart on these young children were modest but significant, averaging across factors 0.45 at $time_1$, 0.50 at $time_2$, and 0.70 at $time_3$.

In the 6-year follow-up study, a peer nomination measure based on a modification and extension of the Pupil Evaluation Inventory (Pekarik et al., 1976) was used. Students were given a matrix of names of classmates on the horizontal margin and attributes on the vertical margin and were asked to put an × under the name of everyone who fit the description of the characteristic. Scores were converted to z scores to remove the effects of differences in class size on total scores. The extended inventory was administered to 320 students. Factor analyzed, it yielded internalizing, externalizing, and competence/likeability factors. Test-retest correlations for all factors a month apart were above 0.80.

Child-self-rating. This rating occurred only at the 6-year follow-up and involved the child rating the same items as on the peer nomination inventory on a 3-point scale, ranging from "not at all like me," and "sometimes like me," to "very like me." The test-retest correlations for the three factors across a 1-month interval were above 0.72.

Twenty-four-hour behavior checklists. On 10 different occasions, residential parents and children were asked to record and report in a telephone interview whether 40 behaviors had occurred in the past 24 hours. Using a split-half reliability of temporal stability for the first 5 days versus the second 5 days, reliabilities average 0.71 for fathers, 0.73 for mothers, and 0.69 for children. Average agreement between mothers and fathers across the three dimensions was 0.70. Agreement between parents and children was lower: 0.62 for mother and child and 0.60 for father and child. Children filled out this checklist only at the 6-year follow-up (time$_4$).

Home observations. Observations in the home were made on six occasions for a minimum of 3 hours. On three of these occasions, recording was done with raters present, and on three occasions the family interactions were videotaped and coded later. This method was used in order to study methods of observation. It was fortunate, however, that some of the interactions had been videotaped, since it was decided that the earlier coding system was not adequate to measure the three dependent child variables of interest in this follow-up study. A new code was developed to include more detailed measures of the three categories. For internalizing, these included such behaviors as crying, self-criticism, staring into space, wandering, expressing fear or worry, passive watching of other's activities, alone inactive, and seeking reassurance. For externalizing, they include such behaviors as aversive opposition, destruction of property, verbal aggression (negative commands, teasing, humiliating, sarcasm, threats, criticism), and physical aggression. For social competence, they included such behaviors as positive initiation, sharing, helping, sympathy, praising, and expressions of affection. Coders were asked to code the tapes as if they were an ongoing interaction. A focal subject coding system was used, where each family served as the focal subject for 10-minute periods in rotation. The behavior of the child of interest in this study was oversampled, so that he or she served as the focal subject three times more often than did the other family members. All behaviors of the focal subject and all the reactions and interactions from other family members to the focal subject were coded at 6-second intervals. In the follow-up study, only three videotaped sets of observations were obtained.

Reliabilities which averaged 0.79 for agreement between categories in each 6-second unit were obtained from two coders coding 20% of the tapes. Cohen's kappas were always significantly above change levels of agreement. Rate per minute of internalizing and externalizing and socially competent behavior was used as the unit of analysis.

School observations. In the first three time periods, each child had been observed in the classroom for 18 10-minute sessions. The child's behavior and the behavior of the person with whom the child was interacting were recorded every 6 seconds. In addition, affect during play had been assessed. The same code used in the original study combined with affect codings was used in the follow-up study. See Hetherington et al. (1979b) for more details on this procedure.

Life experiences survey (LES). An extension of the Sarason et al. (1978) Life Experiences Survey with 10 items added to more intensively study changes in family relations was administered to parents at time$_4$. Parents were asked to indicate the occurrence of certain events in the past year and in the past 6 years time since divorce, followed by separate subjective ratings of the event as positive or negative on 7-point scales. A similar, shorter survey was constructed for children and administered at time$_4$. This measure was read to the children.

RESULTS

Stability of Problem Behavior and Competence

How predictable is the long-term adjustment of children at 6 years following divorce from their adjustment in the first 2 years, or in what has been called the crisis period following divorce? In order to answer this question, composite scores of internalizing, externalizing, and socially competent behaviors were calculated. This involved averaging the scores on each measure across $time_1$ (2 months after divorce), $time_2$ (1 year after divorce), and $time_3$ (2 years after divorce), thus yielding a composite measure for the first 2-year period for each measure. One of the problems in this compositing is that it masks some of the adaptation that is occurring over the course of the first year. In general, correlations between $time_1$ and $time_2$ measures are higher than those between $time_2$ and $time_3$ when accelerated coping is occurring, and correlations between $time_3$ and $time_4$ are higher than those between $time_1$ or $time_2$ and $time_4$.

Pearson product moment correlations were calculated for never-divorced and ever-divorced boys and girls separately. In addition, correlations for boys and girls across family types were calculated. All correlations discussed in the following presentation were significant at at least $p < 0.05$. When the significance of differences between correlations are discussed, the differences have been tested and also found to be significant at at least $p < 0.05$.

Tables 1, 2, 3, and 4 present the significant correlations between the composite scores across $time_1$, $time_2$, and $time_3$ for each measure and the $time_4$ scores for boys and girls in ever-divorced and never-divorced families. Since the number of subjects varies across some cells because of missing data, the probability levels may not appear consistent.

The stability of externalizing behavior is greater for boys and of internalizing behavior is greater for girls. It should be noted, however, that early externalizing behavior also is significantly correlated with later internalizing for both boys and girls on many measures. The relation between social competence and aggression differs for boys and girls. For girls, early aggressive behavior is the best predictor of later low social competence. This relationship is higher than that between early and later social competence. In contrast, early deficits in prosocial behavior show considerable stability across time for boys. Later prosocial behavior is better predicted for boys by early prosocial behavior than by early aggression. In addition, this pattern of sex differences is found more consistently in ratings than in either the 24-hour behavior checklists or observed behavior in the home or in the school, which might be viewed as more objective measures.

Moreover, consistency seems to run across domains or situations and across the source of information. Thus there are more significant correlations across time among measures from the school, such as teacher ratings, peer nominations, and observed behavior in the school, than between school and home measures. It should be noted that, since such

TABLE 1

Significant Correlations between Early and Later Internalizing, Externalizing, and Social Competence Measures for Sons in Divorced Families

Time, Criteria

Composite T₁, T₂, T₃ Predictors	1. MR			2. FR			3. TR			4. PN			5. 24 M			6. 24 F			7. OHB			8. OSB			9. CR			10. 24 C		
	I	E	C	I	E	C	I	E	C	I	E	C	I	E	C	I	E	C	I	E	C	I	E	C	I	E	C	I	E	C
1. MR — I	.41*	.49**	-.39*				.37*	.40*	-.41*				.37*	.44**	-.36*				.39*	.36*	.39*									
E					.42*						.41*	.40*			.36*								.41*	.43*					.38*	
C			.61**						.45*																					
2. FR — I																														
E		.38*			.38*			.37*			.39*															.39*				
C						.39*																								
3. TR — I	.38*						.41*	.46**	.56**	.41*												.38*	.40*	.51**						
E	.37*	.39*	-.38*								.41*	.48*		.42*			.42*	.38*			.37*									
C			.54**																											
4. PN — I																						.43*	.42*							
E											.57**						.39*													
C																														
5. 24 M — I													.39*	.42**	.52**															
E	.37*	.42**	.49**																.36*	.41*	-.37*			.42*			.36*			
C																														
6. 24 F — I													.37*	.40*			.40*	.40*				.41*								
E																	.39*												.41*	
C																														
7. OHB — I																			.42*	.40*	-.36*									
E	.36*	.39*	-.37*											.39*	.38*					.40*			.38*	.36*						
C			.44**																		.47**									
8. OSB — I																						.40*	-.41*	.42*						
E											.42*	.46*								.40*										
C																														

* p < 0.05, ** p < 0.01.

All measures for sons in divorced families have an N of 30, with the exception of those involving peer nominations and school observations (N = 25), teacher ratings (N = 27), father ratings (N = 28), and 24-hour checklist (N = 26).

MR = mother ratings, FR = father ratings, TR = teacher ratings, PN = peer nominations, 24 M = 24-hour checklist by mother, 24 F = 24-hour checklist by father, OHB = observed home behavior, OSB = observed school behavior, CR = child rating, 24 C = 24-hour checklist by child; I = internalizing, E = externalizing, C = social competence.

TABLE 2

Significant Correlations between Early and Later Internalizing, Externalizing, and Social Competence Measures for Sons in Nondivorced Families

Composite T1, T2, T3 Predictors	1. MR			2. FR			3. TR			4. PN			5. 24 M			6. 24 F			7. OHB			8. OSB			9. CR			10. 24 C		
	I	E	C	I	E	C	I	E	C	I	E	C	I	E	C	I	E	C	I	E	C	I	E	C	I	E	C	I	E	C
1. MR I	.43**		-.40*	.36*		-.42**			-.42**				.45**																	
E		.55**	-.49*		.48**			.43**			.43*			.49**	-.37*		.43**			.41**	-.40*		.40*						.37*	
C			.63**			.52**			.57**						.50**			.37*			.45**									
2. FR I	.45**			.45**		-.36*																								
E		.37*			.58**			.46**			.44**						.50**			.49**			.41*						.36*	
C			.46**			.59**			.44**			.46**			.50**		.39*			.39*			.40*						
3. TR I	.40*						.38*																							
E		.46**			.50**			.52**			.40*			.39*			.39*			.36*			.40*						
C			.57**						.41*			.65**			.40*			.37*			.46**									
4. PN I									-.37*																					
E					.42**						.61**									.42*			.40*							
C						.46**			.65**			.41*											.42*							
5. 24 M I	.36*												.36*			.37*														
E		.44**			.42**			.36*			.40*			.49**			.42**			.43**			.41*							
C			.50**						.40*						.43**			.36*			.38*									
6. 24 F I																			.40**											
E		.37*			.49**			.44**			.43*			.39*			.41*			.37*			.36*							
C			.36*			.37*			.37*						.36*			.37*			.38*									
7. OHB I	.36*			.37*												.40**			.40**			.37*								
E		.44**	-.40*		.43**			.37*			.43*			.44**			.39*			.49**	-.36*		.42*						.40*	
C			.45**			.39*			.46**						.37*			.38*			.47**			.41*						
8. OSB I																.37*			.37*											
E		.36*				.36*			.38*		.42*	.40*					.39*			.39**			.47**						.43**	
C																							.41*							

* $p < 0.05$, ** $p < 0.01$.

All measures for sons in nondivorced families have an N of 30, with the exception of those involving peer nominations and school observations ($N = 24$), and teacher ratings ($N = 28$).

MR = mother ratings, FR = father ratings, TR = teacher ratings, PN = peer nominations, 24 M = 24-hour checklist by mother, 24 F = 24-hour checklist by father, OHB = observed home behavior, OSB = observed school behavior, CR = child rating, 24 C = 24-hour checklist by child; I = internalizing, E = externalizing, C = social competence.

TABLE 3

Significant Correlations between Early and Later Internalizing, Externalizing, and Social Competence Measures for Daughters in Divorced Families

Composite T₁, T₂, T₃ Predictors		1. MR I	1. MR E	1. MR C	2. FR I	2. FR E	2. FR C	3. TR I	3. TR E	3. TR C	4. PN I	4. PN E	4. PN C	5. 24 M I	5. 24 M E	5. 24 M C	6. 24 F I	6. 24 F E	6. 24 F C	7. OHB I	7. OHB E	7. OHB C	8. OSB I	8. OSB E	8. OSB C	9. CR I	9. CR E	9. CR C	10. 24 C I	10. 24 C E	10. 24 C C
1. MR	I	.49**			.48**			.53**			.44*			.46**						.45**			.46*								
	E		.37*			.36*			.41*			.40*									.36*			.40*							
	C			-.57**			-.45**			-.41*			-.40*			-.49**						-.50**			-.45*						
2. FR	I	.43**			.31*			.37*						.39*			.37*						.49*								
	E					.36*			.41*															.40*							
	C			-.51**			-.47**			-.40*			-.42*			-.42**						-.39*			-.38*						
3. TR	I	.38*						.53**															.46*								
	E		.36*						.41*			.44*			.36*			.36*						.40*							
	C			-.42**						-.62**			-.42*												-.49*						
4. PN	I							.42*						.39*			.37*			.37*			.42*								
	E		.36*						.37*			-.40*												.40*							
	C																					-.41*			-.41*						
5. 24 M	I	.42**			.36*			.39*						.39*			.36*														
	E	.36*			.36*			.41*						.41*			.39*			.37*											
	C			-.44**			-.38*			.39*						-.42**			-.37*			-.39*									
6. 24 F	I	.37*			.37*									.39*						.36*											
	E					.39*												.36*													
	C						-.36*									-.37*			-.45**												
7. OHB	I	.38*												.42*			.39*			.39*											
	E								.41*			.40*						.38*			.36*										
	C			-.49**						.37*						-.37*			-.39*			-.41*									
8. OSB	I				.46**						.49*			.42*									.42*								
	E				.39*			.38*			.41*									.38*			.40*								
	C									-.41*			-.38*						-.39*						-.50**						

* p < 0.05, ** p < 0.01.

All measures for daughters in divorced families have an N of 30, with the exception of those involving peer nominations and school observations (N = 25), teacher ratings (N = 29), father ratings (N = 26), and 24-hour checklist (N = 24).

MR = mother ratings, FR = father ratings, TR = teacher ratings, PN = peer nominations, 24 M = 24-hour checklist by mother, 24 F = 24-hour checklist by father, OHB =

TABLE 4

Significant Correlations between Early and Later Internalizing, Externalizing, and Social Competence Measures for Daughters in Nondivorced Families

Composite T$_1$, T$_3$ Predictors		1. MR			2. FR			3. TR			4. PN			5. 24 M			6. 24 F			7. OHB			8. OSB			9. CR			10. 24 C		
		I	E	C	I	E	C	I	E	C	I	E	C	I	E	C	I	E	C	I	E	C	I	E	C	I	E	C	I	E	C
1. MR	I	.56**	.43*		.50*			.46*						.43*	.41*	-.52**				.44*	.42*	-.53**			-.46*						
	E	.47*		-.65**	.42*			.41*		-.42*						.41*				.43*											
	C			.47*			-.49*																								
2. FR	I	.49*			.55*	.41*		.43*			.45*			.44*	.44*		.41*			.43*		-.42*			.42*						
	E	.41*		-.58**	.51*	.41*	-.63**			-.44*	.51**		-.43*				.42*		-.49*	.41*											
	C						.41*									.41*															
3. TR	I	.44*			.41*			.57**	.41*	-.55**	.43*		-.47*	.43*		-.44*	.45*			.43*		-.42*			-.45*						
	E	.41*		-.42*	.43*		-.42*	.47*		.42*			.42*		.41*			.41*	-.41*	.41*											
	C						-.43*				.46*																				
4. PN	I										.46*		.43*	.43*			.41*			.41*		-.48*									
	E												.40*	.46*		-.45*				.43*		.42*									
	C																														
5. 24 M	I	.47*			.43*							.41*		.44*		-.49**	.41*		-.45*	.42*		-.47*									
	E	.43*	.41*	-.49*	.41*		-.46*			-.44*		.41*		.46*	.43*		.43*			.46*					-.45*						
	C																			.45*											
6. 24 F	I	.43*			.42*									.44*		-.46*	.43*		-.49*	.45*		-.43*			-.45*						
	E	.41*		-.46*	.41*	.41*	-.46*			-.44*				.42*	.41*		.46*	.41*	-.42*												
	C																														
7. OHB	I	.44*		-.53**	.47*			.46*			.49*			.42*		-.45*		.41*	-.46*	.41*		-.48*	.52**	.47*							
	E	.42*			.42*	.42*	-.43*	.44*		-.41*	.43*		-.46*							.43*		.42*			-.45*						
	C									.43*			.41*																		
8. OSB	I			-.41*																					-.43*						
	E																					.42*			.41*						
	C																														

*p < 0.05, ** p < 0.01.

All measures for daughters in nondivorced families have an N of 23, with the exception of those involving teacher ratings, peer nominations, and school observations where the N = 21.

MR = mother ratings, FR = father ratings, TR = teacher ratings, PN = peer nominations, 24 M = 24-hour checklist by mother, 24 F = 24-hour checklist by father, OHB = observed home behavior, OSB = observed school behavior, CR = child rating, 24 C = 24-hour checklist by child; I = internalizing, E = externalizing, C = social competence.

school measures involve different teachers, peers, and observers at the two points in time, the results cannot be attributed to a response bias, such as might occur in maternal reports when the same individual is reporting on two occasions, albeit widely spaced ones. In addition to the home and school situations playing an important role in consistency across time, the source of information (mother, father, peers, and teacher) and type of measure also influence stability. Thus it can be seen that maternal and teacher measures more often correlate with criterion measures than do nonresidential fathers or peer measures.

The paternal measures in the divorced families must be viewed with caution, since they involve noncustodial fathers, many of whom are seeing their children infrequently and who may have little opportunity to observe their children's behavior. It can be seen that there are few significant correlations involving time$_4$ divorced father measures as the criterion variables. In addition, the test-retest reliabilities of the early peer nomination measures tested at a 1-month interval for 60 children at each age level were significant but modest, and this lower reliability may contribute to the dearth of findings involving early peer nominations. It must be remembered that the time$_1$ children were only 4 years old, whereas time$_4$ children were 10 and more able to respond reliably to the peer nomination measures. However, it should be noted that there are more significant correlations than would be expected by chance between early and later peer nominations and that the pattern of greater stability in externalizing for boys and in internalizing for girls is found in these measures.

The child's self-ratings and 24-hour behavior checklist were available only at the 6-year follow-up. Early teacher, parent, and peer reports did not predict the child's later self-reported internalizing or social competence. Only divorced and nondivorced maternal and nondivorced paternal ratings and 24-hour checklists were modestly correlated with the son's later reports of externalizing on the child's 24-hour checklist. It has been argued (Cairns and Cairns, 1984) that children's self-evaluations represent a type of "private" information that differs from the "public information" used in such measures as parent and teacher ratings, observed behavior, or peer nominations. This particularly may be the case in measures of internalizing, where such things as anxiety and depression may be less obvious to others than are externalizing behaviors such as aggression and noncompliance. Several studies have found low agreement among raters when self-other ratings are involved (Cairns and Cairns, 1984; Ledingham, 1981). Moreover, Ledingham (1981) also found that self-other agreement was higher for aggression than for withdrawal or likeability.

Finally, there are more significant correlations among early predictor and later outcome criteria for nondivorced than divorced families.

Life Change and Instability in Behavior

What factors might contribute to the greater instability of behavior in divorced than in nondivorced families? It has been suggested that divorce increases the probability of children and families encountering life changes, particularly stressful life changes (Hetherington, 1981; Stolberg and Anker, 1983). Separate multivariate analyses of variance followed by univariate analyses of significant effects were performed on the maternal and child reports on the Life Stress Inventory, involving family type and sex of child as independent variables and positive and negative life changes since divorce as dependent measures. Since the measures in these analyses involved only time$_4$ measures, the larger, expanded sample was used in these analyses. This sample included 30 sons and daughters in each of three groups (a nondivorced group, a mother-custody/nonremarried group, and a remarried mother-stepfather group). It is interesting that there is a sex-by-family-type interaction for both maternal and child measures for both the 1- and 6-year measures. Divorced mothers and their sons perceive more negative life changes having occurred since divorce than do mothers and children in nondivorced families. This is true for the 1- and 6-year appraisal. However, daughters in remarried families perceive more negative life changes as having occurred in the last year than any group except sons in the divorced, nonremarried group. A reverse pattern holds for positive life changes.

How are these life changes related to the adjustment of children at time$_4$? The mother's and child's reports of positive and negative life changes over the past year and past 6 years were correlated with the child outcomes. Negative life events tended to be associated with both internalizing and externalizing for boys and girls, and with social competence for boys in divorced families, although the effects were most marked for externalizing in boys and internalizing in girls. The pattern of findings for mothers and children was similar. These effects of negative life events were less marked in nondivorced families, perhaps because of a more restricted range of negative life events. There were no more correlations that would be expected by change between positive changes and children's adjustment. When they did occur, they tended to be related to competence and internalizing. In addition, although there were few differences between the correlations for the past year and the past 6 years, when they did occur they tended to occur in the divorced and remarried families.

Long-Term Outcomes of Divorce and Remarriage

Multivariate analyses, followed by univariate analysis of significant multivariate effects were performed for each of the time$_4$ data sets separately, with family type and sex of child as independent variables and internalizing, externalizing, and competence as dependent variables. The remarried stepfather group was further broken down into a remarried less than 2 years group (early remarriage, ER) and remarried more than 2 years group (late remarriage, LR); thus, there were four family groups. This was based on the assumption that families who were in the first 2 years of a remarriage would be adapting to another life transition, in contrast to families who had been in their current marital situation for more than 2 years. The analyses for residential fathers involved only three family types (early remarriage, later remarriage, and nondivorced). the MANOVAs for noncustodial father measures involved three family types (early remarriage, $N = 44$; later remarriage, $N = 32$, and divorced families, $N = 49$) and involved incomplete data. Noncustodial fathers on the 24-hour behavior checklist evaluated behavior that had occurred only over a 3-hour period spent in visitation. Tables 5, 6, and 7 present the means for the 6-year measures. Significant main effects and interactions are noted. When a significant interaction occurs, letters are appended to the means. Means with common subscripts are not significantly different.

The general pattern of results suggests that daughters in families with a divorced, nonremarried mother are very similar in adjustment to those in nondivorced families. In contrast, even 6 years after divorce, sons in divorced families are showing more externalizing behavior and are sometimes reported to be showing more internalizing behavior and less social competence than sons in nondivorced families. The greater externalizing in divorced male subjects is consistently reported by sons, mothers, teachers, and peers. In addition, this greater antisocial behavior emerges in the observations in the home and in mothers' and sons' 24-hour behavior checklists. Differences in internalizing behavior and social competence are less consistent. Mothers, sons, and noncustodial parents rate the boys in divorced families to be more depressed and withdrawn; teachers and peers do not. Moreover, although high internalizing is reported by these boys on their 24-hour behavior checklists, it is not found on maternal checklists or in observational measures.

The picture that emerges for children in remarried families is very different. Boys and girls with mothers who have been remarried less than 2 years are viewed by themselves and their parents as having more

TABLE 5
Mean Internalizing Measures for Boys and Girls in Nondivorced (ND), Divorced (D), Early Remarried (ER), and Late Remarried (LR) Families

T_4 Measures	Boys (B)				Girls (G)				Significant Effects*
	ND	D	ER	LR	ND	D	ER	LR	
1. MR	50.6_a	59.8_b	51.1_a	50.7_a	52.4_a	51.5_a	54.5_a	52.3_a	F × S
2. RFR	52.9_a		53.0_a	51.4_a	50.1_a		60.6_b	55.0_c	F × S
3. NFR		56.3	52.6	53.4		51.3	54.8	51.7	NS
4. TR	40.4_a	45.7_a	42.1_a	39.3_a	51.2_b	48.6_b	59.9_c	52.9_b	S(G > B) F × S
5. PN	-0.16_a	0.32_a	0.11_a	-0.12_a	-0.06_a	-0.10_a	2.10_b	1.10_b	F × S
6. CR	15.6_a	20.7_b	16.7_a	16.8_a	21.3_b	23.4_b	27.3_c	23.1_b	S(G > B) F × S
7. 24 M	16.0	17.9	19.4	16.3	18.3	21.1	17.6	19.7	NS
8. 24 RF	17.8		16.9	14.8	18.3		14.7	15.6	NS
9. 24 NF		9.0	10.6	11.3		10.8	12.6	9.4	NS
10. 24 C	14.1	19.6	13.2	14.9	17.7	18.5	16.9	19.6	S(G > B)
11. OHB	0.09	0.10	0.03	0.08	0.10	0.09	0.11	0.12	NS
12. OSB	0.12_a	0.09_a	0.06_a	0.11_a	0.16_b	0.19_b	0.36_c	0.13_{ab}	S(G > B) F × S

* Significant effects are indicated by F for family type and S for sex of child. G indicates girl and B boy. When a significant interaction occurs, means with common subscripts are not significantly different.

MR = mother ratings, RFR = residential father ratings, NFR = nonresidential father ratings, TR = teacher ratings, PN = peer nominations, CR = child ratings, 24 M = 24-hour checklist by mother, 24 RF = 24-hour checklist by residential father, 24 NF = 24-hour checklist by nonresidential father, 24 C = 24-hour checklist by child, OHB = observed home behavior, OSB = observed school behavior.

TABLE 6

Mean Externalizing Measures for Boys and Girls in Nondivorced (ND), Divorced (D), Early Remarried (ER), and Late Remarried (LR) Families

T_4 Measures	Boys (B)				Girls (G)				Significant Effects*
	ND	D	ER	LR	ND	D	ER	LR	
1. MR	54.1_a	66.7_b	63.1_b	56.2_a	50.3_a	49.6_a	62.0_b	53.3_a	S(B > G) F × S
2. RFR	53.3_a		64.5_{bc}	60.1_b	48.8_a		66.8_c	59.4_b	F × S
3. NFR		58.3_a	59.7_a	52.4_b		51.6_b	57.9_a	56.7_a	F × S
4. TR	47.4_a	61.5_d	56.2_d	49.9_a	33.6_a	34.1_b	40.3_c	37.3_{bc}	S(B > G) F × S
5. PN	0.17_a	2.08_b	1.89_b	1.73_b	-0.13_a	-0.18_a	2.1_b	1.2_c	S(B > G) F × S
6. CR	17.1_b	23.9_a	22.9_a	16.8_b	11.5_c	12.4_c	18.6_b	16.1_b	S(B > G) F × S
7. 24 M	21.3_{ad}	30.9_b	28.2_b	23.6_a	11.7_c	12.9_c	17.1_d	14.3_c	S(B > G) F × S
8. 24 RF	16.1_a		21.3_c	16.3_a	8.4_b		16.2_a	10.1_b	S(B > G) F × S
9. 24 NF		13.1	14.8	16.0		10.5	14.1	11.2	NS
10. 24 C	20.3_a	32.0_c	26.1_d	20.8_a	13.7_b	14.6_b	19.2_a	11.5_b	S(B > G) F × S
11. OHB	0.11_a	0.40_c	0.29_c	0.14_{ab}	0.07_a	0.09_a	0.19_b	0.07_a	S(B > G) F × S
12. OSB	0.09_a	0.21_{cd}	0.17_b	0.11_a	0.06_a	0.07_a	0.16_a	0.09_a	S(G > B) F × S

* Significant effects are indicated by F for family type and S for sex of child. G indicates girl and B boy. When a significant interaction occurs, means with common subscripts are not significantly different.

MR = mother ratings, RFR = residential father ratings, NFR = nonresidential father ratings, TR = teacher ratings, PN = peer nominations, CR = child ratings, 24 M = 24-hour checklist by mother, 24 RF = 24-hour checklist by residential father, 24 NF = 24-hour checklist by nonresidential father, 24 C = 24-hour checklist by child, OHB = observed home behavior, OSB = observed school behavior.

TABLE 7

Mean Social Competence Measures for Boys and Girls in Nondivorced (ND), Divorced (D), Early Remarried (ER), and Late Remarried (LR) Families

T_4 Measures	Boys (B)				Girls (G)				Significant Effects*
	ND	D	ER	LR	ND	D	ER	LR	
1. MR	54.7ab	42.2c	52.6ab	56.3a	54.9ab	53.6ab	51.9b	50.0b	F × S
2. RFR	55.2a		52.1a	55.6a	60.1b		46.3c	48.4c	F × S
3. NFR		50.3	48.2	51.7		54.5	49.3	49.7	NS
4. TR	39.3	35.4	36.8	37.5	46.6	44.7	42.3	43.9	S(G > B)
5. PN	0.42	−0.38	−0.23	−0.13	0.30	0.27	−0.14	0.26	NS
6. CR	17.3	14.1	13.5	13.7	23.8	22.6	18.9	19.7	S(G > B)
7. 24 M	16.8	14.2	13.9	14.0	18.4	20.9	17.3	19.6	S(G > B)
8. 24 RF	14.3		12.6	13.5	19.9		15.1	18.7	S(G > B)
9. 24 NF		12.7	9.1	11.6		13.4	12.1	14.1	NS
10. 24 C	17.9	16.4	18.1	17.3	22.3	21.8	20.1	23.7	S(G > B)
11. OHB	0.13	0.09	0.11	0.14	0.16	0.19	0.10	0.18	S(G > B)
12. OSB	0.17a	0.06b	0.08b	0.15a	0.19a	0.22a	0.09b	0.15a	S(G > B) F × S

* Significant effects are indicated by F for family type and S for sex of child. G indicates girl and B boy. When a significant interaction occurs, means with common subscripts are not significantly different.

MR = mother ratings, RFR = residential father ratings, NFR = nonresidential father ratings, TR = teacher ratings, PN = peer nominations, CR = child ratings, 24 M = 24-hour checklist by mother, 24 RF = 24-hour checklist by residential father, 24 NF = 24-hour checklist by nonresidential father, 24 C = 24-hour checklist by child, OHB = observed home behavior, OSB = observed school behavior.

externalizing problems than children in nondivorced families. Stepfathers also perceive their stepdaughters to be higher in internalizing and lower in social competence; the stepdaughters agree in reporting themselves to be higher on internalizing but also rate themselves as higher on social competence. The boys from families in which the remarriage occurred more than 2 years before do not differ from boys in nondivorced families, except for a rating of greater externalizing by stepfathers. However, stepdaughters continue to be viewed by their stepfathers and to view themselves as having more problems than girls in nondivorced families. Some adaptation appears to be occurring, however, because they generally are viewed as better adjusted than those in families in the early stages of remarriage. The 24-hour checklists and behavioral observations in general agree with the findings on the ratings measuring externalizing, but show fewer differences on internalizing and socially competent behavior.

The school measures confirm the findings in the home of greater externalizing and less socially competent behavior for boys in divorced families and for boys and girls whose parents are in the early years of remarriage. These girls during early remarriage are also rated by teachers as higher in internalizing. Again, some adaptation occurs to remarriage, since, in the children of the longer remarried mothers, peers but not teachers view sons as still showing more externalizing behavior than those in nondivorced families but less than those in divorced families or in families which had been remarried less than two years. Again, peers report less internalizing and externalizing in the girls from longer remarried families. The observational data in the school indicate more externalizing behavior and less socially competent behavior in sons in divorced families than in other families. More internalizing, externalizing, and less socially competent behavior is observed in the stepdaughters in the first 2 years of remarriage than in the nondivorced or divorced groups.

DISCUSSION

In agreement with the findings of earlier studies, divorce has more adverse, long-term effects on boys (Hetherington et al., 1982; Guidubaldi et al., 1983, 1984; Peterson and Zill, 1983; Zill and Peterson, unpublished manuscript), and the remarriage of a custodial mother is associated with an increase in behavior problems in girls and some decrease in problems in boys (Peterson and Zill, 1983; Santrock et al., 1982). In contrast to Santrock et al. (1982), the findings in this study do not show that stepsons are as well adjusted as sons in nondivorced families, although they are better adjusted in the long run than those who remain in divorced mother-headed households. Divorced mothers and sons who are often involved in mutual patterns of coercion have much to gain from the addition of a responsive, authoritative stepfather, who offers support to both the mother and son (Hetherington et al., 1982). Children benefit from the presence of an involved same-sex parent or parent surrogate. In contrast, divorced mothers and their daughters often form close relationships which the intrusion of a stepfather may disrupt. Stepfathers view the relationships with stepchildren as a major problem in their marriages (Hetherington et al., 1985), and it can be seen that stepfathers report more problem behaviors in their stepchildren, especially their stepdaughters, than is reported by the mothers or children.

The adjustment to remarriage gradually improves as new family roles and relationships are established. The most successful stepfathers are those who establish a positive relationship with the child before taking an active role in discipline and decision making. However, even after this relationship is established, the most successful stepfathers appear to be those who offer emotional support to the mother and support her in her disciplinary role, rather than those who try to take over the role of disciplinarian or who remain uninvolved (Hetherington et al., 1982, 1985).

Do the children who have problems in the preschool years and in the 2 years following divorce continue to show the same problems 4 years later when they are 10? This seems to depend on the sex of the child, the ensuing family reorganization, and the negative life experiences encountered by the child. There is less continuity in the adjustment of children from divorced families than nondivorced families because of the greater probability they have of encountering multiple negative life changes in such things as family relationships, mental and physical health of family members, child care, geographic mobility, and economic status. It should be noted that, although some investigators have emphasized the role of decline in financial status as a major contributor to the adjustment of divorced children, in this study of middle-class families, economic factors did not relate to measures of parent-child relations or child adjustment (Hetherington et al., 1982). Negative life changes play a significant role in sustaining or precipitating the development of behavior disorders in children.

This study supports the findings in a number of other studies that externalizing behavior is more stable over time for boys (Ledingham, 1981; Roff and Wirt, 1984) and internalizing for girls (Ledingham,

1981). Early aggressive and antisocial behavior is more predictive of later behavior problems and lack of social competence than is early withdrawal and anxiety. Moreover, early externalizing behavior in girls, perhaps because it is less frequent and viewed as less sex appropriate, is the best predictor of later socially inept behavior. In contrast, early social competence shows only a modest relationship to later social skills in female subjects. Much greater stability in social competence is found for boys. Preschool boys who are viewed by peers, teachers, and parents as socially unskilled and insensitive are less competent and show more antisocial behavior as 10-year-olds.

In summary, children do adjust to their parents' marital rearrangements, although children who go through divorce and remarriage show at least more short-term problems than do children in nondivorced families. Long-term problems in adjustment differ for boys and girls, with boys showing more long-term problems in response to divorce and girls in response to remarriage. The stability of problem behaviors also varies with sex of child.

Although this paper examines life changes only as a mediator of developmental outcomes for children, other studies have shown that the quality of family relationships may be more important than life changes in moderating the outcomes of divorce and remarriage. Future papers on this follow-up study and the expanded 6-year cohort will examine these relationships.

REFERENCES

Achenbach, T. M. & Edelbrock, C. (1983), *Manual for the Child Behavior Checklist*. New York: Queen City Printers.

Adams, B. (1984), Longitudinal Effects of Divorce on Children. Paper presented at the annual convention of the American Psychological Association, Toronto, Canada (August).

Bloom, B. L., Asher, S. J. & White, S. W. (1978), Marital disruption as a stressor: a review and analysis. *Psychol. Bull.*, 85:867-894.

Cairns, R. B. & Cairns, B. D. (1984), Predicting aggressive patterns in girls and boys: a developmental study. *Aggr. Behav.*, 10:227-242.

Guidubaldi, J., Cleminshaw, H. K., Perry, J. D. & McLoughlin, C. S. (1983), The Impact of Parental Divorce on Children: Report of the Nationwide NASP Study. Paper presented at the annual convention of the National Association for School Psychologists, Detroit (March).

Hetherington, E. M. (1972), Effects of father absence on personality development in adolescent daughters. *Developm. Psychol.*, 7:313-326.

——— (1981), Children and divorce. In: *Parent-Child Interaction: Theory, Research and Prospect*, ed. R. Henderson. New York: Academic Press, pp. 33-58.

——— & Camara, K. A. (1984), Families in transition: the process of dissolution and reconstitution. In: *Review of Child Development Research: The Family*, Vol. 7, ed. R. D. Parke. Chicago: University of Chicago Press, pp. 398-439.

———— Cox, M. & Cox, R. (1978), The aftermath of divorce. In: *Mother-Child, Father-Child Relations*, ed. J H. Stevens, Jr. & M. Matthews. Washington, D.C.: National Association for the Education of Young Children, pp. 110-155.

———— ———— ———— (1979a), Family interaction and the social, emotional and cognitive development of children following divorce. In: *The Family: Setting Priorities*, ed. V. Vaughn & T. Brazelton. New York: Science and Medicine Publishing Co., pp. 89-128.

———— ———— ———— (1979b), Play and social interaction in children following divorce. *J. Soc. Issues*, 35:26-49.

———— ———— ———— (1982), Effects of divorce on parents and children. In: *Nontraditional Families: Parenting and Child Development*, ed. M. E. Lamb. Hillsdale, N.J.: Lawrence Erlbaum, pp. 233-288.

———— Camara, K. A. & Featherman, D. (1983), Achievement and intellectual functioning of children in one-parent households. In: *Assessing Achievement*, ed. J. Spence. San Francisco: W. H. Freeman, pp. 206-284.

———— Arnett, J. & Hollier, A. (1985), The effects of remarriage on children and families. In: *Family Transition*, ed. P. Karoly & S. Wolchick. New York: Garland Press (in press).

Kurdek, L. A. (ed.) (1983), *Children and Divorce*. San Francisco: Jossey-Bass.

Ledingham, J. E. (1981), Developmental patterns of aggressive and withdrawn behavior in childhood: a possible method for identifying preschizophrenics. *J. Abnorm. Child Psychol.*, 9:1-22.

Pekarik, E. G., Prinz, R. J., Liebert, D. E., Weintraub, S. & Neale, J. M. (1976), The Pupil Evaluation Inventory. *J. Abnorm. Child Psychol.*, 4:83-97.

Peterson, J. L. & Zill, N. (1983), Marital Disruption, Parent/Child Relationships and Behavioral Problems in Children. Paper presented at the annual meetings of the Society for Research in Child Development, Detroit, (April).

Roff, J. D. & Wirt, R. D. (1984), Childhood aggression and social adjustment as antecedents of delinquency. *J. Abnorm. Child Psychol.*, 12:111-126.

Santrock, J. W., Warshak, R. A. & Elliott, G. L. (1982), Social development and parent-child interaction in father-custody and stepmother families. In: *Nontraditional Families: Parenting and Child Development*, ed. M. E. Lamb. Hillsdale, N.J.: Lawrence Erlbaum, pp. 289-331.

Sarason, I. G., Johnson, J. & Siegel, J. (1978), Assessing the impact of life changes: development of the Life Experiences Survey. *J. Consult. Clin. Psychol.*, 46:932-946.

Stolberg, A. L. & Anker, J. M. (1983), Cognitive and behavioral changes in children resulting from parental divorce and consequent environmental changes. *J. Divorce* 7:23-41.

Wallerstein, J. S. (1982), Children of Divorce: Preliminary Report of a Ten-Year Follow-up. Paper presented at the 10th international congress of the International Association for Child and Adolescent Psychiatry and Allied Professions, Dublin (July).

———— & Kelly, J. B. (1980), *Surviving the Breakup: How Children Actually Cope with Divorce*. New York: Basic Books.

Warshak, R. A. & Santrock, J. W. (1983), The impact of divorce in father-custody and mother-custody homes: the child's perspective. In: *Children and Divorce*, ed. L. A. Kurdek. San Francisco: Jossey-Bass, pp. 29-46.

Zill, N. & Peterson, J. L. Marital Disruption and Children's Need for Psychological Help. Unpublished manuscript.

24

Children of Divorce: Preliminary Report of a Ten-Year Follow-up of Older Children and Adolescents

Judith S. Wallerstein

Center for the Family in Transition
Corte Madera, California

Preliminary findings from a 10-year longitudinal study of 113 children and adolescents from a largely white, middle-class population of divorced families in Northern California suggest that some psychological effects of divorce are long lasting. Forty young adults who range in age from 19 to 29 at the 10-year mark regard their parents' divorce as a continuing major influence in their lives. A significant number appear burdened by vivid memories of the marital rupture, by feelings of sadness, continuing resentment at parents, and a sense of deprivation. They are as a group strongly committed to the ideals of a lasting marriage and to a conservative morality. Young men and women, and especially young women, are apprehensive about repeating their parents' unhappy marriage during their own adulthood, and they appear especially eager to avoid divorce for the sake of their future children.

Reprinted with permission from the *Journal of the American Academy of Child Psychiatry*, 1985, Vol. 24, 545–553. Copyright 1985 by the American Academy of Child Psychiatry.

This paper is an expanded version of a paper presented at the Tenth International Congress of the International Association for Child and Adolescent Psychiatry and Allied Professions in Dublin, July 1982.

This work is supported by the Zellerbach Family Fund, the San Francisco Foundation, and the Marion E. Kenworthy-Sarah H. Swift Foundation.

This is a preliminary report from a 10-year longitudinal study of the responses of children and their parents to divorce. The study, which began in 1971, and subsequently became widely known as the California Children of Divorce project, was designed to explore the experience of divorce in a nonclinical population of 60 California families whose 131 children were between 2 and 18 years old at the time of the decisive marital separation.

Observations in this paper are based on 40 young people who were 9 years old or older at the time of their parents' decisive separation and who were located for follow-up during a 2-year period beginning in 1981. They are 16 young men and 24 young women who ranged in age from 19 to 29 at the 10-year mark. They comprise a group of young adults who are well past high school, likely to have made some important career and relationship decisions, and to have achieved or consolidated a particular perspective regarding their parents, and perhaps, also, to have formed reasonably stable attitudes regarding the divorce experience of their own childhood and its implications for their own lives. Full data regarding the course of the children and adults over the 10-year period are currently in the process of analysis. This paper represents some of the patterns that emerge on initial clinical inspection of the 40 young people who are entering or have already entered young adulthood.

METHOD AND SAMPLE

To review briefly the population and method of the project at its inception, in 1971 each of 131 children and adolescents, together with their parents, were studied intensively during a 6-week period close to the marital separation (Wallerstein and Kelly, 1980). Each family member was reexamined again at 18 months post-separation and once again at 5 years post-separation. The 131 children were divided roughly equally between male and female (48% boys, 52% girls), slightly more than half were 8 years old or less, 47% were between 9 and 18 years old. At the 5-year mark, the final sample for whom there was sufficient data, including extended interviews at each of the three points in time to permit a full psychological and social assessment, consisted of 96 children from 56 families.* At the 10-year mark, 54 (90%) of the original 60

---

*Analysis of the families who were lost to follow-up at the 18-month and 5-year mark indicates that these families did not differ from the population that remained in the study in their race or socioeconomic status nor along psychological dimensions which we were able to ascertain. Fifty-eight families were located at each of the 3 points in the study, but 2 families with 5 children reconciled and therefore were excluded from this analysis.

families were located, and members in 52 families (87%) were interviewed. Of the children, 110 were interviewed directly, and extensive data regarding another 6 were obtained from family members, surpassing the numbers reached at the 5-year mark. Of all the children reached, 113 met the criteria for inclusion in the analysis. These included 50 male and 63 female subjects, seen over the 2-year period 1981-1983. The mean length of time since the separation was 10.9 years with a range of 9.6-13.1 years.

Our ability to locate these youngsters after a lapse of so many years was unexpectedly aided by the finding that a full 41% of the young people continued to reside in the county in which the initial study was done. An additional 36% moved out of the immediate geographical area to neighboring San Francisco Bay Area counties or elsewhere within the state, so that 77% of the young people in the study had remained in California. Of the remainder, half live in neighboring states. None are living outside of the country. Overall this represents an unanticipated stability in residence.

All of the subjects, the young people and their parents, were seen separately in semistructured clinical interviews of several hours' duration. The interviews were supplemented by questionnaires. We were fortunate in obtaining the participation of 3 of the 5 clinicians who participated in the initial study. The participation of this initial clinical team may well account for the high level of response.

In their initial socioeconomic distribution, the families reflected the population of the Northern California county in which they resided. The families were largely, but not entirely, within the middle-class range. Of the 60 families, 88% were white, 3% were black, and 9% were interracial with one Asian spouse. They were a well-educated group; one-quarter of the men held advanced degrees in medicine, law, or business administration. The average age of the men at separation was 36.9; the mean age for the women was 34.1. They had been married an average of 11.1 years prior to the decisive separation. The couples averaged 2.2 children per family.

It is important in assessing the 10-year findings, as well as those of the earlier checkpoints of the study, to recall that the children were screened initially for chronic psychological problems. Prior to the family rupture, all of the children in the study had reached appropriate developmental milestones in the view of their parents and teachers. They were performing at age-appropriate levels within the school. Children who had ever been referred for psychological or psychiatric treatment were excluded from the study. The study group represented, therefore, young people probably skewed in the direction of psychological health since they had been able by all accounts to maintain their developmental pace within the failing marriage.

Findings from the initial assessment at the time of the breakup showed widespread acute distress among the children accompanied by an almost universal wish to undo the divorce and restore the intact family. Children and adolescents alike suffered with anxiety, depression, worry over one or both parents, rising anger at parents, loyalty conflicts, and guilt. These responses, while occurring at every age, were experienced and expressed largely in accord with the age of the child and his or her place along the developmental continuum. The dominant content of the child's underlying fantasies, the child's perceptions of family events, the coping configurations used, the changed patterns of behavior that emerged (including symptomatic behavior), and the child's dominant response to the departure of one parent were all governed during the early period primarily by factors of age and developmental maturity rather than the individual family history or the specific dynamics of the family relationships.

Youngsters who had been between the ages of 9 and 18 at the initial assessment included two groups, those who were still in latency or preadolescence and those who had already reached adolescence. There were distinguishable differences between these two groups. The later latency or preadolescent youngsters felt especially powerless, as well as frightened, at the marital rupture. Most striking, however, was their intense anger at one or both parents for precipitating the divorce. They were more inclined at this age to align with one parent, to take sides in the parental conflict, and to join with one parent in a bitter, even mischievous harrassment of the other parent. About half of the boys and girls in this group suffered a severe drop in their school work that lasted during the year following the marital rupture (Wallerstein and Kelly, 1976). Responses in the adolescent group were of concern because of the vulnerability of so many youngsters to acute depression, to acting out, to a regression that included emotional and social withdrawal from involvement with friends and investment in school. The anxiety of almost all of the adolescents with regard to their own future ran very high. A significant number of the adolescent young people also showed an impressive developmental spurt. Many were mature, compassionate, and genuinely helpful to one or both parents during and after the marital crisis (Wallerstein and Kelly, 1974).

The second stage of the study, 18 months following the marital separation, revealed psychological decline among children and adolescents who at first seemed to have survived the failing marriage and the conflicts surrounding the marital breakup without significant psychological dysfunction. Differences between the sexes emerged strikingly at this time. Young boys below the age of adolescence were significantly more troubled in their performance and behavior at school, playground, and home than the girls; and, in fact, many of the girls seemed to be well on their way to recovery from their initial distressed reactions. It should, of course, be noted that almost all of these youngsters were in the custody of their mothers. Few differences between the sexes in the incidence of new or continuing distress were noted in the adolescent group at that time.

Conclusions at the 5-year mark showed strong connection between good psychological adjustment in the children and the overall quality of life within the post-divorce family. Neither the age of the child at the time of the marital separation nor the sex of the child was significant in outcome at that time. These and other factors associated with the response to the marital rupture had faded. Instead, the overriding importance of the youngster's experience within the post-divorce family emerged strongly. And while no single factor was associated with good outcome, the quality of the parenting within the post-divorce family, the continuity of relationships with the visiting parent, and the extent to which the conflict between the divorcing partners had subsided all contributed to the well-being of the child. In effect, the extent to which the divorced or the remarried family had been able to create a richer, more emotionally satisfying life that included the children had become salient (Wallerstein and Kelly, 1980).

GOALS AT THE 10-YEAR MARK

The decision to return to the same population at 10 years was stimulated by adolescent youngsters at the 5-year mark who called attention to some of their grave concerns regarding their capacity to establish and maintain an enduring love relationship. As they looked ahead toward adulthood, they were frightened by the long shadows that they perceived to be cast by their parents' divorce. Their worry was that they might be doomed to repeat their parents' divorce during their own adulthood. It seemed very important to follow these young people in their entry into young adulthood and to ascertain whether the anxiety which they had expressed during adolescence had persisted and whether indeed this had translated into difficulty in forging relationships and making commitments. It also seemed important to determine how widespread such concerns might be.

A great many related questions emerged quickly as the research plan developed. To name only a few: To what extent had the divorce experience been consigned to the distant past at the 10-year mark? We had been surprised during the 5-year assessment at the persistence of anger at the parent who had initiated the divorce, at the intensity of longing for the absent or erratically visiting parent, at the persistence of the youngster's wish to reconstitute the pre-divorce family. Had these feelings and wishes been maintained by young people entering adulthood? To what extent, if at all, does having experienced divorce in one's family as a child remain an important part of the young adult's identity? Is it an experience that remains central to the young person's view of him or herself and stance vis-à-vis the world, or does it get pushed to an unimportant periphery? Which issues are more likely to find resolution with increasing maturity? Are there issues which are more likely to remain unresolved, and for whom and under what circumstances?

Additionally, a significant number of children and adolescents were considered psychologically troubled at the 5-year mark. We had diagnosed moderate to severe clinical depression in over a third of the original sample at that time. It appeared important to know whether these youngsters had rallied during the intervening years, with or without psychological intervention, and whether they had been able to resolve some of the conflicts which had preoccupied them at that time. Alternatively, we were interested in the young people who had become more mature and more independent in response to the family crisis and had provided sustained help and emotional support to one or both parents during the trying period of the divorce and the several-year aftermath. Had these young people been able to maintain their mature stance, and had they moved into young adulthood with the same vigor and forthrightness that had characterized their early response to the marital rupture and to their parents' need?

On a more theoretical level, I have, in an earlier paper (Wallerstein, 1983), conceptualized adolescence as a natural restorative period within the developmental process which, while it carries the potential for serious decline, also presents the young person with an opportunity for a full dress reworking of the divorce experience. And I have suggested, as well, that therefore adolescence may have special importance for children who have experienced serious distress during their earlier years. Thus, in extension of the conception put forth by Blos (1962) of adolescence as a "second chance," we observed at the 5-year study that many youngsters were in the process of revising their earlier views of the divorce. Their attitudes and relationships with parents and stepparents seemed to be undergoing shifts at that time. Young people who had been estranged from a parent for many years actively sought out that parent. Others were able for the first time to recognize severe mental illness or deviance in a parent and to understand the basis for the divorce of which they had earlier strongly disapproved (Wallerstein and Kelly, 1980). It seemed important to follow the course of these young people and to find out whether psychological changes evident at the close of adolescence reflected resolution of conflicts which had been stirred or exacerbated by the family ordeal and whether the changes that we observed in adolescence were holding through the young adult years. Finally, of course, a longitudinal study of a population that has sustained a particular stress, in this instance divorce, would lend itself to an examination of patterns of continuity and discontinuity throughout the 10-year period. These and many other questions guided our efforts.

SCHOOL AND EMPLOYMENT

Of the 40 young men and women who were between 9 and 18 at the time of their parents' divorce, and between 19 and 29 at the 10-year follow-up, almost half were full time in school at the 10-year mark. Additionally, 2 young men were full time at work and continued to maintain a full-time commitment to school. Of those entirely out of school, half had dropped out, 5 from college-level programs (1 from a 4-year college and 4 from junior college) and 5 from high school. All of the youngsters who dropped out of high school before graduation were girls.

Of the young people entirely out of school, almost a third (30%) were unemployed, of whom only a very few had marketable skills. The remainder had a history of low-level jobs and frequent change in employment. Of the 14 young people who had left school and were fully in the employment market, only 4 held professional or career-oriented jobs. The troublesome finding is that, of the 14 who had opted for employment and left school, most were employed in itinerant, relatively unskilled jobs, such as waitressing or temporary sales positions. Additionally, one married young woman with 2 children had left her chronically unemployed husband and was subsisting on welfare. The inescapable conclusion, therefore, is that except for a minority of these young people, those who had entered the employment market were poorly equipped to enter that market and were doing so at the lower levels. This is a striking finding considering the middle-class status or upper middle-class status of the families of their origin.

We were struck by the finding that only two-thirds of these young people were attending or had graduated from college or were seeking advanced degrees in a community where 85% of the high school graduates go on directly to junior college or 4-year college programs. It may well be that this lower incidence of college enrollment among this group is related, at least in part, to the fact that in the majority of the families child support stopped abruptly when the youngsters reached 18. Certainly those who were at the university at the time of the follow-up were often carrying jobs or sometimes even alternating school semester with full-time work in order to earn tuition and living expenses. Of those 8 who had dropped out of college after entering, 5 had been struggling financially and were receiving no financial help from their fathers. Of the 20 young people who were in college or graduate school at the time of the study, 5 received no help at all from wealthy fathers whose income at the time was a hundred thousand dollars a year or more. Four of these 5 young people were no longer living at home and required independent support. Overall, the burdening of the opportunity for post-secondary education for children in divorced families, if found to exist in a wide population, represents a grave issue, not only for these youngsters but for society as a whole in the potential for educational and economic disadvantaging of these young people.

DELINQUENCY

Of the 40 young people 27 (68%) of the group—11 male and 16 female subjects—had engaged in mild to serious illegal activity during their adolescence or young adulthood. The delinquency of more than half of these young people consisted only of underage alcohol consumption or recreational drug use. The remaining 12 (30% of those who were 9–18 years old at the initial assessment) had engaged in moderately serious or serious illegal activities, including assault, burglary, arson, drug dealing, theft, and serious traffic violations, such as drunk driving. Seven of these 12 youngsters were involved in these activities after reaching age 18; and of these, 4 were recidivists with multiple arrests to the point of seemingly chronic behavior. Two young men had served jail sentences. One had been in and out of jail for burglary on several occasions, while another at 21 had been involved in many delinquent acts, including theft, drug dealing, drunk driving, assault, and beating up his girlfriend.

The type of offense differed considerably between the sexes as expected. Only 3 of the girls had engaged in serious delinquent activity, including prostitution, burglary, and physical assault. Clearly, although men and women were equally represented in the group of young people who had at some time broken the law, the young men were more often involved in more serious offenses, and it was only among the young men that chronicity appeared.

MARRIAGE AND PREGNANCY

Of the 40 young people, 6 women and 3 men were married. Three women married at 17, 18, and 19 years old, respectively. One woman who married at 18, divorced by age 21, and remarried at age 22.

A third ($N = 8$, 33%) of the women had been pregnant outside of marriage. Three women had children of their own. One had her first child out of wedlock and subsequently married another man who fathered her second child. Another miscarried but married her lover and went on to bring her next pregnancy to term. The remainder, or one-quarter of the women, elected to have abortions. Two women had second abortions.

THEIR RESPONSE TO THE INTERVIEWS

Although 5 years had elapsed since our last meeting, most of the young people came willingly to see us. The greater number by far stayed well beyond the 2 hours that we had allotted for the interview. As a group, they were willing to talk not only about their current situation, but many were eager, as well, to employ the opportunity provided in order to review the years that had elapsed and especially to return to their experience at the time of the divorce. Thus, one young woman whom we interviewed early in the study alerted us to what might follow. Entering the office, she announced with a dramatic flourish, "I just turned 21. You called me at just the right time." She remained to talk for 3½ hours.

As these young people spoke with us, they revealed how often and how soberly they had thought and rethought their parents' divorce over the intervening years. They had considered and reconsidered the reasons that led to the marital rupture. They had reflected on the behavior of their parents at that time and since and on the consequences of the experience for them and for their siblings. And they had drawn sobering conclusions for their own use in the present and the future. By and large, they expressed themselves thoughtfully and carefully, wanting to make sure that their exact meaning had been conveyed and correcting us when we failed to grasp nuances of their thoughts and feelings. Often they were moving and eloquent.

DOMINANT MOOD AND FEELINGS

We were struck by the ready availability of strong feelings, especially feelings of sadness. Tears were not infrequently shed as these youngsters recalled the marital rupture and other events from their past. With a few exceptions of cynicism, striking a "cool" pose, and some rigidity and constriction among the young men, they did not consciously attempt to conceal or deny feelings. We were impressed with their candor, their openness, and by their eagerness to confide after the initial reluctance was overcome.

Perhaps the most striking was the accessibility of memory, especially memories of the separation, which for 40% of these young people had remained surprisingly fresh as if, in fact, the incidents had occurred very recently. It may well be, in fact, that we have altogether overestimated the effect of time in muting experiences and painful feelings and that memories or perhaps some memories do not fade.

Thus, Dana, age 19, told us, "The hardest thing for me was my mother's pain. I remember the night when my dad left and how my mother sat up all night rocking and crying in the red rocking chair. I cried, too." In listening to her, it was hard to believe that she was describing an experience that had occurred 10 years earlier. Or Betty, who said, "I'm 19 years old, but I still wake up when I hear loud talking or yelling. And I cry." Many youngsters remembered the day of the marital separation in exact detail, including their feelings at the time. Greta, age 21, said, "The day my mom left my dad she didn't tell him we were leaving, and all I could think of all day was how much it hurt him." Or two sisters, aged 23 and 21, each of whom remembered separately the shock of a chance meeting at a county fair with their father together with the woman who subsequently became his wife. The distress and embarrassment that each conveyed would have placed the encounter yesterday.

And, finally, parting from us and perhaps from the opportunity which our meeting provided was sometimes not easy for these young people. Several asked as they left whether we planned another round of interviews and when that might be. A number had trouble bringing the interview to a close. One young woman in her 20s stood tearfully on the sidewalk, slowly waving as the interviewer drove off. The responsiveness of these young people and their pleasure with our interest and concern were profoundly moving. It may be that we have tapped into the widespread existential loneliness of young people in our society. Or it may be that the loneliness of these youngsters is special.

VIEW OF THE DIVORCED FAMILY

The predominant mood that attached to looking backward was one of regret, restrained sadness, and yearning. Overall, they were in agreement that they had sustained an important loss. Close to two-thirds of the young people felt that, as a consequence of the divorce, their childhood and their adolescence had been significantly burdened. What had they lost? This is a relevant question since most of these young people had maintained sporadic or regular contact with the parent who had left the home. Additionally, 20% of the youngsters had during adolescence gone to live with the departed parent for a period of time, and an additional 12% had moved back and forth several times between the mother's home and the father's home during adolescent years. Yet, they had, in their view, lost the experience of growing up within the protection and the rich emotional nurturance which the intact family at its best can provide. Undoubtedly this was an idealized family for these youngsters, an inner vision of Jerusalem that they carried and preserved separate from their real experience in family life. And, indeed, the greater number distinguished the longing that they experience as a wish for the family that they had never had. Nevertheless, whether these youngsters were doing well or poorly, and whether they defended, praised, or criticized their parents' divorce, and *unrelated* to the contact with both parents over the years, most of them shared the sense of having been deprived or needy, which they related to having missed the important experience of the intact, together family. Their dominant feeling about this was sorrow. Their shared sense was that life had been for them more difficult, more hazardous, and less pleasurable than for their peers whose families had remained intact. These feelings appeared to have remained close to the surface and were readily accessible, and, in fact, for over 80% of these young men and women, it appeared to us that the divorce continued to hold a moderately or highly central position in their psychological functioning. They told us, "My life would have been happier if my parents hadn't divorced." "Divorce was better for them but not for me. I lost my family." "I lost the experience of growing up in a family unit." "I wish my mom and dad had not divorced. It would have been easier to be a regular family." "I was really hurt. The hardest thing was watching my family break up." "It was only when I was a student in an AFS family abroad that I got to see parents who quarrel and resolve the argument."

There were, as expected, some differences in attitude. A significant subgroup estimated at 30% of this sample, and incidentally a much larger group that we had observed at the time of the marital rupture, reported relief that they had experienced, as they said, from the outset at having been separated by the divorce from a tyrannical parent. Dora, at age 22, said, "I get mad at all these programs about how bad divorce is for children. They should tell both sides of the story. I felt pretty happy after the divorce. At least my mom and dad weren't going to be fighting anymore. The divorce changed my life for the better because I got away from Dad." Then she added, "I don't think the effect of the divorce was very good. I could have been more of a person. Some people, after divorce, became more careful in their relationships with men. I became careless." She told us ruefully that she had married at 18 after a several-week courtship and divorced her first husband at 21.

ANGER

The anger at one or both parents that emerged at the time of the marital rupture and continued in a significant number of the youngsters at the 5-year mark had dissipated in intensity by 10 years, although almost one-half of the youngsters still retained some anger. This diminution of anger went hand in hand with a reassessment of the parental decision to divorce. By the 10-year mark, two-thirds of the young people had concluded that their parents were ill suited to each other and approved the divorce at this time as both inevitable and necessary. This attitude represented for most of these young people an important shift from the view that they had held earlier at the 5-year mark post-divorce. Most of the reversal of earlier thinking occurred during adolescence when they reached the conclusion that the divorce decision was wise and inevitable given their parents' differences.

Of those who remained angry, a significant number were, despite the passage of many years, severely critical of their parents for what they considered their parents' immoral behavior during the marriage. Many of these young people had embraced a morality that was more traditional than that of their parents. They continued to condemn their parents for what they viewed as irresponsible or immoral conduct in the past. They told us vehemently, "My parents lied and cheated on each other." "Dad was irresponsible. That's why I hate irresponsibility so much. I haven't forgiven him. I still feel distaste and bitterness." "I saw my dad beat up my mom. That is a scar I think of every day." "Some day I will say to my father," said a 26-year-old man who had been his father's favorite child, reflecting on his father's repeated infidelity throughout the marriage and his father's promiscuity during the post-divorce period, " 'Are you proud of what you have done with your life?' But," he added bitterly, "what can he answer me?" Others were resentful of the continuing conflict between their parents. One 20-year-old said, "I am bitter about all the turmoil in my life. I wish it hadn't happened. I was hurt."

Although most of these young people had arrived at the understanding that the divorce of their parents had been a wise decision, many of them remained critical of both parents for having made the mistake of a misguided marriage. They were especially critical of their parents for not having rectified the mistake before the children were born. Their anger at their parents for not having divorced prior to the decision to have children was clear and direct. They said, "A child should not be subjected to divorce. Why didn't they divorce before they had kids?" "I wish it had never happened. You can undo a marriage, but you can't undo a child." "If you have kids, it's stupid to get a divorce."

Out of their criticism and their pain these young people drew implications for a future that they hoped would enable them to avoid their parents' mistake. They were concerned with how to select a marital partner more carefully and had spent uncounted hours thinking about these issues. They said, "I learned from my parents' mistakes. I want a long-term relationship because sex without love is animal passion. I want to be in love. There is more to be gained from a long-term relationship." "I wouldn't divorce. It hurts other people." "Divorce is terrible, the worst thing there is. It damages people for life." "Marriage is good. Fidelity is good. Don't cheat. Talk about everything. Don't split up." "I want to have a child, but I don't want to be a single parent. Ideally I would like to find someone to settle down with forever. It's a lot of work, but I think I can, and I have to. I have to be willing to put temptation in anyone else aside. I think it would be fulfilling to have one relationship, but divorce is so frequent. I believe that marriage should be a permanent thing." "I am in awe of relationships where people are together."

Most of these young people were eager for a lasting marriage. The greater majority, in fact over three-quarters of the group, had retained their enthusiasm for marriage, and most held a romantic view of love. Of those who were still unmarried, almost three-quarters fully expected to marry in the future. Most agreed, as if they had consulted with each other, that marriages should not occur early and that impulsive marriages should be avoided. By and large, they strongly eschewed infidelity which they referred to as "cheating." They stressed the importance of choosing correctly the first time around. The solution they envisioned most was that of living with a lover for several years prior to marriage and knowing that person very well. They planned a second delay after marriage to be absolutely sure of the relationship before children were conceived.

We were interested to find that these young people did not take emotional comfort or find intellectual reassurance in the high incidence of divorce in their society. They did not conclude that the divorced familiy represented a new norm in family relationships. On the contrary, the high incidence of divorce intensified their anxiety about the hazards of love and commitment. Two-thirds of the group expressed conscious fear of marriage despite their wish to marry. A smaller number (26%) were intensely fearful of repeating their parents' mistakes in a relationship of their own, and another 40% of the group were at least moderately worried.

In their hopes and their fears regarding marriage, these young people differ little, if at all, from other young people in their generation who share their anxiety regarding the high likelihood of divorce, although it may be that the concern among these youngsters was more intense and more pervasive. What distinguished these young people, however, was their intense wish to avoid divorce for the sake of their children. Their identification was with these projected unborn children despite their own adulthood. In a profound way, they continued to see themselves as children of divorce as if this had become a fixed identity that would not change although they had shed their own childhood.

A SUBGROUP OF YOUNG WOMEN

A significant minority consisting of one-third of the young women ($N = 8$, 33%) had drawn another set of conclusions as guidelines for their own lives. Several of these young women left home at high school graduation or before graduation to live with a man. They seemed to be drifting from job to job and from man to man. Others had graduated from college and were uncertain and frightened about the next step. Several had selected older men as lovers. Their interest was not primarily in economic support, since they did not choose wealthy men, and they continued to work at mostly poor paying jobs. They sought men who would be caring and would treat them well. They told us: "He treats me like a queen." "I like older men. Some of it is a father complex. I've had many surrogate fathers." Referring to her 45-year-old lover, one 20-year-old said, "He takes care of me, and he cares about me." And still another, "I prefer older men. Younger men are always falling in love with you. My boyfriend is older than my father." A young woman of 25 told us, "Don't get too attached. If you don't build up a relationship, you don't fall so hard. I'm on a roller coaster. I fall in and out of love and in and out of relationships." Or, as one 20-year-old whose life story sounded like an excerpt from *Fanny Hill* told us, "I've had no limits and no control. I'm prepared for anything. I don't expect a lot. I just want to stay alive. Love is a strange idea to me. Life is a chess game, and I'm a pawn. I've always been a pawn." Or a 24-year-old who was living with a divorced man almost twice her age, "I'm afraid to use the word love. Relationships are too uncertain. You can hope that a relationship is going to be permanent, but you can't expect it." Or still another, "I'm scared to get married because I don't want to divorce." Or another, "I'm so afraid that I'll marry someone like my father."

These young women are attractive and intelligent. Yet they are worried, even despairing, fearful of being rejected in their search for a man who would care for them and burdened by anxieties which *they* relate directly to their parents' divorce. Their difficulties extend to making commitments about a career, as well as to an education appropriate to their intellectual capacity. Some of these youngsters had been sexually promiscuous and wild during their adolescent years. Others, however, who remained conservative and restrained, sometimes protective of a distressed parent throughout their adolescence, seemed to have lost their way after graduation from high school.

Two-thirds of the young women of the sample were fearful of betrayal in their relationships with men as compared with one-half of the young men who shared this preoccupation. A few of the young women were consumed with fear of betrayal to the extent that they feared that relationships could not even be trusted from minute to minute. One 22-year-old said, "I'm always afraid if my boyfriend is 30 minutes late that he is with another woman." Another 23-year-old told us, "My problem is that I'm jealous. My boyfriend has a female employee who he works with, and I wonder all the time whether sex would be better with her and whether he will fall in love with her, and whether they will fall in love with each other. I never feel sure of him." Or still another, "I guess it's a rare couple that goes through life without one of them being sexually involved with somebody else. I wouldn't want it to happen, and yet it's important to survive. I guess I'm afraid of being exploited. My father's relationship and his using my mother is still on my mind." And finally, one 21-year-old said despairingly, "How can you expect commitment when anyone can change his mind any time? Divorce destroyed my fantasy of love and life."

GREATER INDEPENDENCE AND MATURITY

Many of these youngsters describe themselves as having emerged stronger and more independent as a consequence of their parents' divorce. They affirmed that the divorce had thrust them earlier into positions of responsibility, and they, in turn, had benefited from the opportunity and their own response. And, indeed, many of these youngsters had spent much of their time during adolescence and childhood contributing to the care of the household, taking care of younger children, taking responsibility for themselves at a very young age. There has been much interest in recent years in this phenomenon of children of divorce growing up faster with a greater sense of determination and a firm, clear grasp of reality (Weiss, 1979). Sometimes their statements reflected their perception of themselves as having walked through and survived an extraordinary life-threatening ordeal. They told us with pride, "The outcome of the divorce was to survive. I had to be independent to supervise myself." "Divorce tore up my life, but I came out stronger." "I'm a capable person. There's always opportunity. I guess I can make it. I know I can make it. I'm a survivor." "I gained responsibility and independence from the divorce. I took care of myself." "I have the attitude I don't need anyone, that I can take care of myself any time."

Yet, there was a bittersweet quality to their prideful pronouncements. Despite pride and achievement, many of these youngsters perceived that the price had been too high. Side by side with the enhanced maturity was the rueful sense of having missed out on childhood, of having been pushed or even been exploited by a parent, of having worked too hard and grown up too fast. They said, "If my parents hadn't divorced, it would have been better. I was working so hard by the time I was 18." "I had to give up a lot of freedom because of my mom's divorce decision."

Several complained that a significant part of their play and school time had been sacrificed to their parents' divorce. One 22-year-old said, "I had to take care of my brothers and sisters, and I got blamed for everything." Others spoke of loneliness and lack of supervision during their adolescence. One young woman of 19 said, "I never had any rules. I wouldn't have gotten into so much trouble if there had been someone at home." Another 19-year-old told us, "The worst thing about divorce was that my mom wasn't home. There was no discipline and no rules, just an empty feeling. That's how I got into sex." Perhaps the most poignant was the wistfully expressed gentle wish of a young man, "I wish that I had been more of a child."

SOME SIBLING RELATIONSHIPS

We were impressed with the solidarity between siblings in a subgroup of these families—with the love, intimacy, and loyalty among brothers and sisters and the candor and pride with which this was acknowledged. "My brother and I are unusually close," Theresa, age 27, volunteered. "I don't know what I would have done without him. The divorce left a mark, but he's my other half. If I lost him, I would be alone with the family." "The divorce was better for my mom but horrible for my brother and for me. Divorce forced my brother and me to grow up and to be close to each other. My brother and I are the closest. We talk about everything, even sex, together." "My relationship with my sister has been the saving of our emotional and physical selves. We have always been close. Without the other our chances of turning out as we are would have been very different. If I'd been an only child, I might have lost my sanity. We have always been faithful to each other. Always." And, finally, as one 18-year-old said, "I rely a lot on my brother. We're intimate in our discussions. A few months ago he came into my room and said to me, 'Did you know that you were an unwanted child? All of us were unwanted children,' he told me. We sit every night and talk together."

It seems that when the relationship between the parents weakens and disrupts that siblings can turn toward each other to huddle together, to protect each other, to remain intimate with each other, and perhaps most of all to remain faithful to each other. In a subgroup of families, it appears that the most enduring and the richest relationship during the childhood and adolescent years was that among the siblings, and that this relationship had survived the centrifugal pulls of adolescence and young adulthood.

SUMMARY

Preliminary findings from a 10-year longitudinal study of 113 children and adolescents from a largely white, middle-class population of divorced families in Northern California suggest that some psychological effects of divorce are long lasting. Forty young people from 26 of the families who range in age from 19 to 29 at the 10-year mark regard their parents' divorce as a continuing major influence in their lives. A significant number are burdened by vivid memories of the unhappy events at the time of the marital rupture. Their predominant feelings as they look backward are restrained sadness, some remaining resentment at their parents, and a wistful sense of having missed out on the experience of growing up in an intact family. And although many are proud of their enhanced maturity, they regret the ways in which the divorce cut into the play and school time of their growing-up years.

One-half of these young people are still full time at school; one-third are fully self-supporting; and the greater majority are law abiding. Nevertheless, a significant number of men and women, and especially women, appear troubled and drifting. A minority consisting of one-third of the women appear especially wary of commitment and fearful of betrayal and seem caught up in a web of short-lived sexual relationships. The greater number, however, are strongly committed to the ideals of a lasting marriage and to values that include romantic love and fidelity. They are apprehensive about repeating their parents' unhappy marriage during their own adulthood and especially eager to avoid divorce for the sake of their own still unborn children. This relatively fixed identification with being a child of divorce may be one of the lasting sequelae of the experience of parental divorce during childhood.

Finally, in a subgroup of families, the sibship emerges as a powerful supportive network with the capacity not only to buffer the family ordeal but also to provide the significant nutriments of family relationships and to actualize for these young people their otherwise battered conceptions of fidelity, enduring love, and intimacy.

REFERENCES

Blos, P. (1962), *On Adolescence: A Psychoanalytic Interpretation*. New York: Free Press of Glencoe.

Wallerstein, J. (1983), Children of divorce: stress and developmental tasks. In: *Stress, Coping and Development*, ed. N. Garmezy & M. Rutter. New York: McGraw-Hill, pp. 265-302.

———— & Kelly, J. (1974), The effects of parental divorce: the adolescent experience. In: *The Child in His Family*, ed. E. J. Anthony & C. Koupernik. New York: John Wiley & Sons, pp. 479-505.

———— ———— (1976), The effects of parental divorce: experiences of the child in later latency. *Amer. J. Orthopsychiat.*, 46:256-269.

———— ———— (1980), *Surviving the Breakup: How Children and Parents Cope with Divorce*. New York: Basic Books.

Weiss, R. S. (1979), *Going It Alone*. New York: Basic Books.

Part VII
DEPRESSION IN CHILDHOOD AND ADOLESCENCE

It is only in the past 10 to 15 years that the frequency of depressive symptoms in childhood has been recognized. In the short period of years since increasing attention has been paid to this issue, a number of research studies have explored etiologic questions, diagnostic considerations, and treatment approaches from various different points of view. Several excellent reviews have appeared that have summarized systematically much of our present knowledge of the syndrome of childhood depression.

Many questions remain unanswered, including the relationship of childhood to adult depression. The paper by Digdon and Gotlib presents another review which is noteworthy for its major emphasis on the relationship between childhood depression and normal developmental processes. The review assesses the major theories of depression, as well as epidemiological data, and diagnostic issues from this developmental perspective. They find that developmental issues are relevant to the study of childhood depression, and spell out their reasons for this judgment in detail. This conclusion may appear obvious, but it is still true that many investigators of normal childhood behavior or clinical syndrome ignore the basic issue—their research data must take into account that the same behavior may have different meanings for children at different developmental levels. Digdon and Gotlib conclude by pointing out the implications of a developmental approach for the design of investigations on the syndrome of childhood depression, including its relationship to adult depression.

The study of childhood and adolescent depression is significant for a number of reasons. One of the most important is the risk of suicide in such cases, which has become one of the leading causes of death among adolescents. The paper by Robbins and Alessi addresses this issue by assessing depressive symptoms and suicidal behaviors in a group of

64 adolescent psychiatric patients. Their findings are of importance to clinicians working with adolescent patients. Adolescents appear to be reliable reporters of their suicidal feelings when they have some degree of rapport with the interviewer. More intense suicidal feelings are associated with more dangerous suicidal behavior, and alcohol and other substance abuse increase the danger of suicide.

25

Developmental Considerations in the Study of Childhood Depression

Nancy Digdon and Ian H. Gotlib

The University of Western Ontario, London

Although a great deal of research has been conducted examining biological and psychological factors related to adult depression, relatively little attention has been given to the study of depression in children. The purpose of the present article is to illustrate the importance of considering normal developmental processes in the study of childhood depression. Epidemiological data, diagnostic issues, and methods of assessment in childhood depression are discussed from a developmental perspective, and the role of developmental issues in both the manifestation of depression and its assessment is outlined. Four major theories of depression—biological, psychoanalytic, behavioral, and cognitive—are presented, and developmental issues are discussed in relation to each theory's formulation of the etiology, maintenance, and treatment of depression. Finally, alternative methodologies for the study of childhood depression are considered, and directions for future research, particularly for investigations examining the relationship between childhood and adult depression, are advanced.

Reprinted with permission from *Developmental Review*, 1985, Vol. 5, 162–199. Copyright 1985 by Academic Press, Inc.

Preparation of this article was facilitated by Grant MA-8574 from the Medical Research Council of Canada to the second author. The authors express their appreciation to Grover J. Whitehurst and an anonymous reviewer for their helpful comments on an earlier draft of this article.

451

Depression was one of the first mental disorders to be recognized and studied by psychiatrists and psychologists, the first well-documented case predating the time of Hippocrates. Since that time, there has been a plethora of research examining the etiology, symptomatology, and treatment of depression in adults, and a number of often diverse theories and models have been formulated to establish frameworks in which to view the depressed adult (e.g., Abramson, Seligman, & Teasdale, 1978; Beck, Rush, Shaw, & Emery, 1979; Coyne, 1976b; Lewinsohn, 1974).

In sharp contrast to the abundance of research on depression in adults, relatively little research examining depression in children was evident until the past 10 or 15 years. Prior to this time, even the possibility that depression could exist in children was questioned (cf. Rie, 1966). This reluctance to accept the concept of childhood depression was due in part to the pervasive influence of early psychoanalytic theory, in which depression was conceptualized as a superego phenomenon. Since children were not regarded to possess a well-internalized superego before adolescence, they were not thought capable of experiencing depression; childhood depression, therefore, was a theoretical impossibility.

Whatever the reasons for the paucity of research on childhood depression, the fact remains that a wide discrepancy exists between what is known about adult depression and our understanding of depression in childhood. Since there is already a considerable knowledge base in adult depression, some researchers have advocated taking the established findings from these studies and extrapolating downward in an effort to understand childhood depression (e.g., Nowels, 1977), essentially an example of "adultomorphism" (cf. Ausubel, Sullivan, & Ives, 1980). Although this strategy appears efficient and logical, it faces at least one major problem: the failure to consider the depression in relation to what is normal for a particular state of development. For example, while frequent crying may be indicative of depression in a 20-year-old, this same behavior could hardly be regarded as depressive in a 2-year-old. Implicit in the position to understand childhood depression in terms of the adult disorders is the assumption that the manifestation and significance of depression are constant across ages. This paper represents an attempt to demonstrate that this assumption may not be justified.

Are childhood depressions essentially the same disorders as their adult counterparts, or are they distinct clinical entities? A major controversy pervades the literature, focusing on just this question (see, for example, Cytryn, McKnew, & Bunney, 1980; Kashani et al., 1981; Lefkowitz & Burton, 1978). The purpose of this paper is not to address this debate, but to illustrate the importance of considering normal developmental processes in studying depression, whether one uses developmental considerations to modify the adult models or to reject these models and formulate new models of childhood depression.

In recent years there have been several excellent reviews of childhood depression. Kovacs and Beck (1977) and Kazdin (1981), for example, presented an overview of symptoms of depression in children and described instruments and procedures used in the assessment of these symptoms. Puig-Antich (1980) provided a comprehensive review of manic-depressive and major depressive disorders in children, with a major emphasis on studies conducted within a biological perspective. Cantwell and Carlson (1979) organized their review around five distinct headings: clinical picture, family studies, follow-up studies, treatment, and laboratory studies, and from this framework described affective disorders both in adults and in children. Finally, Kashani et al. (1981) presented a very broad review of childhood depression, discussing such topics as the historical background of the disorder, diagnostic criteria and classifications, conceptual models relevant to etiology and treatment, and studies of interventions. Although it may appear in the face of these recent reviews that another is not needed, it is important to note that the present paper is unique in its major emphasis on the relationship between childhood depression and normal developmental processes, and consequently overlaps to only a small extent with these reviews.

This paper is divided into three sections. In the first section childhood depression is described in terms of symptoms and syndromes, and the implications of adopting a developmental framework within which to understand both of these concepts are outlined. Although there are several theoretical perspectives in developmental psychology concerning the nature of developmental differences and the processes underlying developmental change (see Miller, 1983, for a discussion of various approaches to this issue), we are essentially using the term "developmental" in this paper to describe age-related differences in cognitions, emotions, physical development, or behaviors that affect the way in which depression is manifested in different age groups. In the second section, which constitutes the main focus of the paper, four major theories of depression are presented, and the role of developmental issues is discussed in relation to each theory's formulation of the etiology, maintenance, and treatment of depression. Finally, alternative methodologies for examining childhood depression which are particularly relevant to controlling for and incorporating developmental issues are considered, and directions for future research are advanced.

SYMPTOMS AND SYNDROMES

One would be hard put to present a universal picture of the "depressed child." A vast array of symptoms has been ascribed to depressed children. Ling, Oftedal, and Weinberg (1970) found mood change, social withdrawal, sleep disturbance, decreased school performance, and somatic complaints to be the most common symptoms exhibited by a group of 4- to 16-year-old depressed children. Lopez (1972) focused on the somatic complaints associated with depression and listed headaches, dizziness, cephalalgias, nausea, abdominal pain, encopresis, and anorexia nervosa as the most common signs of depression in children. Pearce (1977) cited a considerable list of signs of depression, including such symptoms as phobias, refusal to go to school, obsessions, and altered perceptions, and Kuhn and Kuhn (1972) concluded that morning tiredness was the cardinal symptom of preadult depression.

Considering all of the various lists of symptoms of depression, one must acknowledge that virtually any type of problem behavior could be included under the rubric of depression. Lefkowitz and Burton (1978) note that any disturbing behavior could potentially result in a child receiving a label of depressed. Whereas numerous behaviors and symptoms have been ascribed to depressed children, there have been few attempts to relate these behaviors and symptoms to the particular ages and developmental levels of the children. Certain behaviors may not be symptomatic of depression at all ages. The significance of a particular behavior will be influenced by its prevalence in nondepressed as well as in depressed children. According to a statistical definition of pathology, a behavior is abnormal if it occurs in no more than 10% of nonpathological people within the age range of interest (Quay, 1979; Shepherd, Oppenheim, & Mitchell, 1971). Interestingly, Achenbach and Edelbrock (1981) reported that depressive affect, as rated by parents, occurred in 13% of a group of 4- to 13-year-old children with no psychiatric referral; depressive affect in this age group, therefore, would fail to meet the criterion for a label of "pathological." Although it may be argued that 13% is not significantly different from 10%, the point remains that at least some of the many behaviors described as symptomatic of depression may be too prevalent in certain age groups to warrant a diagnosis of depression.

Epidemiological studies have assessed the frequency of various behaviors across age (e.g., MacFarlane, Allen, & Honzik, 1954), and, interestingly, some of the behaviors examined in these studies have been listed in other investigations as symptoms of depression. It has been shown from the epidemiological studies that these behaviors may be very common in normal children, and that their frequency tends to decrease with increasing age. MacFarlane et al., for example, found that insufficient appetite was manifested by 33% of 6-year-olds, but by only 7.5% of 9-year-olds. A statistical definition of depression would lead to the inclusion of insufficient appetite as a symptom of depression in 9-year-olds, but not in 6-year-olds. Thus, the question of whether particular behaviors should be regarded as symptoms of depression must entail a consideration of age. The prevalence of the behaviors in nondepressed children must be thoroughly examined before one can ascertain the status of the behaviors as symptoms of depression. As Wenar (1982) states, "clearly the study of normal and deviant development should go hand in hand." (p. 199).

Although numerous symptoms have been attributed to depressed children, researchers downplay the importance of each symptom in isolation. Instead, they emphasize an examination of groups of co-occurring symptoms, or syndromes. Thus, it is not sufficient for a child to exhibit only one of the previously mentioned symptoms; she/he must manifest a constellation of the symptoms in order to be labeled depressed. Unfortunately, there is not good agreement concerning the particular symptoms that comprise the syndrome of depression. Different researchers have postulated different and often conflicting groups of symptoms to comprise a depressive syndrome in children (cf. Achenbach, 1978; Dweck, Gittelman-Klein, & McKinney, 1977; Ling et al., 1970; Weinberg, Rutman, Sullivan, Penick, & Deitz, 1973). Beck (1967), for example, has categorized symptoms of depression into four groups, each focusing on one specific area of functioning. The four areas are cognitive functioning, attitudes and motivation, psychomotor functioning, and mood state. According to Beck, a diagnosis of depression is contingent on the manifestation of symptoms from *each* of the four areas. Beck's diagnostic criteria, however, were established from research on adult depressives, and it is not clear that these criteria are appropriate in understanding the manifestation of depression in children.

The conceptualization of childhood depression as a syndrome is largely due to the precedent of the similar practice in conceptualizing depressions in adults. Since depressions in adults are characterized as syndromes, it apparently was difficult for researchers to generate a priori reasons why syndromes should not also be evident in childhood depressions (Kovacs & Beck, 1977). From a developmental perspective, however, there are a number of issues which must be explored before adopting this position. In order for *syndrome* to be a useful concept, for example, it must be amenable to reliable and valid psychological assessment. As Jacobson (1957) has noted, however, the measurement of emotions in children is more restricted than it is in adults, and consequently, it is likely that a particular display of emotion by a child can be taken to represent a broader number of inner states than would a similar display of emotion by an adult. Corroborating this position, Borke (1971) found that young children experience considerable difficulty in distinguishing between sadness and anger. While it is important to note that children's difficulties in expressing and distinguishing among different emotions does not necessarily mean that they cannot clearly convey their emotions, it does seem that a diagnosis of depression in children must nonetheless remain more tenuous than the same diagnosis in adults.

In addition to the problems associated with assessment, the concept of a syndrome suggests that there are interrelationships among the areas of functioning impaired by depression. It is not clear whether these interrelationships are as well defined in the developing child as they are in the older child and adult. Immaturities in some areas of functioning may differentially prevent the expression of certain depressive symptoms. Anthony (1967), for example, argued that children differ from adults in their ability to verbalize affective states, in their superego development, and in their self-representation. These differences may influence whether depressive syndromes are manifested and, if they are, what form they might take. For instance, children may be too immature cognitively to experience the depressive symptoms of severe self-doubt and repudiation (cf. Glasberg & Aboud, 1982). Self-doubt and repudiation, in turn, may be causally related to other symptoms comprising the syndrome of depression (such as lack of interest in work or school).

Another difficulty in identifying depressive symptoms in children involves children's natural mood state, which may mask the depressive symptoms. There is evidence to indicate that children's mood is naturally elevated compared to that of adults (Gittelman-Klein, 1977). Because sadness is typically included in lists of syndromes of depression (see, for example, DSM-III), it is important to realize that children may not appear as sad as adults when depressed simply because they seem happier than the adults initially. The children's natural exuberance may counteract the state of sadness associated with depression. Thus, it may be unwarranted to expect the same depth of sadness in depressed children as is evident in depressed adults. In contrast to adults, a serious or neutral mood may be sufficient to indicate depression in children.

Finally, if syndromes of depression are to be used in describing depressed children, it is not clear that they should be identical to those used to describe the depressed adult. In an analysis of responses to a 15-item questionnaire, McConville, Boag, and Purohit (1973) found that depressive syndromes took three different forms in 6- to 13-year-old children. Each form of syndrome was found to correspond to a particular age range of children and was distinguishable from the other forms by the particular symptoms manifested. Children with affectual depression, the first form, were characterized by such symptoms as expressions of sadness and helplessness, as well as by occasional hopelessness. This form of depression was most common in the 6- to 8-year-olds. Children with negative self-esteem depression predominantly experienced thoughts and feelings about depression, and were often obsessed with feelings of worthlessness, of being unloved, and of being used by other people. This form of depression was most common in the 8-year-olds, although it was still relatively common in children between the ages of 8 and 11 years. Finally, the children with guilt depression felt that they were inherently wicked and that they should be put to death. Although this third form of depression tended to be rare relative to the other two forms, it was most prevalent in the 12- and 13-year-olds. Findings such as these strongly indicate the existence of developmental differences in the manifestation of depressive symptoms in children.

The position that the manifestation of depression may be different in children and adults is currently reflected in DSM-III. Although the essential features of a major depressive episode are considered identical for children and adolescents, there are also age-specific features described for different ages and developmental levels (e.g., separation anxiety for prepubertal children, and antisocial behavioral for adolescents). It is important to realize, however, that since DSM-III was developed primarily as an instrument for practicing clinicians, these latter features are derived not from empirical research but entirely from clinical experience. As Cantwell (1982) notes, therefore, it is not yet clear whether operational criteria for depressive disorders derived from research with adult depressives should be modified for use with children.

The position that there are different manifestations of depression at different ages is consistent with research indicating that children of different ages tend to use different criteria in conceptualizing and recognizing emotions and affect. Harris, Olthof, and Terwogt (1981), for example, asked nondepressed 6-, 11-, and 15-year-olds general questions about emotions. In responding to the questions, the 6-year-olds tended to focus solely on publicly observable components of emotion, such as the eliciting situation and overt behavioral reactions, whereas the older children in addition considered several mental, internal aspects of emotion. It appears that there is a relationship, then, between people's concepts of emotions and their display of affect. Since children of different ages have different concepts of emotions, it is reasonable to postulate that they may also exhibit different symptoms of depression.

Glaser (1967) used developmental level as a criterion for organizing types of depression, and specified two levels of depressive reaction. Infants and small children were postulated to have deprivation reactions manifested in developmental retardation, affecting physical, intellectual, and emotional development, and older children and adolescents were postulated to exhibit behavior problems such as delinquency, temper tantrums, disobedience, and truancy. It is important to note, however, that Glaser's organization does not differentiate children who demonstrate these symptoms and are depressed from children who manifest these symptoms in the absence of depression.

Finally Jacobsen, Lahey, and Strauss (1983) examined depressed moods in normal children to determine whether they were correlated with other problems or behaviors. Depressed mood was found to be associated with unpopularity and conduct problems in boys in Grades 2–7. Furthermore, in girls in the same grade range, depressed mood was associated with somatic complaints, unpopularity, and behavioral problems. It is interesting to observe that the correlates of depressed affect appear to be similar in nondepressed and depressed children, a finding that lends support to the position that knowledge of the nature of depressed moods in normal children will augment our understanding of affect in clinically depressed children.

From the preceding discussion, it should be apparent that although there are differences in the expression of depression between children and adults, the nature and extent of these differences is unclear at present. In any case, however, these differences will necessitate changes in assessment techniques, and certain developmental characteristics of children in general will likely render some traditional adult assessment measures inappropriate for use with this population.

Self-report measures are the most widely used devices for the assessment of depression (Kazdin, 1981). A number of the adult instruments (such as the Beck Depression Inventory) have been modified for use with children. Although these modified self-report instruments may be appropriate for use with children as young as those in the fifth grade in terms of vocabulary and language level (cf. Berndt, Schwartz, & Kaiser, 1983), the use of self-report measures in general may be inappropriate for use with younger depressed children. On self-report measures, children are required to state whether certain behaviors and descriptions are characteristic of themselves. Included in the descriptions are statements of sad affect and emotion. Glasberg and Aboud (1982) found that young children (5-year-olds) denied known sad experiences and were not likely to perceive sadness as part of their emotional disposition. Thus, self-report measures may not detect sad affect in young children simply because they tend to distance themselves from this emotion.

A promising alternative to self-report measures is a peer nomination technique, in which children are presented with descriptions, such as "this child likes to play alone," and are then asked to name the classmate who best suits the description. Young children will ascribe sad affect to others, even though they will not ascribe it to themselves (Glasberg & Aboud, 1982), and many of the symptoms of depression are likely to be detected by peers, who usually see each other on a daily basis. This technique has been found to be more sensitive and reliable than self-rating procedures (Lefkowitz & Tesiny, 1980) and is more stable over a 6-month period than either teacher ratings or self-ratings of depression (Tesiny & Lefkowitz, 1982). Finally, the peer nomination technique is relatively free from response biases (Kane & Lawler, 1978).

In summary, developmental issues are important in determining the manifestation of both the individual symptoms and the syndromes of depression. The categories of symptoms comprising a syndrome appear to be contingent in large part on the developmental level of the depressed individual, and both the presence or incidence of depressive symptomatology and the ease with which these symptoms can be reliably assessed are developmentally dependent. Finally, labeling a particular behavior as symptomatic of depression requires a knowledge of the incidence of that behavior in nondepressed as well as in depressed children. Results from a number of epidemiological studies suggest that several behaviors indicative of depression in adults may occur too frequently in some age groups of children to be considered pathological.

THEORIES OF DEPRESSION

In this section, four major theories of depression are reviewed, and the role of normal development in each theory is considered. No attempt is made either to evaluate the efficacy of these theories or to determine which theory is most valid. The literature has yet to provide one theory sufficiently comprehensive to account for all relevant aspects of depression. Rather, the purpose of this section is to integrate developmental concerns into the theoretical frameworks discussed.

Biological Theories

Biological theories of depression attribute the symptoms and affect of depression to chemical or molecular physical irregularities. The nature of the particular irregularities postulated to be responsible for depression varies with different biological theories. Theories of depression have variously implicated characteristics of the X chromosome (Van Eerdewegh, Gershon, & Van Eerdewegh, 1979) arousal level (Molinoff & Axelrod, 1971), the presence or absence of certain hormones or minerals (Sachar, 1973), brain receptor sensitivity (Mobley & Sulser, 1981), and the amount of neurotransmitters in the brain (Maas, 1975) in the etiology of this disorder. No conclusive data support any one of these theories over the others (see, for example, Garvey, Tuason, Johnson, & Valentine, 1982). Rather, there is growing evidence suggesting that the theories are describing different types of depressives (cf. Rosenbaum et al., 1983). A variety of studies have demonstrated that adult depressives do not comprise a biologically homogeneous population. For example, whereas some depressives manifest irregular EEG patterns during their sleep, others do not (Kupfer, Foster, & Coble, 1978). Furthermore, those depressives with irregular EEG patterns are more likely not to have a family history of depression, whereas those depressives with no irregular EEG patterns are more likely to have a positive family history of depression (Kadrmas & Winokur, 1979). Thus, these studies seem to have identified two biologically distinct groups of depressives: those with EEG disturbances and those with a positive family history of depression.

The biogenic amine theory of depression attributes depression to a deficiency in monoamine neurotransmitters at functionally important synapses in the brain (Richelson, 1979). Although research on the brain metabolism of adult depressives is progressing, there are problems in extending this line of research to children. In addition to the technical difficulties associated with urine monitoring and lumbar punctures in children, many of the metabolic indices examined in adult populations have been found to be highly correlated with age in child populations (Leckman et al., 1980), thereby complicating interpretation of the significance of the measures. Leckman et al. suggest that brain neurotransmitter systems (and specifically those involving dopamine) mature relatively late, typically during latency and adolescence. Consequently, it may not be possible at this time to extend the adult methodologies and findings in this area to research with young children.

In any case, research on adult depression has established that depression can result from multiple biological causes and, furthermore, that depressives do not seem to constitute a homogeneous group. These findings may be particularly relevant to childhood depression. Considerable variability exists in the biological causes of depression in adults, and it is likely that variability also exists across age groups. Research to date has not examined whether particular biological causes of depression are more frequent in or are restricted to particular age groups. It may be that one group of biological factors is responsible for depression in adults, whereas other biological irregularities are implicated in childhood depression.

There have been an increasing number of studies of the biological indices of childhood depression (see Kazdin, Rancurello, & Unis, in press, for a comprehensive review of this literature). The results from many of these investigations, however, are difficult to interpret because the criteria for the diagnosis of depression either were not well specified or were not objective. Thus, the homogeneity of samples within studies and the comparability of samples across studies are questionable. Some of the more recent studies, however, have used more clear-cut and objective diagnostic criteria (e.g., Research Diagnostic Criteria [RDC], DSM-III), and the results of these studies suggest biological similarities between adult and child depressives.

Neuroendocrinological investigations conducted by Carroll and his associates, for example, have led to the development of a laboratory procedure, the dexamethasone suppression test (DST), that effectively discriminates among adults with endogenous depression, those with nonendogenous depression, and those who are nondepressed (e.g., Carroll, Feinberg, & Greden, 1981; Carroll, Feinberg, & Steiner, 1980). The diagnostic utility of the DST has also been demonstrated in a group of 6- to 12-year-old children. Poznanski, Carroll, Banegas, Cook, and Grossman (1982) found that 56% of the children in their study who were diagnosed as depressed according to RDC criteria had abnormal DST results, a figure that compares favorably with the 49% of depressed adults in the Carroll et al. (1980) study. Similarly, Poznanski reported that 89% of her nondepressed children had normal DST results, compared with 96% of nondepressed adults in the Carroll et al. study.

Similar results were reported by McKnew and Cytryn (1979), who found that depressed children excrete lower levels of urinary metabolites (specifically MHPG), a replication of similar findings obtained with certain subgroups of adult depressives (cf. Schildkraut et al., 1978). Although the results of these studies appear to support the notion of biological similarity between adult and child depressions, they are not without controversy. In addition to the group of depressed children in their study, for example, McKnew and Cytryn used two control groups: a group of normal, active 10-year-old boys, and a group of 6- to 12-year-old children who were bedridden due to lower limb fractures. Interestingly, the depressed children had lower MHPG urine levels than did the control group of active 10-year-olds, but higher MHPG levels than did bedridden controls, and there is some question concerning whether the MHPG urine levels reflect the depressive disorder per se or, rather, are influenced primarily by activity level, and as such are not central to childhood depression.

Another developmental issue with respect to etiology of depression from a biological perspective is that the same biological factor may result in different symptoms in adults and children. For example, children and adults react differently to changes in the level of corticosteroids in the blood (Fawcett & Bunney, 1967). Adults react to excessive blood levels of corticosteroids by showing classic symptoms of depression such as dysphoria (Williams, Dulhy, & Thorn, 1974), whereas children more commonly become irritable and hyperactive (Eberlain & Winter, 1969). This finding is important because it lends credibility to the existence of different symptomatology in children: the same factors that lead to classic depressive symptoms in adults may result in different symptoms in children.

Finally, many adult depressives manifest sleep irregularities such as a decreased interval between the onset of sleep and the transition into rapid eye movement (REM) sleep, decreased delta sleep, fits of wakefulness during a sleeping period, and an increase in the frequency of eye movements during REM sleep (see Kupfer & Foster, 1972, for a review of this literature). Interestingly, none of these sleep irregularities are common in childhood depression (cf. Puig-Antich et al., 1982). Although one may be tempted to interpret this discrepancy as evidence supporting the view of adult and childhood depressions as separate and distinct syndromes, it is important to be cognizant of the distinction between central and epiphenomenal symptoms. If sleep irregularities in adult depressives are found to be central, one must then ascertain whether the irregularities can be explained in terms of maturational differences in normal sleep that interact with the depressive disorder. If this is the case, adult and childhood depressions could be conceptualized as the same syndrome, with the expression of this syndrome being modified by developmental differences that interact with the depression. The conceptualization of separate depressive syndromes for adults and children, consequently, would be unnecessary. It is clear from this discussion that a comprehensive examination of developmental differences in normal sleep patterns is necessary in order to determine the status of sleep irregularities in depression.

From a biological perspective, treatment for depression typically involves the administration of various antidepressant medications. One class of commonly used medications is tricyclic antidepressants (imipramine, doxepin, amitriptyline, etc.). The efficacy of these drugs has been established by research on adult depressives (e.g., Kupfer & Spiker, 1981; Risch, Huey, & Janowsky, 1979a). The actual mechanisms of these drugs, however, are still unclear. Although the determination of blood plasma levels of tricyclic antidepressants may be important in assessing clinical usefulness, in monitoring treatment, and in predicting drug side effects, it is important to note that plasma levels may be influenced by age, sex, race, and concurrent medications (Risch et al., 1979a). Children ages 3–10 years, for example, have been found to obtain higher plasma levels than do adults at the same dosage per kilogram of body weight (Risch, Huey, & Janowsky, 1979b). Risch et al. (1979b) hypothesize that this may be related to the fact that children have a relatively larger ratio of liver mass to total body mass than do adults. Since the liver is involved in metabolizing the drug, children may have a higher ratio of metabolites to active drug. In any case, it is clear that the significance of various blood levels of active drug will vary depending on whether the patient is an adult or a child.

Drug metabolism in general may differ in adults and children, and the presence of different distributions in children may arise from their higher total body and extracellular water content, their reduced capacity for protein binding of drugs, and the bidirectional effect of growing tissue on drug uptake (Briant, 1978). In addition, dose calculations of drugs excreted mainly by the kidneys may need to be adjusted for differences in body surface area values between children and adults, and it has been suggested that children are able to tolerate higher drug:body weight doses than are adults. Indeed, despite their lower body weights, the children often require adultlike maintenance doses (Briant, 1978).

Several studies in the early 1970s suggested that approximately 75% of all children treated with tricyclics respond positively (e.g., Connell, 1972; Kuhn & Kuhn, 1972; Stack, 1972; Weinberg et al., 1973). These results are difficult to interpret, however, because of various methodological problems with the studies, including the use of heterogeneous diagnostic groups, the lack of objective means of making diagnostic decisions, the absence of outcome measures, the lack of placebo controls, the use of nonblind raters, the presence of other concurrent treatments, and the great variability in drug dosage and duration. A recent study by Puig-Antich (1982) was free of many of these methodological limitations and provides more conclusive evidence that tricyclics are useful in treating childhood depression. Puig-Antich examined prepubertal boys, all of whom met RDC criteria for major depressive disorder. In addition, approximately one-third of this sample also met DSM-III criteria for conduct disorder. All children had a full antidepressant response between the 5th and 18th week after initiating the drug treatment. Moreover, in 85% of the boys with conduct disorders the problem behaviors were absent following the antidepressant response. Unfortunately, however, in 70% of those children for whom long-term follow-up was reported depressive episodes recurred after treatment was discontinued. These data suggest that although tricyclics may be effective, they will not protect the child from later episodes of depression. It is imperative that future research pursue the prospect of more long-term treatment regimes with an eye toward the prevention of later depressive episodes.

Within the class of tricyclics, research has demonstrated that different types of tricyclics exert different effects on behaviors associated with depression. Phenelzine, for example, has a drive-enhancing effect and may lead to aggression, whereas imipramine alleviates aggression and hostility (Davidson, McLeod, Turnbull, & Miller, 1981). Therefore, although both drugs successfully treat depression, they have different effects on aggression. This has important implications for depression in children. Childhood depressions are frequently accompanied by conduct disorders or aggression (Puig-Antich, 1982), which are rare in depressed adults. Effects of tricyclics on aggression in children may not become apparent, based solely on drug research with adult depressives. If phenelzine is administered to an adult depressive, an increase in aggression may not be notable, particularly if the adult is initially passive and unassertive. If, however, phenelzine is administered to a depressed child who is also overtly aggressive, the child's condition may worsen. According to Pallmeyer and Petti (1979), for example, some children treated with tricyclics become more aggressive, angry, and hostile as their lethargy, depression, and dejection improves.

Although the efficacy of tricyclic antidepressants has been well established, there are certain individuals who do not respond to these drugs (Davidson et al., 1981). Predictors of positive response to tricyclics include insidious onset of the depression, the presence of anorexia or weight loss, the presence of insomnia, and psychomotor disturbance; predictors of negative response to tricyclics include the presence of neurotic behavior, the presence of hypochondriacal and hysterical traits, and a history of multiple prior episodes of depression (Kupfer & Spiker, 1981). Kupfer and Spiker's findings of differential responsivity to tricyclics were based on research conducted with adult depressives. It is not clear whether the same predictors would be relevant to childhood depression. In fact, Pallmeyer and Petti (1979) found that symptoms most likely to improve in children who respond positively to tricyclics include dysphoria, anhedonia, and suicidal ideation, whereas other behaviors such as irritability and crying may emerge or worsen.

Although the use of tricyclics has received the most research attention, the effects of other antidepressant medications have also been examined. Frommer (1967) studied the effects in 32 depressed children of a combination of monoamine oxidase (MAO) inhibitor and Librium compared to phenobarbitol, each given over 2 weeks in a double-blind crossover design study. More than 75% of the children improved in the MAO/Librium condition, compared to only about 50% on phenobarbitol. Unfortunately, the design of this study does not allow definite conclusions concerning the effects of either MAO inhibitors or Librium alone and, perhaps more importantly, diagnostic criteria for the diagnosis of depression in the subjects were not presented.

Even if MAO inhibitors do effectively alleviate depression, there are drawbacks to their use with children that are of only minor concern with adults. The use of MAO inhibitors, for example, must entail certain dietary restrictions in order to prevent dangerous side effects (see Kazdin et al., in press, for a discussion of this concern). These dietary restrictions may be difficult to enforce in pediatric populations, and if they are not enforced the child may suffer serious repercussions. In general, the use of any type of antidepressant medication may pose special concerns in pediatric populations. It is not clear whether or not the side effects of the drugs will interfere with ongoing cognitive, academic, and social development. Children may be more prone than adults to accidental overdoses or misuses of medication. And perhaps most serious, children may be more prone to toxic effects from the drugs. In their review of pharmacologic and clinical effects of cyclic antidepressants, for example, Kazdin et al. (in press) note that there is reason to believe that children run a greater risk of cardiotoxic metabolites such as 2-OH-imipramine during the course of drug treatment.

In sum, the abundance of research supporting the use of antidepressants in the treatment of depression in adults cannot be cited with confidence in support of their efficacy and safety in the treatment of depression in children. A number of authors, in fact, have argued that drugs are of little benefit in treating depressed children (e.g., Eaton, Sells & Lucas, 1977; Krakowski, 1970). Although several investigators have found tricyclic antidepressants to be effective in treating various other childhood behavior disorders (e.g., Gittelman-Klein & Klein, 1973), there may be serious side effects, and in at least one case tricyclics may have caused the death of a 6-year-old (Saraf, Klein, Gittelman-Klein, & Grof, 1974). At best, as Conners and Werry (1979) argue, no unequivocal antidepressant drug effect in children with primary depression has yet been demonstrated.

Psychoanalytic Theories

Early psychoanalytic theories of depression, such as those of Freud (1957/1917) and Rado (1928), did not deal with explaining the disorder in children. Instead, these theories concentrated on explaining depression in adults and used knowledge of childhood events to predict the adult's current emotional state. Certain childhood traumata were thought responsible for a person's later manifestation of depression. For example, Rado (1928) viewed depression as a result of a loss of self-love. The time at which this loss occurs, however, was considered to be crucial. The first blow to self-love must have occurred during childhood (more precisely, before the resolution of the Oedipal conflict) if the person were later to become depressed. Thus, although early psychoanalytic theories did take developmental issues into consideration when postulating the *causes* of depression, they did not do so when explaining the *manifestations* of this disorder. There was thought to be only one state of development when depression could be manifested—during adulthood, when the superego is sufficiently developed. As Mahler (1961) stated, "We know that the systematized affective disorders are unknown in childhood. It has been conclusively established that the immature personality structure of the infant or older child is not capable of producing a state of depression" (p. 342). Given this theoretical climate, a consideration of developmental issues in child depression would have been inconsequential.

The more recent psychoanalytic theories, however, do consider developmental differences in the manifestation of depression (Bemporad, 1970). These theories attribute depression to ego rather than to superego problems. The ego develops before the superego and is sufficiently formed in children for depression to occur. Thus, more recent psycho-analytic theorists recognize depression in children, with its particular manifestation varying with the child's developmental stage of ego functioning (Malmquist, 1977). Changes in ego functioning result in changes in the perception and interpretation of events, and in changes in the ability to contain emotions and inhibit motor expressions of affect. For example, whereas a young child with immature ego functioning may react to a depressing situation by crying, an older child might react to the same unpleasant situation by withdrawing. The expression of depression, therefore, changes as the ego develops.

Reactions of children in various age groups to depressing situations and the presence of age-related depressive states have frequently been described in the psychoanalytic literature (see Arieti & Bemporad, 1978, for a review). Infants react to maternal and sensory deprivation by crying, losing weight, and generally deteriorating (Spitz, 1946). There is a temptation to think of these phenomena as constituting a form of depression, but within the ego-analytic framework, if one considers these behaviors in terms of the level at which the infant is functioning cognitively and affectively, this temptation is no longer compelling. Ego functioning is virtually nonexistent in infants (cf. A. Freud, 1953); rather, infant behavior is governed primarily by the id, the most primitive component of personality. Behaviors driven by the id are simple and impulsive, including such activities as kicking and grasping. Actual emotions are not manifested until after infancy (Blumberg, 1981). The existence of "depressivelike" symptoms in infants demonstrates that the behaviors are not functionally equivalent across age. Crying, weight loss, and general deterioration may be indicative of depression in adults but from this perspective, not in infants. Developmental considerations come to bear, therefore, on both the external expression of depressive behaviors and the postulated internal processes underlying the behaviors.

Preschool and elementary school children may also react to certain situations with depressive types of symptoms, but the precipitating causes and the duration of the depressive behaviors change with the age of the child (Bemporad, 1978). Preschoolers strive for independence and individuation, and if these strivings are thwarted, the preschooler may develop depressive symptoms. The preschoolers will appear sad, frightened, and overly serious but yet will not have an awareness of their feelings. In addition, although preschoolers are capable of speech, they are not typically able to describe their emotions through language (Anthony, 1975). While some aspects of the depressed preschooler's behaviors may be comparable to those exhibited by an older depressive, the underpinnings of these behaviors are very different. They do not hold the same significance, since the children are not as aware of the feelings beneath the behaviors. Finally, compared to older depressives, depressed preschoolers are more able to alter their feelings and mood states as situations change. For example, when around people who encourage their quest for independence and individuation, depressed preschoolers will seem happier (Schulterbrandt & Raskin, 1977).

Elementary school children are less able to readily change their moods. There is evidence of prolonged periods of sadness in elementary school age children (cf. Arieti & Bemporad, 1978). Children of this age range are prone to depression if they are rejected by others, deprived of gratification, or rewarded for behaviors that inhibit their individuation. With respect to overt behavior, depressed elementary school age children resemble older depressives. This is not necessarily true, however, of the cognitive correlates of the depressive behavior. For example, whereas the behavior of older depressed children is accompanied by guilt and lowered self-regard (Arieti, 1978), younger children are not able cognitively to assimilate or accommodate guilt and lowered self-regard; they lack the prerequisite ego functions of self-observation and self-criticism (Malmquist, 1977; recall the similar findings of McConville et al., 1973). Thus, the child's depression appears not to be as all encompassing as that of an adult.

The differences noted in depression described at various ages are consistent with theorized age differences in ego development. Loevinger (1976), for example, describes the infant's ego stage as presocial and symbiotic, and accordingly, depressive sympathology in infants is conceptualized as resulting from a loss of maternal stimulation and well being, thereby emphasizing the primary importance of the relationship between the infant and the caregiver. Loevinger describes preschooler's ego stage as being characterized by self-protectiveness, externalization of blame, and opportunism. All of these characteristics are consistent with the preschooler's rapid recovery from depression as conditions change. Whereas the preschooler is largely externally governed, elementary school age children have more internalized ego functions such as conformity to rules and experience shame and guilt for breaking rules. The ability to feel guilt brings them closer to the depressions of adults, whose depressions typically involve cognitions about internal processes.

Psychoanalytic treatment of depression in adults typically focuses on resolving the depressive conflict. Psychoanalysis requires a strong, personal relationship between the patient and the therapist. When psychoanalysis is conducted with depressed adults or adolescents, the focus of the therapy is on unconscious motivations, with the goal of obtaining abreaction and catharsis (Blumberg, 1981). This form of psychotherapy, however, must be modified when used to treat children. The focus of treatment in this case must be extended to include children and their families rather than remaining solely on the children themselves and their unconscious motivations. Children's depressions may be reflections of their identification and symbiosis with parental moods, attitudes, and disappointments (Malmquist, 1977). A depressed child, then, may have a depressed parent who is contributing to his/her depression. Consistent with this position, the incidence of depression in the children of depressed adults has been found to be remarkably high (e.g., Cytryn, McKnew, Bartko, Lamour, & Hamovitt, 1982; Decina et al., 1983). It is important, therefore, to determine whether or not one (or both) parents of a depressed child need to be treated. In sum, the focus of psychoanalytic treatment varies with the age of the depressed patient. If the patient is an adult, treatment is concentrated on the patient; if the patient is a young child, treatment focuses on the environment; and if the patient is an older child or adolescent, treatment focuses on both the patient and his/her environment.

Psychoanalytic treatment must also be extended to explore factors in the depressed child's present as well as past situation. Although psychoanalytic therapy with adults involves an almost exclusive focus on events that have occurred in the past, this approach may not be appropriate with young children. Many of the factors contributing to the child's depression may still be present at the time of treatment. Consequently, the focus of the psychotherapy must encompass both the child's past and present.

An alternative to treating depression by resolving the depressive conflict is to provide the depressed person with substitute gratifications. Problems associated with classical psychoanalysis, therefore, can be avoided. Mahler, Pine, and Bergman (1975) suggest that this may be an appropriate form of treatment for depressed children who have acquired object permanence (which occurs sometime between 18 and 36 months of age). Given that traditional psychoanalysis is not recommended for children younger than six years (Blumberg, 1981), provision of substitute gratifications may be a particularly relevant form of treatment for younger depressed children, who lack the verbal skills necessary for psychoanalysis.

Behavioral Theories

Behavioral theories of depression, like behavioral theories in general, are concerned primarily with the analysis of overt behavior (cf. Costello, 1972; Ferster, 1973; Lazarus, 1968; Lewinsohn, 1974). Rather than postulating underlying mental causes of behavior, these theories focus on understanding behavior in terms of environmental events that either precede or follow the behavior. With respect to depression, behavioral theories focus both on the presence of depressive symptoms and on the absence or reduced frequency of normal behaviors. Behavioral changes, such as the emergence of depressive symptoms or the attenuation of normal behaviors, are seen as being caused by changes in reinforcement. Although virtually all of the behavioral theories recognize changes in reinforcement as the primary etiological factor in depression, the theorists do not necessarily agree on the type of reinforcement changes that are critical for depression to occur. Ferster (1973) and Lazarus (1968), for example, hypothesize that it is a loss in the number of reinforcers that leads to depression. Lewinsohn (1974) more specifically postulates that depression results from a loss of response-contingent positive reinforcement. Costello (1972) focuses not on the number of reinforcers but on their effectiveness. An individual becomes depressed, therefore, when previously effective reinforcers become ineffective. Finally, Seligman (1975) views the main cause of depression as the loss of contingency between reinforcement and behavior. When behaviors no longer adequately elicit reinforcement, or when reinforcement is perceived to be independent of behavior, depression will result.

There are numerous situations and factors that could be involved in reinforcement changes. One common factor involves the loss of the person or persons who previously supplied the reinforcement. From a developmental perspective, it is important to note that the types of people providing reinforcement to an individual will vary as the person grows older. For example, the loss of the mother does not result in the same reinforcement loss for a 6-month-old as for a 20-year-old. The 6-month-old's loss is usually particularly traumatic and devastating, unless a mother replacement is offered (cf. Spitz, 1946). The 20-year-old's loss of a mother is not usually as life shattering, but whatever reinforcement the mother was providing is not as likely to be replaced. A second factor that may result in reinforcement change involves the ineffectiveness of the depressed person's own skills in obtaining reinforcement or in making reinforcers available (cf. Gotlib, 1982; Lewinsohn, 1974). This situation seems particularly relevant to children, given their continual development. What was acceptable behavior at one state of development soon becomes unacceptable as the child progresses (Gut, 1982), and the child's behavior must develop as quickly as people's tolerance for it diminishes. A child may lose reinforcement if his behavior becomes disturbing to other people (cf. Algozzine, 1977).

One recent theory of depression, in fact, ascribes considerable importance to the negative effects induced by the depressed person in those with whom she/he interacts. Coyne (1976b) posits that depressed persons repond to stress by seeking support from other people. Depressive symptoms, in fact, are seen functionally as a means of soliciting this support. Although others in the depressive's environment may initially respond with support, in the absence of improvement these individuals themselves soon begin to feel depressed and frustrated. The depressed person becomes aware of these negative reactions from others, and becomes even more needy and symptomatic in an attempt to regain the support she/he had received earlier. Coyne suggests that this "deviation-amplifying process" continues until, in the extreme, members of the social environment withdraw completely from the depressive or have him withdrawn through hospitalization.

Although this model of depression has been formulated only recently, it has already received empirical support from a number of investigations (e.g., Coyne, 1976a; Gotlib & Beatty, 1985; Gotlib & Robinson, 1982; Strack & Coyne, 1983). All of these studies, however, have examined this model as it relates to depression in adults, and it is not clear that this formulation can readily be extended to account for childhood depression. For example, if children turn to their peers for support, it is not likely that they would be rejected. Moore (1967) found that young children do not react negatively to a peer's solicitation for support. In fact, they react more positively. As Moore concluded, "a child's need or desire to seek help, affection, and support from companions may actually enhance him in their eyes. Young children may be somewhat flattered at having a young companion come to them for attention" (p. 224). Similarly, if children seek support from adults, it is not clear that adults would find the depressive symptoms aversive. In all likelihood, adults would be more tolerant of symptoms in children than of symptoms in other adults simply because children are normally perceived and accepted as being more dependent than are adults. An individual's attraction and acceptance of another person is related to perceptions of the potential for a positive interpersonal relationship (Huston, 1973), and it is likely that the types of "positive interpersonal relationships" that adults anticipate with children are different from those that they anticipate with other adults. For instance, adults may desire a child to be dependent in a relationship, and if this were the case, depressed children would not be rejected as often as would depressed adults. If and when treatment approaches for childhood depression based on Coyne's (1976b) model arise, they will undoubtedly be influenced by developmental differences in communication, in person perception, and in interpersonal interaction.

If the behavior of particular children does become consistently disturbing to others, these children may find themselves to be soccially isolated. The literature suggests that there are two distinct types of socially isolated children: those who do not interact frequently with peers and those who do interact with peers but are rejected (Gottman, 1977a). Moreover, these two types of social isolates are not necessarily related. For example, Gottman, Gonso, and Rasmussen (1975) found that the dispensing of positive reinforcement was related to peer acceptance; the dispensing of negative reinforcement, however, was not found to be related to peer rejection. Furthermore, Gottman (1977b) found that total frequency of interaction was not correlated with measures of peer acceptance and suggested that these measures do not assess the same constructs. Although a number of treatment studies of socially isolated and withdrawn children have been reported (see Conger & Keane, 1981, for a review of this literature), it is not entirely clear how to ameliorate rejection and isolation and replace them with acceptance. As Gottman et al. (1975) state:

> Despite the fact that most intervention programs teach isolated children how to gain entry into a peer group, these programs are not based upon the knowledge of how non-isolated children at a specific developmental level gain entry. Children's style of gaining entry may be very different from that of adults or from what we imagine it to be (p. 71)

The importance of determining how different age groups gain peer acceptance is underscored by studies suggesting that inability during childhood to gain peer acceptance is related to subsequent depression in adulthood. Kohn and Clausen (1955), for example, found that almost one-third of a sample of adult manic–depressives had been social isolates as children, whereas in a normal control group this proportion was close to zero. Thus, peer rejection and/or the lack of adequate interpersonal skills in childhood may be intimately related to the later emergence of depressive symptoms.

Behavioral theories also focus on reinforcement changes in their approaches to the treatment of depression. Treatment is carried out in large part by manipulating reinforcements. Therapy programs range from social skills and assertion training to trying to increase the depressed individual's involvement in rewarding activities. The effectiveness of these various programs in the treatment of depression in adults is not clear from the literature (see Blaney, 1981, for a review). While some studies show positive effects, others find no effects, and the differences across studies do not seem to be readily attributable to methodological differences or to flaws in the studies. One factor that may account for discrepant findings is ambiguity in the diagnosis of depression. In several studies a diagnosis of depression was based on BDI scores (e.g., Sanchez, 1978), whereas in other studies diagnostic criteria involved other measures, such as MMPI-D scores and RDC criteria (e.g., Maish, 1972). Although type of diagnostic criteria used was not directly related to treatment outcome (i.e., studies using the same diagnostic criteria were found to differ with respect to outcome), the issue of uniformity and objectivity in the diagnosis of depression is underscored, and it is clear that diagnostic comparability across studies is sorely needed in this area. Liberman (1981) stressed that in order to make a diagnosis from a behavioral framework, one needs to specify the actions, verbal and nonverbal expressions, and behavioral deficits and excesses that serve as criteria necessary to determine the presence of depression.

One behavioral treatment technique involves the differential reinforcement of appropriate behaviors (Ferster, 1973). When appropriate behaviors are continually reinforced, they should occur more often. Since a person has the capacity for only a finite amount of behavior, an increase in the amount of appropriate behavior should result in a decrease in the amount of inappropriate or depressive behavior. This treatment technique seems relatively easy to apply and appears equally applicable with both adults and children. The only major developmental considerations in utilizing this form of treatment would be in defining both age-appropriate reinforcers and age-appropriate behavior.

Frame, Matson, Sonis, Fialkov, and Kazdin (1982) reported a case study of the behavioral treatment of a depressed 10-year-old boy. Inappropriate body position, lack of eye contact, poor speech quality, and bland affect constituted the target behaviors, and were assessed during baseline, treatment, and follow-up. The treatment program followed a multiple-baseline design. The first six treatment sessions were devoted to the joint treatment of body position and eye contact, the next five sessions to the treatment of speech quality, and the last nine sessions to the teaching of appropriate affective expression. The treatment itself consisted of a skills-training package involving instructions, modeling, role play, and performance feedback. After treatment, changes in the target behaviors were immediate, substantial, and durable. The use of multiple baseline design ensured that improvement was not attributable to extraneous factors, since each target behavior did not decrease until it was the focus of treatment.

It is not clear from the Frame et al. (1982) report, however, whether changes in the target behaviors were attributable to the treatment package as a whole or whether a subset of the treatment components would have been sufficient. Furthermore, all treatment was carried out in a treatment center, and it is not clear whether changes in the target behaviors generalized to other environments, such as the child's home and school. Although this study is notable because of the careful pretreatment assessment of depression (Frame et al. used DSM-III criteria and self-, mother-, and observer ratings on the CDI to make a diagnosis of depression), only the target behaviors were reassessed following the end of treatment. Thus, there was no indication that the depressive disorder itself was reduced or eliminated. In sum, then, this study provides evidence that some depressive symptoms respond well to behavioral treatment, but does not address the broader issue of treating a depressive syndrome.

The applicability of other more radical behavioral treatments for use with children is less clear. Lazarus (1968), for example, reviewed three such treatments, one of which involved time projection with constant positive reinforcement. During this treatment the patient is either hypnotized or extremely relaxed, and is then instructed to imagine himself or herself at particular times in the future engaging in rewarding activities. All of the patients successfully treated by this method were adults, and all were able to picture vivid mental images in their minds. The reliance of this method on the ability to adequately utilize mental imagery has important developmental implications. Children younger than 8 years old are not adept enough at using mental imagery to be able to imagine future situations (Pressley, 1977). Furthermore, children are more tuned to the here-and-now than are adults (Nowels, 1977), and enticement of future reinforcement may therefore be ineffective with children simply because they cannot think or plan far ahead. A final problem with applying this technique to children involves the difference between children and adults in the ability to relax and in their susceptibility to hypnosis. Children are not as receptive as adults to relaxation induction or hypnosis (see Redd, Porterfield, & Andersen, 1979, for a review of similar problems in using systematic desensitization with children), and this treatment approach would have to be altered accordingly.

Cognitive Theories

The main proponents of a cognitive conceptualization of depression have been Beck (e.g., Beck, 1967, 1976; Kovacs & Beck, 1977) and Seligman (e.g., Abramson et al., 1978; Seligman, 1975). Although Beck's cognitive distortion model and Seligman's learned-helplessness model share a number of conceptual underpinnings, for the purposes of the present paper they are discussed separately. (See Coyne & Gotlib, 1983, for a critical review of these two models presented in greater detail.)

Cognitive distortion model. Beck (1967, 1976) has formulated a cognitive distortion model of depression based on his observations of depressed adults. Although he did not explicitly study depression in children, Beck suggested that his model could, in fact, be appropriate for the study of childhood depression (cf. Kovacs & Beck, 1977). After examining the dreams and free associations of depressed adults, Beck (1967) postulated that depression is a disorder of thinking rather than of affect, and argued that the behavioral and affective manifestations of depression result from the activation of particular patterns of cognitions. Specifically, Beck proposed that the depressed person maintains a negative conception of the self, a negative interpretation of life experiences, and a nihilistic view of the future. The self is viewed as deficient or unworthy; the world is seen as demanding and as often presenting insurmountable obstacles; and the future is anticipated as a continuation of current negative experiences. This "negative cognitive triad" is proposed to affect the depressed individual's interactions with his environment, causing him to distort and misinterpret environmental feedback in a negative direction in order to make it congruent with his negative schema. These distortions of the environment, according to Beck, "can be postulated to be the first link in the chain of symptoms" (Beck et al., 1979, p. 19), resulting in such expressions of depression as sad mood and psychomotor retardation.

A number of investigations with depressed adults have provided empirical support for Beck's model (e.g., De Monbruen & Craighead, 1977; Gotlib, 1981, 1983; Gotlib & McCann, 1984; but see also Alloy & Abramson, 1979; Golin, Terrell, & Johnson, 1977, for discrepant findings). It is not clear, however, that the results of these studies can simply be extrapolated downward in the study of childhood depression. In examining the role of developmental factors in the negative triad, one must consider whether the skills involved in forming a negative triad are evident across various stages of development. Are children capable of forming a negative triad? Would a negative triad, even if present in children, maintain the same relationship with emotions and behaviors as it does in adults? Although Beck did not focus explicitly on the etiology of the negative triad, he did suggest that it may emerge in response to perceived loss or rejection (Arieti & Bemporad, 1978). Whatever the cause, the actual construction of the negative triad assumes certain prerequisite cognitive skills. First, it assumes ability to abstract common themes (e.g., the theme that life is terrible) across a variety of situations. Second, it involves the generation of a negative schema or set through which to interpret new events. Third, the formation of a negative cognitive triad involves the ability to think beyond the present, to speculate about the future.

According to Piaget (cf. Mussen, Conger, & Kagan, 1974), children younger than 7 years of age should not be capable of forming a negative triad. These children do not have firmly articulated concepts and do not have well-defined mental representations of things that go together (i.e., a set). Thus, it is doubtful whether these young children would be able to abstract a common theme of pessimism from their life experiences (cf. Ausubel et al., 1980). Furthermore, children are more sensitive to external cues than are adults (Diamond, 1982). This sensitivity to external cues would weaken the effect of a negative cognitive set or schema in guiding their perceptions and behaviors. Finally, children up to age 8 or 9 have a "here and now" or present orientation, and it has been suggested that this tendency to not reason about the future precludes the development of true affective disorder (Campbell, 1983).

Information-processing theorists disagree with Piaget and maintain that young children are in fact capable of adult cognitive skills, although they are less efficient at using them (see for example, Dempster, 1981). According to these theorists, young children should be as capable as adults of forming a negative triad, although they would have more difficulty in doing so. For example, they would have fewer life experiences from which to abstract a common theme, and even though they are capable of abstracting a theme, they may not do so spontaneously. Abstraction involves retrieving past experiences from memory and comparing them with present experiences. Although young children are capable of retrieval when given sufficient prompting (cf. Ruch & Levin, 1979), they are inefficient retrievers and have difficulty retrieving memories spontaneously. Thus, the likelihood that a child will formulate a negative triad may be considerably less than that of an adult.

The second major point open to developmental consideration concerns the variability of the impact of the negative triad across age. Even if children formulate a cognitive triad, it is not clear that it will influence their emotions and behaviors as profoundly and pervasively as it does those of adults. Studies have been conducted that examine to what degree individuals' thoughts and verbalizations direct and control their behavior. Children have difficulty using thoughts to mediate behavior (Camp, Blom, Herbert, & Van Doornick, 1977). However, when they are taught to verbalize their thoughts (i.e., to "think aloud"), they are able to successfully use their thoughts to mediate their behavior. With respect to depression, therefore, children may not spontaneously use their negative distorted thoughts to guide their behavior unless explicitly trained to do so.

The first step in cognitive therapy from Beck's perspective is an assessment of the negative cognitions that are influencing the depressed person, a procedure which involves verbalization of the thoughts. The second step in therapy entails encouraging the depressed person to reflect on his/her negative thoughts and to replace them with more positive cognitions. The final component of this treatment is self-monitoring of thoughts. The major difficulty with using this procedure with children, of course, is the almost exclusive reliance on verbal communication. Young children are not effective communicators when talking about such abstract topics as thoughts and feelings, and as Hobbs, Moguin, Tyroler, and Lahey (1980) have noted, cognitive therapy with children may prove to be a difficult endeavor.

Learned-helplessness model. The phase "learned-helplessness" was first invoked to explain the debilitated escape–avoidance responding demonstrated by dogs exposed to prior inescapable shock. The concept was subsequently extended to account for the debilitated task performance of humans exposed to experimenter-induced failure and was then advanced as an explanatory model of depression (cf. Seligman, 1975). The original learned-helplessness theory proposed that a state of helplessness develops from the perception of an independence between responding and outcome in a situation, resulting in a belief in uncontrollability. The learned expectation that outcomes are uncontrollable lowers the individual's motivation to make new coping responses (the motivational deficit), which in turn impairs the learning that other outcomes can be controllable (the cognitive deficit) and results in negative affect and depression (the emotional deficit).

In this formulation of learned helplessness, little attention needed to be given to the role of developmental factors. Essentially, all that was necessary for a state of learned helplessness to be possible was that an organism have the capacity to learn that outcomes are uncontrollable. Theoretically, therefore, learned helplessness (and analogously, depression) could be observed in very young children. A recent reformulation of the learned-helplessness model, however, has complicated this theoretical position considerably. Abramson et al. (1978) argued that mere exposure to current uncontrollability is not sufficient for a state of learned helplessness to be produced; rather, persons must come to expect that future outcomes are uncontrollable. Abramson et al. emphasize the importance of causal attributions in the development of learned helplessness: "When a person finds that he is helpless, he asks *why* he is helpless. The causal attributions he makes determine the generality and chronicity of his helplessness deficits as well as his later self-esteem" (p. 50). According to this reformulation, persons who are prone to becoming helpless or depressed tend to attribute negative outcomes to internal, stable, and global factors. Attributions of negative events to internal factors lead to lowered self-esteem; stability attributions lead to a persistence of deficits over time; and attributions to global factors lead to a generalization of deficits across situations.

As was the case with Beck's cognitive distortion model, the reformulated learned-helplessness model of depression has received empirical support from a number of investigations of depressed adults (e.g., Metalsky, Abramson, Seligman, Semmel, & Peterson, 1982; Raps, Peterson, Reinhard, Abramson, & Seligman, 1982; but see also Gotlib & Olson, 1983; Lewinsohn, Steinmetz, Larson, & Franklin, 1981, for discrepant results, and Coyne & Gotlib, 1983, for a detailed critique of this literature). In addition, several studies have examined the relationship between attributions and learned helplessness in children. Most notable in this area has been, perhaps, the work of Dweck and her colleagues. In an early study Dweck and Reppucci (1973) found that children whose performance deteriorated most following experimenter-induced failure made more external attributions (i.e., attributing both failure and success less to effort) for the outcome than did children who maintained or improved their performance. Other studies have corroborated this finding, reporting that helplessness-related deficits are often associated with external attributions (e.g., Diener & Dweck, 1980). Moreover, Dweck (1975) reported that an attribution retraining procedure which emphasized the importance of making effort attributions was effective in reducing the performance deterioration following failure experiences in a sample of fifth-grade helpless children.

This line of research represents a promising step in the elucidation of psychological processes underlying childhood depression. There are, however, a number of limitations to these studies. For example, while Abramson et al. (1978) emphasize the importance of the three additional dimensions of internality, stability, and globality in the development of learned helplessness. Dweck and her colleagues have typically restricted their focus to a few very specific causal attributions (i.e., effort, ability, and the agent of evaluation). Furthermore, because investigators have not examined explicitly the relationship between learned helplessness and depressive symptomatology in children, it is not clear that the helplessness-associated attributions that have been reported are in fact characteristic of depressed children. Finally, and for the purposes of the present paper, most importantly, the research examining learned helplessness in children has paid little attention to developmental issues in this formation and utilization of various types of attributions. Given the etiological significance to depression accorded causal attributions by the learned-helplessness model, it is clear that an understanding of developmental patterns of attributions is an imperative prerequisite to the understanding of childhood depression.

Although not explicitly discussed with reference to depressive symptomatology, the development of attributions in children has been the focus of a considerable body of research. A number of consistent findings have emerged from this literature, two of which have particularly important implications for the study of depression in children. First, young children generally overestimate the degree of contingency between outcomes and behavior, attributing noncontingent outcomes to factors such as skill and concentration that would actually affect only contingent outcomes (cf. Weisz, 1980); furthermore, this illusory perception of contingency declines as children mature (Piaget, 1976). Given this early tendency of children to perceive contingency where there actually is none, it would be especially difficult for younger children to become helpless (or depressed) as a result of their attributions regarding perceived *noncontingency* (see Schwartz, 1981, for a similar argument concerning the development of learned helplessness in adults). Consistent with this postulation, Rholes, Blackwell, Jordan, and Walters (1980) reported that following failure, fifth-grade children were more likely than kindergarteners, or first or third graders to manifest helplessness-related attributions and behaviors.

The second relevant finding is that younger children have more positive self-evaluations than do older children and appear to respond differently to failure feedback. Glasberg and Aboud (1982), for example, note that younger children are unable to see themselves as possessing socially undesirable or negative qualities. Ruble, Parsons, and Ross (1976) found that failure feedback affected the self-evaluations of children between 8 and 11 years of age, but not the self-evaluations of 6- and 7-year-olds. Ruble et al. suggest that the self-concept of the younger child is not yet well-enough developed to be affected by failure information, a formulation consistent with Nicholls' (1978) finding of a developmental decline in the positivity of children's self-evaluations. The results of these studies, considered collectively, suggest that the "negative self-concept" of the adult depressive may be nonexistent in children younger than approximately 8 years of age.

In summarizing the literature examining children's attributions, Guttentag and Longfellow (1978) state that

> In sum, the work suggests that before the age of 6 or 7, children have a notion of a psychological motivational force, but the concept is global and undifferentiated, applied indiscriminantly to the animate and inanimate world. At the age of 6 or 7, they begin to distinguish between the possible causes for physical and social phenomena. . . . The youngest children studied (5- and 6-year-olds) had only a partial scheme of causal attributions. . . . By the time children are 9 years old, they can clearly coordinate information on possible causes in an interrelated way because of their ability to decenter. (pp. 308–311)

Similar conclusions have been reached by Ruble and Rholes (1981) regarding children's attributions for interpersonal behavior:

> In general, like the achievement studies mentioned earlier, these studies report that 5 to 6-year-old children do not regularly use complex causal schemata . . . in their attributions, but that . . . principles gradually emerge and reach maximum development at the approximate age of 9 to 11. (p. 17)

It appears, then, that until the age of about 9 years, children are unsystematic in their attributions, if in fact they make them at all. In any case, it is clear, as Flavell (1977) states, that young children's attributions are dramatically different from those of older children and adults, and that the same attributions are likely to be interpreted differently by young children and adults (cf. Hymel et al., 1983). It is important that these developmental differences must be taken into consideration in applying learned helplessness as an explanatory model for childhood depression.

CONCLUDING COMMENTS

Throughout the course of this paper, various developmental issues have been examined as they affect such aspects of depression as etiology, symptoms and syndromes, and treatment. A number of developmental issues were found to be relevant only to certain theoretical orientations. From a biological perspective, for example, developmental concerns were considered in examining drug responsivity and metabolic functioning. Similarly, from a psychoanalytic perspective, developmental issues were raised with respect to the delineation of the various depressive reactions. From a behavioral orientation, developmental issues were considered with respect to the significance of the role of reinforcement and the concept of social isolation. Finally, from a cognitive framework, attention was given to the determination of the likelihood of forming a cognitive triad, to the significance of such a triad, and to the development of attributional processes.

Other developmental issues were found to be common to several of the different theoretical orientations. One such issue, for example, involves age-related differences in verbal skills. The use of verbal reports plays an important, albeit implicit, role in a number of conceptualizations of depression in adults. Verbal facility is implicated in depressed patients' reports of their feelings of sadness, in their overt displays of pessimistic attitudes, and in their ascription of negative events to internal, stable, and global factors. Furthermore, most diagnostic instruments rely heavily on self-report measures. Patients are instructed to describe their depressive affect or to recognize which of a number of feelings and behaviors are self-descriptive. The lack of adequately developed verbal skills in young children may render many of these diagnostic instruments relatively insensitive in detecting depression in this population. Children's comparatively poor verbal skills necessitates a change in the conceptualization and assessment of depression in younger populations. Emphasis must be redirected to the children's overt behavior and to assessment approaches that do not rely solely on self-report measures. In this regard, the peer nomination method discussed earlier appears to be a particularly promising technique for the assessment of depression in children.

Investigations of childhood depression must also consider the incidence of "depressive" behaviors in nondepressed children. Knowledge of normative behavior is crucial if one is to determine whether certain behaviors are sufficiently rare to be regarded as symptoms of depression. It is important to be cognizant, however, of the fact that the prevalence of many normative behaviors varies with age. Consequently, a particular behavior may be indicative of depression at one age range, but not at another (cf. MacFarlane et al., 1954). Considerable research has been conducted in an attempt to discriminate among various subtypes of depressives (e.g., Kupfer et al., 1978; Sabelli, Fawcett, Javaid, & Bagri, 1983). Developmental issues may ultimately prove to be particularly relevant to this task, with age being one of the variables along which various types of depressives differ significantly (cf. McConville et al., 1973).

Childhood depression may also be more likely than adult depression to be accompanied by various antisocial behaviors that present unique problems in terms of intervention. Treatment of depression in children may require dealing with antisocial behaviors accompanying the depression (e.g., hyperactivity, aggression), many of which put strains on the psychotherapeutic situation. Friend (1972), for example, noted that a therapeutic relationship with adolescents was extremely difficult to establish because many adolescents had problems of acting out. Moreover, even if a therapeutic relationship is successfully formed, gains made in treatment may be difficult to maintain. Lewis and Lewis (1981) found that although depressed adolescents became increasingly animated and related more easily over the course of the therapy hour, these positive changes did not last much longer than the therapy session itself. A further difficulty involves determining whether changes apparent in depressed children following treatment are due to the therapeutic intervention, to developmental reorganization and maturation, to environmental influences, or to some combination of these three factors. Because of the rapid and continual growth of young children, evaluation of treatment for childhood disorders is particularly difficult.

The acknowledgment that developmental issues are relevant to the study of depression has implications for the design of investigations of this disorder. The most effective approach in examining the relationship between child and adult depression would seem to be the use of longitudinal investigations, in which age-correlated effects are examined by sampling the same individuals across different points in time. Longitudinal studies would address most directly the question of whether depressed children become depressed adults (cf. Crook & Eliot, 1980). The importance of this methodological approach is underscored by a longitudinal study reported by Poznanski, Krahenbuhl, and Zrull (1976), who found that after 6 years 50% of their subjects who could be located were still clinically depressed. Age-related differences do exist between younger and older depressives, however, and depending on whether these differences are believed to be quantitative or qualitative in nature, investigators may have to incorporate this finding in the type of measures they use to assess depression across age groups. If quantitative differences are expected, then similar measures may be adequate with various age groups. If changes of a more qualitative nature are predicted, however, age-specific measures must be developed and used.

In a recent review of the childhood depression literature, Kashani et al. (1981) concluded that

> Since there are probably many etiological factors in this disorder, it will be important to study childhood depression using the various frameworks of biochemical, genetic, psychosocial stress, behavioral reinforcement, and cognitive theories. Although the literature on adults reaches into each of these areas, the research on children is still at the preliminary stage of mostly descriptive study. (p. 151)

There is now ample evidence that developmental differences in the manifestation of depression do exist. It is time to focus our efforts toward an understanding of the role that these differences play in defining the relationship between childhood depression and depression in adults.

REFERENCES

Abramson, L. Y., Seligman, M. E. P., & Teasdale, J. D. (1978). Learned helplessness in humans: Critique and reformulation. *Journal of Abnormal Psychology*, **87**, 49-74.

Achenbach, T. M. (1978). Psychopathology of childhood: Research problems and issues. *Journal of Consulting and Clinical Psychology*, **46**, 759-776.

Achenbach, T. M., & Edelbrock, C. S. (1981). Behavioral problems and competencies reported by patients of normal and disturbed children aged 4 through 16. *Monographs of the Society for Research in Child Development*, **46**, (Serial No. 188).

Algozzine, B. (1977). The emotionally disturbed child: Disturbed or disturbing? *Journal of Abnormal Child Psychology*, **5**, 205-211.

Alloy, L. B., & Abramson, L. Y. (1979). Judgment of contingency in depressed and nondepressed students: Sadder but wiser? *Journal of Experimental Psychology: General*, **108**, 441-485.

Anthony, E. J. (1967). Psychoneurotic disorders. In A. M. Freedman & H. G. Kaplan (Eds.), *Comprehensive textbook of psychiatry* (pp. 1387-1406). Baltimore: Williams & Wilkins.

Anthony, E. J. (1975). Childhood depression. In E. J. Anthony & T. Benedek (Eds.), *Depression and human existence*. Boston: Little, Brown.

Arieti, S. (1978). The basic questions and the psychological approach. In S. Arieti & J. Bemporad (Eds.), *Severe and mild depression* (pp. 3-10). New York: Basic Books.

Arieti, S., & Bemporad, J. (1978). *Severe and mild depression.* New York: Basic Books.

Ausubel, D. P., Sullivan, E. V., & Ives, W. S. (1980). *Theory and problems of child development.* New York: Grune & Stratton.

Beck, A. T. (1967). *Depression: Causes and treatment.* Philadelphia: Univ. of Pennsylvania Press.

Beck, A. T. (1976). *Cognitive therapy and the emotional disorders.* New York: International Universities Press.

Beck, A. T., Rush, A. J., Shaw, B. F., & Emergy, G. (1979). *Cognitive therapy of depression.* New York: Guilford.

Bemporad, J. (1970). New views on the psychodynamics of the depressive character. In S. Arieti (Ed.), *The world biennial of psychiatry and psychotherapy* (Vol. 1). New York: Basic Books.

Bemporad, J. (1978). Manifest symptomatology of depression in children and adolescents. In S. Arieti & J. Bemporad (Eds.), *Severe and mild depression* (pp. 87-108). New York: Basic Books.

Berndt, D. J., Schwartz, S., & Kaiser, C. F. (1983). Readability of self-report depression inventories. *Journal of Consulting and Clinical Psychology, 51,* 627-628.

Blaney, P. H. (1981). The effectiveness of cognitive and behavioral therapies. In L. P. Rehm (Ed.), *Behavior therapy for depression* (pp. 1-32). New York: Academic Press.

Blumberg, M. L. (1981). Depression in abused and neglected children. *American Journal of Psychotherapy, 35,* 342-355.

Borke, H. (1971). Interpersonal perception of young children: Egocentrism or empathy? *Developmental Psychology, 5,* 263-269.

Briant, R. H. (1978). An introduction to clinical pharmacology. In J. S. Werry (Ed.), *Pediatric psychopharmacology: The use of behavior modifying drugs in children.* New York: Brunner/Mazel.

Camp, B. W., Blom, G. E., Herbert, F., & Van Doornick, W. J. (1977). "Think aloud": A program for developing self-control in young aggressive boys. *Journal of Abnormal Child Psychology, 5,* 157-169.

Campbell, S. B. (1983). Developmental perspectives in child psychopathology. In T. H. Ollendick & M. Hersen (Eds.), *Handbook of child psychopathology.* New York: Plenum.

Cantwell, D. P. (1982). Childhood depression: A review of current research. In B. B. Lahey & A. E. Kazdin (Eds.), *Advances in clinical child psychology* (Vol. 5, pp. 39-93). New York: Plenum.

Cantwell, D. P., & Carlson, G. (1979). Problems and prospects in the study of childhood depression. *Journal of Nervous and Mental Disease, 167,* 522-529.

Carroll, B. J., Feinberg, M., & Greden, J. F. (1981). A specific laboratory test for the diagnosis of melancholia: Standardization, validation and clinical utility. *Archives of General Psychiatry, 38,* 15-22.

Carroll, B. J., Feinberg, M., & Steiner, M. (1980). Diagnostic application of the dexamethasone suppression test in depressed outpatients. *Advances in Biological Psychiatry, 5,* 107-116.

Conger, J. C., & Keane, S. P. (1981). Social skills intervention in the treatment of isolated or withdrawn children. *Psychological Bulletin, 90,* 478-495.

Connell, H. M. (1972). Depression in childhood. *Child Psychiatry and Human Development, 4,* 71-85.

Conners, C. K., & Werry, J. S. (1979). Pharmacotherapy. In H. C. Quay & J. S. Werry (Eds.), *Psychopathological disorders of childhood* (pp. 336-386). New York: Wiley.

Costello, C. G. (1972). Depression: Loss of reinforcers or loss of reinforcer effectiveness? *Behavior Therapy*, **3**, 240-247.

Coyne, J. C. (1976a). Depression and the response of others. *Journal of Abnormal Psychology*, **85**, 186-193.

Coyne, J. C. (1976b). Toward an interactional description of depression. *Psychiatry*, **39**, 14-27.

Coyne, J. C., & Gotlib, I. H. (1983). The role of cognition in depression: A critical appraisal. *Psychological Bulletin*, **94**, 472-505.

Crook, T., & Eliot, J. (1980). Parental death during childhood and adult depression: A critical review of the literature. *Psychological Bulletin*, **87**, 252-259.

Cytryn, L., McKnew, D. H., Bartko, J. J., Lamour, M., & Hamovitt, J. (1982). Offspring of patients with affective disorders: II. *Journal of the American Academy of Child Psychiatry*, **21**, 389-391.

Cytryn, L., McKnew, D. H., & Bunney, W. E. (1980). Diagnosis of depression in children: A reassessment. *American Journal of Psychiatry*, **137**, 22-25.

Davidson, J. R. T., McLeod, M. N., Turnbull, C. D., & Miller, R. D. (1981). A comparison of phenelzine and imipramine in depressed inpatients. *Journal of Clinical Psychiatry*, **42**, 395-397.

Decina, P., Kestenbaum, C. J., Farber, S., Kron, L., Gagan, M., Sackeim, H., & Fieve, R. (1983). Clinical and psychological assessment of children of bipolar probands. *American Journal of Psychiatry*, **140**, 548-553.

DeMonbreun, B. G., & Craighead, W. E. (1977). Selective recall of positive and neutral feedback. *Cognitive Therapy and Research*, **1**, 311-329.

Dempster, F. N. (1981). Memory span: Sources of individual and developmental differences. *Psychological Bulletin*, **89**, 63-100.

Diamond, N. (1982). Cognitive theory. In B. B. Wolman (Ed.), *Handbook of developmental psychology* (pp. 3-22). Englewood Cliffs, NJ: Prentice-Hall.

Diener, C. I., & Dweck, C. S. (1980). An analysis of learned helplessness: II. The processing of success. *Journal of Personality and Social Psychology*, **39**, 940-952.

Dweck, C. S. (1975). The role of expectations and attributions in the alleviation of learned helplessness. *Journal of Personality and Social Psychology*, **31**, 674-685.

Dweck, C. S., Gittelman-Klein, R., & McKinney, W. T. (1977). Summary of the Subcommittee on Clinical Criteria for Diagnosis of Depression in Children. In J. G. Schulterbrandt & A. Raskin (Eds.), *Depression in children: Diagnosis, treatment, and conceptual models*. New York: Raven Press.

Dweck, C. S., & Reppucci, N. D. (1973). Learned helplessness and reinforcement responsibility in children. *Journal of Personality and Social Psychology*, **25**, 109–116.

Eaton, M., Sells, C. J., & Lucas, B. (1977). Psychoactive medication and learning disabilities. *Journal of Learning Disabilities*, **10**, 403-410.

Eberlain, W. R., & Winter, J. S. (1969). Cusing's syndrome in childhood. In L. I. Gardner (Ed.), *Endocrine and genetic diseases of childhood* (pp. 428-436). New York: Harper & Row.

Fawcett, J. A., & Bunney, W. E. (1967). Pituitary adrenal function and depression. *Archives of General Psychiatry*, **16**, 517-535.

Ferster, C. B. (1973). A functional analysis of depression. *American Psychologist*, **28**, 857-869.

Flavell, J. H. (1977). *Cognitive development.* Englewood Cliff, NJ: Prentice-Hall.

Frame, C., Matson, J. L., Sonis, W. A., Fialkov, M. J., & Kazdin, A. E. (1982). Behavioral treatment of depression in a prepubertal child. *Journal of Behavior Therapy and Experimental Psychiatry, 3,* 239-243.

Freud, A. (1953). Some remarks on infant observation. *The Psychoanalytic Study of the Child, 8,* 9-19.

Freud, S. (1957). Mourning and melancholia. In J. Strachey (Ed. and Trans.), *The standard edition of the complete psychological works of Sigmund Freud* (Vol. 14). London: Hogarth Press. (Original work published 1917).

Friend, M. R. (1972). Social service information in child psychiatry. In A. M. Freedman & H. I. Kaplan (Eds.), *The child: His psychological and cultural development.* New York: Atheneum.

Frommer, E. A., Mendelson, W. B., & Reid, M. A. (1972). Differential diagnosis of psychiatric disturbance in preschool children. *British Journal of Psychiatry, 121,* 71.

Garvey, M. J., Tuason, V. B., Johnson, R. A., & Valentine, R. (1982). RDC depressive subtypes: Are they valid? *Journal of Clinical Psychiatry, 43,* 442-444.

Gittelman-Klein, R. (1977). Definitional and methodological issues concerning depressive illness in children. In J. G. Schulterbrandt & A. Raskin (Eds.), *Depression in childhood: Diagnosis, treatment and conceptual models.* New York: Raven Press.

Gittelman-Klein, R., & Klein, D. F. (1973). School phobia: Diagnostic considerations in the light of imipramine effects. *Journal of Mental Diseases, 156,* 199-215.

Glasberg, R., & Aboud, F. (1982). Keeping one's distance from sadness: Children's self-reports of emotional experience. *Developmental Psychology, 18,* 287-293.

Glaser, K. (1967). Masked depression in children and adolescents. *American Journal of Psychotherapy, 21,* 565-574.

Golin, S., Terrell, F., & Johnson, B. (1977). Depression and the illusion of control. *Journal of Abnormal Psychology, 86,* 440-442.

Gotlib, I. H. (1981). Self-reinforcement and recall: Differential deficits in depressed and nondepressed psychiatric inpatients. *Journal of Abnormal Psychology, 90,* 521-530.

Gotlib, I. H. (1982). Self-reinforcement and depression in interpersonal interaction: The role of performance level. *Journal of Abnormal Psychology, 91,* 3-13.

Gotlib, I. H. (1983). Perception and recall of interpersonal feedback: Negative bias in depression. *Cognitive Therapy and Research, 7,* 399-412.

Gotlib, I. H., & Beatty, M. E. (1985). Negative responses to depression: The role of attributional style. *Cognitive Therapy and Research, 9,* 91-103.

Gotlib, I. H., & McCann, C. D. (1984). Construct accessibility and depression: An examination of cognitive and affective factors. *Journal of Personality and Social Psychology, 47,* 427-439.

Gotlib, I. H., & Olson, J. M. (1983). Depression, psychopathology, and self-serving attributions. *British Journal of Clinical Psychology, 22,* 309-310.

Gotlib, I. H., & Robinson, L. A. (1982). Responses to depressed individuals: Discrepancies between self-report and observer-rated behavior. *Journal of Abnormal Psychology, 91,* 231-240.

Gottman, J. M. (1977a). The effects of a modeling film on social isolation in preschool children: A methodological investigation. *Journal of Abnormal Child Psychology, 5,* 69-78.

Gottman, J. M. (1977b). Toward a definition of social isolation in children. *Child Development, 48,* 513-517.

Gottman, J., Gonso, J., & Rasmussen, B. (1975). Social interaction, social competence, and friendship in children. *Child Development*, **46**, 709-718.

Gut, E. (1982). Cause and function of the depressed response: A hypothesis. *International Review of Psychoanalysis*, **63**, 179-189.

Guttentag, M., & Longfellow, C. (1978). Children's social attributions: Development and change. In H. E. Howe, Jr., & C. B. Keasy (Eds.), *Nebraska symposium on motivation, 1977*. Lincoln: Univ. of Nebraska Press.

Harris, P. L., Olthof, T., & Terwogt, M. M. (1981). Children's knowledge of emotion. *Journal of Child Psychology and Psychiatry and Allied Disciplines*, **22**, 247-261.

Hobbs, S. A., Moguin, L. E., Tyroler, M., & Lahey, B. (1980). Cognitive behavior therapy with children: Has clinical utility been demonstrated? *Psychological Bulletin*, **87**, 147-165.

Huston, T. L. (1973). Ambiguity of acceptance, social desirability and dating choice. *Journal of Experimental Social Psychology*, **9**, 32-42.

Hymel, S., Freigang, R., Franke, S., Both, L., Bream, L., & Borys, S. (1983, June). *Children's attributions for social situations: Variations as a function of social status and self-perception variables*. Paper presented at the meeting of the Canadian Psychological Association, Winnipeg.

Jacobsen, R. H., Lahey, B. B., & Strauss, C. C. (1983). Correlates of depressed mood in normal children. *Journal of Abnormal Child Psychology*, **11**, 29-40.

Jacobsen, E. (1957). On normal and pathological moods. *Psychoanalytic Study of the Child*, **12**, 73-113.

Kadrmas, A. K. & Winokur, G. (1979). Manic depressive illness and EEG abnormalities. *Journal of Clinical Psychiatry*, **40**, 306-307.

Kane, J. S., & Lawler, E. E., III. (1978). Methods of peer assessment. *Psychological Bulletin*, **85**, 555-586.

Kashani, J. H., Husain, A., Shekim, W. O., Hodges, K. K., Cytryn, L., & McKnew, D. H. (1981). Current perspectives on childhood depression. An overview. *American Journal of Psychiatry*, **138**, 143-153.

Kazdin, A. E. (1981). Assessment techniques for childhood depression: A critical appraisal. *Journal of the American Academic of Child Psychiatry*, **20**, 358-375.

Kazdin, A. E., Rancurello, M. D., & Unis, A. S. (in press). Childhood depression. In G. D. Burrows & J. S. Werry (Eds.), *Advances in human psychopharmacology* (Vol. 4). Greenwich, CT: JAI Press.

Kohn, M., & Clausen, J. (1955). Social isolation and schizophrenia. *American Sociological Review*, **20**, 265-273.

Kovacs, M., & Beck, A. T. (1977). An empirical clinical approach towards a definition of childhood depression. In J. G. Schulterbrandt & A. Raskin (Eds.), *Depression in children: Diagnosis, treatment and conceptual models* (pp. 1-25). New York: Raven Press.

Krakowski, A. J. (1970). Depressive reactions of childhood and adolescence. *Psychosomatics*, **11**, 429-433.

Kuhn, V., & Kuhn, R. (1972). Drug therapy for depression in children: Indications and methods. In A. L. Annell (Ed.), *Depressive states in childhood and adolescence* (pp. 455-459). Stockholm: Almquist & Wiksell.

Kupfer, D. J. & Foster, F. G. (1972). Interval between onset of sleep and rapid-eye-movement sleep as an indicator of depression. *Lancet*, **11**, 684.

Kupfer, D. J., Foster, F. G., & Coble, P. (1978). The application of EEG sleep for the differential diagnosis of affective disorder. *American Journal of Psychiatry*, **135**, 69-74.

Kupfer, D. J., & Spiker, D. G. (1981). Refractory depression: Prediction of nonresponse by clinical indicators. *Journal of Clinical Psychiatry*, **42**, 307-312.

Lazarus, A. (1968). Learning theory and the treatment of depression. *Behavior Research Therapy*, **6**, 83-89.

Leckman, J. F., Cohen, D. J., Shaywitz, B. A., Caparulo, B. K., Heninger, G. R., & Bowers, M. B. (1980). CSF monoamine metabolites in child and adult psychiatric patients. *Archives of General Psychiatry*, **37**, 677-681.

Lefkowitz, M. M., & Burton, N. (1978). Childhood depression. *Psychological Bulletin*, **85**, 716-726.

Lefkowitz, M. M., & Tesiny, E. P. (1980). Assessment of childhood depression. *Journal of Consulting and Clinical Psychology*, **48**, 43-50.

Lewinsohn, P. M. (1974). A behavioral approach to depression. In R. J. Freidman & M. M. Katz (Eds.), *The psychology of depression: Contemporary theory and research* (pp. 157-186). New York: Wiley.

Lewinsohn, P. M., Steinmetz, J. L., Larsen, D. W., & Franklin, J. (1981). Depression-related cognitions: Antecedent or consequence? *Journal of Abnormal Psychology*, **90**, 213-219.

Lewis, M., & Lewis, D. (1981). Depression in childhood: A biopsychosocial perspective. *American Journal of Psychotherapy*, **35**, 323-329.

Liberman, R. P. (1981). A model for individualizing treatment. In L. P. Rehm (Ed.), *Behavioral therapy for depression* (pp. 231-254). New York: Academic Press.

Ling, W., Oftedal, G., & Weinberg, W. (1970). Depressive illness in childhood presenting as severe headache. *American Journal of Diseases of Children*, **120**, 122-124.

Loevinger, J. (1976). *Ego development*. San Francisco: Jossey-Bass.

Lopez, I. J. (1972). Masked depression. *British Journal of Psychiatry*, **120**, 245-258.

Maas, J. W. (1975). Biogenic amines and depression: Biochemical and pharmacological separation of two types of depression. *Archives of General Psychiatry*, **32**, 1357-1361.

MacFarlane, J. W., Allen, L., & Honzik, M. P. (1954). *A developmental study of the behavioral problems of normal children between 21 months and 14 years*. Berkeley: Univ. of California Press.

Mahler, M. S. (1961). On sadness and grief in infancy and childhood. *Psychoanalytic Study of the Child*, **16**, 332-354.

Mahler, M., Pine, F., & Bergman, A. (1975). *The psychological birth of the human infant*. New York: Basic Books.

Maish, J. I. (1972). The use of an individualized assertive training program in the treatment of depressed inpatients. *Dissertation Abstracts International*, **33**, 2816.

Malmquist, C. P. (1977). Childhood depression: A clinical and behavioral perspective. In J. Schulterbrandt & A. Raskin (Eds.), *Depression in childhood: Diagnosis, treatment and conceptual models* (pp. 33-60). New York: Raven Press.

McConville, B. J., Boag, L. C., & Purohit, A. P. (1973). Three types of childhood depression. *Canadian Psychiatric Association Journal*, **18**, 133-318.

McKnew, D. H., & Cytryn, L. (1979). Urinary metabolites in chronically depressed children. *Journal of the American Academy of Child Psychiatry*, **18**, 608-615.

Metalsky, G. I., Abramson, L. Y., Seligman, M. G. P., Semmel, A., & Peterson, C. (1982). Attributional styles and life events in the classroom: Vulnerability and invulnerability to depressive mood reactions. *Journal of Personality and Social Psychology*, **43**, 612-617.

Meyer, A. (1908). The problems of mental reaction-types, mental causes and diseases. *Psychological Bulletin*, **5**, 265.

Miller, P. H. (1983). *Theories of developmental psychology*. San Francisco: Freeman.

Mobley, P. L., & Sulser, F. (1981). Down-regulation of the central noradrenergic receptor system by antidepressant therapies: Biochemical and clinical aspects. In S. J. Enna, J. B. Malick, & E. Richelson (Eds.), *Antidepressants: Neurochemical, behavioral and clinical perspectives.* New York: Raven Press.

Molinoff, P. B., & Axelrod, J. (1971). Biochemistry of catecholamines. *American Review of Biochemistry,* **40,** 465-500.

Moore, S. G. (1967). Correlates of peer acceptance in nursery school children. In W. W. Hartup & N. L. Smothergill (Eds.), *The young child* (pp. 229-247). Washington, DC: National Association for the Education of Young Children.

Mussen, P. H., Conger, J. J., & Kagan, J. (1974). *Child development and personality* (4th ed.). New York: Harper & Row.

Nicholls, J. G. (1978). The development of the concepts of effort and ability, perception of academic attainment, and the understanding that difficult tasks require more ability. *Child Development,* **49,** 800-814.

Nowels, A. (1977). Discussion of the chapter by Drs. Kovacs and Beck. In J. Schulterbrandt & A. Raskin (Eds.), *Depression in childhood: Diagnosis, treatment and conceptual models* (pp. 27-32). New York: Raven Press.

Pallmeyer, T. P., & Petti, T. A. (1979). Effects of imipramine on aggression and dejection in depressed children. *American Journal of Psychiatry,* **11,** 1472-1473.

Pearce, J. (1977). Depressive disorders in childhood. *Journal of Child Psychology and Psychiatry,* **18,** 79-83.

Petti, T. A. (1981). Active treatment of childhood depression. In J. F. Clarkin & H. I. Glazer (Eds.), *Depression: Behavioral and directive intervention strategies.* New York: Garland STPM Press.

Petti, T. A., Bornstein, M., Delamater, A., & Conners, C. K. (1980). Evaluation and multimodality treatment of a depressed pre-pubertal girl. *Journal of the American Academy of Child Psychiatry,* **19,** 690-702.

Piaget, J. (1976). *The grasp of consciousness.* Cambridge, MA: Harvard Univ. Press.

Poznanski, E. O., Carroll, B. J., Banegas, M. C., Cook, S. C., & Grossman, J. A. (1982). The dexamethasone suppression test in prepubertal children. *American Journal of Psychiatry,* **139,** 321-324.

Poznanski, E. O., Krahenbuhl, V., & Zrull, J. P. (1976). Childhood depression: A longitudinal perspective. *Journal of the American Academy of Child Psychiatry,* **15,** 491-501.

Pressley, M. (1977). Imagery and children's learning: Putting the picture in developmental perspective. *Review of Educational Research,* **47,** 585-622.

Puig-Antich, J. (1980). Affective disorders in childhood: A review and perspective. *The Psychiatric Clinics of North America,* **3,** 403-424.

Puig-Antich, J., Goetz, R., Hanlon, C., Davies, M., Thompson, J., Chambers, W. J., Tabrizi, M. A., & Weitzman, E. D. (1982). Sleep architecture and REM sleep measures in prepubertal children with major depression. *Archives of General Psychiatry,* **31,** 932-939.

Quay, H. C. (1979). Classification. In H. C. Quay & J. S. Werry (Eds.), *Psychopathological disorders of childhood* (pp. 1-42). New York: Wiley.

Rado, S. (1928). The problem of melancholia. *International Journal of Psychoanalysis,* **9,** 420-438.

Raps, C. S., Peterson, C., Reinhard, K. E., Abramson, L. Y., & Seligman, M. E. P. (1982). Attributional style among depressed patients. *Journal of Abnormal Psychology,* **91,** 102-108.

Redd, W. H., Porterfield, A. L., & Anderson, B. L. (Eds.). (1979). *Behavior modification:*

Behavioral approaches to human problems. New York: Random House.

Rholes, W. S., Blackwell, J., Jordan, C., & Walters, C. (1980). A developmental study of learned helplessness. *Developmental Psychology,* **16**, 616-624.

Richelson, E. (1979). Tricyclic antidepressants and neurotransmitter receptors. *Psychiatric Annals,* **9**, 186-194.

Rie, H. E. (1966). Depression in childhood: A survey of some pertinent contributions. *Journal of American Academy of Child Psychiatry,* **5**, 653-685.

Risch, S. C., Huey, L. Y., & Janowsky, D. S. (1979a). Plasma levels of tricyclic antidepressants and clinical efficacy: Review of the literature: Part I. *Journal of Clinical Psychiatry,* **40**, 4-16.

Risch, S. C., Huey, L. Y., & Janowsky, D. S. (1979b). Plasma levels of tricyclic antidepressants and clinical efficacy: Review of the literature: Part II. *Journal of Clinical Psychiatry,* **40**, 58-69.

Rosenbaum, A. H., Maruta, T., Schatzberg, A. F., Orsvlak, P. J., Jiang, N., Cole, J. O., & Schildkraut, J. J. (1983). Toward a biochemical classification of depressive disorders: VII. Urinary free cortisol and urinary MHPG in depressions. *American Journal of Psychiatry,* **140**, 314-318.

Ruble, D. N., Parsons, J. E., & Ross, J. (1976). Self-evaluative responses of children in an achievement setting. *Child Development,* **47**, 990-997.

Ruble, D. N., & Rholes, W. S. (1981). The development of children's perceptions and attributions about their social world. In J. H. Harvey, W. Ickes, & R. F. Kidd (Eds.), *New directions in attribution research* (Vol. 3, pp. 3-36). Hillsdale, NJ: Erlbaum.

Ruch, M. D., & Levin, J. R. (1979). Partial pictures as imagery-retrieval cues in young children's prose recall. *Journal of Experimental Child Psychology,* **28**, 268-279.

Sabelli, H. C., Fawcett, J., Javaid, J. I., & Bagri, S. (1983). The methylphenidate test for differentiating desipramine responsive from nortriptyline-responsive depression. *American Journal of Psychiatry,* **140**, 212-214.

Sachar, E. J. (1973). Endocrine factors in psychopathological states. In J. Mendels (Ed.), *Biological Psychiatry* (pp. 175-198). New York: Wiley.

Sanchez, V. C. (1979). Assertion training: Effectiveness in the treatment of depression. *Dissertation Abstracts International,* **39**, 5085.

Saraf, K., Klein, D., Gittleman-Klein, R., & Grof, S. (1974). Imipramine and side effects in children. *Psychopharmacologia,* **37**, 265-275.

Schildkraut, J. J., Orsulak, P. J., LaBrie, R. A., Schatzberg, A. F., Gudeman, J. E., Cole, J. O., & Rohde, W. A. (1978). Toward a biochemical classification of depressive disorders: II. Application of multivariate discriminant function analysis to data on urinary catecholamines and metabolites. *Archives of General Psychiatry,* **35**, 1436-1439.

Schildkraut, J. J., Orsulak, P. J., Schatzberg, A. F., Gudeman, J. E., Cole, J. O., Rohde, W. A., & LaBrie, R. A. (1978). Toward a biochemical classification of depressive disorders: I. Differences in urinary MHPG and other catecholamine metabolites in clinically defined subtypes of depressions. *Archives of General Psychiatry,* **35**, 1427-1433.

Schulterbrandt, J. G., & Raskin, A. (Eds.) (1977). *Depression in childhood: Diagnosis, treatment and conceptual models.* New York: Raven Press.

Schwartz, B. (1981). Does helplessness cause depression, or do only depressed people become helpless? Comment on Alloy and Abramson. *Journal of Experimental Psychology; General,* **110**, 429-435.

Seligman, M. E. P. (1975). *Helplessness: On depression, development and death.* San Francisco: Freeman.

Shepherd, M., Oppenheim, B., & Mitchell, S. (1971). *Childhood behavior and mental health.* New York: Grune & Stratton.

Spitz, R. (1946). Anaclitic depression. *The Psychoanalytic Study of the Child,* 5, 113-117.

Stack, J. J. (1972). Chemotherapy in childhood depression. In A. L. Annell (Ed.), *Depressive states in childhood and adolescence.* New York: Wiley.

Strack, S., & Coyne, J. C. (1983). Social confirmation of dysphoria: Shared and private reactions to depression. *Journal of Personality and Social Psychology,* 44, 798-806.

Tesiny, E. P., & Lefkowitz, M. M. (1982). Childhood depression: A 6-month follow-up study. *Journal of Consulting and Clinical Psychology,* 50, 778-780.

Van Eerdewegh, Gershon, E. S., & VanEerdewegh, P. M. (1979). X-chromosome threshold models of bipolar manic–depressive illness. *Journal of Psychiatric Research,* 15, 215-338.

Weinberg, W. A., Rutman, J., Sullivan, L., Penick, E. C., & Dietz, S. G. (1973). Depression in children referred to an educational diagnostic center. *Journal of Pediatrics,* 83, 1065-1072.

Weisz, J. R. (1981). Illusory contingency in children at the state fair. *Developmental Psychology,* 17, 481-489.

Wenar, C. (1982). Developmental psychology: Its nature and models. *Journal of Clinical Child Psychology,* 11, 192-201.

Williams, G. H., Dulhy, R. G., & Thorn, G. W. (1974). Diseases of the adrenal cortex. In M. W. Wintrobe, G. W. Thorn, & R. D. Adams (Eds.), *Harrison's principles of internal medicine* (7th ed., pp. 499-505). New York: McGraw Hill.

PART VII: DEPRESSION IN CHILDHOOD AND ADOLESCENCE

26

Depressive Symptoms and Suicidal Behavior in Adolescents

Douglas R. Robbins and Norman E. Alessi

University of Michigan, Ann Arbor

Depressive symptoms and suicidal behavior in 64 adolescent psychiatric patients were assessed by a structured interview and the Schedule for Affective Disorders and Schizophrenia. The medical seriousness of suicidal behavior was associated with conscious intent to die and with the number of previous nonlethal suicide attempts. Suicidal behavior was associated with depressed mood, negative self-evaluation, anhedonia, insomnia, poor concentration, indecisiveness, lack of reactivity of mood, psychomotor disturbance, and alcohol and drug abuse. The results suggest that adolescents can be reliable reporters of their suicide potential and that clinicians need to be sensitive to symptoms of major depressive disorder in assessing potentially suicidal adolescents.

Suicide is the third leading cause of death in adolescents, and the rate appears to have doubled between 1961 and 1975 (1). Clinicians face difficult dilemmas, however, in identifying those who are at greatest risk for medically serious suicide attempts. Many more adolescents make nonlethal attempts than make lethal attempts, and even more express

Reprinted with permission from the *American Journal of Psychiatry*, 1985, Vol. 142, 588–592. Copyright 1985 by the American Psychiatric Association.

suicidal thoughts. Presumably, not all of these adolescents are at risk for potentially lethal attempts, and we have no clear indices to guide efforts at prevention and treatment. It would be helpful if we could more clearly define clinical and biological features associated with risk for serious suicide attempts.

Much work has been done on the clinical and sociodemographic correlates of suicide in adults (2-6). Although correlations can be demonstrated between variables such as the presence of psychiatric illness, depressive diagnoses, age, sex, ethnic group, and suicidal behavior, researchers who made a careful attempt to use such factors in a large prospective study (7) concluded that it was not currently feasible to identify individuals who would later commit suicide. The ability to predict suicide in individuals is limited by the low base or prevalence rate of the disorder and the consequent number of false-positive or false-negative identifications by any of the methods tried.

Nevertheless, the identification of factors associated with greater risk is valuable to the clinician, who must integrate such factors with many variables that may be unique to the particular patient when making decisions about how to intervene therapeutically. Certain factors have been identified by investigators studying suicide in adolescents. Age appears to be important, since suicide is unusual before puberty but increases in frequency with increasing age through adolescence (1, 8). Disturbed family environment has been identified as a factor (9-11), and angry affect and substance abuse have also bee noted (11). Although the relationship between depression and suicide is not simple or linear (12), diagnoses of affective disorders are quite frequent among suicidal adolescents. Friedman et al. (13) observed that 27 of 28 inpatient adolescents who had made suicide attempts had an affective disorder, while one had schizophrenia. Crumley (14) found that 33 of 40 outpatient adolescent suicide attempters had affective diagnoses according to *DSM-III*. It has further been noted that many adolescents with major depressive disorders also have borderline personality disorders (15) and that this subgroup is particularly at risk for suicide attempts (13, 14).

Questions the clinician commonly confronts in dealing with adolescents include whether those who make nonlethal attempts go on to make more dangerous attempts, whether an adolescent's statements about mood and suicidal intent are useful indicators, and whether the identification of certain symptoms may be helpful in anticipating suicidal behavior. This paper examines the associations between symptoms assessed in structured interviews and suicidal behavior in psychiatrically hospitalized adolescents.

METHOD

Sixty-four adolescents (27 male and 37 female), 13-18 years of age, consecutively hospitalized in the adolescent psychiatry service of the University of Michigan Hospital were evaluated by two child psychiatrists in a structured interview that followed the format of the Schedule for Affective Disorders and Schizophrenia (SADS) (16), as part of an ongoing study of affective disorders in adolescents. Diagnoses according to the Research Diagnostic Criteria (RDC) (17) and *DSM-III* were made by consensus on the basis of the SADS interview and other clinical observations. The use of the RDC with adolescents has been described elsewhere (18, 19).

The SADS assesses suicidal tendencies, expressed intent to die, number of previous gestures or attempts, and the lethality of the most recent attempt; Pearson correlation coefficients of these four dimensions with each other were determined. In addition, correlations between each of 38 SADS items related to depression and each of the four suicide items were analyzed, and multiple regression analyses were done to identify the symptom cluster most highly associated with the suicide items.

RESULTS

Of the 64 patients, 31 made no suicide attempts, 15 made two or more attempts, and six made attempts of significant medical dangerousness. Significant medical danger is defined as a rating on SADS medical lethality of 4 (brief unconsciousness) to 6 (respiratory arrest). While more girls (N = 22) than boys (N = 11) made suicide attempts and more girls (N = 10) than boys (N = 5) made multiple attempts, more boys (N = 4) than girls (N = 2) made medically dangerous attempts. Those who attempted suicide tended to be older than the nonsuicidal patients (mean age = 16, range 14.5–17.5 years, for those who made two or more attempts; mean = 16.6, range = 16–17.5 years, for those who made serious attempts; mean = 15, range = 13–17.5 years, for nonsuicidal patients). Those who made the more dangerous attempts were slightly older than the multiple attempters (mean = 16.6 versus 16 years).

Table 1 shows the diagnoses of these patients. Five (83%) of the six patients who made medically serious suicide attempts had diagnoses of major depressive disorder, melancholic (four unipolar and one bipolar, depressed). The remaining patient had a dysthymic disorder.

The relationships of the four SADS items describing suicidal feelings and behavior are presented in table 2. "Suicidal tendencies" on the SADS

TABLE 1. Diagnoses[a] of 64 Hospitalized Adolescent Psychiatric Patients

| | | | Patient Group | | | | | |
| | All Patients (N=64) | | No Suicide Attempts (N=31) | | Two or More Suicide Attempts (N=15) | | Medically Serious Suicide Attempts (N=6)[b] | |
Diagnosis	N	%	N	%	N	%	N	%
Major depressive disorder, melancholic	17	27	3	9	5	33	5	83
Major depressive disorder, nonmelancholic	13	20	3	9	2	13	0	
Bipolar disorder	6	9	2	6	2	13	1	17
Dysthymic disorder	9	14	7	22	1	6	1	17
Cyclothymic disorder	4	6	0		2	13	0	
Conduct disorder	11	17	8	25	0		0	
Anorexia, bulimia	5	8	2	6	0		0	
Attention deficit disorder	3	5	3	9	0		0	
Schizophrenia	5	8	3	9	0		0	
Anxiety disorders	2	2	0		0		0	
Other	10	16	2	6	0		0	

[a]Both primary and secondary diagnoses are included.
[b]SADS score of 4 or more.

TABLE 2. Correlations Between Aspects of Suicidal Feelings and Behavior in 64 Hospitalized Adolescent Psychiatric Patients

SADS Suicide Items	Correlation
Suicidal tendencies vs. seriousness of intent	.6711[a]
Suicidal tendencies vs. number of gestures	.5982[a]
Suicidal tendencies vs. medical lethality	.6476[a]
Number of gestures vs. seriousness of intent	.7136[a]
Number of gestures vs. medical lethality	.7234[a]
Seriousness of intent vs. medical lethality	.8981[a]

[a]$p < .00001$.

is a global assessment of preoccupation with suicide, ranging from vague thoughts of wishing one were dead to serious suicidal behavior. The other items describe different aspects of suicidal experience. "Seriousness of intent" assesses the intended result of the behavior, ranging from purely communicative intent to serious intent to die. "Number of gestures" refers to the number of suicidal behaviors, irrespective of intent or actual physical dangerousness. "Medical lethality" rates the physical seriousness of the most recent behavior, ranging from minimal to potentially lethal. All four suicide items were highly correlated with each other ($p < .00001$ for all pairs).

The associations between the four suicide items and the 38 symptoms of depression noted in the SADS are presented in table 3. Suicidal tendencies were highly associated ($p < .001$) with depression, negative self-evaluation, hopelessness, insomnia, initial insomnia, poor concentration, and anhedonia. Significant associations ($p < .05$-.005) were also seen with specific (depressive) concerns, worrying, guilt, low energy, poor appetite, indecisiveness, social withdrawal, alcohol abuse, and lack of reactivity of mood.

The number of self-destructive gestures or attempts was highly associated with depression and alcohol abuse and was also significantly associated with specific concerns, negative self-evaluation, and drug abuse.

The seriousness of intent was highly associated with depression and negative self-evaluation. It was also significantly associated with hopelessness, psychic anxiety, indecisiveness, anhedonia, psychomotor agitation, lack of reactivity, insomnia, and alcohol abuse.

The medical lethality of the suicidal behavior was highly associated with depression and also significantly associated with negative self-evaluation, anhedonia, psychomotor agitation, alcohol abuse, and drug abuse.

Multiple regressions were calculated to assess which combinations of the variables listed in table 3 could best predict suicidal tendencies, num-

TABLE 3. Correlations of Specific Symptoms With Suicidal Features in 64 Hospitalized Adolescent Psychiatric Patients

Symptom	Correlation			
	Suicidal Tendencies	Number of Gestures	Seriousness of Intent	Medical Lethality
Depression	.5749[a]	.4498[b]	.5572[a]	.4913[c]
Distinct quality of mood	.2047	-.0037	.0061	-.0985
Association with specific concerns	.3717[d]	.3594[d]	.2515	.1282
Worrying	.3597[e]	.2805	.3764	.2497
Guilt	.3157[e]	.1940	.2146	.1134
Negative self-evaluation	.4865[c]	.3839[d]	.4693[c]	.3389[d]
Hopelessness	.5261[a]	.2262	.3423[d]	.2367
Somatic anxiety	.1995	.1438	.2517	.2060
Psychic anxiety	.2264	.0815	.2721[e]	.2331
Insomnia	.4048[b]	.2065	.3179[e]	.2122
Initial insomnia	-.4187[b]	-.0491	-.2077	-.1660
Middle insomnia	-.0832	-.1308	-.1120	-.0215
Terminal insomnia	-.2490	-.0963	-.1685	-.1063
Hypersomnia	.1816	-.0244	.0526	.0359
Low energy	.4003[d]	.1400	.2423	.1346
Poor appetite	.3321[d]	.1769	.0877	.0549
Weight loss	.0862	.0334	-.0677	-.1557
Increased appetite	.0461	-.0361	.1065	.1361
Weight gain	.0330	-.0872	.0337	.1513
Concern with bodily functions	.1043	.0229	.0302	-.0110
Indecisiveness	.3540[d]	.2225	.3366[d]	.2396
Poor concentration	.4657[c]	.0861	.1654	.1342
Anhedonia	.5980[a]	.2144	.3695[d]	.3185[e]
Social withdrawal	.3322[d]	.0295	.1575	.1371
Depersonalization	.1552	.2044	.2015	.1760
Subjective anger	.1595	.0945	.1103	.0773
Overt irritability	.1286	.0404	.0741	.1013
Psychomotor agitation	.2232	.1567	.2796[e]	.3077[e]
Psychomotor retardation	.0892	.1406	.1378	.0729
Lack of reactivity	.4601[d]	.2410	.2979[e]	.1713
Feeling worse in the morning	.0087	.0475	.2251	.1733
Feeling worse in the evening	.0625	.0793	.1249	.0440
Alcohol abuse	.2845[e]	.4246[b]	.3500[d]	.3569[d]
Drug abuse	.1737	.3154[e]	.2395	.2546[e]
Antisocial behavior	.0079	-.0180	.0455	.0088
Distrustfulness	.2110	.1729	.2212	.2123
Delusions	-.0672	.0853	.0424	.0030
Hallucinations	-.2085	-.0355	-.0081	-.0058

[a]$p<.00001$.
[b]$p<.001$.
[c]$p<.0001$.
[d]$p<.01$.
[e]$p<.05$.

ber of gestures, seriousness of intent, and medical lethality. These data are presented in table 4. Depression accounted for 25%–35% of the variance in three of the four analyses. Alcohol abuse accounted for 25% of the variance in the number of gestures and for 4%–11% in the other three analyses.

DISCUSSION

The correlations presented here should not be construed as defining a reliable profile of adolescents at risk for suicide. Indeed, the question of risk factors was not directly addressed, since the patients studied were already identified as psychiatrically ill by their hospitalization and thus were not a sample of all adolescents at risk for suicidal behavior, and the ratings of depressive symptoms were made after rather than before the suicidal behavior. The data do suggest, however, several issues of importance to the clinician.

The high correlations of the four dimensions of suicidal ideation and behavior with one another suggest a degree of reliability in the assess-

TABLE 4. Stepwise Multiple Regression Analyses of Suicidal Features in 64 Hospitalized Adolescent Psychiatric Patients

Dependent and Predictor Variables	p	Total Percent Variance Accounted For at Each Step
Suicidal tendencies		
Depression	.0030	35.5
Anhedonia	.0034	41.8
Feeling worse in the morning[a]	.0068	48.8
Alcohol abuse	.0442	52.8
Number of gestures		
Alcohol abuse	.0001	25.1
Depression	.0039	36.5
Seriousness of intent		
Depression	.0000	34.6
Alcohol abuse	.0026	45.6
Psychomotor retardation[a]	.0378	50.2
Negative self-evaluation	.0427	54.3
Social withdrawal	.0338	58.5
Overt irritability	.0368	62.3
Insomnia	.0361	65.9
Medical lethality		
Depression	.0001	25.5
Alcohol abuse	.0055	36.1
Weight loss[a]	.0285	42.0

[a]Negative correlation.

ment of a suicidal adolescent that some may have doubted. The high association between the adolescent's expressed seriousness in his or her intent to die and the lethality of the behavior should be noted. It is our experience that adolescents may minimize or exaggerate suicidal and other symptoms in the context of the family, but these distortions appeared to be minimal in the interviews with the adolescents alone, and their statements regarding depressed mood and suicidal intent correlated highly with their actual behavior. This suggests that adolescents should be interviewed directly, separate from family members, to assess this component of suicidal risk, irrespective of suspicions about manipulativeness or attention seeking. This finding is consistent with observations by others that children and adolescents are reliable reporters of their own affective symptoms (20). It also suggests, as one might expect, that unlike prepubertal children, who may be unable to devise effective self-destructive methods despite real suicidal intent, adolescents with serious intent are likely to be genuinely dangerous to themselves.

The association between the number of instances of self-destructive behavior and the medical lethality of the most recent behavior is noteworthy. All of those who made very serious attempts (SADS medical lethality rating of 4 or more) had made previous less medically serious attempts. This association with previous attempts judged to be more communicative than serious has been observed in adults (6) and suggests that those who make nonlethal attention-seeking attempts may be at higher risk for more serious attempts.

The recurrence of associations between suicide and depression, feelings of worthlessness, anhedonia, insomnia, poor concentration, indecisiveness, lack of reactivity of mood, and psychomotor disturbance should be noted. These appear to be symptoms that the clinician should inquire about and take seriously. Depressed mood, as was directly evident in the interviews with the adolescents, is clearly an important symptom. Others have noted that the relationship between depression and suicidal feelings or behavior is not simple or linear (12), and certainly other factors such as family and social supports, impulsiveness, and anger may be involved in the determination of suicidal behaviors, but depressed mood is clearly significant.

This association of suicidal feeling and behavior with depressed mood and with all the symptoms contributing to the *DSM-III* diagnosis of major depressive disorder indirectly suggests the validity and clinical importance of this diagnosis in adolescents. The occurrence of suicidal behavior could be considered to be a validator external to the diagnostic criteria—analogous to etiology, treatment response, or prognosis—by which the validity of the designation of a symptom cluster as a syndrome could be judged. To test this more appropriately, all patients should be rediagnosed with suicidal feelings and behavior excluded from the criteria for major depressive disorder. This was not done in our study.

The negative correlations in the multiple regressions of the suicide items with three symptoms usually thought of as components of a major depressive disorder, namely, worse mood in the morning, psychomotor retardation, and weight loss, are puzzling. These will be reexamined as more data are gathered.

It is interesting that overt irritability was significant only in the multiple regression analysis of seriousness of intent and that subjective anger was not significantly associated with any of the suicide items. Others have commented on the importance of anger in suicide (11, 21, 22), and the concept of depression as rage turned inward has been a part of our thinking for decades (23). It was anticipated, therefore, that subjective and expressed anger would be more commonly seen. It is possible that the elapse of 1 or more weeks between the suicidal behavior and our interview was sufficient for anger not to be recalled. Furthermore, Freud's original concept was that this transformation of rage to depression was unconscious, and so the lack of conscious anger is not a refutation of that hypothesis and might, in fact, be predicted by it.

It is noteworthy that alcohol abuse was significantly associated with all four dimensions of suicidal ideation and behavior (table 3). Alcohol abuse also appeared in the multiple regression analyses of all four suicide items, accounting for 25% of the variance in the number of suicidal gestures and for 4%–11% of the variance of the other three dimensions. Substance abuse may be an important additional symptom contributing to suicidal risk. Substance abuse in a depressed adolescent appears both to increase the risk of multiple attempts and to add to the risk of a medically serious attempt. Our cross-sectional data do not allow us to know whether the substance abuse or the affective disorder was primary. It was our clinical impression that for many of our patients the substance abuse was secondary to the affective disorder, but longitudinal study or careful retrospective histories with corroboration by parents or schools would be needed to establish this. Substance abuse may be an indicator of adolescents at higher risk, such as those with a particular maladaptive response to depressive affect or those with a less supportive family and inadequate social supports. Alternatively, substance abuse itself, with its own destructive effects, may make the abusing adolescent more likely to be suicidal. These data do not allow us to understand the exact nature of the association, but substance abuse appears to be an important complication or concomitant of affective disorder in adolescents, which may increase the risk for suicide.

In summary, these data suggest several points that should be helpful to clinicians working with potentially suicidal adolescents. Adolescents appear to be reliable reporters of their suicidal feelings when they are interviewed directly by someone with whom they have some degree of rapport. More intense suicidal feelings are associated with more dangerous suicidal behavior. Serious attempts are likely to be preceded by nonlethal, more communicative attempts. Depressed mood and most of the associated symptoms with which adult psychiatrists are familiar—feelings of worthlessness, hopelessness, insomnia, inappropriate guilt, psychomotor agitation or retardation, loss of energy, poor concentration, indecisiveness, and a lack of reactivity of mood—all appear to be associated with one or more dimensions of suicide in adolescents. And finally, alcohol and other substance abuse is associated with both suicidal feelings and behavior.

REFERENCES

1. Holinger, P. C.: Violent deaths among the young: recent trends in suicide, homicide, and accidents. Am J Psychiatry 136:1144-1147, 1979.
2. Beck, A. T., Kounes, M., Weissman, A.: Hopelessness and suicidal behavior: an overview. JAMA 234:1146-1149, 1975.
3. Brown, T. R., Shevan, T. J.: Suicide prediction: a review. Suicide Life Threat Behav 2:67-98, 1972.
4. Murphy, G. E.: The clinical identification of suicidal risk, in The Prediction of Suicide. Edited by Beck, A. T., Resnik, H. L. P., Lettieri, P. J. Barrie, Md Charles Press, 1924.
5. MacKinnon, D., Farberow, N.: An assessment of the utility of suicide prediction. Suicide Life Threat Behav 6:86-91, 1975.
6. Pallis, D. J., Barraclough, B. M., Levey, A. B., et al.: Estimating suicide risk among attempted suicides, 1: the development of new clinical scales. Br J Psychiatry 141:37-44, 1982.
7. Pokorny, A. D.: Predictions of suicide in psychiatric patients: report of a prospective study. Arch Gen Psychiatry 40:249-257, 1983.
8. Schaffer, D., Fisher, P.: The epidemiology of suicide in children and young adolescents. J Am Acad Child Psychiatry 20:545-565, 1981.
9. McIntire, M. S., Angle, C. R., Wikoff, R. L., et al.: Recurrent adolescent suicidal behavior. Pediatrics 60:605-608, 1977.
10. Dorpat, T. L., Jackson, J. K., Ripley, H. S.: Broken homes and attempted and completed suicide. Arch Gen Psychiatry 12:213-216, 1965.
11. Garfinkel, B. D., Froese, A., Hood, J.: Suicide attempts in children and adolescents. Am J Psychiatry 139:1257-1261, 1982.
12. Carlson, G. A., Cantwell, D. P.: Suicidal behavior and depression in children and adolescents. J Am Acad Child Psychiatry 21:361-368, 1982.
13. Friedman, R. C., Clarkin, J. F., Corn, R., et al.: *DSM-III* and affective pathology in

hospitalized adolescents. J Nerv Ment Dis 170:511-521, 1982.
14. Crumley, F.: Adolescent suicide attempts. JAMA 241:2404-2407, 1979.
15. McManus, M., Lerner, H., Barbour, C., et al.: Assessment of borderline symptomatology in hospitalized adolescents. J Am Acad Child Psychiatry 23:685-694, 1984.
16. Spitzer, R. L., Endicott, J.: Schedule for Affective Disorders and Schizophrenia (SADS), 3rd ed. New York, New York State Psychiatric Institute, Biometrics Research, 1977.
17. Spitzer, R. L., Endicott, J., Robins, E.: Research Diagnostic Criteria: rationale and reliability. Arch Gen Psychiatry 35:773-782, 1972.
18. Robbins, D. R., Alessi, N. E., Cook, S., et al.: The use of the Research Diagnostic Criteria (RDC) for depression in adolescent psychiatric patients. J Am Acad Child Psychiatry 21:251-255, 1982.
19. Strober, M., Green, J., Carlson, G.: The reliability of psychiatric diagnosis in hospitalized adolescents. Arch Gen Psychiatry 38:141-145, 1981.
20. Puig-Antich, J.: Affective disorders in childhood: a review and perspective. Psychiatr Clin North Am 3:402-424, 1980.
21. Weissman, M., Fox, K., Klerman, G. L.: Hostility and depression associated with suicide attempts. Am J Psychiatry 130:450-455, 1973.
22. Vinodna, K. S.: Personality characteristics of attempted suicides. Br J Psychiatry 112:1143-1150, 1966.
23. Freud, S.: Mourning and melancholia (1917), in Complete Psychological Works, standard ed, vol 14. Translated and edited by Strachey, J. London, Hogarth Press, 1955.

Part VIII
AUTISM

The malignant childhood psychiatric disorder of autism has been the object of intensive research activity on many fronts in a number of centers in this country and abroad for the past quarter century. Much has been learned and there is a consensus that the syndrome represents a pervasive developmental disorder rather than a condition with a psychogenic etiology. However, the basic etiology of this disorder still remains unclear, and trials of a variety of therapeutic measures have not as yet revealed any therapy with definitive successful results. The three studies of autism in this section by prominent investigators make their contribution on different levels—neurophysiologic, clinical, and genetic.

Ornitz provides a comprehensive review of the neurophysiology of autism. He delineates the two major neurophysiologic hypotheses that have been offered by past and present research efforts and then describes some recently completed studies from his own research unit on vestibular nystagmus in autistic children. He then compares the two major hypotheses and concludes by suggesting some possible complementary effects of the pathophysiologic mechanism proposed in each of these two hypotheses.

Rumsey and her coworkers explore the outcome of autistic children as adults, pointing out that in previous studies done by other investigators the mean age at follow-up was only 15 years. The authors recruited 14 men, varying in age from 18 to 39 years, through organizations and school programs that serve children and adults with autism. The childhood diagnosis of autism in each case appeared to be well documented. An intensive psychiatric evaluation was done in all cases and supplementary data were obtained from the parents. Residual social impairments and various residual symptoms were identified in all cases, but none showed positive schizophrenic symptoms or qualified for any adult psychiatric diagnosis other than autism or autism, residual state.

These findings provide evidence to support Kanner's position that autism is a unique syndrome, distinct from schizophrenia. However, as the authors point out, their sampling procedure was not designed to yield a representative sample of the adult outcome of children with autism. It may be that if certain autistic children become schizophrenic they might be under the care of organizations or institutions that would not be reached by the authors' sampling procedure. This possibility is suggested by the report by Petty and her associates, reprinted in our 1985 Annual Progress volume, of three autistic children who appeared definitely to have become schizophrenic by middle childhood. Thus, there may be a subgroup of autistic children in which this transformation occurs, although we do not have any markers that can predict such an outcome. In any case, the study by Rumsey and her associates provides valuable evidence that in some, if not all cases of childhood autism, the disorder persists as such into adult life.

The paper by Ritvo and his associates explores the genetic issue in autism by the traditional method of comparing a group of monozygotic twins with a group of dizygotic twins. The authors found a concordance for autism in 22 of 23 MZ twins, as contrasted to a concordance of only 4 out of 17 of the DZ twins. The authors point out that autism has heterogeneous etiologies, but this twin study indicates that pathogenic genes are involved in some as yet undetermined proportion of cases.

27

Neurophysiology of Infantile Autism

Edward M. Ornitz

Brain Research Institute, UCLA

Neurophysiologic hypotheses of infantile autism fall into two broad categories. One is a caudally directed sequence of pathophysiologic influence originating in telencephalic structures. The other is a rostrally directed sequence of pathophysiologic influence originating in brainstem and diencephalic structures. This paper relates each hypothesis to relevant aspects of autistic behavior, reviews neurophysiologic research relevant to each hypothesis, and describes recently completed studies of vestibular nystagmus, relating these new findings to the brainstem-diencephalic hypothesis. Those studies that delineate subgroups of autistic children are distinguished from those that characterize the entire group of autistic children. Those results that point toward maturational delays are distinguished from those that characterize deviant neurophysiologic abnormalities.

Infantile autism is a behavioral syndrome consisting of specific disturbances of social relating and communication, language, response to objects, sensory modulation, and motility. The uniqueness of this syndrome suggests one underlying pathophysiologic mechanism, although

Reprinted with permission from the *Journal of the American Academy of Child Psychiatry,* 1985, Vol. 24, 251–262. Copyright 1985 by the American Academy of Child Psychiatry.

This research was supported by the generosity of Mrs. Harriet Striker, and in part by NIMH grant MH-26798, the Alice and Julius Kantor Charitable Trust, NIMH Grant MH-30897 to the Clinical Research Center for the Study of Childhood Psychosis, UCLA, and (in respect to normal subjects) by NEI Grant EY-02612.

multiple etiologies, which could activate or replicate such a mechanism, have been demonstrated. Neurophysiologic hypotheses of this pathophysiologic mechanism fall basically into two categories. One is a caudally directed sequence of pathophysiologic influence originating in telencephalic structures, particularly the mesolimbic cortex, including the temporal lobes, and the neostriatum. This hypothesis emphasizes the autistic disturbances of language and communication, and assumes an underlying specific cognitive disorder, presumably of cortical origin. Research relevant to this telencephalic hypothesis has included cognitive and linguistic studies, EEG studies, radiologic studies, including several CT investigations, and event-related potential studies. The other hypothesis is a rostrally directed sequence of pathophysiologic influence originating in brainstem and diencephalic structures, particularly the pontine and midbrain reticular formation, the substantia nigra, and the nonspecific thalamic nuclei. This hypothesis emphasizes the autistic disturbances of sensory modulation and motility, and recognizes the role of the brainstem in the initiation of complex adaptive and motivated behavior. Research relevant to this hypothesis has included autonomic studies, brainstem auditory evoked response studies, and vestibular studies.

There are five sections to this paper. The first two review past and present neurophysiologic research relevant to each hypothesis and indicate to what extent each is supported by experimental evidence as opposed to analogies with models from clinical neurology or experimental animal preparations. The third section describes recently completed studies of vestibular nystagmus in autistic children, and relates these new findings to the brainstem-diencephalic hypothesis. The fourth section compares the two hypotheses, distinguishing studies that have been successful in indicating subgroups of autistic children from those that have been successful in demonstrating neurophysiologic findings that statistically characterize the entire population of autistic children in the study. The first type of result may delineate one or more of the many etiologies of infantile autism, while the second may point toward a common neurophysiologic mechanism underlying autistic behavior. This section also distinguishes between those results that point toward maturational delays, i.e., findings characteristic of younger normal children, and those that characterize neurophysiologic abnormalities that are *deviant*, i.e., not found in younger normal children. The final section of this paper suggests some possible complementary effects of the pathophysiologic mechanisms proposed in each of the neurophysiologic hypotheses.

NEUROPHYSIOLOGIC STUDIES RELEVANT TO THE TELENCEPHALIC HYPOTHESIS

The telencephalic hypothesis of autism has stimulated investigations of hemispheric lateralization and other cortical phenomena. The possibility of a disorder of hemispheric lateralization, affecting particularly linguistic functions, has been considered because of the profound language disorder in autism. Intuitively, the severe delays and deviances in language development would seem to imply pathophysiologic cortical mechanisms, although the mesencephalic and tectal portions of the reticular core within the brainstem have been implicated in the inability of autistic children to perceive those features in speech which are prerequisite to the use of language for social communication (Simon, 1975), and more generally, any inadequate modulation of sensory input during subcortical processing would compromise its value as information during cortical processing (James and Barry, 1980a; Ornitz, 1974, 1983). While the latter considerations would relegate disturbances of cortical processing to the status of secondary consequences, a primary cortical dysfunction in autism has remained a compelling hypothesis. Rutter (1978a) approached this issue by defining a cognitive disturbance specific to autism and fundamental to the autistic language disorder. Such a formulation implies cortical dysfunction. Others have attempted to define the notion of cortical dysfunction more specifically as pathophysiology of the temporal lobes (DeLong, 1978) or, more broadly, as dysfunction of mesolimbic cortex and associated neostriatal structures (Damasio and Maurer, 1978). Both of these formulations have been derived solely from analogies between autistic behavior and that of neurologically damaged adults and experimentally lesioned animals (see review in Ornitz (1983)). To what extent have experimental observations supported these hypotheses?

Experimental studies of cerebral lateralization have included monaural ear advantage, dichotic listening, EEG lateralization and radiologic investigations. Indirect evidence that autistics do not have the same degree of cerebral hemispheric specialization for linguistic functions as normals comes from listening preference, monaural ear advantage, and dichotic stimulation studies. Autistic children preferred nonverbal (music) to verbal auditory stimuli (Blackstock, 1978), an observation which might reflect only their lack of interest in speech. Using reaction times to monaural presentation of tones in a study controlled for age, James and Barry (1983) have demonstrated a significant developmental delay in ear advantage, and (by inference) the establishment of cerebral lateralization, in autistic children. In a dichotic listening task, autistics did not show the normal right ear advantage in one investigation (Prior and Bradshaw, 1979). This finding appeared to be limited to those autistics who are echolalic (Wetherby et al., 1981) and could not be confirmed at all in a more recent study which was designed to avoid confounding laterality with the more general linguistic disadvantage of autistics (Arnold and Schwartz, 1983).

EEG studies have suggested a deficiency in hemispheric lateralization. In autistic children, the mean integrated EEG voltage over the left hemisphere did not show the normal increment over the right hemisphere (Small, 1975). During linguistic tasks, 7 of 10 older autistics showed a lack of left hemispheric EEG activation (reduction of alpha activity), indicating deficient left hemispheric specialization for linguistic functions (Dawson et al., 1982). In a recent sleep study (Ogawa et al., 1982), autoregressive analysis of the EEG during Stage II sleep in 2–8-year-old children revealed a lack of hemispheric lateralization in the autistics (and significant lateralization in normal controls).

The attempt to move from functional to structural investigations of cerebral laterality in autism, using radiologic techniques, has generated a conflicting literature. Hauser et al. (1975) examined pneumoencephalograms (PEG) and reported enlarged left temporal horn lateral clefts in 14 of 16 children who were considered autistic, suggesting loss or lack of development of left temporal lobe tissue. A conservative analysis of both the reported case histories and the quantitative PEG measurements suggested that only 13 of the children were unequivocally autistic and that left temporal horn lateral cleft enlargement clearly occurred in only 10 of these cases. Since 3 of 4 nonautistic cases also had the left lateral cleft enlargement, using the same criteria, this finding could have occurred by chance (Ornitz, 1978a). Hier et al. (1979) used computerized tomography (CT) to measure the parieto-occipital width in 16 autistics. In 57% (9 cases) of these autistics, the right parieto-occipital width was wider than the left, a pattern which occurred only in 23% and 25%, respectively, of larger groups of mentally retarded and neurologic patients. This finding was not replicated in another CT study of autistics (Damasio et al., 1980). These investigators also could not confirm the left temporal lateral cleft enlargement observed by Hauser et al. (1975). They found reversal of the normal lateral ventricular asymmetry in only 6 of 17 cases. More recently, comparisons between autistic and neurologic patients (Tsai et al., 1982, 1983) failed to reveal any significant increase in unfavorable brain asymmetries in autism.

In summary, there is evidence from quantitative EEG studies (Dawson et al., 1982; Ogawa et al., 1982; Small, 1975), and from one study of the maturation of ear advantage, for unfavorable cerebral lateralization in autism. This concept does not receive support from either dichotic listening studies or CT scan studies.

Clinical EEG abnormalities, event related potentials and CT scans have been used to look for possible cerebral abnormalities other than those associated with unfavorable brain asymmetries. The extensive literature on clinical EEG studies in infantile autism has been reviewed repeatedly (James and Barry 1980a; Ornitz, 1973, 1983; Ornitz and Ritvo, 1976). It can be concluded that abnormal EEGs do occur in some autistic children, reflecting the extent to which infantile autism occurs in association with various organic syndromes (Finegan and Quarrington, 1979; Ornitz, 1983; Ornitz et al., 1977), and thereby broadening our appreciation of the multiple etiologic factors underlying autism. It can also be concluded that the presence of abnormal EEGs adds little to our understanding of the neurophysiologic mechanisms underlying autistic symptoms; therefore clinical EEG studies will not be considered further in this paper.

Lelord et al. (1973) has reported that when clicks and flashes were coupled, autistics failed to show the normal enhancement of auditory evoked responses from occipital EEG derivations. However, this finding could not be replicated by the same laboratory (Martineau et al., 1980). In a pilot study, 5 autistic patients showed small or absent late auditory evoked responses (wave P300) to signal stimuli, even when a behavioral response indicated detection of the signal stimuli (Novick et al., 1980). Niwa et al. (1983) recently reported similar results in a no-task situation: 4 autistics showed smaller P300 waves in response to signal stimuli than did 4 normal controls. Abnormal CT scans have been found in only a minority of autistic patients (Damasio et al., 1980; Delong et al., 1981; Campbell et al., 1982; Gillberg and Svendsen, 1983). It is noteworthy that the two studies which included relatively large numbers of autistics, 45 (Campbell et al., 1982) and 27 (Gillberg and Svendsen, 1983), both found almost the same percentage of abnormal CT scans, 25% and 26%, respectively. These figures are remarkably close to the 23% of a sample of 74 unselected autistic children reported by Ornitz et al. (1977) to suffer from a major concomitant organic brain condition. Most of those 17 autistics had an associated condition in which an abnormal CT scan would be likely to occur.

In summary, the telencephalic theory of autism has received limited support from neurophysiologic experiments. Most promising are the quantitative EEG studies which both during wakefulness, without (Small, 1975) and with tasks (Dawson et al., 1982), and sleep (Ogawa et al., 1982) suggest abnormal patterns of cerebral lateralization. These findings receive no consistent support from dichotic listening studies or CT scans. One study of ear advantage (James and Barry, 1983) suggests that abnormal patterns of cerebral lateralization may represent a maturation delay rather than a neurophysiologic deviancy. However, Ogawa et al. (1979) have observed the normal development of EEG hemispheric lateralization from 36 weeks postconceptual age. Therefore, the failure of EEG lateralization in 2–8-year-old autistics (Ogawa et al., 1982) represents a very profound maturational delay, of a degree of magnitude which may have the significance of a deviancy. Other evidence supporting the telencephalic theory comes from two reports of small P300 waves in response to target stimuli (Niwa et al., 1983; Novick et al., 1980) but the combined population of the two studies is only 9 autistics. Other event related potential studies have failed to demonstrate cortical abnormalities. CT scans have shown abnormal structural configurations in only about one-quarter of autistic subjects (Campbell et al., 1982; Gillberg and Svendsen, 1983), suggesting a subgroup of autistics in which the autism is associated with a structural brain abnormality (Ornitz, 1983; Ornitz et al., 1977).

NEUROPHYSIOLOGIC STUDIES RELEVANT TO THE BRAINSTEM-DIENCEPHALIC HYPOTHESIS

Unlike the telencephalic hypothesis which is supported primarily by analogies between the behavior of autistic children and that of neurologic patients and lesioned animals (Damasio and Maurer, 1978; Delong, 1978), the brainstem-diencephalic hypothesis (Ornitz, 1983) has been developed to explain the behavior of autistic children per se. While the telencephalic hypothesis was postulated to account for the autistic linguistic and cognitive disturbances, the brainstem-diencephalic hypothesis has been developed to explain the inability of young autistic children to modulate their own responses to sensory input and consequently their own motor output (Ornitz, 1974, 1983). The complete autistic behavioral syndrome is complex. It can, however, be understood by organization into functional subclusters of symptomatology (Ornitz, 1973; Ornitz et al., 1977, 1978). Figure 1 suggests a simplified scheme. The disturbances of relating to people and objects include emotional remoteness, lack of eye contact, indifference to being held, stereotypic ordering and arranging of toys, general intolerance of change in surroundings and routines, and the absence of imaginative play. The disturbances of communication and language include the absence of both verbal and nonverbal communicative intent, severe delays in the acquisition of language, and deviant forms of language, such as delayed echolalia and pronoun reversal (Simon, 1975). These areas of symptomatology have been recognized as essential elements of the autistic syndrome in all serious descriptive schemes (e.g., Kanner (1943), Ornitz (1973), Ornitz and Ritvo (1976), Rutter (1974, 1978a), and DSM-III), although different investigators have emphasized different components of the syndrome.

Less attention has been paid to the disturbances of sensory modulation and motility, and these disturbances have not been explicitly recognized in DSM-III. However, parental reports indicate that such behaviors, e.g., absence of response to sounds and hand flapping, occur in over 70% of autistic children, and their occurrence correlates strongly with disturbances of social relating (Ornitz et al., 1978). These symptom clusters have been described as an inadequate modulation of sensory input and motor output (Ornitz, 1974). Although overlooked by some authorities (Rutter, 1974, 1978b), the inability to modulate sensory input is a striking

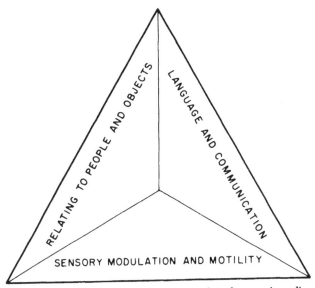

FIG. 1. Autistic behavior falls into three broad categories—disturbances of relating, communication and language, and sensory modulation and motility.

aspect of autistic symptomatology (Bergman and Escalona, 1949; Ornitz, 1969, 1973; Ornitz and Ritvo, 1968, 1976). All sensory modalities can be affected, and the faulty modulation is manifest as either underreactivity or overreactivity to sensory stimuli. The latter manifestation is often associated with a tendency to seek out and induce sensory input, as in the preoccupation with spinning objects (Ornitz, 1974). Some of the motility disturbances, e.g., hand flapping, may provide such input through proprioceptive and visual channels.

The disturbances of sensory modulation and motility have been overlooked in some descriptive systems because of developmental factors. They occur predominantly, though not exclusively, in the 2–4-year-old autistic child. If autistics are examined after the preschool years, and if parents are not carefully questioned regarding earlier behavior, then the frequency of occurrence of these behaviors will be missed. When autistic children are carefully examined before the age of 5 years, the behavioral profiles for the disturbances of motility and sensory modulation are very similar to those for the disturbances of relating to people and objects (Ornitz et al., 1977).

The predominance of the disturbances of sensory modulation necessitates consideration of the several levels of the neuraxis at which sensory input is processed. Most of these points of transfer of sensory input are in the brainstem and contiguous diencephalic structures (see review of neurophysiologic data in Ornitz (1983)). To what extent is the brainstem-diencephalic hypothesis supported by experimental data? This hypothesis has stimulated investigations of autonomic responses, brainstem auditory evoked responses (BAER), and vestibular responses in autistic children.

Autonomic response studies have focused on the regulation of cardiovascular and respiratory responses mediated by the vagus nerve and originating at its source within the brainstem. MacCulloch and Williams (1971), drawing on the experiments of Bonvallet and Allen (1963), have argued that the increased heart rate variability of autistic children may reflect reticular formation responses to insignificant stimuli. They drew attention particularly to the nucleus of the tractus solitarius which lies close to the vestibular nuclei in the brainstem. Also, increased heart rate variability is greatest when autistics engage in stereotyped behaviors (Hutt et al., 1975), linking the dysmodulation of autonomic responsivity to the motility disturbances. Failure to habituate respiratory responses, and enhancement of vascular responses to visual stimuli, indicating incapacity to reduce stimulus novelty and therefore bombardment with sensory stimuli (James and Barry, 1980b), links the abnormal autonomic responses to the disturbances of sensory modulation. Additional reports of elevated peripheral blood flow (Cohen and Johnson, 1977) and heart rate (Kootz and Cohen, 1981) in autistics provide further evidence of abnormal autonomic responsivity.

The BAER would seem to be the most direct measure of brainstem function, particularly as it is relatively free from modulating cortical influences. The brainstem transmission time (BSTT) for click evoked auditory responses measures the function of a subset of neurons within the auditory pathway through the brainstem as rostral as the inferior colliculus. However, the results of BAER studies have been equivocal. While three laboratories have reported significantly prolonged BSTT (Rosenblum et al., 1980; Skoff et al., 1980; Taylor et al., 1982) in autistics, five others did not find consistent group differences between autistics and controls (Gillberg et al., 1983; Novick et al., 1980; Ornitz and Walter, 1975; Ornitz et al., 1980; Student and Sohmer, 1978, 1979; Tanguay et al., 1982), particularly when autistics and normals were matched for both age and sex (Tanguay et al., 1982). Although significant differences characterizing the autistic population have not been found, several studies have identified subgroups (ranging from 33 to 56% of the populations under study) of autistics with prolonged BSTTs (Fein et al., 1981; Gillberg et al., 1983; Tanguay et al., 1982).

Vestibular reflexes also provide a measure of brainstem function, and there have been a number of studies of vestibular nystagmus induced by acceleration of autistic children. Most of these studies, while demonstrating abnormal responses, have suffered from diagnostic imprecision (Piggott et al., 1976; Pollack and Krieger, 1958; Zlotnik et al., 1971), failure to control for the effects of visual fixation (Colbert et al., 1959), or the use of idiosyncratic response measures (Ornitz, 1978b; Ornitz et al., 1974; Ritvo et al., 1969) which are difficult to interpret in terms of current models of the vestibulo-ocular response (VOR) (Baloh and Honrubia, 1979; Honrubia et al., 1982; Robinson, 1981). One of these studies did demonstrate, however, that even with fixation precluded by the use of frosted goggles, visual influence can evoke abnormal responses (reduced duration of postrotatory nystagmus) to vestibular stimulation in autistic children (Ornitz et al., 1974). This report was partially replicated in a recent pilot study of 8 autistic children, 4 of whom showed "almost complete lack of postrotatory nystagmus during a Bárány test behind Frenzel glasses" (Gillberg et al., 1983). Of particular interest, "Three of the 4 children with pathologic results . . . showed pathologic BAER results as well," suggesting brainstem pathophysiology manifest in multiple sensory responses (auditory and visual-vestibular).

The abnormal visual-vestibular interaction is important since the influence of vision provides stabilization of gaze at frequencies too low for the vestibular system to function effectively (Henn et al., 1980). Autistic children show pronounced peculiarities of behavior, e.g., staring both at fixed and spinning objects, which could reflect disturbances in such visual-vestibular interactions (Ornitz, 1973; Ornitz and Ritvo, 1976).

RECENTLY COMPLETED VESTIBULAR STUDIES

In our most recent experiments, we have evaluated nystagmus data from autistic children in terms that are consistent with current models of the vestibulo-ocular response (VOR). Although visual-vestibular interaction appears to be of considerable importance, we have simplified the model in these initial experiments by studying the VOR to constant angular (ramp) acceleration *in absolute darkness* (to eliminate any visual input). The response consists of nystagmus with an increasing slow component velocity (SCV) during acceleration (primary peracceleration nystagmus), a decaying SCV following acceleration (primary postacceleration nystagmus), and a subsequent reversal of nystagmus direction (secondary nystagmus). The VOR is an open-loop control system (Miles and Lisberger, 1981) subject to control system analysis (Robinson, 1981) and is best characterized by its gain and time constant of decay (Baloh and Honrubia, 1979; Honrubia et al., 1982). In response to very low frequency rotation, or to the ramp acceleration used in these experiments, the gain is the output of the system (measured as the peak slow component velocity) relative to the head acceleration. The time constant of decay reflects the mechanical deflection of the cupula (peripheral time constant) and the effect of a central integrator which prolongs the peripheral time constant to that of the primary postacceleration nystagmus (Koenig and Dichgans, 1981).

In this study, we have calculated the gain and the time constant of the primary nystagmus reponse to acceleration in a clinically thoroughly described group of young autistic children under conditions which completely precluded the influence of the visual system during the experiments. Modification of gain and time constant of the *primary* nystagmus has been attributed to transmission through the vestibular nuclei and the brainstem reticular formation, respectively (Blair and Gavin, 1979, 1981). Modification of these measures in autistic children should be relevant to the hypothesis of brainstem dysfunction in this syndrome.

In these experiments, nystagmus was evoked by a ramp acceleration of a remotely controlled chair maintained for 18 sec at 10°/sec² *in absolute darkness*; constant velocity at 180°/sec was continued for 200 sec *in absolute darkness*. The autistic children were gradually adapted to the experimental conditions (sitting still, maintaining proper head position, accepting electrodes, darkness) during several sessions prior to those in which the rotations were given. After dark adaptation, ocular displacement was calibrated while the subject followed the instantaneous movement of a pinpoint red light through 10° of arc. Horizontal eye movements were recorded bipolarly from silver-silver chloride electrodes at the outer canthi, using DC amplification. An infrared TV system rotating with the child, permitted observation of head and eye movements and facial expression *in absolute darkness* through 360° of rotation. Changes from an alert to drowsy state were monitored by visual observation of facial expression and posture, by changes in concomitantly recorded EEG and blinking, and by the development of slow rolling movements in the oculogram. Trials were discarded if drowsiness, eye closure, head movement, or facial movement were detected visually or by electrophysiologic recording. Every 0.1 sec of the horizontal oculogram was coded for the presence or absence of nystagmus beats or artifact. A *nystagmus beat* was defined as a slow component characterized by constant velocity until termination by a fast component in the opposite direction. The slow and fast component amplitudes (*a*) and durations (*d*) were measured for each beat and the slow component velocity (*v*) was computed every 3 sec as $v = a_1 + a_2 + \ldots + a_n/d_1 + d_2 + \ldots + d_n$.

During the primary response, the VOR gain and the time constant of the response were computed. Since the maximum velocity of the slow component increases proportionally to the magnitude of head acceleration during constant angular acceleration, the VOR gain during primary nystagmus was expressed as the ratio of maximum slow component velocity (usually occurring 15–18 sec after onset of acceleration) to head acceleration (Baloh and Honrubia, 1979). Since the slow component velocity decays from its maximum deviation exponentially, with its characteristic time constant (Baloh and Honrubia, 1979), the method of Blair and Gavin (1979) was used to compute the time constant of the response. The time constant, the time required for the nystagmus velocity to decrease to 37% of the velocity it had at any previous time, is derived from the least square regression line computed from the log transformation of the slow component velocity during the primary postacceleration nystagmus. Further details of data measurement and data sampling can be found in Ornitz et al. (1979).

Nystagmus recordings were obtained from 25 normal children, 22–84 months old, and 22 autistic children, 29–71 months old, who met the diagnostic criteria which have been incorporated into DSM-III for infantile autism. These data were compared to responses recorded under identical conditions from a larger group of normal infants and children spanning an age range from 2 to 130 months and normal adults. The regression on (log) age for this larger normal population ($N = 84$, $r = 0.40$, $p < 0.001$) showed that the time constants increased across this age range from 7.7 sec to 11.0 sec (Fig. 2). The time constants of the 42 youngest infants (2–14 months) were 8.76 ± 1.86 sec. The time constants of the 25 normal children who were age matched to the autistic children were longer (9.83 ± 2.26 sec) than those of the infants, and compared to these age matched children, the time constants of the 22 autistics (11.3 ± 3.00) were significantly ($p = 0.035$, one-way analysis of variance and covariance with age as the covariate) prolonged (Figs. 3 and 4). Thus, the time constants of the autistics could not be attributed to immaturity, which is associated with shorter time constants. Additional data analyses ruled out developmental retardation, differences in arousal level, or habituation as possible explanations of the prolonged time constants. Prior habituation due to possible excess experiences with vestibular stimulation could also be ruled out, since habituation leads to shorter, not longer, time constants.

Brainstem lesion (Blair and Gavin, 1981) and pharmacologic (Blair and Gavin, 1979, Gavin and Blair, 1981) studies suggest that lengthening of nystagmus time constants can be attributed to inhibitory mechanisms in the brainstem reticular formation (BSRF). Studies of the transfer characteristics of vestibular neurons associate prolonged time constants with feedback loops involving sequences of several synapses within the BSRF (Buettner et al., 1978). Therefore, the experimental finding of prolonged time constants in the autistic group suggests dysfunction of a multisynaptic path in the BSRF in the autistics, a path that might involve reverberating neuronal circuits. Such a hypothesis might explain, in part, the perseverative stereotypic, driven behaviors, e.g., hand flapping, that are so characteristic of many autistic children. The gain was within normal limits in the autistic children. Since the locus of modification of gain is probably within the vestibular nuclei (Blair and Gavin, 1979), the combined experimental findings, normal gain and prolonged time constants, reinforce the suggestion of dysfunction of a multisynaptic neuronal network in the BSRF in the autistics.

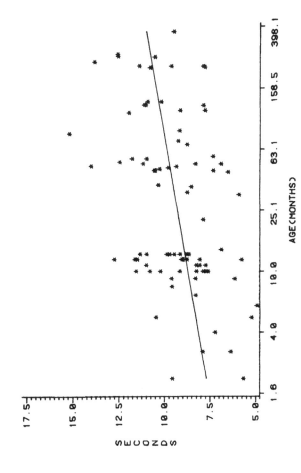

FIG. 2. The time constants of decay of primary nystagmus plotted against age (on a log scale) for 84 normal subjects from 2 months to 31 years of age. The *solid line* is the regression on log age. Prolongation of time constant with (log) age is significant across these normal subjects ($r = 0.40$, $p < 0.001$, two-tailed).

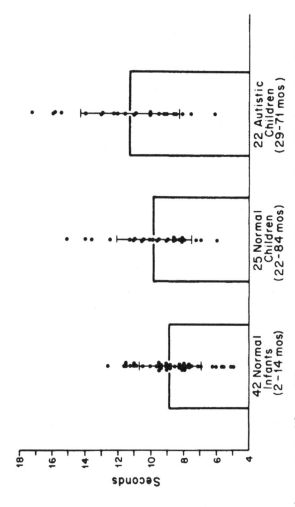

FIG. 3. The time constants of decay of the nystagmus response (including means ±1 S.D.) for the autistic children compared to those of age-matched normal children and the youngest infants from the normal population shown in Figure 2.

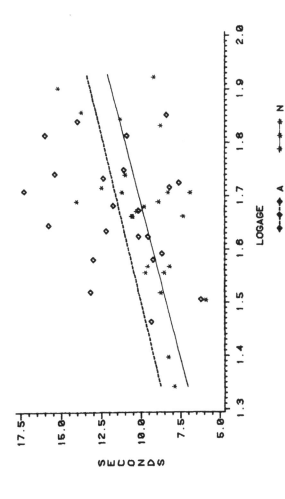

FIG. 4. Time constants of decay of the nystagmus response plotted against logage for the 22 age-matched autistic and 25 normal children. The *solid* and *dashed lines* indicate the regressions on log age. For the normal children, the prolongation of time constant with (log) age is significant ($r = 0.55$, $p < 0.01$, two-tailed).

519

COMPARISON OF THE BRAINSTEM-DIENCEPHALIC AND TELENCEPHALIC HYPOTHESES: POPULATION CHARACTERISTICS OR SUBGROUPS; DEVIANT RESPONSES OR DEVELOPMENTAL DELAYS

In this paper, the experimental evidence for two contrasting neurophysiologic hypotheses of autism has been compared. The hypothesis of telencephalic pathophysiology is supported by quantitative EEG findings of diminished cerebral lateralization (Dawson et al., 1982; Ogawa et al., 1982; Small, 1975), and by event related potential studies suggesting diminished late evoked responses to signal stimuli (Niwa et al., 1983; Novick et al., 1980). However, the latter studies have involved only a combined total of nine autistic subjects, and one study of behavioral responses to monaural stimulation suggests that inadequate cerebral lateralization may be a developmental delayed rather than a deviant neurophysiologic finding in autistics (James and Barry, 1983). These EEG and event-related potential studies of cortical lateralization and signal processing distinguish autistic from control populations. CT scans have not identified cortical pathology characteristics of autistic populations, but have revealed abnormal structure only in individual autistics or subgroups (Campbell et al., 1982; Damasio et al., 1980; Delong et al., 1981; Gillberg and Svendsen, 1983), a finding consistent with the known association between CNS organicity and about one-quarter of autistic cases (Ornitz, 1983; Ornitz et al., 1977).

The hypothesis of brainstem-diencephalic pathophysiology is supported by autonomic response (Hutt et al., 1975; James and Barry, 1980a; Kootz and Cohen, 1981; MacCulloch and Williams, 1971) and vestibular response (Ornitz (1978b), Ornitz et al. (1974), and this paper) studies. The autonomic response studies discriminate between populations of autistics and controls. The increased reactivity of autonomic responses has been linked by James and Barry (1980a, b) to the autistic disturbances of sensory modulation (Ornitz, 1974); the deficiency in autonomic habituation leads to (or perhaps reflects) the autistic inability to "gate" or "filter" trivial sensory stimuli, thereby compromising appropriate selective attention. The vestibular response studies also distinguish autistic from control populations. They have demonstrated abnormal visual-vestibular interactions, even in the absence of the influence of visual fixation (Ornitz et al., 1974). The prolonged time constants reported in this paper occur independent of visual input, suggest the influence of excessive reverberation of multisynaptic brainstem pathways, and are deviant responses, not related to maturational effects. Thus, the aberrant vestibular responses do not reflect the general maturational lag which is characteristic of many features of autistic behavior and development (see discussion in James and Barry (1981)). The BAER studies, on the other hand, have not consistently supported the brainstem hypothesis; prolonged BSTTs have been limited to subgroups of autistics (Fein et al., 1981; Gillberg et al., 1983; Tanguay et al., 1982). This may reflect the fact that the BAER is the response to a subset of neurons within the brainstem. In contrast, the vestibular and autonomic responses probably involve widespread interconnecting neuronal fields within the brainstem. The mechanism underlying the autistic behavioral syndrome is likely to involve a system dysfunction rather than a pathologic change in tissue or a specific group of neurons. The minority of autistics who do show prolonged BSTT may, in fact, represent instances of brainstem structural lesions which could be added to the long list of pathologic conditions associated with autism. In contrast, the vestibular and autonomic abnormalities are more likely to reflect a common brainstem mechanism which could be activated by many different etiologies, including, on occasion, brainstem structural lesions (Ornitz, 1978a, 1983). The results of the BAER and vestibular studies of autism are contrasted in Figures 5 and 6. Figure 5 is adapted from the BAER study of Gillberg et al. (1983) to show the distribution of BSTTs in autistics and normals. Twenty-five percent of the autistics had BSTT values which were 3 standard deviations greater than the normal mean. The distribution clearly shows that these constitute an abnormal subgroup, while the majority of autistics had a distribution similar to that of the normal controls. Figure 6 shows the distribution of time constants from the vestibular experiments described in this paper. Only 1 autistic child out of 22 (4.5%) has a value more than 3 standard deviations greater than the normal mean. The distributions indicate a statistically significant tendency for the autistics as a group to have longer time constants than the normal controls; no subgroup is indicated.

In summary, there is neurophysiologic evidence for both the telencephalic and brainstem-diencephalic hypotheses. These hypotheses parallel the behavioral components of the autistic syndrome which suggest both cortical dysfunction (cognition and language) and subcortical dysfunction (sensory modulation and motility). To a degree, the evidence for one or the other hypothesis will appear more compelling, depending on which of the clinical facets of the syndrome appears more important. In the older autistic individual, the cognitive and language deficits loom larger and have obvious therapeutic and prognostic significance. From a developmental perspective, however, the disturbances of sensory modulation and motility appear early, at which time they dominate the clinical

scene, and they may have explanatory value in respect to the total behavioral syndrome. The autistic syndrome consists of three major clusters of behavioral disturbances: relating to people and objects; language
and communication; and sensory modulation and motility (Fig. 1). These
symptom subclusters might occur independently, or any one might influence one or more of the others. Assuming some interrelationships,
it is difficult to imagine how the disturbances of relating and of language
might evoke those of sensory modulation and motility. On the other
hand, a number of clinical investigations, reviews, and theoretical pro-
posals have stressed that social awareness, motivation, and use of language in autistics seem to be dominated by disordered perceptual

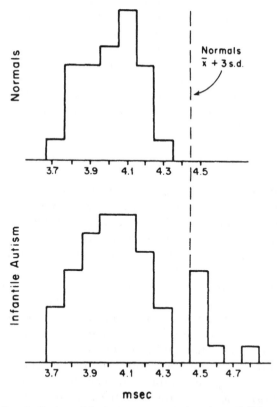

FIG. 5. Prolonged brainstem transmission times (I–V latency)
(Gillberg et al., 1983) identify a subgroup of autistic children, but
do not characterize the total population, 75% of the autistics having
a frequency distribution similar to that of the normals (no mean
shift).

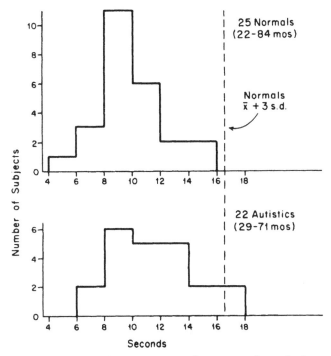

FIG. 6. Prolonged time constants of nystagmus decay do characterize the total population of autistic children (there is a significant mean shift of the frequency distribution relative to the normals) but do *not* indicate a subgroup with extreme values (compare Fig. 5).

processes (James and Barry, 1980a; Ornitz, 1969, 1973, 1974, 1983; Reichler and Schopler, 1971; Simon, 1975). Thus, disturbances of relating, language, and communication can be considered consequences of inconstancy of perception due to faulty modulation of sensory input. The autistic child cannot relate to or imitate that which he cannot reliably preceive. Cognitive deficits could similarly be explained in terms of distorted sensory input: the autistic child cannot make *sense* out of *sensation*.

POSSIBLE RELATIONSHIPS BETWEEN THE BRAINSTEM-DIENCEPHALIC AND TELENCEPHALIC HYPOTHESES

The disturbance of sensory modulation suggests a pathoneurophysiologic process likely to take place in brainstem and diencephalic structures where sensory input is gated (Ornitz, 1983). However, the possibly mutual relationship between these subcortical structures and telencephalic influence must be considered. For example, the inadequate cortical lateralization demonstrated in several quantitative EEG studies (Dawson et al., 1982; Ogawa et al., 1982; Small, 1975) could be secondary to dysfunction of normal asymmetric sensory transmission mechanisms at the level of the brainstem (Levine and McGaffigan, 1983). On the other hand, attentional mechanisms, perhaps of telencephalic origin, can modify brainstem reflexes (Anthony and Graham, 1983); thus, telencephalic influence could potentially contribute to the abnormal autonomic and vestibular responses found in autistic children.

The anatomical relationships between brainstem-diencephalic centers and telencephalic centers that bear on these clinical and experimental considerations have been discussed in detail (Ornitz, 1983). Various brainstem centers project to higher levels of the neuraxis and, in return, receive input from higher centers. There is a strong projection of neurons responsive to multimodal sensory stimuli to nonspecific thalamic nuclei, and there are vestibular projections to specific thalamic nuclei. Cortical centers and the neostriatum in turn can modify vestibular, midbrain, and diencephalic function, but only by engaging rostrally directed sensory influences at diencephalic gates. Thus, cortical or neostriatal dysfunction can be replicated, or in fact, initiated by brainstem or diencephalic dysfunction. Thus, the brainstem, including the vestibular nuclei, and related nonspecific thalamic centers could be the primary loci of the system dysfunction in autism. This conclusion is consistent with much of the experimental evidence reviewed in this paper as well as the clinical observations suggesting that the disturbances of social relating, communication, and language are secondary to a disorder of sensory modulation. Thus, experimental evidence and clinical observation point toward dysfunction of a cascading series of neurophysiologic levels or interacting neuronal loops in the brainstem and diencephalon which subserve modulation of sensory input (see Fig. 7 and review in Ornitz (1983)). Other experimental evidence reviewed in this paper implicates cortical centers. Thus, both a rostrally and a caudally directed sequence of pathophysiologic events could contribute to the system dysfunction in autism. A suggested approach to this issue is based on the principle of John Hughlings Jackson that higher levels of the nervous system represent and re-represent all lower centers (Jackson, 1884), i.e., the functions of lower systems are re-represented and controlled by, but are not replaced by, phylogenetically newer structures. Berntson and Micco (1976) have reviewed a broad base of data which argues strongly for the role of the brainstem in the generation of adaptive behavior. Stimulation and lesion studies suggest that brainstem mechanisms cannot only integrate complex behavior but also influence the function of more rostral levels. Prosencephalic systems, including the limbic system, are "involved more in the further elaboration and control rather than the fundamental organization of adaptive behaviors" generated in the brainstem. Thus, there has developed a system of "reciprocal interactions between brainstem systems and other levels of the neuraxis" (Berntson and Micco,

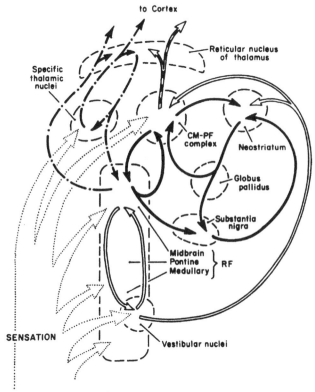

FIG. 7. Schematic representation of the modulation of the rostral flow of sensation through three interacting neuronal loops in the brainstem and diencephalon. A vestibulo-midbrain reticular formation (*RF*) loop (*open lines*) impinges on a midbrain RF-thalamic loop (*dot-and-dash lines*) and a midbrain-striatal-nonspecific thalamic (represented by the centro-median-parafascicularis complex, *CM-PF*) loop (*solid lines*) at midbrain RF, striatal, and thalamic junctions. The latter two modulating loops also impinge on each other at midbrain RF and thalamic levels. The relevant neuroanatomic and neurophysiologic data have been reviewed by Ornitz (1983).

1976). Such a phylogenetic development of re-representation of older behavioral mechanisms offers an alternative to a dichotomy between rostrally and caudally directed influence. From this perspective, the symptoms of autism can be explained in terms of dysfunction of brainstem behavioral systems *and* further distortion by selected higher neural structures which are themselves influenced by the brainstem and its dysfunction.

REFERENCES

Anthony, B. J. & Graham, F. K. (1983), Evidence for sensory-selective set in young infants. *Science*, 220:742-743.

Arnold, G. & Schwartz, S. (1983), Hemispheric lateralization of language in autistic and aphasic children. *J. Aut. Develpm. Disord.*, 13:129-139.

Baloh, R. W. & Honrubia, V. (1979), *Clinical Neurophysiology of the Vestibular System*. Philadelphia: F. A. Davis.

Bergman, P. & Escalona, S. K. (1949), Unusual sensitivities in very young children. *The Psychoanalytic Study of the Child*, 3-4:333-353.

Berntson, G. G. & Micco, D. J. (1976), Theoretical review: organization of brainstem behavioral systems. *Brain Res. Bull.*, 1:471-483.

Blackstock, E. G. (1978), Cerebral asymmetry and the development of early infantile autism. *J. Aut. Childh. Schizo.*, 8:339-353.

Blair, S. & Gavin, M. (1979), Modifications of vestibulo-ocular reflex induced by diazepam. *Arch. Otolaryngol.*, 105:698-701.

———— ———— (1981), Brainstem commissures and control of time constant of vestibular nystagmus. *Acta Otolaryngol.*, 91:1-8.

Bonvallet, M. & Allen, M. B., Jr. (1963), Prolonged spontaneous and evoked reticular activation following discrete bulbar lesions. *Electroenceph. Clin. Neurophysiol.*, 15:969-988.

Buettner, U. W., Büttner, U. & Henn, V. (1978), Transfer characteristics of neurons in vestibular nuclei of the alert monkey. *J. Neurophysiol.*, 41:1614-1628.

Campbell, M., Rosenbloom, S., Perry, R., George, A. E., Dricheff, I. I., Anderson, L., Small, A. M. & Jennings, S. J. (1982), Computerized axial tomography in young autistic children. *Amer. J. Psychiat.*, 139:510-512.

Cohen, D. J. & Johnson, W. T. (1977), Cardiovascular correlates of attention in normal and psychiatrically disturbed children. *Arch. Gen. Psychiat.*, 34:561-567.

Colbert, E. G., Koegler, R. R. & Markham, C. H. (1959), Vestibular dysfunctions in childhood schizophrenia. *Arch. Gen. Psychiat.*, 1:600-617.

Damasio, A. R. & Maurer, R. G. (1978), A neurological model for childhood autism. *Arch. Neurol.*, 35:778-786.

Damasio, H., Maurer, R. G., Damasio, A. R. & Chui, H. C. (1980), Computerized tomographic scan findings in patients with autistic behavior. *Arch. Neurol.*, 37:504-510.

Dawson, G., Warrenburg, S. & Fuller, P. (1982), Cerebral lateralization in individuals diagnosed as autistic in early childhood. *Brain Language*, 15:353-368.

DeLong, G. R. (1978), A neuropsychologic interpretation of infantile autism. In: *Autism: A Reappraisal of Concepts and Treatment*, ed. M. Rutter & E. Schopler. New York: Plenum Press.

—— Bean, S. C. & Brown, F. R., III (1981), Acquired reversible autistic syndrome in acute encephalopathic illness in children. *Arch. Neurol.*, 28:191-194.

Fein, D., Skoff, B. & Mirsky, A. F. (1981), Clinical correlates of brainstem dysfunction in autistic children. *J. Aut. Develpm. Disord.*, 11:303-315.

Finegan, J. & Quarrington, B. (1979), Pre-, peri-, and neonatal factors in infantile autism. *J. Child Psychol. Psychiat.*, 20:119-128.

Gavin, M. & Blair, S. (1981), Modification of the Macaque's vestibulo-ocular reflex by picrotoxin. *Arch. Otolaryngol.*, 107:372-376.

Gillberg, C. & Svendsen, P. (1983), Childhood psychosis and computed tomographic brain scan findings. *J. Aut. Develpm. Disord.*, 13:19-32.

—— Rosenhall, U. & Johansson, E. (1983), Auditory brainstem responses in childhood psychosis. *J. Aut. Develpm. Disord.*, 13:181-195.

Hauser, S. L., DeLong, G. R. & Rosman, N. P. (1975), Pneumographic findings in the infantile autism syndrome: a correlation with temporal lobe disease. *Brain*, 98:667-688.

Henn, V., Cohen, B. & Young, L. R. (1980), Visual-vestibular interaction in motion perception and the generation of nystagmus. *Neurosci. Res. Prog. Bull.*, 18:459-651.

Hier, D. B., LeMay, M. & Rosenberger, P. B. (1979), Autism and unfavorable left-right asymmetries of the brain. *J. Aut. Develpm. Disord.*, 9:153-159.

Honrubia, V., Jenkins, A., Baloh, R. W. & Lau, C. G. Y. (1982), Evaluation of rotary vestibular tests in peripheral labyrinthine lesions. In: *Nystagmus and Vertigo*, ed. V. Honrubia & M. A. B. Brazier. New York: Academic Press, pp. 57-77.

Hutt, C., Forrest, S. J. & Richer, J. (1975), Cardiac arrhythmia and behavior in autistic children. *Acta Psychiat. Scand.*, 51:361-372.

Jackson, J. H. (1958), Evolution and dissolution of the nervous system. In: *Selected Writings of John Hughlings Jackson* (Croonian Lectures, 1884), ed. J. Taylor. New York: Basic Books.

James, A. L. & Barry, R. J. (1980a), A review of psychophysiology in early onset psychosis. *Schizo. Bull.*, 6:506-525.

—— —— (1980b), Respiratory and vascular responses to simple visual stimuli in autistics, retardates, and normals. *Psychophysiology*, 17:541-547.

—— —— (1981), General maturational lag as an essential correlate of early-onset psychosis. *J. Aut. Develpm. Disord.*, 11:271-283.

—— —— (1983), Developmental effects in the cerebral lateralization of autistic, retarded and normal children. *J. Aut. Develpm. Disord.*, 13:43-54.

Kanner, L. (1943), Autistic disturbances of affective contact. *Nerv. Child*, 2:217-250.

Koenig, E. L. & Dichgans, J. (1981), Aftereffects of vestibular and optokinetic stimulation and their interaction. *Ann. N.Y. Acad. Sci.*, 374:434-445.

Kootz, J. P. & Cohen, D. J. (1981), Modulation of sensory intake in autistic children. *J. Amer. Acad. Child Psychiat.*, 20:692-701.

Lelord, G., Laffont, F., Jusseaume, P. & Stephant, J. L. (1973), Comparative study of conditioning of averaged evoked responses by coupling sound and light in normal and autistic children. *Psychophysiology*, 10:415-425.

Levine, R. A. & McGaffigan, P. M. (1983), Right-left asymmetries in the human brain stem: auditory evoked potentials. *Electroencephalog. Clin. Neurophysiol.*, 55:532-537.

MacCulloch, M. J. & Williams, C. (1971), On the nature of infantile autism. *Acta Psychiat. Scand.*, 47:295-314.

Martineau, J., Laffont, F., Bruneau, N., Roux, S. & Lelord, G. (1980), Event related potentials evoked by sensory stimulation in normal, mentally retarded and autistic children. *Electroencephalog. Clin. Neurophysiol.*, 48:140-163.

Miles, R. A. & Lisberger, S. G. (1981), Plasticity in the vestibulo-ocular reflex. *Annual Rev. Neurosci.*, 4:273-299.

Niwa, S., Ohta, M. & Yamazaki, K. (1983), P300 and stimulus evaluation process in autistic subjects. *J. Aut. Develpm. Disord.*, 13:33-42.

Novick, B., Vaughan, H. G., Jr., Kurtzberg, D. & Simon, R. (1980), An electrophysiologic indication of auditory processing defects in autism. *Psychiat. Res.*, 3:107-114.

Ogawa, T., Baba, C., Nakashita, Y. & Hiramatsu, K. (1979), The ontogeny of functional asymmetry of EEG in preterm infants (in Japanese). *No To Shinkei*, 31:1105-1110.

———— Sugiyama, A., Ishiwa, S., Suzuki, M., Ishihara, T. & Sato, K. (1982), Ontogenic development of EEG-asymmetry in early infantile autism. *Brain Develpm.*, 4:439-449.

Ornitz, E. M. (1969), Disorders of perception common to early infantile autism and schizophrenia. *Comprehensive Psychiat.*, 10:259-274.

———— (1973), Childhood autism: a review of the clinical and experimental literature. *Calif. Med.*, 118:21-47.

———— (1974), The modulation of sensory input and motor output in autistic children. *J. Aut. Childh. Schizo.*, 4:197-215.

———— (1978a), Biological homogeneity or heterogeneity? In: *Autism: A Reappraisal of Concepts and Treatment*, ed. M. Rutter & E. Schopler. New York: Plenum Press, pp. 243-250.

———— (1978b), Neurophysiologic studies. In: *Autism: A Reappraisal of Concepts and Treatment*, ed. M. Rutter & E. Schopler. New York: Plenum Press, pp. 117-139.

———— (1983), The functional neuroanatomy of infantile autism. *Int. J. Neurosci.*, 19:85-124.

———— & Ritvo, E. R. (1968), Perceptual inconstancy in early infantile autism. *Arch. Gen. Psychiat.*, 18:76-98.

———— ———— (1976), The syndrome of autism: A critical review. *Amer. J. Psychiat.*, 133:609-621.

———— & Walter, D. O. (1975), The effect of sound pressure wave-form on human brain stem auditory evoked responses. *Brain Res.*, 92:490-498.

———— Brown, M. B., Mason, A. & Putnam, N. H. (1974), Effect of visual input on vestibular nystagmus in autistic children. *Arch. Gen. Psychiat.*, 31:369-375.

———— Guthrie, D., & Farley, A. J. (1977), The early development of autistic children. *J. Aut. Childh. Schizo.*, 7:207-229.

———— ———— ———— (1978), The early symptoms of childhood autism. In: *Cognitive Defects in the Development of Mental Illness*, ed. G. Serban. New York: Brunner/Mazel, pp. 24-42.

———— Atwell, C. W., Walter, D. O., Hartmann, E. E. & Kaplan, A. R. (1979), The maturation of vestibular nystagmus in infancy and childhood. *Acta Otolaryngol.*, 88:244-256.

———— Mo, A., Olson, S. T. & Walter, D. O. (1980), Influence of click sound pressure direction on brain stem responses in children. *Audiology*, 19:245-254.

Piggott, L., Purcell, G., Cummings, G. & Caldwell, D. (1976), Vestibular dysfunction in emotionally disturbed children. *Biol. Psychiat.*, 11:719-729.

Pollack, M. & Krieger, H. P. (1958), Oculomotor and postural patterns in schizophrenic children. *Arch. Neurol. Psychiat.*, 79:720-726.

Prior, M. R. & Bradshaw, J. L. (1979), Hemisphere functioning in autistic children. *Cortex*, 15:73-81.

Reichler, R. J. & Schopler, E. (1971), Observations on the nature of human relatedness. *J. Aut. Childh. Schizo.*, 1:283-296.

Ritvo, E. R., Ornitz, E. M., Eviatar, A., Markham, C. H., Brown, M., & Mason, A. (1969), Decreased postrotatory nystagmus in early infantile autism. *Neurology*, 19:653-658.

Robinson, D. A. (1981), The use of control systems analysis in the neurophysiology of eye movements. *Annual Rev. Neurosci.*, 4:463-503.

Rosenblum, S. M., Arick, J. R., Krug, D. A., Stubbs, E. G., Young, N. B. & Pelson, R. O. (1980), Auditory brainstem evoked responses in autistic children. *J. Aut. Develpm. Disord.*, 10:215-225.

Rutter, M. (1974), The development of infantile autism. *Psychol. Med.*, 4:147-163.

——— (1978a), Language disorder and infantile autism. In: *Autism: A Reappraisal of Concepts and Treatment*, ed. M. Rutter & E. Schopler. New York: Plenum Press, pp. 85-104.

——— (1978b), Diagnosis and definition of childhood autism. *J. Aut. Childh. Schizo.*, 8:139-161.

Simon, N. (1975), Echolalic speech in childhood autism: consideration of underlying loci of brain damage. *Arch. Gen. Psychiat.*, 32:1439-1446.

Skoff, B. F., Mirsky, A. F. & Turner, D. (1980), Prolonged brainstem transmission time in autism. *Psychiat. Res.*, 2:157-166.

Small, J. G. (1975), EEG and neurophysiological studies of early infantile autism. *Biol. Psychiat.*, 10:385-397.

Student, M. & Sohmer, H. (1978), Evidence from auditory nerve and brainstem evoked responses for an organic brain lesion in children with autistic traits. *J. Aut. Childh. Schizo.*, 8:13-20.

——— ——— (1979), Erratum (Evidence from auditory nerve and brainstem evoked responses for an organic brain lesion in children with autistic traits). *J. Aut. Childh. Schizo.*, 1978, 8:13-20). *J. Aut. Develpm. Disord.*, 9:309.

Tanguay, P. E., Edwards, R. M., Buchwald, J., Schwafel, J. & Allen, V. (1982), Auditory brainstem evoked responses in autistic children. *Arch. Gen. Psychiat.*, 39:174-188.

Taylor, M. J., Rosenblatt, B. & Linschoten, L. (1982), Auditory brainstem response abnormalities in autistic children. *Canad. J. Neurol. Sci.*, 9:429-433.

Tsai, L., Jacoby, C. G., Stewart, M. A. & Beisler, J. M. (1982), Unfavorable left-right asymmetries of the brain and autism. *Brit. J. Psychiat.*, 140:312-319.

——— ——— ——— (1983), Morphological cerebral asymmetries in autistic children. *Biol. Psychiat.*, 18:317-327.

Wetherby, A. M., Kogel, R. L. & Mendel, M. (1981), Central auditory nervous system dysfunction in echolalic autistic individuals. *J. Speech Hear.*, 24:420-429.

Zlotnik, G., Iverson, P. B., Tolstrup, K. & Zilstorff, K. (1971), Vestibular function of patients in a child psychiatric department. *Danish Med. Bull.*, 18:152-156.

PART VIII: AUTISM

28

Autistic Children as Adults: Psychiatric, Social, and Behavioral Outcomes

Judith M. Rumsey, Judith L. Rapoport, and Walter S. Sceery

National Institute of Mental Health, Bethesda

The psychiatric, social, and behavioral outcomes of 14 men ($\bar{X}$ age = 28 years, S.D. = 6.8), with well-documented histories of infantile autism, 9 of whom were unusually high functioning, were studied in the longest term, systematic follow-up on autism to date. Residual social impairments and varied residual psychiatric and behavioral symptoms were seen in all subjects and are described. Especially frequent were stereotyped movements and concrete thinking. No subject showed positive schizophrenic symptoms or qualified for any DSM-III adult diagnosis other than autism or autism, residual state.

Autism is a relatively new syndrome, having first been identified by Professor Leo Kanner of Johns Hopkins School of Medicine in 1943. Initially viewed as continuous with adult schizophrenia, the term "childhood schizophrenia" was also applied to this syndrome. Kanner's (1943)

Reprinted with permission from the *Journal of the American Academy of Child Psychiatry,* 1985, Vol. 24, 465–473. Copyright 1985 by the American Academy of Child Psychiatry.

The authors thank the National Society for Autistic Adults and Children and the Linwood Center in Ellicott City, Maryland, for their invaluable assistance in announcing our study to families and the families who participated in this research.

530

position that autism was unique and distinct from schizophrenia stimulated controversy concerning the continuity of these disorders (Bender and Faretra, 1973; Fish, 1977).

Follow-up studies of autistic children (DeMyer et al., 1973; Eisenberg, 1956, 1957; Eisenberg and Kanner, 1956; Kanner et al., 1972; Lotter, 1974; Rutter, 1970; Rutter and Lockyer, 1967) have shown that the natural course of autism is gradual symptomatic improvement with persistent, residual social impairments. Despite great variability in intellectual and linguistic functioning across patients, there is continuity within individuals, and IQ and the presence of communicative speech by age 5 years are good prognostic indicators. These studies have also shown that autistic children do not develop hallucinations and delusions, but frequently develop seizures, findings which support Kanner's view of discontinuity. However, the mean age at follow-up in these more systematic studies is 15 years, which falls short of the age of greatest risk for major adult psychiatric disorders.

In addition, comparative studies of children with early onset (under 2 years) versus late onsets (above 11 years) of illness (Kolvin 1971; Kolvin et al., 1971) have found differences in clinical symptoms, thus providing additional validation of discontinuity. Kolvin (1971) and Kolvin et al. (1971) found that only those psychotic children with late onsets showed delusions, hallucinations, and thought disorder, as seen in schizophrenia, while early onset cases showed gaze avoidance, abnormal preoccupations, self-isolating behavior, echolalia, and hyperactivity more often than did late onset cases.

Influenced by these studies, the DSM-III reflects the notion of discontinuity held by the majority of workers in this field. Infantile autism is classified as a pervasive developmental disorder, and early onset and absence of hallucinations, delusions, and incoherence are required for its diagnosis. A DSM-III diagnosis of schizophrenia or other psychosis in children requires that the patient meet criteria for the diagnosis of those disorders in adults; no unique set of criteria is used for diagnosing schizophrenia or other psychoses in childhood.

The present study examined psychiatric and behavioral outcomes in 14 men with clearly documented early childhood diagnoses of autism compatible with DSM-III criteria. Nine subjects were unusually high functioning, a factor which facilitated satisfactory examinations of mental status. This paper reports on the long-term continuity in symptoms and disability, of particular interest because of the advanced age of this sample as compared with other systematically studied groups. Given the high levels of functioning in our sample, we also attempted to glean retrospective, subjective accounts of the disorder, including reports about delusions and the quality of relationships with parents.

METHOD

Subjects

Autistic men were sought nationwide through organizations and school programs which serve children and adults with autism for participation in a PET scan study which required subjects to be at least 18 years of age and in good physical health (Rumsey et al., 1985). Only patients with clearly documented histories of autism compatible with DSM-III were considered as potential participants. Exclusionary criteria were: (1) known infectious, metabolic, or neurological disease; (2) seizures; (3) inability to discontinue any medications; (4) inability to cooperate with medical tests; (5) history of highly invasive medical procedures to the head (e.g., neurosurgery); and (6) hard neurological findings (e.g., frank hydrocephalus), focal signs, and any gross neurological deficits other than mental retardation. (See one exception below.) "Soft" neurological signs and isolated abnormalities of tone, reflexes, or movement, characteristic of developmental disorders, were expected and did not constitute a basis for exclusion. Evaluations included a medical history, general physical and neurological examinations, including routine blood and urine chemistry determinations, EEG, and CT scan.

Fourteen men, 18–39 years of age ($\bar{X}$ = 28, S.D. = 6.8), were admitted to the study. All were evaluated by a psychiatrist not associated with the study to determine their ability to give informed consent. Dependent upon the outcome, patients and/or parents discussed research procedures with an investigator and signed a consent form which described the purposes of the study and testing procedures.

Thirteen were seen as inpatients, and one as an outpatient, over 5 days. Seven had been diagnosed as autistic by Professor Leo Kanner, one by a student of his, and five by other physicians. One subject had suffered a sudden loss of sight in one eye as a teenager, which was attributed to thrombosis of the retinal artery, but was otherwise healthy and free of other major neurological findings. His unusually good outcome and the clear independence of the partial sensory impairment from his autism led us to include him in the clinical follow-up.

This sample was heterogeneous despite the application of these specific selection criteria. Therefore, they are subgrouped as follows for descriptive purposes: Nine patients with verbal and performance IQs above 80 and good language skills constitute our "high functioning subgroup." Our "lower functioning subgroup" consists of two patients with some mental retardation and three with specific language deficits (mutism or limited speech) with approximately average or higher performance IQs. (Specific test scores follow.)

Structured Psychiatric Interviews

Patients were interviewed by a child psychiatrist using the NIMH Diagnostic Interview Schedule (DIS) (Robins et al., 1981) and portions of the Diagnostic Interview for Children and Adolescents (DICA) (Herjanic and Campbell, 1977). In addition, subjects with good language were questioned about early memories and specifically about "why" they engaged in rituals, resisted change, and the like and about the quality of their relationship with each parent. Together these interviews provided comprehensive information on lifetime and current symptoms. Current DSM-III diagnoses were made on the basis of these interviews, behavioral observations, and the patient's history.

Parent Interviews

Mothers of 13, fathers of 7, and an advocate-trainer of 1 subject were interviewed regarding the patient's history and current status, thus providing validating and supplemental information. In addition, parents were interviewed for information about themselves and other family members with a modified version of the Schedule for Affective Disorders and Schizophrenia (SADS)-Form L (Mazure and Gershon, 1979). Parental social class was rated on the basis of occupation and education of the head of household with a modification of the Hollingshead index (Watt, 1976).

The Vineland Social Maturity Scale (1965) was completed by a psychologist using parents and the advocate-trainer as informants. This widely used clinical measure of social-adaptive functioning includes items that tap communication, socialization, locomotion (e.g., independent travel), occupational pursuits and achievements, self-direction, and self-help skills from infancy to adulthood. It yields a global social age score, which is divided by the patient's chronological age up to a ceiling of 25 years and multiplied by 100 to yield a social quotient (SQ). An average score is 100 ± 5, and standard deviations range from 6 to 12 within the age range studied here (Doll, 1953). The SQ is less sophisticated psychometrically and not precisely comparable to Wechsler IQ scores. However, some general comparisons of the two are possible.

Additional Measures

The 5-day period of admission and extensive study allowed staff to observe behaviors within the social context of the ward and various laboratories that were not necessarily observed in the psychiatric interview situation. A written record of unusual behaviors seen throughout the week was made for each patient, usually adding information on motor symptoms and abnormal social behaviors.

Patients were also tested with the Wechsler Adult Intelligence Scale (WAIS) and Wide Range Achievement Test (WRAT).

Symptom Patterns and Behavioral Characteristics

Table 1 lists the number of patients showing various symptoms identified in psychiatric interviews and/or direct observations. Parental reports sometimes suggested that symptoms were present which were not observed by us. This supplemental information is included in the following descriptions, but excluded from Table 1 because it represents a less systematic data base.

Social relatedness and interactions. As seen in Table 1, all patients continued to exhibit social impairments. All would certainly be viewed as peculiar by the layman, a factor which affected their ability to function independently. Parents generally described their sons as loners, and only one patient reported any current friendships. This individual, who was gregarious and underinhibited, related primarily to church groups. Others had found social outlets through school clubs and social activities organized by community mental health centers or religious groups, but had difficulty maintaining relationships when the organizations' structure was absent. None were married or had contemplated marriage. Several patients resembled young children in their general demeanor. Some high functioning men exhibited highly stereotyped and/or inappropriate social behaviors. Examples include repetitions of a fixed script when meeting people and inappropriate touching of others' clothing.

While some desired friendships, but lacked social competencies, others lacked social motivation either currently or historically. High functioning subjects' memories concerning childhood interactions with parents were concrete and unelaborated. They universally reported feeling that their parents were "on their side" and trustworthy and attributed their un-affectionate childhood behavior to "lack of interest," denying conflict and anxiety. Several, however, voiced feelings of resentment and jealousy toward siblings. Some previously "disinterested" individuals expressed current social motivation, while others remained aloof.

Marked social improprieties, such as inappropriate nudity or partial undress on the ward and inappropriate comments, were also noted, even in some high functioning patients. Such behaviors appeared to stem from poor social awareness and immaturity in all cases, rather than sexual interest.

Affect and anxiety. Although none met DSM-III criteria for affective disorder, several showed various affective symptoms. Half the sample showed affective flattening, manifested in monotonous intonation, re-stricted facial expression, and other nonverbal behavioral deficits (e.g., little body movement). Chronic, generalized anxiety was seen in half of the group.

In addition, caretakers of six patients, five of whom were high func-tioning, reported infrequent temper outbursts, stimulated by frustration and an inability to cope with environmental demands. These incidents involved aggression against others, destruction of property, and, in some cases, stereotyped movements such as arm flapping. In all cases, they appeared "out of character." Precipitating events included absent-mind-edness on the part of the patient (e.g., forgetting an airline ticket or one's driver's license), pressure induced by having to make independent decisions, and, in one case, trivial frustrations or environmental changes, such as a lack of soap in a bathroom.

Thought processes. A majority of patients (approximately ¾) were con-crete in their thinking. Other more variable features included persev-erative, impoverished, circumstantial, and obsessional thinking. None were incoherent, and even those with limited speech were comprehen-sible. While no patient showed formal thought disorder (e.g., loose as-sociations, blocking), some parents reported immature beliefs and naivete (e.g., beliefs in fictional characters like Santa Claus until late adolescence).

Positive schizophrenic symptoms. Hallucinations, delusions, and incoher-ence, which constitute positive symptoms of schizophrenia, were absent at follow-up. However, two high functioning patients reported childhood memories which raised some question about the former presence of delusions. One stated that, at approximately age 7, he believed that poison gas came out of the wall plugs. This resulted in a drive to cover up all electrical outlets. Another recalled that, at age 14, he thought his

TABLE 1

Psychiatric and Behavioral Characteristics of Autistic Men, as Assessed by Psychiatric Interviews[a] and Behavioral Observations Made Over 5-Day Hospitalizations

Characteristic	No. and Type of Subjects Showing Symptom				Total Sample
	High functioning subgroup	Lower functioning subgroup			
	WAIS VIQ and PIQ 82-126[b]	Language-impaired WAIS PIQ 88-129[b]	Mentally retarded WAIS VIQ and PIQ 48-77[b]		
	(N = 9)	(N = 3)	(N = 2)		(N = 14)
	N (%)	N (%)	N (%)		N (%)
Social relating:					
Lacks friends	8 (89)	3 (100)	2 (100)		13 (93)
Aloof	4 (44)	1 (33)	1 (50)		6 (43)
Marked social improprieties[c]	3 (33)	0 (0)	1 (50)		4 (29)
Oppositional	3 (33)	0 (0)	0 (0)		3 (21)
Affect and anxiety:					
Flat affect	5 (56)	1 (33)	1 (50)		7 (50)
Generalized anxiety	6 (67)	0 (0)	1 (50)		7 (50)
Depression	2 (22)	0 (0)	0 (0)		2 (14)
Silly, immature, teasing	2 (22)	0 (0)	0 (0)		2 (14)
Separation anxiety	1 (11)	0 (0)	1 (50)		2 (14)
Phobic	0 (0)	1 (33)	0 (0)		1 (7)
Mania	0 (0)	0 (0)	0 (0)		0 (0)
Thought processes:					
Concrete	7 (78)	1 (33)	2 (100)		10 (71)
Perseverative	4 (44)	0 (0)	1 (50)		5 (36)
Impoverished (*content* of speech)	3 (33)	0 (0)	2 (100)		5 (36)
Circumstantial or irrelevant	3 (33)	0 (0)	1 (50)		4 (29)
Obsessional thinking	4 (44)	0 (0)	0 (0)		4 (29)
Racing thoughts, pressured speech	1 (11)	1 (33)	0 (0)		1 (7)
Positive schizophrenic symptoms:					
Hallucinations	0 (0)	0 (0)	0 (0)		0 (0)

	A	B	C	D
Delusions	0 (0)	0 (0)	0 (0)	0 (0)
Incoherence	0 (0)	0 (0)	0 (0)	0 (0)
Motor symptoms:				
Stereotyped repetitive movements:	7 (78)	3 (100)	2 (100)	12 (86)
Arm, hand, or finger movements	6 (67)	3 (100)	2 (100)	11 (79)
Pacing	1 (11)	2 (67)	1 (50)	4 (29)
Rocking	2 (22)	1 (33)	0 (0)	3 (21)
Vocal tics	1 (11)	2 (67)	1 (50)	4 (29)
Compulsions	3 (33)	0 (0)	0 (0)	3 (21)
Hyperactivity	1 (11)	0 (0)	1 (50)	2 (14)
Speech and language:				
Peculiar uses of speech and language:	5 (56)	1 (33)	1 (50)	7 (50)
Talks to self	4 (44)	0 (0)	1 (50)	5 (36)
Uses words or phrases with special meanings	2 (22)	0 (0)	1 (50)	3 (21)
Perseveration, repetitive questions or phrases	4 (44)	1 (33)	2 (100)	7 (50)
Poverty of speech (little spontaneous speech)	3 (33)	1 (33)	2 (100)	6 (43)
Monotone, lack of normal vocal inflections	4 (44)	1 (33)	1 (50)	6 (43)
Word or phrase repetition[d]	4 (44)	0 (0)	0 (0)	4 (29)
Highly stereotyped	1 (11)	0 (0)	2 (100)	3 (21)
Occasional stuttering	1 (11)	0 (0)	0 (0)	1 (7)
Sensory/perceptual:				
Smells objects	1 (11)	0 (0)	0 (0)	1 (7)
Hypersensitive to light	1 (11)	0 (0)	0 (0)	1 (7)
Hypersensitive to sound	0 (0)	0 (0)	0 (0)	0 (0)
Other:				
Attentional deficits	2 (22)	0 (0)	1 (50)	3 (21)
Somatization	1 (11)	0 (0)	0 (0)	1 (7)

[a] Psychiatric interviews were the NIMH Diagnostic Interview Schedule (DIS) and the Washington University School of Medicine's Diagnostic Interview for Children and Adolescents (DICA).

[b] WAIS VIQ and PIQ are Verbal and Performance IQs, respectively.

[c] Marked social improprieties refer to behaviors such as inappropriate nudity or undress on the ward and socially inappropriate comments.

[d] This refers to repetitions of a word or several words, which resemble stuttering in that the subject appears motorically "stuck" and unable to move on to the next word. This contrasts with language perseveration, which involves use of stereotyped utterances without such motor difficulty, and which may reflect ideational perseveration.

clothing was too small and believed that others knew of this thought. While neither of these two retrospective reports presents certain evidence of delusions, they do raise questions about the complete absence of delusions in autism.

Motor symptoms. Stereotyped, repetitive movements were highly prevalent and were directly observed in 12 patients (86%), including 7 high functioning patients. High functioning patients seemed to intentionally suppress these movements in social situations, and some appeared embarrassed when seen engaging in such movements. When parental reports are included, *all* patients continued to show some stereotyped movements. In some instances, such movements were reported by parents to occur in response to stress or emotional upset.

The movements, both observed and reported, most frequently involved the hands or arms. Individual finger movements, rotating movements of the hand, arm flapping, and shaking of the hands or arms were characteristic. Hand-biting was reported by several parents and rhythmic movements of whole body—rocking and pacing—were also seen. In addition to these more bizarre movements, several patients repetitively tapped papers and table surfaces and interrupted their writing to repetitively tap pencils and pens against their fingers. Individuals generally had a repertoire of one or two particular movements, but these varied among individuals.

Other motor symptoms included vocal tics (grunts, squeaks, hissing sounds), seen primarily in lower functioning patients, compulsions, and hyperactivity. Compulsions included putting objects in their proper places, handwashing, and stereotyped touching of clothing and other objects. Peculiar gaits and limb postures (e.g., flexed arm posture) were also noted.

Speech and language. Language status ranged from normal to complete mutism. Impairments included very limited, dysphasic speech, as well as highly deviant speech. A single mildly retarded patient showed fluent and grammatical, but repetitive and nonsensical speech ("language deviance," rather than deficit). He repetitively asked hospital staff questions about his childhood acquaintances.

The most common abnormalities, particularly in the high functioning subgroup, involved speech and its social use. Speech was often monotonous, lacking normal intonational contours. Several patients repeated words or phrases within a sentence, appearing motorically "stuck" and unable to move on to the next word, giving their speech a stammering quality.

Several patients mumbled to themselves when with others or talked to themselves when alone. Some held idiosyncratic meanings for conventional words and phrases, seemingly for self-amusement or -stimulation. Poverty of speech and stereotyped speech were also seen with some frequency.

Sensory-perceptual. Although there was little evidence of sensory-perceptual disturbance, this category was coded because of theories which emphasize such features (Ornitz, 1974, 1983). A single patient showed an unusual tendency to smell objects, while another showed some sniffing movements when exploring a room. One patient also kept his room dim and complained about sunlight when his draperies were open. No behavior suggesting hyperacusis was observed. Some parents reported that their sons still cover their ears with their hands and show other stereotyped behavior in reaction to stress, rather than auditory stimulation. One patient insisted on keeping his room very warm and generally wore excessive clothing to keep warm.

Other. Varying "attentional deficits" were coded in three patients. These included unusual slowness in responding, as well as difficulties in attending to the examiner which may have stemmed from anxiety. Two individuals showed some unusual staring and inappropriate smiling. Although several parents reported their sons had unusually good memories, particularly for factual information like calendar dates, there were also reports of absentmindedness, or failure to adaptively draw upon stored memories to meet practical needs.

DSM-III Diagnoses

While all patients displayed residual symptoms, these varied considerably. The three patients who displayed specific language deficits as well as the one with highly deviant (repetitive) speech met DSM-III criteria for Infantile autism, full syndrome present (299.00). The remaining 10 patients, 9 of whom were high functioning, met DSM-III criteria for Autism, residual state (299.01). The presence of good language was the major disqualifying factor for a current diagnosis of "autism, full syndrome." All had shown severe language impairments in early childhood, which included delayed onsets of speech and immediate and delayed echolalia, and, in fact, three showed little or no communicative speech until after 5 years of age, according to parental reports. Their current linguistic abilities were good although abnormalities of speech (e.g., dysprosodies) were apparent. Varying degrees of social deficits and other phenomena that might be regarded as "bizarre responses to the environment" (e.g., stereotyped behavioral patterns) remained.

Because most current symptoms appeared to be residuals of early autism, no additional DSM-III diagnoses were warranted. However, in the absence of such a history, one might have considered the diagnoses of Generalized anxiety disorder (300.02), Schizoid personality (301.20), and Simple phobia (300.29) for some of these individuals. Obsessional preoccupations and compulsive phenomena were also present but lacked an ego-dystonic quality and thus would not support the diagnosis of Obsessive-compulsive disorder (300.30). A diagnosis of Compulsive personality disorder (301.40), on the other hand, would not have encompassed additional symptoms displayed by these patients. None of these patients showed current evidence of delusions, hallucinations, or incoherence, the features which differentiate between DSM-III diagnoses of Pervasive developmental disorder, residual state (299.01, 299.91) and Schizophrenia (295.x).

Adaptive Functioning

Table 2 lists each subject's Vineland SQ, level of educational attainment, employment status, and living situation, as well as age and verbal and performance IQs. As shown here, two high functioning patients completed a year or more of junior college, while most others completed high school with or without receiving diplomas. All of the lower functioning patients received special education into late adolescence or early adulthood. Basic reading, spelling, and math skills, as assessed by the Wide Range Achievement Test (WRAT), were generally consonant with education and IQ scores. Therefore, as measured by the most basic of academic skills, these individuals received considerable benefits from their educations. According to parents, two high functioning subjects also had done well in foreign language courses. This was notable in light of their early language impairments. Several showed relative strengths in math.

However, social-adaptive functioning, as reflected in employment status, living arrangements, and Vineland SQs, fell below expectations based on IQs. As shown in Table 2, even those few individuals who lived apart from parents received some professional or parental support and supervision. Lower functioning patients, of course, were more dependent on others. Only four of the nine high functioning patients were competitively employed (see Table 2); and these, in routine jobs with

TABLE 2

Social-Adaptive Functioning of Autistic Men

ID	Age (yr)	WAIS IQs		Vineland Social Quotient	Education	Employment	Residence
		Verbal	Performance				
1	39	108	108	68	Regular high school diploma	Sheltered workshop	With parents
2	36	110	113	80	High school equivalency	Janitor	Supervised apartment[a]
3	31	106	111	88	Regular high school diploma	Cab driver	With parents
4	30	99	102	72	Eighth grade	Unemployed	Apartment
5	27	103	81	80	One year junior college	Library aid	Supervised apartment[a]
6	22	117	115	64	Associate degree, junior college	Key punch operator	With parents
7	21	97	97	57	High school, with part-time special education	Special job train-program	With parents
8	20	82	86	80	High school equivalency	Part-time vocational training	With parents
9	18	109	126	56	Special education through high school	Part-time special college student	With parents
10	37	Severe deficit	129 (3 subtests)	32	Special education	Sheltered workshop	With parents
11	32	No speech	88 (4 subtests)	32	Special education	Sheltered workshop	State hospital
12	22	62	93	45	Special education through high school	Unemployed	With parents
13	32	77	55	56	Special education through high school	Attends day program at state hospital	With parent
14	25	48	60	30	Special education	Special job program	Group home

[a] Supervision is minimal and consists of weekly visits by a counselor, who troubleshoots and helps patient plan.

limited decision making and minimal social interaction. One exception to this was the position of cab driver, which requires more social interaction and independence than did the other jobs held. One high functioning patient was fired from a job because of his compulsive touching of other people and other inappropriate, intrusive social behavior. Another high functioning patient worked in a sheltered workshop for retardates because of limitations imposed by his rigidity, obsessional preoccupations, and anxiety about schedules.

The three youngest high functioning patients, ages 18–21, were all receiving some additional education or job-training and might be capable of holding competitive jobs in the future. One patient's compulsive habits (e.g., handwashing), obsessional questioning, oppositional personality, and rigidity constituted interfering factors for job success at the time he was seen. Another generally worked slowly and had some time-consuming compulsions (e.g., hand and arm washing) that could limit his job opportunities. A third demonstrated a talent for math and computer programming, but displayed poor initiative, a factor which might be compensated for by considerable supervision.

In addition to patient-related factors (e.g., competencies, maladaptive behaviors), "parent factors" were influential in determining employment outcome. Only two high functioning patients obtained their current jobs on their own, and one of these had received help obtaining his first jobs. Parents and agencies, but particularly parents, played a major role in finding employers willing to give their sons a chance.

The Vineland SQs were generally low, relative to IQs, sometimes strikingly so. Low SQs seen in high functioning patients primarily reflected deficits in areas of self-direction, socialization, and occupational achievements. This is illustrated in the sample Vineland profile shown in Figure 1.

As shown here, the emphasis of this scale shifts from self-help items to self-direction, socialization, and occupational skills with increasing age. The failures of this group occur on higher level items and reflect poor initiative, restrictions in social relationships, stereotyped behavioral patterns, and, in some instances, restricted independent travel. Even those patients who function well on their jobs may follow inflexible routines with respect to dress (e.g., wearing an established set of clothing each day of the week) and may be restricted to routine routes in traveling to and from work. Most of these individuals require help with nonroutine matters, e.g., financial planning, dealing with the phone company. Though basic self-help skills are present, some need reminders and feedback from parents about grooming and dress. While these limitations are prevalent, an exception is again seen in one individual who obtained several jobs on his own, files his own taxes, purchased his own automobile, directs his own financial affairs, and vacations alone out of state, showing good self-direction and isolated deficits in social relating.

Lower functioning patients showed more pervasive deficits involving self-direction, socialization, communication, occupational achievements, and independence of travel (locomotion). Of the five lower functioning patients, two were unemployed, while three worked in highly supervised settings. Those with high nonverbal IQs were able to use their visuospatial skills to do work such as disassembling and sorting machine parts.

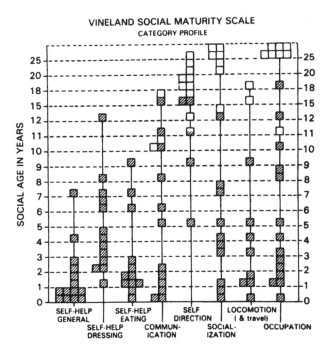

PATIENT # 10
CHRONOLOGICAL AGE 22
WAIS VERBAL IQ 117
WAIS PERFORMANCE IQ 115
SOCIAL AGE 14.4
SOCIAL QUOTIENT 64

FIG. 1. Item composition of Vineland Social Maturity Scale and sample profile of a high functioning adult male with autism, residual state. *Shaded boxes* reflect positive item scores, or competencies, while *blank boxes* reflect failed items.

Parental Status and Experiences

No history of major psychiatric illness was identified in parents or first degree relatives, although parents did suffer emotional distress because of difficulties inherent in the raising of handicapped children. Parental social class was as follows: 6 upper-upper, 2 lower-upper, 3 upper-middle, and 2 lower-middle. This bias toward higher socioeconomic status was likely a function of biased sampling procedures.

Without exception, parents reported early experiences of going from clinic to clinic in an attempt to get a diagnosis they could accept. The usual diagnosis was mental retardation, which did not "fit" with parents' impressions. When these patients were young, autism was still unfamiliar to many people in the mental health field. When autism was diagnosed, parents came away feeling that they were being held responsible and accused of poor parenting. Once able to work through their feelings, these parents made intensive, persistent efforts to obtain help for their children. Support of national organizations such as those established for many chronic diseases was unavailable. Thus, these parents found themselves part of a small group laboring to establish resources for their autistic children. One common feature of the families was a relative lack of long-term planning for the patients, a possibility attributable to several factors. Several parents expressed longstanding denials of the irreversible nature of the disorder. Demands of everyday living also seemed to infringe on long-term planning. And finally, most parents were unsure of how to proceed. Some set up trusts to provide for financial and day-to-day support they knew would eventually be needed. Others made plans for other family members to accept this responsibility in the future. Casework with this group involved facilitating these plans and involving social agencies that work with handicapped adults.

In summary, the parents of these subjects were highly committed to helping their children achieve their maximum potential. We found them to be warm, dedicated, and unrelenting in their efforts.

DISCUSSION

Each of the patients studied had retained autistic symptoms. While certain "negative," or deficit, symptoms of schizophrenia—most notably flat affect and concrete thinking—were prevalent, no patient showed positive symptoms of schizophrenia. In addition, individual symptoms (but not full syndromes) of anxiety, schizoid, and obsessive-compulsive disorders were seen. Thus, no specific links to schizophrenia were suggested.

In contrast to this, two recent follow-up reports on "psychotic" children have suggested possible associations between autism and later-developing schizophrenia. Howells and Guirguis (1984) followed up 10 childhood psychotics with onsets before 30 months and 10 with onsets between 30 months and 11 years. The entire group showed residual symptoms and "schizophrenic states" characterized by negative symptoms (Kraepelin's simple schizophrenia, DSM-III schizophrenia residual state, and Crow's type III schizophrenia). None showed any of Schneider's "first-rank" symptoms—hallucinations and delusions, although they were "suspected" in 10 patients, 2 of whom were from the early onset group.

The findings of residuals and negative symptoms in 10 early onset "psychotics" are consistent with our findings, whereas the suspicion of positive symptoms is not. This latter difference may reflect differences in the incidence and/or degree of mental retardation and language impairment in the two samples. Howells and Guirguis' subjects were not described with respect to IQ or language status, so that intellectual or linguistic impairments may have made these determinations difficult. Our most retarded subject was at worst moderately retarded, and the largest proportion of our subjects showed average intelligence and good language. Thus, psychiatric examinations may have yielded clearer results in our sample. In addition, conditions associated with autism—mental retardation, language impairment, and seizure disorder—are themselves associated with increased incidences of psychiatric disorder, independent of their associations with autism (Rutter et al., 1970).

Some of our high functioning subjects did recall holding false beliefs at some time during their development, raising some question concerning the absence of delusions in autism. However, these beliefs were relatively unelaborated and may have reflected concrete thinking, social immaturity, and naivete. They may have been similar to "childish fantasies" reported in autistic adolescents by Rutter and Lockyer (1967). Delusions in schizophrenia are elaborate and complex; and productions (language, drawings), symbolic and imaginative. These qualities were lacking in the productions of our subjects, just as they are characteristically lacking in the play of autistic children (Cantwell et al., 1978; Wing et al., 1977). The ability to engage in complex imaginative, creative, or symbolic thought may be a feature that differentiates the two disorders and the sorts of false beliefs seen in them.

Petty et al. (1984) has recently described schizophrenic disorders in three children, ages 8, 12, and 17 years, with histories suggestive of autism. All had approximately average Wechsler Verbal IQs, suggesting relatively good language function, which would facilitate psychiatric examination. The early diagnoses of autism were, however, retrospective in two cases, while the age of diagnosis and type of professional making the diagnosis was unspecified in the third. Low performance IQs relative to verbal IQs were seen in Petty's sample and are believed to be uncharacteristic of autism (Lockyer and Rutter, 1970). However, sizable differences (22 points) in this direction were also seen in two of our subjects, suggesting heterogeneity in patterns of neuropsychological deficits associated with autism.

Similarities between autism and disorders other than schizophrenia have received little attention. The high incidence of stereotyped movements and other motor symptoms, obsessional and compulsive phenomena, and anxiety symptoms would suggest avenues for future behavioral and biological comparisons.

The high prevalence of stereotyped movements, particularly involving hands or arms, in this relatively high functioning sample was surprising. Freeman et al. (1981) and Bartak and Rutter (1976) found hand and finger stereotypies to be more prevalent in autistic children with IQs under 70, as compared to those with higher IQs. Freeman et al. (1981) suggested such movements, not required in DSM-III, might be of diagnostic importance independent of IQ. Our experience suggests that such movements occur with a higher frequency and public visibility in more impaired autistic adults but may be equally prevalent in high functioning adults, who might intentionally suppress such movements. Motoric features may well be of diagnostic and neurobiological significance.

Methodological techniques are likely to significantly affect prevalence estimates of movements and other features. Naturalistic observations over 5 days yielded higher estimates of stereotyped movements than did psychiatric interviews. Parental reports yielded even higher estimates, a phenomenon seen in Bartak and Rutter's (1976) study as well.

Generalizations from these findings are of course limited by our sampling procedures. Our procedures were not designed to yield a sample representative of the growing autistic adult population. Data from previous follow-up studies (DeMyer et al., 1973; Lotter, 1974; Rutter and Lockyer, 1967) suggest that our sample was a relatively high functioning one overall and that our high functioning subgroup was drawn from among the 5–15% of those with the best clinical outcomes. Excluded were the 20–30% of autistic patients who develop epilepsy (Deykin and MacMahon, 1979; Rutter, 1970) and many autistic patients with substantial language impairments and retardation. In addition, the 1–2% of individuals with the best outcomes might have been less likely to learn of our study, reluctant to miss time from work, or reluctant to volunteer for a study that would identify them as deviant.

SUMMARY

Continuing social impairments and varied psychiatric and behavioral symptoms were seen in our entire sample of 14 men with childhood histories of autism. Three continued to meet DSM-III criteria for autism, while 10 met criteria for autism, residual state. None showed positive schizophrenic symptoms or qualified for an additional DSM-III diagnosis. Stereotyped movements and concrete thinking were highly prevalent (present in at least 70%). Flat affect, generalized anxiety, a lack of normal vocal inflections, peculiar uses of speech and language, language perseveration, and poverty of speech were moderately prevalent (present in 40–50%). Few were competitively employed, and few enjoyed a degree of independence typically associated with adulthood. These findings would suggest that autistic children do not generally, with any great frequency, develop schizophrenia or other adult psychiatric disorders, but rather display continuing, less severe symptoms of their original autism, which significantly limit their social and economic independence. Generalizations are, however, limited by our sampling procedures.

REFERENCES

Bartak, L. & Rutter, M. (1976), Differences between mentally retarded and normally intelligent autistic children. *J. Aut. Childh. Schizo.*, 6:109-120.

Bender, L. & Faretra, G. (1973), The relationship between childhood schizophrenia and adult schizophrenia. In: *Genetic Factors in Schizophrenia*, ed. A. R. Kaplan. Springfield, Ill.: Charles C. Thomas.

Cantwell, D., Baker, L. & Rutter, M. (1978), A comparative study of infantile autism and specific developmental receptive language disorder; IV. Analysis of syntax and language function. *J. Child Psychol. Psychiat.*, 19:351-362.

DeMyer, M., Barton, S., DeMyer, W. E. et al. (1973), Prognosis in autism: a follow-up study. *J. Aut. Childh. Schizo.*, 3:199-246.

Deykin, E. Y. & MacMahon, B. (1979), The incidence of seizures among children with autistic symptoms. *Amer. J. Psychiat.*, 136:1310-1312.

Doll, E. A. (1953), *Measurement of Social Competence*. Circle Pines, Minn.: American Guidance Service, p. 376.

Eisenberg, L. (1956), The autistic child in adolescence. *Amer. J. Psychiat.*, 12:607-612.

——— (1957), The course of childhood schizophrenia. *Arch. Neurol. Psychiat.*, 78:69-83.

——— & Kanner, L. (1956), Childhood schizophrenia: early infantile autism, 1943–55. *Amer. J. Orthopsychiat.*, 26:556-564.

Fish, B. (1977), Neurobiologic antecedents of schizophrenia in children: evidence for an inherited congenital neurointegrative defect. *Arch. Gen. Psychiat.*, 34:1297-1313.

Freeman, B. J., Ritvo, E. R., Schroth, P. C. et al. (1981), Behavioral characteristics of high- and low-IQ autistic children. *Amer. J. Psychiat.*, 138:25-29.

Herjanic, B. & Campbell, J. W. (1977), Differentiating psychiatrically disturbed children on the basis of a structured interview. *J. Abnorm. Child Psychol.*, 5:127-135.

Howells, J. G. & Guirguis, W. R. (1984), Childhood schizophrenia 20 years later. *Arch. Gen. Psychiat.*, 41:123-128.

Kanner, L. (1943), Autistic disturbances of affective contact. *Nerv. Child*, 2:217-250.

—— Rodriquez, A. & Ashenden, B. (1972), How far can autistic children go in matters of social adaptation? *J. Aut. Childh. Schizo.*, 2:9-33.

Kolvin, I. (1971), Studies in the childhood psychoses: I. Diagnostic criteria and classification. *Brit. J. Psychiat.*, 118:381-384.

—— Ounsted, C., Humphrey, M. & McNay, A. (1971), II. The phenomenology of childhood psychoses. *Brit. J. Psychiat.*, 118:385-395.

Lockyer, L. & Rutter, M. (1970), A five to fifteen year follow-up study of infantile psychosis; IV. Patterns of cognitive ability. *Brit. J. Soc. Clin. Psychol.*, 9:152-163.

Lotter, V. (1974), Social adjustment and placement of autistic children in Middlesex: a follow-up study. *J. Aut. Childh. Schizo.*, 4:11-32.

Mazure, C. & Gershon, E. (1979), Blindness and reliability in lifetime psychiatric diagnosis. *Arch. Gen. Psychiat.*, 36:521-525.

Ornitz, E. M. (1974), The modulation of sensory input and motor output in autistic children. *J. Aut. Childh. Schizo.*, 4:197-215.

—— (1983), The functional neuroanatomy of infantile autism. *Int. J. Neurosci.*, 19:85-124.

Petty, L. K., Ornitz, E. M., Michelman, J. D. et al. (1984), Autistic children who become schizophrenic. *Arch. Gen. Psychiat.*, 41:129-135.

Robins, L., Helzer, J., Croughan, J. & Ratcliffe, K. (1981), National Institute of Mental Health Diagnostic Interview Schedule. *Arch. Gen. Psychiat.*, 38:381-389.

Rumsey, J. M., Duara, R., Grady, C. et al. (1985), Brain metabolism in autism: resting cerebral glucose utilization as measured with positron emission tomography (PET). *Arch. Gen. Psychiat.*, 42:448-455.

Rutter, M. (1970), Autistic children: infancy to adulthood. *Seminars in Psychiatry*, 2:435-450.

—— & Lockyer, L. (1967), A five to fifteen year follow-up study of infantile psychosis; I. Description of Sample. *Brit. J. Psychiat.*, 113:1169-1182.

—— Graham, P. & Yule, W. (1970), *A Neuropsychiatric Study in Childhood.* London: Heineman.

Vineland Social Maturity Scale (1965), Circle Pines, Minn.: American Guidance Service.

Watt, N. M. (1976), Two factor index of social position: Amherst modification. Unpublished manuscript; available from Norma Watt, Ph.D., Department of Psychology, Child Study Center, 2460 S. Vine St., Denver, Colorado.

Wing, L., Gould, J., Yeates, S. R. et al. (1977), Symbolic lay in severely mentally retarded and in autistic children. *J. Child Psychol. Psychiat.*, 18:351-362.

29

Concordance for the Syndrome of Autism in 40 Pairs of Afflicted Twins

Edward R. Ritvo, B. J. Freeman,
Anne Mason-Brothers, Amy Mo, and Anne M. Ritvo
Neuropsychiatric Institute, UCLA School of Medicine

The UCLA Registry for Genetic Studies in Autism was established in 1980 to test the hypothesis that genetic factors may be etiologically significant in subsets of patients. To date 61 pairs of twins have enrolled and 40 meet research diagnostic criteria for autism. The authors found a concordance for autism in these 40 pairs of 95.7% in the monozygotic twins (22 of 23) and 23.5% in the dizygotic twins (four of 17).

Since the syndrome of autism was first described by Kanner in 1943 (1), a consensus has been reached that the symptoms express underlying neuropathology of various etiologies. Earlier theories of psychological causes have been discarded (2). The syndrome has been identified in all

Reprinted with permission from the *American Journal of Psychiatry*, 1985, Vol. 142, 74–77. Copyright 1985 by the American Psychiatric Association.

Presented at the 137th annual meeting of the American Psychiatric Association, Los Angeles, May 5–11, 1984.

Supported by the Max and Lottie Dresher Research Fund, the Bennin Fund, NIMH grants MH-31274 and MH-30897 (from the Clinical Research Center for the Study of Child Psychosis), and National Institute of Child Health and Human Development grants HD-04612 and MCH-927.

The authors thank the National Society for Autistic Children, George Realmuto, M.D., Magda Campbell, M.D., Steve Funderburk, M.D., Lynn Jorde, Ph.D., and Mary Coleman, M.D., for assistance. Bernice Heyert provided editorial assistance and typing.

parts of the world and in all social classes and races without special distribution (3). It occurs three to four times more often in males and is frequently found in association with other syndromes such as epilepsy and mental retardation. Longevity is normal, and while certain patients may also have neuropathology and/or hyperserotonemia, no specific biomedical markers have been uniquely associated with an etiologic subtype (4, 5).

Previous twin studies in which zygosity was documented reported 15 pairs of monozygotic twins in which nine pairs (60%) were concordant for autism and 15 pairs of dizygotic twins in which two pairs (15%) were concordant (see references 6 and 7 and table 1). All of these studies were conducted before a consensus was established concerning the diagnostic criteria for the syndrome of autism (18, *DSM-III*). Thus, it is impossible to combine these earlier reports for statistical purposes or to draw conclusions from the limited number of cases in each study.

TABLE 1. Studies of Autism in Twins With Confirmed Zygosity[a]

Study	Total Pairs	Concordant[b] Pairs	Sex	
			Male	Female
Monozygotic pairs	15	9	24	6
Bakwin, 1954 (8)	1	1	2	0
Kamp, 1964 (9)	1	0	2	0
McQuaid, 1975 (10)	1	1	2	0
Folstein and Rutter, 1977 (7)[c]	9	4	12	6
Eshkevari, 1979 (11)	1	1	2	0
Campbell et al., 1980 (unpublished)	2	2	4	0
Dizygotic pairs	13	2	14	12
Ward and Hoddinott, 1962 (12)[a]	1	1	0	2
Böök et al., 1963 (13)	1	0	1	1
Vaillant, 1963 (14)	1	0	2	0
Havelkova, 1967 (15)	1	0	1	1
Kotsopoulos, 1976 (16)	1[d]	1	1	1
Folstein and Rutter, 1977 (7)[c]	4	0	6	2
Sloan, 1978 (17)	1	0	1	1
Campbell et al., 1980 (unpublished)	3	0	2	4

[a]Zygosity confirmed by blood group tests or opposite sex except for the study by Ward and Hoddinott (12) in which it was confirmed by separate placentas and different appearance.
[b]Concordance rate: monozygotic, 60%; dizygotic, 15%.
[c]Eight patients from this study are not included here because they did not have blood typing.
[d]Has a cousin with autism.

METHOD

The scientific rationale for forming the UCLA Registry for Genetic Studies in Autism and the methods for recruiting patients have been published (19, 20). In summary, families of 16 monozygotic and 12 dizygotic pairs of twins answered an advertisement in *The Advocate*, the newsletter of the National Society for Autistic Children. Seven families of monozygotic and five families of dizygotic twins were identified from the UCLA outpatient department or personal referrals. All patients enrolled were diagnosed independently by two of us (E.R.R., B.J.F.) in accordance with the diagnostic criteria of the National Society for Autistic Children and *DSM-III*. This required a review of obstetrical, birth, pediatric, psychiatric, psychological, and educational records to document the presence of pathognomonic symptoms before 30 months of age. Similar medical and professional records were obtained on all siblings of autistic patients who were reported to have had developmental disturbances. In addition, two of us (E.R.R., B.J.F.) conducted neuropsychiatric evaluations on 11 monozygotic and seven dizygotic pairs and concurred on all diagnoses in the 40 families.

Sixty-one families with twins enrolled in the registry between January 1980 and April 1984. Forty-seven provided sufficient records so that their children could be diagnosed in accordance with the research protocol. Seven of the pairs of twins were diagnosed as not being autistic, leaving 40 pairs with one or two autistic children. Figure 1 displays the age, sex, and birth order of each offspring in the 40 families.

To meet the research diagnostic criteria all patients were documented as having 1) onset before 30 months of age, 2) pervasive lack of response to other people, 3) gross deficits in language development, 4) if speech was present, peculiar speech problems such as immediate and delayed echolalia, metaphorical language, proniminal reversal, 5) bizarre responses to the various aspects of the environment, e.g., resistance to change, peculiar interest in or peculiar interest in or attachment to animate or inanimate objects, and 6) absence of delusions, hallucinations, loosening of associations, and incoherence as in schizophrenia (18, *DSM-III*).

Blood samples from 17 pairs (12 monozygotic, five dizygotic) were analyzed for gene markers, serum proteins, red cell enzymes, red cell antigens, and HLA typing. These tests assure zygosity assignment with greater than 99% accuracy. Five more dizygotic pairs were opposite sex, which assures dizygosity. These 22 pairs were labeled "zygosity confirmed," and the remaining 18 of the 40 pairs were awaiting blood testing

FIGURE 1. Age, Sex, and Birth Order for 23 Pairs of Monozygotic Twins and 17 Pairs of Dizygotic Twins

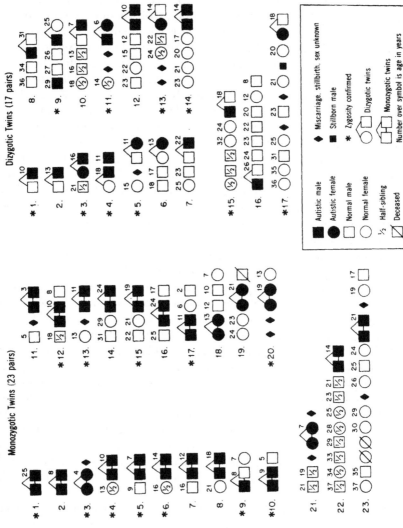

(11 monozygotic, seven dizygotic, same sex) and were labeled "zygosity presumed" (table 2) on the basis of obstetrical and pediatric records and parental and independent observations of similar or dissimilar appearances.

RESULTS

Table 2 shows concordance rates in 23 monozygotic and 17 dizygotic pairs of twins. The rates in confirmed and presumed zygosity pairs were not significantly different (Fisher's exact test). The only monozygotic twin pair discordant for autism was originally diagnosed by Dr. George Realmuto at the University of Minnesota and was interviewed by one of us (E.R.R.).

Of the 23 monozygotic pairs 18 are male and five are female (78.3% male); of the 17 dizygotic pairs nine are male, one is female, and seven are mixed sex (73.5% of all siblings of the dizygotic pairs are male and 71.4% of the dizygotic autistic patients are male) (see figure 1).

DISCUSSION

The limited data available from our study do not permit extensive statistical testing or drawing definitive conclusions concerning genetic modes of inheritance. However, the results to date are compatible with autosomal recessive inheritance, which predicts 100% concordance in monozygotic pairs and 25% concordance in dizygotic pairs. A binomial significance test revealed that the concordance rate in the dizygotic pairs

TABLE 2. Concordance for Autism in 40 Pairs of Twins

Zygosity	Total Pairs	Concordant Pairs	Noncon- cordant Pairs	Concordance (%)[a]
Monozygotic	23	22	1	95.7
Confirmed	12	11	1	91.7
Presumed	11	11	0	100
Dizygotic	17	4	13	23.5
Confirmed	10	3	7	30[b]
Presumed	7	1	6	14.3

[a]No significant differences between confirmed and presumed groups for monozygotic or dizygotic pair (Fisher's exact test) and between expected frequencies for recessive model prediction of 100% for monozygotic pairs and 25% for dizygotic pairs. Significant difference found between the dominant model prediction of 50% in dizygotic pairs and that observed (binomial distribution, $p < .05$).

is significantly different (p > .05) from the 50% concordance rate predicted by a dominant model of inheritance with full penetrance. The recessive model of heritability does not account for the excessive number of males in our twins; however, the excess found is very close to the ratio noted in other surveys of autistic patients (21) and other diseases attributed to recessive heritability (22). It is also quite plausible that the excess of males is due to other etiological subgroups in our twin sample. Other investigators have reviewed the methodological problems and limitations of twin studies (6, 7, 17, 22).

To assess the proportion of all twins with autism in the United States enrolled in the registry to date we followed the model published by Folstein and Rutter (7). They estimated that between 18 and 26 same sex autistic children were born from twin births in Great Britain over a 13-year time span. The United States has approximately four times the population of Great Britain, and the age range we sampled spanned approximately 26 years. From these figures we can estimate that the number of same sex autistic persons from twin births in the United States available for our study is between 144 and 208—18 to 26 (autistic persons from twin births) × 4 (population correction) × 2 (age span correction). Thus, the 57 same sex autistic persons from twin births we have diagnosed to date present approximately 27% to 40% of all autistic persons from twin births in the United States on the basis of Folstein and Rutter's method of estimation. Other means of estimating our percentage of ascertainment reveal similar figures (e.g., by estimating the total number of autistic persons in the United States and dividing by the estimated numbers of monozygotic and dizygotic twins in the population).

It has been proposed by Folstein and Rutter (7) that autism could represent the severest form of a continuum of inherited pathology of cognitive processing. August et al. (23) studied this possibility; they observed cognitive processing pathology in 15% (11 of 71) of siblings of autistic probands, a percentage significantly different from the 2.8% rate in their comparison group of siblings of Down's syndrome probands (1 of 38). Campbell et al. (24) also reported similar findings in families of autistic probands. Although our project did not systematically address this issue, all parents were asked to report if any developmental language problems had occurred in their nonautistic children. Our 17 dizygotic families had a total of 45 nonautistic full siblings, seven (15%) of whom were reported to have had such problems; our 23 monozygotic families had a total of 33 nonautistic nontwin full siblings, one (3%) of whom was reported to have had a possible developmental language problem.

Combining these data yields an incidence of possible cognitive processing pathology among all our nonautistic siblings of 10.3% (78 nonautistic siblings, eight possibly pathologic), a figure remarkably close to those previously reported by Folstein and Rutter (7) (10% in siblings of dizygotic twins) and by August et al. (23) (15% in nontwin siblings). Further research is warranted by these intriguing observations, which tend to support the presence of genetic factors.

Although it is generally agreed that autism is a behaviorally defined syndrome that may be genetically linked to other cognitive disorders (7) and has heterogeneous etiologies (2), it remains to be determined what, if any, proportion of cases are caused by pathogenic genes. However, the assumption that pathogenic genes are present poses the fascinating task of determining where on the gene map they reside, precisely what pathologic ciphers they transmit, and whether we can deduce their presence from clinical clues.

REFERENCES

1. Kanner, L.: Autistic disturbances of affective contact. Nervous Child 2:217-250, 1943.
2. Ritvo, E. R.: The syndrome of autism: a medical model. Integrative Psychiatry 1:103-122, 1983.
3. Ritvo, E. R., Cantwell, D., Johnson, E., et al.: Social class factors in autism. J Autism Childhood Schizo 1:297-310, 1971.
4. DeMyer, M. K., Hingtgen, J. N., Jackson, R. K.: Infantile autism reviewed: a decade of research. Schizophr. Bull 7:387-452, 1981.
5. Freeman, B. J., Ritvo, E. R.: The syndrome of autism: establishing the diagnosis and principles of management. Pediatr Ann 13:285-295, 1984.
6. Hanson, D. R., Gottesman, I.: The genetics, if any, of infantile autism and childhood schizophrenia. J Autism Child Schizo 6:269-274, 1976.
7. Folstein, S., Rutter, M.: Infantile autism: a genetic study of 21 twin pairs. J Child Psychol Psychiatry 18:297-321, 1977.
8. Bakwin, H.: Early infantile autism. J Pediatr 45:492-497, 1954.
9. Kamp, L. N.: Autistic syndrome in one of a pair of monozygotic twins. Psychiatr Neurol Neurochir 67:143-147, 1964.
10. McQuaid, P. E.: Infantile autism in twins. Br J Psychiatry 127:530-534, 1975.
11. Eshkevari, H. S.: Early infantile autism in monozygotic twins. J Autism Dev Disord 9:105-109, 1979.
12. Ward, T. F., Hoddinott, B. A.: Early infantile autism in fraternal twins. Can Psychiatr Assoc J 7:191-195, 1962.
13. Böök, J. A., Nichtern, S., Gruenberg, E.: Cytogenetical investigation in childhood schizophrenia. Acta Psychiatr Scand 39:309-323, 1963.
14. Vaillant, G.: Twins discordant for early infantile autism. Arch Gen Psychiatry 9:163-167, 1963.
15. Havelkova, M.: Abnormalities in siblings of schizophrenic children. Can Psychiatr Assoc J 12:363-369, 1967.

16. Kotsopoulos, S.: Infantile autism in dizygotic twins: a case report. J Autism Child Schizo 6:133-138, 1976.
17. Sloan, J. L.: Differential development of autistic symptoms in a pair of fraternal twins. J Autism Child Schizo 8:191-202, 1978.
18. Ritvo, E. R., Freeman, B. J.: National Society for Autistic Children definition of the syndrome of autism. J Am Acad Child Psychiatry 17:565-576, 1978.
19. Ritvo, E. R., Ritvo, E. C., Brothers, A. M.: Genetic and immunohematologic factors in autism. J Autism Dev Disord 12:109-114, 1982.
20. Ritvo, E. R., Ritvo, E. C.: Genetic and immunohematologic factors in autism, in Biological Psychiatry 1981: Proceedings of the IIIrd World Congress of Biological Psychiatry. Edited by Perris, C., Struwe, G., Jansson, B. New York, Elsevier, 1981.
21. Tsai, L., Steward, M. A., August, G.: Implication of sex differences in the familial transmission of infantile autism. J Autism Dev Disord 11:165-174, 1981.
22. Thompson, J. S., Thompson, M. W.: Genetics in Medicine. Philadelphia, Saunders, 1980.
23. August, J., Stewart, M. A., Tsai, L.: The incidence of cognitive disabilities in the siblings of autistic children. Br J Psychiatry 138:416-422, 1981.
24. Campbell, M., Minton, J., Green, W. H., et al.: Siblings and twins of autistic children, in Biological Psychiatry: Proceedings of the IIIrd World Congress of Biological Psychiatry. Edited by Perris, C., Struwe, G., Jansson, B. New York, Elsevier, 1981.

Part IX
OTHER CLINICAL ISSUES

Rutter and Sandberg discuss a number of key conceptual and substantive issues in child psychiatry epidemiology, including the definition of a disorder and the steps taken to identify cases. The latter issue involves strategies of sampling and measurement, and the authors review the use of administrative statistics, hospital/clinic data, questionnaire surveys and two-stage interview surveys. Problems of diagnosis and classification are also reviewed. Rutter and Sandberg then discuss the use of epidemiological/longitudinal data for the study of causal mechanisms in specific syndromes and with risk factors. The paper is far-reaching in its scope as contrasted to narrowly focused epidemiological studies of estimates of prevalence. Each point in the paper is illuminated by relevant concrete examples, and the authors conclude by emphasizing the need for both the imaginative application of epidemiological techniques and the use of other specified research strategies if we are to make further progress in delineating the ways in which risk processes operate.

The paper by Kraemer and her associates challenges the strong claims that have been made regarding the adverse effects of obstetric drugs on the behavioral development of children. They analyze the inadequacies of the studies that have formed the basis for these claims and cite several controlled studies that have failed to find any significant association between obstetric drug use and infant behavior. They conclude that the issue is an open one, and well-designed and well-executed studies are necessary. Pregnant women should not be denied the benefits of useful obstetric drugs, because of a sweeping generalization about their harmful effects, until adverse effects are substantiated by adequate studies.

Spurlock discusses the issues involved in the assessment and therapeutic intervention of black children. She warns against the two opposite stereotypic approaches that may lead the clinician astray. On the one hand, the black child may be assessed only as a victim of racism and little or no effort is made to evaluate individual intrapsychic factors. On the other hand, the clinician may be blinded to the effects of differences of

557

race or class. Spurlock also emphasizes the need to identify the strengths of the black child and family, which may easily be overlooked if they do not correspond to the standard white middle-class models. She presents rich clinical material to illustrate these issues. While they apply most sharply to the evaluation and treatment of black children, and especially those from poor families, the principles she enunciates also apply to other minority groups, and even to white middle-class children whose families have special idiosyncratic features that deviate from the standard cultural norms. Spurlock's theme on the need to look at the individual child without present stereotypic judgments may not appear to be a new one, but it still needs the kind of emphasis and illumination that she gives to it.

Gualtieri and Hicks present a sophisticated and valuable review of the research literature and their own research findings on the neuropharmacology of methylphenidate (ritalin) in childhood schizophrenia. It appears from this review that the effects of stimulant drugs on different outcome measures are variable, unpredictable, and nonintercorrelated. These findings lead them to propose a theory of hyperactivity as a dysregulatory disorder based on frontal-striatal dysfunction or dysmaturation. Their data are presented incisively, and the logic of their hypothesis as it flows from the data is spelled out clearly and thoughtfully.

The paper by Finkelhor and Browne proposes a framework for the systematic understanding of the psychological effects of child sexual abuse. Based on a review of the literature, the authors identify four dynamic responses that are productive of the traumatic impact of the child victim—traumatic sexualization, betrayal, stigmatization, and powerlessness. They make the important point that the extent of the traumatic impact of these four factors depends not only on the experience of the sexual abuse itself, but also on the child's life experience both prior to and subsequent to the abuse. This theme is spelled out with pertinent specific examples. The authors conclude by suggesting approaches to both research and therapeutic intervention based on their conceptual model.

Drotar and Crawford discuss the issue of the psychological adaptation of siblings of chronically ill children. For the healthy child, the presence of a chronically ill sibling in the family is stressful. Different children cope with different degrees of success with this stress, and the authors emphasize that there is no one-to-one correspondence between the presence of a chronically ill child or the type of illness and risk for psychological disturbance in the healthy siblings. A number of variables can influence this risk factor, but further research is necessary to clarify their significance in individual cases. The quality of family functioning and relationships is one variable that can be identified as an important mediating influence.

As a final comment on the papers in this section, a clear theme runs through their presentations. Global generalizations may be useful as preliminary guidelines for the clinician, but the assessment and treatment of a child suffering from stress or trauma or a specific disorder requires an approach that takes into account the specific characteristics and life experiences of that individual child. The danger is always that a fixed generalization will be applied in the same manner to all children, and in the process ignore or misinterpret the special issues and needs of any one specific youngster.

30

Epidemiology of Child Psychiatric Disorder: Methodological Issues and Some Substantive Findings

Michael Rutter and Seija Sandberg

Department of Child and Adolescent Psychiatry
Institute of Psychiatry, London

Key conceptual and substantive issues in child psychiatric epidemiology are reviewed using mainly European studies in terms of methodological problems and causal mechanisms. Attention is paid to issues in the measurement and categorization of disorder, case definition, case identification and classification. Research into causal processes is discussed in relation to organic brain dysfunction, temperamental risk, parental mental disorder and stress associated with multiple hospital admission.

Over the last decade, there has been a major burgeoning of interest within child psychiatry in the use of epidemiological strategies as research tools. This growing appreciation of the wide ranging uses to which epidemiological data may be put has been reflected in a series of systematic reviews[1,2,3,4,5,6,7,8] and two volumes on epidemiological approaches in child psychiatry[9,10] as well as a variety of methodological critiques[11,12,13,14,15] and a host of reports of individual epidemiological studies. In this paper, we make no attempt to cover the whole of this very large field of ideas and

---

Reprinted with permission from *Child Psychiatry and Human Development*, 1985, Vol. 15, 209–233. Copyright 1985 by Human Sciences Press.

empirical findings; rather (using mainly European studies) we selectively focus on a few of the key, conceptual and substantive issues that represent some of the current major points of discussion in child psychiatric epidemiology. In doing so, we highlight the variety of ways in which epidemiological approaches can contribute to knowledge—theoretical, clinical and policy-oriented.

METHODOLOGICAL ISSUES

Epidemiology comprises the study of the distribution of disorders in a defined population, together with an examination of the factors that influence that distribution. Usually, but not always, the defined population is some portion of the general population living in the community. Also, in most cases, 'disorder' is defined in terms of some set of operational criteria rather than in terms of hospital or clinic attendance. Hence, the people said to have disorders are not referred patients. Not surprisingly, therefore, there has been much debate on how to decide who is a 'case' (i.e. a person with a disorder); on how to measure disorder (or 'caseness' to use the awkward jargon that has been introduced); and on how to classify or categorize different types of disorder.

Definition of Disorder

In Psychiatry as a whole, there has been much debate on both the conceptual and methodological issues involved in decisions concerning 'what is a case?'[16]. Thus, for example, arguments have raged over whether the high rates of depression found in inner city working class women represent a disease state or just 'demoralization' in relation to life stresses[17,18,19]. Precisely the same issues apply to the field of child psychiatric disorders, well evidenced by the disputes over the prevalence of depressive disorders in prepubertal children[20]. Sometimes, it is thought that this is a peculiarly psychiatric problem, stemming from confused concepts and a lack of etiological knowledge; but that is not so. The same dilemmas apply to traditional medical diseases[21,22] where there are both 'cut-off' and 'categorical versus dimensional' problems. Thus, should tuberculosis be defined in terms of an immunological response to a tuberculin test even when there are no signs or symptoms or illness, or should 'caseness' require impaired function together with isolation of mycobacteria? Of course, the answer will depend on the purpose—as it does in psychiatry. Similarly, even with indubitable disease states, dimensional approaches may be preferred over categorical distinctions in some circumstances. Scadding[22] gives the example from respiratory diseases in which the evidence from prospective studies shows that separate quantitative estimates of bronchial catarrh and of airflow limitations are better predictors than conventional disease categories such as 'chronic bronchitis' or 'emphysema'.

The lesson, however, is *not* that such decisions are arbitrary, but rather, that empirical data are required in order to provide rational solutions. Several different research approaches have been followed. These include the use of predictive validity, symptom patterning, and psychosocial correlates. Their strengths and limitations are most easily illustrated by reference to a few specific disorders.

Anorexia Nervosa

Anorexia nervosa, as present in hospital clinics, is a severe condition—indeed it is one of the very few psychiatric disorders in childhood and adolescence that carries with it a significant mortality. Yet, there are striking parallels with the psychological changes seen in normal development. Anorexia nervosa is very much commoner in girls than in boys, typically its onset is in adolescence, and it seems to have become more common in recent years[23]. But in the general population, too, severe dieting is very much an adolescent phenomenon; it also is largely seen in girls and it is characteristic that adolescent girls tend to be dissatisfied with the bodily changes of puberty (especially the increased deposition of fat), whereas boys tend to be pleased (especially with their increased height and muscularity)[24]. Is the severe dieting in 'normal' adolescent girls a form of subclinical anorexia nervosa? Abraham *et al*[25] found that some fifteen percent of young women had at some time fulfilled the criteria for anorexia or bulimia nervosa, and some seven per cent had abused laxatives or diuretics in order to lose weight. This was especially so among ballet dancers although none had engaged in the self-induced vomiting so often seen in anorexia nervosa. Garner *et al*[26] found similarly that dieting, a morbid fear of becoming fat, bodily dissatisfaction and a drive for thinness were common among college and ballet students. However, only about a third of the weight-preoccupied women showed other psychological features associated with anorexia nervosa. Szmukler and Eisler[27] found that anorexia nervosa, as diagnosed in a community survey of a ballet school, did *not* have the poor prognosis associated with hospital cases. It seems that there are both continuities and discontinuities between clinic and community cases[28].

This is, of course, a common state of affairs—as shown by the parallel with alcoholism. Factors such as the cost of alcoholic drinks are related to the per capita annual consumption of alcohol, which in turn is related to various indices of alcoholism and alcohol-related diseases[29]. In other words, variables that influence drinking levels in normal individuals also influence rates of alcoholism—an important form of continuity. On the other hand, it appears that there may be genetic factors that apply to some forms of alcoholism but that do not determine individual differences in drinking levels in the general population[30,31]. It may be that the same applies to anorexia nervosa. The answer to the question of case definition in anorexia nervosa, as in so many other psychiatric disorders, does not lie in any setting of arbitrary criteria, but rather, it requires a specific research focus on the 'grey' area of severe dieting and weight preoccupation seen in community surveys that fall short of the gross impairments of hospital in-patient treated anorexia nervosa.

Emotional and Conduct Disorders

Comparable issues arise regarding case definition with the much commoner emotional and conduct disorders that make up the bulk of child psychiatric clinical practice. When does 'normal' rebelliousness, aggression, and petty delinquent behavior become a psychiatrically significant 'conduct disorder'? What is the distinction between 'ordinary' misery and fearfulness and the psychiatric conditions characterized by depression and anxiety? The British epidemiological studies such as the Isle of Wight enquiry[32] and the London surveys of preschool[33] and schoolage children[34,35] have tended to define disorders in terms of indices of persistence and social impairment. By restricting the category of disorder to problems that had been sufficiently marked to interfere with social functioning over a period of at least some months, it was hoped to identify clinically significant conditions. The validity of this assumption was tested mainly in two ways. Firstly, 4 to 5 year follow-up studies[29,33] showed a high level of persistence—especially for conduct disorders. The finding was perhaps particularly striking in the case of the preschool problems because many people had tended to assume that these were a normal part of growing up—transient difficulties that would pass as the children grew older. Accordingly, the high level of disorder at age eight years for the children who showed problems at age three years indicated that this general presumption of transience was incorrect. Secondly, the correlates of disorder as found in these community studies were shown to be closely comparable to those found in clinic series. Thus, psychiatric disorders were more frequent in children with general or specific cognitive disabilities (such as language delay or reading difficulties), in those whose parents had a mental disorder, and in those from discordant, quarrelsome homes. It may be concluded that the prevalence rates of five to ten per cent for child psychiatric disorders do indeed refer to clinically significant conditions.

That conclusion, of course, refers to persistent, socially handicapping problems. The same epidemiological data were useful in further delineating some of the criteria that pointed to the likelihood of a problem being a significant one[7,36,37]. First, the pattern of symptomatology was relevant. Some features, such as poor peer relationships and hyperactivity/inattention, are not only strongly associated with other indicators of psychopathology, but also relate to a worse prognosis. Other features, such as nailbiting and thumbsucking, proved to be of little psychiatric import. Secondly, in general, disorders that are pervasive over situations tend to be more persistent over time. Many childhood problems are largely situation-specific; these may be quite severe and incapacitating at the time, but on the whole, they reflect maladaptive patterns of interpersonal interaction and they respond to changes in such patterns. It is evident that knowledge regarding the situational-specificities in children's problems may have important implications for therapeutic interventions. Nevertheless, it should be noted that child psychiatric disorders associated with severe environmental stressors (such as parental mental disorder or family discord) frequently do generalize across situations and often persist over time[38,39,40]. Thirdly, disorders associated with a wide range of emotional or behavioral difficulties tend to have a worse outcome than those associated with a single 'symptom' or a narrow range of problems. Indeed, isolated transient emotional or conduct problems are very common in normal children; on their own, such problems usually have little clinical significance. Fourthly, on the whole, problems that are out of keeping with normal developmental trends usually have a worse outcome than those that constitute exaggerations of age-appropriate phenomena. Thus, delinquent activities tend to peak in adolescence; delinquency that begins in early or middle childhood is more likely to be associated with recidivism. Conversely, separation anxiety is normal in preschoolers, and exaggerations of this in the form of elective mutism or school refusal about the time of school entry tend to have a good prognosis. Similar problems arising later in childhood are more likely to be persistent and to be associated with generalized psychosocial malfunction. It seems that it is not early or late onset *per se* that matters most, but rather, the developmental inappropriateness of the problems.

It is clear from this brief summary of some of the key epidemiological findings that the data that have been most useful in providing answers to the methodological problem of case definition have also been most informative in clarifying clinical issues. It should also be noted, however, that much of the pay-off has come from the combination of epidemiological and longitudinal research strategies[7].

IDENTIFICATION OF CASES: MEASUREMENT AND SAMPLING

A further methodological issue concerns the steps taken to identify cases; an issue that involves both sampling and measurement. Several quite different research strategies have been employed; each being better adapted for some purposes than others.

Administrative Statistics

Administrative statistics are of very limited value for most epidemiological purposes in child psychiatry, but the statistics on suicide provide an important exception[41]. They have been highly consistent in showing a very dramatic increase in suicide rate across the adolescent age period—with scarcely any suicides under the age of ten years and an increase of several hundred fold between ten and twenty years. These data, combined with comparable (although lesser) increases in parasuicide and in depressive disorders over the same age period,[42] point to the crucial importance of developmental factors in relation to affective disorders.

The reasons for these age changes have yet to be identified. It could be that biological vulnerabilities to depression and mania increase sharply during the teenage years, or that environmental stressors increase over the same age period, or that there are protective factors in childhood that decrease in salience or prevalence during adolescence, or that children's cognitive capacities to experience depression become well developed only after middle childhood. In these cases, as in others, epidemiological data have been crucial in identifying the issue; but other research strategies are needed in order to delineate the causal mechanisms involved.

Hospital/Clinic Data

Because so many children with a psychiatric disorder do not receive hospital care, hospital or clinic data are also of very limited use for epidemiological purposes. However, there are some examples in which the severity of a disorder makes it very likely that the child will have come into contact with some form of services. This applies, for example, to infantile autism. Accordingly, it is possible to obtain a nearly complete tally of all cases of autism through a systematic coverage of all possibly relevant services. However, there are two crucial methodological points. First it would *not* be acceptable to pool all hospital statistics on cases of autism. This is because it is common for children with autism to attend *several* different facilities. A pooling of statistics will lead to counting some children more than once; rather, an unduplicated count is essential. Necessarily, this requires either an entirely reliable system of records linkage (as by means of a psychiatric register—see[43]) or a case by case survey of individual children's records at each hospital or clinic. Secondly, the survey could not be restricted meaningfully to psychiatric clinics or even to hospital services because many autistic children see pediatricians rather than psychiatrists, and because others are dealt with by special schools without direct medical involvement. A comprehensive survey of all relevant services, medical and non-medical, is required.

Given that there has been an unduplicated count of cases derived from a systematic coverage of services, reasonably reliable figures for autism can be obtained. It might be thought that, apart from a prevalence estimate, such epidemiological data would add little to hospital studies if nearly all autistic children attend clinics. However, that is not the case for several different reasons. Most particularly, different clinical facilities are likely to see somewhat different distributions of cases because of both rational and irrational referral biases. In addition, however, epidemiological data facilitate certain sorts of comparisons with other diagnostic groups that may largely attend different services. For example, such data have been important in showing that autistic children differ markedly from non-autistic, mentally retarded children in terms of the high frequency with which epileptic seizures develop in adolescence rather than early childhood[44], but that they differ little from normal children with respect to maternal infections during the pregnancy[45], apart from congenital rubella[46].

Epidemiological data derived from studies of mentally retarded children have also highlighted a rather different sort of issue—namely that many severely retarded children show some features of autism, although not the full syndrome[47]. The finding raises the question as to whether these 'partial' syndromes differ in degree or in kind from 'classical' cases of autism. It may be that family-genetic data will provide an answer to that question, but, so far, no satisfactory answer is available.

QUESTIONNAIRE SURVEYS

For the most part, questionnaires on their own are of limited use for case identification because they cannot give the kind of detailed information needed for psychiatric diagnosis. However, they may be adequate when dealing with single items of behavior that are of significance even when they occur in isolation. For instance, this applied to nocturnal enuresis. There are uncertainties as to whether this should be considered as a syndrome in any sense, but unquestionably, it constitutes a persistent and handicapping behavior that commonly is unassociated with other forms of psychiatric disturbance[48].

Epidemiological/longitudinal data have been vital in the identification of three crucial phenomena. Firstly, the spontaneous remission rate over the next 12 months drops markedly about age four years—from 40% at age two to 20% at three to 6% afterwards. This suggests that 'pathological' varieties of enuresis are largely to be found over the age of four years. Secondly, there is an *increase* in the rate of enuresis between the ages of five and seven years[49], emphasizing that enuresis cannot be considered just as a delay in the developmental acquisition of a particular 'skill'; children can gain bladder control and then lose it. Thirdly, epidemiological data show that although most enuretics do not show any significant emotional or behavioral disturbance, nevertheless, there is a significant association between enuresis and psychiatric disorder. The meaning of this association remains rather obscure, but it constitutes an aspect of enuresis that requires further investigation.

One of the reasons that questionnaires on their own are of limited value for case identification is that the information provided is necessarily rather crude and also reliant on the perceptions of raters who may not have the skills required to make crucial behavioral distinctions. However, further limitations stem from situational specificity, from less than perfect reliability, and from the high frequency of transient emotional/behavioral disturbances—factors that are general in the assessment of individual behavioral characteristics[50]. Several solutions have been adopted. Thus, attention may be confined to questionnaire scores that are deviant in at least two situations (usually home and school)—an approach that has paid off in the study of hyperactivity (see below). Alternatively, or in addition, cases may be defined in terms of scores that remain deviant on a second questionnaire completion a couple of months after the first occasion[51]. Finally, if there are longitudinal as well as epidemiological data, there may be a focus on children who show deviant scores on a majority of ratings made over the course of several years[40,52]. These various approaches all emphasize the general epidemiological finding that transient emotional or behavioral difficulties are very common in childhood, but that pervasive and persistent difficulties are likely to be of much greater psychiatric significance.

Two Stage Interview Surveys

The most common approach in British child psychiatric epidemiological studies has been a two stage inquiry with questionnaire screening of the total population in the first stage, and in the second stage, detailed interviewing of high risk groups identified on the basis of questionnaire scores. The procedure works well for most types of disorder, but it is important to recognize that it relies on several assumptions. Firstly, it assumes that all cases will be picked up by one or other of the screening questionnaires. It is essential that this assumption be tested through inclusion of a random sample in the second intensive stage of the study—in order to calculate the proportion of cases missed. All studies have shown the importance of multiple sources of data. For pre-adolescent children the combination of parent and teacher questionnaires has proved reasonably satisfactory. However, in adolescence it has been found that there is a substantial proportion of (mainly depressive) disorders that are missed by parents and teachers, and hence, require the completion of questionnaires by the young people themselves[53]. Peer group ratings may also be helpful for picking out socially rejected children with psychiatric problems[54]. Secondly, it assumes that high scores, reflecting many different types of difficulties, adequately tap all forms of possible psychiatric disturbance. While that has been shown empirically to be the case in most instances, it follows that such general purpose questionnaires will not be satisfactory for the detection of monosymptomatic disorders—such as enuresis. Also, they may not be very satisfactory for conditions involving symptoms that are relatively rare (and not likely to be included in the screening questionnaire). Hence, this approach is less likely to be effective for the detection of obsessive-compulsive disorders or conversion hysteria. Of course, more focused questionnaires can be devised for these purposes, as they have for the detection of anorexia nervosa[28].

Having used the screening instruments to pick out high risk groups (plus randomly selected controls), the fuller, more detailed interview assessments can be employed more economically with smaller numbers. The approach at this second stage more closely resembles that employed in the clinical setting in its reliance on systematic interviewing; it differs primarily in the need to use standardized interview methods and standardized approaches to coding and diagnosis in order to insure that the data are directly comparable from case to case. At one time, it was assumed that only very indirect, projective play methods could be used to elicit information from the children themselves. However, it has been well demonstrated that direct questioning is both possible and productive with schoolage children; although, there are constraints in young children's abilities to conceptualize and report both emotions and behaviors[55]. Accordingly, this second intensive stage would ordinarily include separate standardized interviews with children and with their parents—possibly supplemented with teacher interviews.

The main alternative to the two stage approach is to utilize a highly structured, questionnaire type interview that can be given by lay interviewers to the whole of the population to be studied (and not just screened high risk groups). Ordinarily, it would be prohibitively expensive to use clinicians on such a large scale; hence, the need to devise a more mechanical interview that does not rely on clinical skills. Such interviews can be devised and have proved satisfactorily reliable for many purposes—although not for the detection of depressive states[56]. However, they give rise to a large number of symptom codings rather than any overall clinical diagnosis. Diagnoses then have to be derived mechanically according to the presence of particular sets of symptoms. The practical consequence of this approach is that each case tends to receive multiple diagnoses because mixed clinical pictures are so very common.

Diagnosis and Classification

This point raises the issue of what should be the 'correct' approach to diagnosis in epidemiological studies. Broadly speaking, four main solutions are possible. Firstly, categorical distinctions can be avoided through the use of dimensions of one kind or another. Thus, epidemiological methods can be used to produce population distributions on extent of delinquent activities (see[37]) or on neuroticism or IQ. These dimensions will be considered separately so that the score on one will not influence the coding on another. Nevertheless, it is often convenient to introduce categorical distinctions into dimensional measurements. For example, IQ is measured in dimensional terms, but for clinical and service-planning purposes, it is usually convenient to subdivide mentally handicapped groups into mild (IQ 50-69) and severe (IQ below 50), as these differ so markedly in both biopsychosocial characteristics and in service requirements (see [57]).

Secondly, as noted above, symptom constellations can be used to derive multiple overlapping diagnoses. Thus, a child may show an attention deficit disorder, a conduct disorder and a major depressive disorder—not an uncommon occurrence with this approach to diagnosis which deals with conditions simply in terms of symptom constellations—an approach that is reflected both in the highly structured questionnaire type interviews and in the American Psychiatric Association[58] DSM-III classification. The approach has the merit of recognizing the frequency of mixed symptom patterns, but it is not at all clear what concept of disorder is being employed if it is usual for children to have several different disorders simultaneously. Moreover, the sheer complexity of describing multiple, overlapping diagnoses means that usually epidemiological data are reported only in terms of the one that constitutes the source of main interest to the investigator. This means that it is quite difficult to know whether the findings mainly concern, for example, the depressive disorders reported or whether they largely stem from the conduct disorders also present but not reported.

Thirdly, the more traditional medical approach can be employed in which there is a prior decision as to whether the child has any disorder and then, if he has, the clinician has to decide which it is. In essence, there has to be a decision as to whether the signs and symptoms indicate measles or scarlet fever, major depression or an attention deficit disorder. Of course, it is possible for someone to have two quite distinct diseases at the same time, but it is expected that this will be the exception rather than the rule. It is accepted that there may be mixed symptom patterns, but it is assumed that they represent different facets of one underlying disorder; it is up to the clinician to decide which diagnosis best fits the clinical picture. The main drawback of this approach is that in many cases, the data needed to decide how to give precedence to one diagnosis over another are lacking. On the other hand, the explicit recognition of this problem has led to the direct use of epidemiological data to test alternative hypotheses on classificatory approaches.

For example, this has been the case with the British research into the attention deficit/hyperactivity syndrome and its major overlap with disturbances of conduct. Both clinical[59] and epidemiological[60] studies showed that there were no substantial differences in familial or neurodevelopmental correlates between conduct disordered boys with and without hyperactivity as assessed on parent or teacher questionnaires. Nevertheless, factor analytic studies show that there is a constellation of overactivity/inattention behaviors that is distinct from antisocial problems[61]. Moreover, that constellation is of some prognostic significance[62].

The question is whether or not it is helpful to consider it as a separate syndrome (rather than as a behavioral dimension). The patient sample data suggested that the small group of boys with pervasive hyperactivity/inattention at home, school and as observed at the clinic did differ from the rest in important ways. Epidemiological/longitudinal data from the Isle of Wight studies[63] confirmed the clinical significance of *pervasive* hyperactivity/inattention in terms of its association with cognitive defects and with a worse prognosis. The linkage between pervasive hyperactivity/inattention and cognitive problems has recently been confirmed in an epidemiological study in Quebec[51]. Thus, the epidemiological data suggest that the presence of situational hyperactivity/inattention is of little clinical significance, but that the rarer syndrome of pervasive hyperactivity/inattention may constitute a valid diagnostic entity that differs from the broad run of conduct disturbances[64,65]. The better response to stimulant drugs shown by this rarer subgroup also serves to differentiate it[66].

The fourth approach to diagnosis and classification adopts the same model as that just described with one important difference—namely the use of multiple axes. This approach is distinctive in terms of its explicit recognition that diagnosis may involve several, conceptually distinct elements each of which need to be separately classified (see[57]). Thus, the psychiatric syndrome axis is separate from the intellectual level axis—reflecting the fact that the two are not only conceptually distinct, but also, that it is inherently foolish to force a false choice between, say, autism and mental handicap when both may be present. It is also clear that this multiaxial approach fits well with clinical practice and is readily adaptable for epidemiological purposes, although the details of the axes may need to be modified.

CAUSAL MECHANISMS

In the introduction, the point was made that epidemiology made use of the study of factors that are associated with variations in the distribution of disorders. Such data are, of course, essential for the planning of services, but they also may be employed to examine causal hypotheses (see[14]). In this latter section of the chapter, we examine the application of epidemiological/longitudinal data to the study of causal processes in relation to four rather different factors: organic brain dysfunction, temperamental risk factors, parental mental disorder and the stresses associated with hospital admission.

Organic Brain Dysfunction

The Isle of Wight studies[32,67] used the total population epidemiological approach for the study of associations between organic brain pathology and psychiatric disorder. The entire child population aged 9 to 12 years was screened using sets of instruments designed to detect a) neuro-epileptic disorders, b) other forms of chronic physical disability (such as asthma, heart disease and diabetes), and c) psychiatric problems. Children for whom the screening instruments suggested possible disorder in any of the three categories were then seen for individual diagnostic assessment—using separate parent and child interviews, pediatric examination, and neurodevelopmental examination. In this way, it was possible both to provide a total count of the three varieties of disorder, and also to examine the overlap between them. The findings showed that the rate of psychiatric disorder was slightly raised in the other chronic physical disability group but greatly increased in the neuro-epileptic group. The difference in psychiatric risk between the two suggested that the main risk arose from the presence of organic brain dysfunction *per se* rather than from non-specific physical disabilities. However, before drawing that causal inference, it was essential to rule out other possibilities stemming from difference between the groups other than the presence of organic brain pathology. Two possibilities stood out. First, the neuroepileptic group were of substantially lower IQ and the cognitive impairment might have constituted the main vulnerability factor. Accordingly, the groups were equated for IQ by excluding all children with neuroepileptic disorders who had an IQ below 80[68]. This reduced the between group difference, but psychiatric disorder was still twice as common in the neuroepileptic group—suggesting that organic brain pathology constituted a specific psychiatric risk factor.

The second possibility was that the psychiatric risk stemmed from visible physical crippling—a feature that was much more frequent in the neuroepileptic group. In order to test that hypothesis adequately, it was necessary to turn to another study population—namely one in which all children had physical crippling, in some cases due to organic brain pathology and in some cases due to neurological lesions below the brain stem—such as poliomyelitis or muscular dystrophy[69]. The design relied on the epidemiological strategy of contrasting high risk groups that differed in terms of the key variable hypothesized as causal, but that were otherwise comparable. The findings showed that psychiatric problems were twice as frequent in the organic brain pathology group.

The pattern of results across studies was consistent in supporting the causal hypothesis, but the causal inference necessarily relied on cross-sectional associations. In science as a whole, it is always desirable to follow such correlational findings with an experimental approach in which *changes* in the hypothesized causal variable can be related to *changes* in the dependent variable. The epidemiologist seeks the 'natural experiment' in which these changes occur in the community, and in which the consequences can be studied longitudinally. Severe head injuries constitute just such a natural experiment of acquired brain damage. Accordingly, systematic coverage of neurosurgical units was obtained in order to collect a complete sample of such injuries (with a post-traumatic amnesia lasting a week or longer). Comparison was made with a group suffering orthopedic injuries that did not involve loss of consciousness or damage to the head, both groups being followed over a 2¼ year period[70]. The findings showed that there was a marked increase in the rate of psychiatric disorder following severe head injury but not after orthopedic injuries. The 'natural experiment' confirmed the causal hypothesis that organic brain pathology substantially increased the risk of psychiatric disorder in childhood.

Two main questions follow. First, does organic brain pathology lead directly to a specific type of psychiatric disorder, or rather are the effects indirect as a result of a generally increased vulnerability? The findings are consistent in suggesting that the latter explanation (of indirect effects) is more usually correct[68]. Of course, occasionally, organic brain dysfunction leads to distinctive organic psychiatric syndromes such as confusional states[71], but in the great majority of cases, it leads to a mixture of emotional and behavioral disorders that do not differ in form from those that are *not* due to brain injury. Moreover, even in brain damaged children, psychosocial factors play an important role in the etiology of psychiatric problems.

'Minimal Brain Dysfunction'

The second question stems from the epidemiological finding that although brain damage greatly increases the psychiatric risk, only a tiny minority of psychiatric disorders are associated with overt organic brain pathology. Hence, the question arises as to whether a higher proportion of psychiatric problems may be a consequence of minimal brain dysfunction (MBD) and, if so, whether there is a distinctive, diagnosable MBD syndrome[72]. Epidemiological studies have tackled this question with at least five different strategies. First, within samples of children with indubitable gross brain injury, there has been investigation of whether the psychiatric risk is increased in children without abnormalities on a clinical neurological examination; the results showed that it was[70]. Second, in studies that have examined associations between neurological 'soft signs' and psychiatric disorder[73,74] substantial associations have been found. Unfortunately, the meaning of this important finding remains unclear in the absence of firm knowledge regarding what it is that 'soft signs' measure[75]. Epidemiological data have shown extremely weak links between perinatal complications and soft signs[76], and it is most dubious that soft signs reflect brain damage, although they may reflect some constitutional feature.

Third, epidemiological investigations have examined the extent to which different indices of cerebral dysfunction overlap together with their associations with psychiatric disorder. Thus, Schmidt *et al*[77] studied 400 eight year old children with a battery of tests of neurological impairment (such as dysdiadokokinesis and choreoathetoid movements), of EEG features (such as retardation in the theta rhythm), of neurodevelopmental features (e.g. visuomotor coordination), and of specific cognitive deficits (as in language or visuospatial skills). Low correlations between these measures were found suggesting that there is no *one* syndrome of cerebral dysfunction. Thirteen per cent of eight year olds showed abnormality on one or other of the indices; of these, nearly two-fifths showed psychiatric disorder—a rate four times that in the rest of the population. Expressed another way, a quarter of the children with psychiatric disorder showed 'cerebral dysfunction' compared with five per cent of the remainder. However, it is important that the psychiatric association was largely accounted for by the neuropsychological measures rather than by the neurological or EEG measures; moreover, psychiatric disorder showed a stronger association with measures of psychosocial adversity, and 'cerebral dysfunction' was not significantly related either to historical indices of possible brain damage or to a specific behavioral pattern.

Fourth, Gillberg[78] used an epidemiological approach to obtain a sample of six year olds with problems in 'motor control, perception, conceptualization, and attention/behavior', in which MBD was diagnosed on the basis of the combination of attentional deficits with the other disabilities. In this approach, the diagnosis of MBD combines the independent and dependent variables to be studied—in other words the definition of MBD includes both neurodevelopmental variables (such as poor motor control) and behavioral variables (such as attention deficits) that may be conceptualized as psychiatric and which have no necessary neurological basis. Not surprisingly, therefore, MBD was found to be associated with psychiatric disorder. However, the results also showed that within the MBD group, psychosocial adversity was the variable most strongly associated with psychiatric disorder.

The fifth approach, adopted by Shen and her colleagues[79,80], is to define the MBD syndrome in behavioral terms, to obtain an epidemiological sample of children with this behavioral syndrome, and then to determine whether the syndrome is associated with organic or psychosocial risk factors. Their results from a study of three communities in mainland China showed a 3 to 8% prevalence rate for MBD. The children with MBD differed from controls in having a somewhat increased rate of organic risk factors but a much increased rate of psychosocial risk factors. It seems that behaviorally defined MBD syndromes do not coincide with organically determined psychiatric disorders.

The overall conclusion with respect to minor neurological dysfunction is that probably it does give rise to an appreciably increased psychiatric risk, but it does not lead to a homogeneous behaviorally recognizable syndrome.

Temperamental Risk Factors

Numerous studies of various specialized samples have shown associations between temperamental risk factors and psychiatric disorder[81]. These same studies have been important in delineating the various mechanisms by which temperamental adversity might give rise to a psychiatric vulnerability. Thus, for example, it is evident that temperamentally difficult children tend to elicit negative reactions from their caregivers[82]. In this way, characteristics that are in part genetically determined may serve to create environments that are maladaptive in their effects[83]. However, it is only recently that the psychiatric risks associated with temperamental features have been studied epidemiologically in general population samples. Maziade *et al*[84] surveyed a thousand seven year old children in Quebec, Canada using the Thomas, Chess and Korn temperament questionnaire completed by parents. Some 12% of boys but only 6% of girls showed a 'difficult' temperament defined in terms of a constellation of low adaptability, withdrawal from new stimuli, intense emotional reactions, negative mood and low distractibility. It was striking that the sex differences for this constellation of temperamental features were greater than for individual features considered in isolation. The finding emphasizes the potential value of composite indices and also suggests that temperamental differences between boys and girls may play a part in the greater psychiatric vulnerability of boys.

The role of temperament in psychiatric vulnerability was tested empirically by taking 24 subjects with high scores ($\leq$70th percentile) on at least four of the five 'difficult' dimensions on *both* of two administrations of the questionnaire four weeks apart[85]. The requirement of deviant scores on both occasions was an important methodological step in increasing reliability of identification of a temperamental group hypothesized to be at high risk. This group was compared with 15 children similarly defined with easy temperament. Follow-up four years later at age 12 was undertaken 'blind' to the temperamental designation. Half of the temperamentally difficult children showed a psychiatric disorder compared with only 1 in 15 of those with easy temperaments—a highly significant difference. There was an additive risk effect from the combination of a dysfunctional family and temperamental adversity, and *superior* family functioning largely mitigated the effects of a difficult temperament. Thus, the epidemiological findings both confirmed the reality of the psychiatric risk associated with a difficult temperament and also supported the suggestion that such a temperament did not lead directly to disorder; rather, it was necessary to take into account the interactions between the child and his family.

Parental Mental Disorder

Several, quite different issues arise with respect to the hypothesized effect by which parental mental illness predisposes to psychiatric disorder in the children. First, it is necessary to rule out the possibility that the association stems from a referral artifact. Numerous clinical studies have noted the link between psychiatric disturbances in parents and their children[86], and the same has been evident in epidemiological studies based on general practice records[87]. In both cases, it is possible that the association stemmed from a tendency for mentally ill parents to be more likely to seek psychiatric aid for their children. This artifact could be dealt with by using direct measures of psychiatric disability (rather than relying on indices of clinic attendance) in relation to epidemiological samples of either psychiatrically disturbed parents (see[40,88,89]) or of children with psychiatric disorder (see[33,34]). The findings from both strategies indicate that the association is real and *not* due to a referral artifact.

The second question concerns the extent to which the psychiatric risk to the children stems from parental mental illness *per se* rather than from factors with which it is associated. The particular need to ask the question arises from the observed frequency with which psychiatric disorder in adults is accompanied by non-illness features, such as marital discord and family disruption which also put the children at risk. This issue may be tackled by comparing rates of psychiatric disorder in epidemiologically based samples of children of mentally ill parents with community samples of children after matching for these other risk factors. Rutter and Quinton[40] found that when this was done, the children of ill parents no longer showed any increase in emotional/behavioral disturbance. Within *both* samples, psychiatric disorder in the children was most frequent when there was a combination of different family adversities. It may be concluded that, for the most part, parental mental disorder does not give rise to an increased risk for the children that is independent of the family's psychosocial circumstances as a whole.

That conclusion raises the further question of just *which* are the key features associated with parental mental disorder that must put the children at risk. The question is highlighted by the universal observation that many of the children of ill parents do *not* develop psychiatric problems. The issue requires a within-group analysis of families of ill parents comparing those in which the children do and those in which the children do not show psychiatric disturbance. Using this research strategy, Rutter and Quinton[40] found that family discord and parental aggression/hostility constituted the most powerful risk factor.

The fourth query is whether this mechanism applies similarly to all forms of parental mental illness and to all types of psychiatric sequelae in the children. So far, there are rather few studies that have examined that issue. Nevertheless, such data as there are suggests the likelihood that several different risk processes are operative. Thus, Emery *et al*[90] found that the presence of discord did not account for the risk to the children of schizophrenics. Also, Weissman *et al's*[89] findings suggest that there may be some specific association between depression in the parent and depression in the children. The matter warrants further study.

The last issue concerns the role of the children: to what extent do the children's disturbances predispose to or aggravate psychiatric problems in their parents? That question, too, has been little investigated up to now. It is not likely that child effects account for the overall association, if only because epidemiological/longitudinal data show that the presence of family discord when the children are very young is associated with the *later* development of psychiatric disorders in the offspring[33]. Nevertheless, it seems that children with a difficult temperament tend to elicit negative behavior from their parents[40], and it is probable that two-way interactions occur in some instances. That possibility requires investigation.

Acute Stressors: Hospital Admission

The last hypothesized causal process to consider, namely the stresses associated with hospital admission, raises both similar and different issues. As with the other variables discussed, the first question concerns the reality of the association between the supposed risk factor and psychiatric disorder in the children. Douglas[91] used longitudinal data from the epidemiologically based British National Survey to examine the matter. The findings showed that children who experienced multiple hospital admissions in which the first admission occurred before five years of age had a significantly increased rate of later emotional/behavioral problems; however, there was no increased risk associated with a single admission lasting less than a week. The key issue that followed was whether the risk stemmed from the admissions *per se* or rather from the physical illness or social circumstances that led to recurrent hospitalization (because children suffering repeated admission to hospital are unlikely to be ordinary members of the general population). Quinton and Rutter[92] using data from two local epidemiological studies showed that part of the risk stemmed from chronic family adversity (such adversity being associated with a higher likelihood of repeated admission); nevertheless, it seemed that part of the risk stemmed from the admission experiences.

The third point stems from the finding in both studies that whereas two admissions increased the psychiatric risk, one admission did not do so at all. The implication is that the first admission may have served in some way to sensitize the children so that they were more likely to react adversely next time, a possibility that arises more generally in relation to people's responses to acute stressors[93]. The sensitization process could involve either altered patterns of parent-child interaction (a feature of the stresses associated with the birth of a sibling—[94]) or some aspect of the child's own perception of and response to hospital admission. A further query concerns the aspects of hospital admission that create the risk, an important issue, as it is clear that both better preparation of children for admission and improved conditions during admission can reduce acute distress reactions[95]. Have improved patterns of paediatric care in recent years significantly reduced the psychiatric risks to the children? The data from the Christchurch (New Zealand) epidemiological/longitudinal study[96] suggest that this may have occurred.

Neither of these last two issues (the hypothesized sensitization process and the risk aspects of hospital admission) has been subjected to much vigorous scrutiny up to now. However, as with so many questions, it is clear that research strategies other than epidemiology will be required to provide a satisfactory answer. Epidemiological studies can go far in delineating possible causal processes but usually some form of experiment, natural or contrived, will be needed to put the causal hypothesis to the crucial test.

CONCLUSION

Traditionally, epidemiological studies have been used most frequently to obtain estimates of the prevalence of particular disorders. In this brief overview of some aspects of epidemiological research in the field of child psychiatry, we have paid little attention to questions of prevalence as these have been well discussed in previous reviews of the topic. Instead, we have focused on some of the key methodological issues that apply to any use of epidemiological data in the field of child psychiatry, and have then gone on to discuss the way such data may be used to tackle the testing of causal hypothesis. It is evident from the four examples of risk factors we have chosen—organic brain dysfunction, 'difficult' temperament features, parental mental disorders and the stresses associated with recurrent hospital admission—that considerable progress has been made in the delineation of the ways in which such risk processes operate. Equally, however, it has been clear that many questions remain to be answered and that their answering requires both the imaginative application of epidemiological techniques and also the employment of other research strategies, especially the intensive study of carefully chosen, small groups and the investigation of the effects of interventions designed to alter the risk features.

REFERENCES

1. Earls, F.: Epidemiological child psychiatry: An American perspective. In Purcell, E. F. (Ed), *Psychopathology of Children and Youth: A Cross-Cultural Perspective.* New York: Macy Foundation, 1980.
2. Earls, F.: Epidemiology and child psychiatry: future prospects. *Comprehensive Psychiatry,* 23:75-84, 1982.
3. Gould, M. S., Wunsch-Hitzig, R. and Dohrenwend, B. P.: Formulation of hypotheses about the prevalence, treatment and prognostic significance of psychiatric disorders in children in the United States. In Dohrenwend, B. P., Dohrenwend, B. S., Gould, M. S., Link, B., Neugebauer, R., and Wunsch-Hitzig, R. *Mental Illness in the United States: Epidemiological estimates.* New York: Praeger, 1980.

4. Graham, P. J.: Epidemiological studies. In Quay, H. C. and Werry, J. S. (Eds) *Psychopathological Disorders of Childhood (2nd edition)* New York: Wiley, 1979.
5. Graham, P. J.: Epidemiological approaches to child mental health in developing countries. In Purcell, E. F. (Ed), *Psychopathology of Children and Youth: A Cross-Cultural Perspective* New York: Macy Foundation, 1980.
6. Links, P. S.: Community surveys of the prevalence of childhood psychiatric disorders: a review. *Child Development, 54*:531-548, 1983.
7. Rutter, M.: Epidemiological-longitudinal approaches to the study of development. In Collins, W. A. (Ed) *The Concept of Development* The Minnesota Symposia on Child Psychology, Hillsdale, New Jersey: Lawrence Erlbaum, 1982.
8. Yule, W.: The epidemiology of child psychopathology. In Lahey, B. B. and Kazdin, A. E. (Eds) *Advances in Clinical Child Psychology, Vol. 4*. New York: Plenum, 1981.
9. Graham, P. J. (Ed): *Epidemiological Approaches in Child Psychiatry*. London & New York: Academic Press, 1977.
10. Schmidt, M. H. and Remschmidt, H. (Eds): *Epidemiological Approaches in Child Psychiatry II*. Stuttgart: Verlag; New York: Thieme-Stratton, 1983.
11. Gould, M. S., Wunsch-Hitzig, R. and Dohrenwend, B.: Estimating the prevalence of childhood psychopathology: a critical review. *Journal of the American Academy of Child Psychiatry, 20*:462-476, 1981.
12. Rutter, M.: Epidemiological strategies and psychiatric concepts in research on the vulnerable child. In Anthony, E. and Koupernik, C. (Eds), *The Child in His Family: Children at Psychiatric Risk, Vol. 3* New York: Wiley, 1974.
13. Rutter, M.: Surveys to answer questions. In Graham, P. J. (Ed) *The Epidemiological Approaches in Child Psychiatry* London and New York: Academic Press, 1977.
14. Rutter, M.: Epidemiological/longitudinal strategies and causal result in child psychiatry. *Journal of the American Academy of Child Psychiatry, 20*:513-544, 1981.
15. Stein, Z. and Susser, M.: Methods in epidemiology. *Journal of the American Academy of Child Psychiatry, 20*:444-461, 1981.
16. Wing, J. K., Bebbington, P. and Robins, L. N. (Eds): *What is a Case? The Problem of Definition in Psychiatric Community Surveys.* London: Grant McIntyre, 1981.
17. Brown, G. W. and Harris, T.: *Social Origins of Depression.* London: Tavistock Press, 1978.
18. Link, B. and Dohrenwend, B. P.: Formulation of hypotheses about the true prevalence of demoralization in the United States. In Dohrenwend, B. P., Dohrenwend, B. S., Gould, M. S., Link, B., Neugebauer, R. and Wunsch-Hitzig, R. (Eds) *Mental Illness in the United States: Epidemiological estimates* New York: Praeger, 1980.
19. Tennant, C. and Bebbington, P.: The social causation of depression: a critique of the work of Brown and his colleagues. *Psychological Medicine 8*:556-576, 1978.
20. Rutter, M.: Depressive feelings, cognitions and disorders: A research postscript. In Rutter, M., Izard, C. and Read, P. (Eds), *Depression in Young People: Developmental and Clinical Perspectives* New York: Guilford Press, (in press).
21. Scadding, J. G.: The concepts of disease: A response. *Psychological Medicine, 10*:425-428, 1980.
22. Scadding, J. G.: Book Review: *What is a Case? The Problem of Definition in Psychiatric Community Surveys.* Wing, J. K., Bebbington, P., and Robins, L. N. (Eds) London: Grant McIntyre, 1981. *Psychological Medicine, 12*, 207-208, 1982.
23. Russell, G. F. M.: Anorexia and bulimia nervosa. In Rutter, M., Hersov, L. (Eds), *Child and Adolescent Psychiatry: Modern Approaches (2nd edition)* Oxford: Blackwell Scientific, 1985.
24. Graham, P. J. and Rutter, M.: Adolescent disorders. In Rutter, M. and Hersov, L.

(Eds) *Child and Adolescent Psychiatry: Modern Approaches (2nd edition)*. Oxford: Blackwell Scientific, 1985.

25. Abraham, S. F., Mira, M., Beumont, P. J. V., Sowerbutts, T. D. and Llewellyn-Jones, D.: Eating behaviours among young women. *Medical Journal of Australia*, 2:225-228, 1983.

26. Garner, D. M., Olmsted, M. P. and Garfinkel, P. E.: Does anorexia nervosa occur on a continuum? Subgroups of weight-preoccupied women and their relationship to anorexia nervosa. *International Journal of Eating Disorders*, 2:11-20, 1983.

27. Szmukler, G. I. and Eisler, I.: Anorexia nervosa in a ballet school: problems of diagnosis. Proceedings of the International Conference on Anorexia Nervosa and Related Disorders. University College, Swansea, September 1984.

28. Szmukler, G. I.: The epidemiology of anorexia nervosa and bulimia. Proceedings of the International Conference on Anorexia Nervosa and Related Disorders. University College, Swansea, September 1984.

29. Rutter, M.: *Changing Youth in a Changing Society: Patterns of Adolescent Development and Disorder*. Nuffield Provincial Hospitals Trust, London 1979 (Cambridge, Mass.: Harvard University Press, 1980).

30. Bohman, M., Sigvardsson, S. and Cloniger, R.: Maternal inheritance of alcohol abuse: cross-fostering analysis of adopted women. *Archives of General Psychiatry*, 38:965-969, 1981.

31. Cloninger, C. R., Bohman, M. and Sigvardsson, S.: Inheritance of alcohol abuse: cross-fostering analysis of adopted men. *Archives of General Psychiatry*, 38:861-868, 1981.

32. Rutter, M., Tizard, J. and Whitmore, K. (Eds): *Education, Health and Behaviour*. London: Longmans, 1970 (Reprinted, 1981, Krieger, Huntington, New York).

33. Richman, N., Stevenson, J. and Graham, P. J.: *Pre-school to School: A Behavioural Study*. London: Academic Press, 1982.

34. Rutter, M., Cox, A., Tupling, C., Berger, M. and Yule, W.: Attainment and adjustment in two geographical areas. I. The prevalence of psychiatric disorder. *British Journal of Psychiatry*, 126:493-509, 1975.

35. Rutter, M., Yule, B., Quinton, D., Rowlands, O., Yule, W. and Berger, M.: Attainment and adjustment in two geographical areas. III. Some factors accounting for area differences. *British Journal of Psychiatry*, 126:520-533, 1975.

36. Rutter, M. and Garmezy, N.: Developmental psychopathology. In Hetherington, E. M. (Ed), *Socialization, Personality, and Social Development, Vol. IV, Mussen's Handbook of Child Psychology (4th edition)* New York: Wiley, 1983.

37. Rutter, M. and Giller, H.: *Juvenile Delinquency: Trends and Perspectives*. Harmondsworth, Middx: Penguin Books, 1983.

38. Emery, R. E.: Interparental conflict and the children of discord and divorce. *Psychological Bulletin*, 92:310-330, 1982.

39. Hetherington, E. M., Cox M. and Cox, R.: Effects of divorce on parents and children. In Lamb, M. (Ed) *Non-traditional Families* Hillsdale, New Jersey: Lawrence Erlbaum, 1982.

40. Rutter, M. and Quinton, D.: Parental psychiatric disorder: Effects on children. *Psychological Medicine 14*:853-880, 1984.

41. Shaffer, D.: Child and adolescent suicide: Developmental factors. In Rutter, M., Izard, C. and Read, P. (Eds), *Depression in Young People: Developmental and Clinical Perspectives* New York: Guilford Press, (in press), 1985.

42. Rutter, M.: The developmental psychopathology of depression. In Rutter, M., Izard,

C. and Read, P. (Eds), *Depression in Young People: Developmental and Clinical Perspectives* New York: Guilford Press, (in press), 1985.

43. Wing, J. K. and Hailey, A. M.: *Evaluating a Community Psychiatric Service: the Camberwell Register 1964-1971.* London: Oxford University Press, 1972.
44. Deykin, E. Y. and MacMahon, B.: The incidence of seizures among children with autistic symptoms. *American Journal of Psychiatry, 136*:1310-1312, 1979.
45. Deykin, E. Y. and MacMahon, B.: Viral exposure and autism. *American Journal of Epidemiology, 109*:628-638, 1979.
46. Chess, S., Fernandez, P. B. and Korn, S. J.: Behavioral consequences of congenital rubella. *Journal of Pediatrics, 93*:699-703, 1978.
47. Wing, L. and Gould, J.: Severe impairments of social interaction and associated abnormalities in children: Epidemiology and classification. *Journal of Autism and Developmental Disorders, 9*:11-30, 1979.
48. Shaffer, D.: Enuresis. In Rutter, M. and Hersov, L. (Eds), *Child and Adolescent Psychiatry: Modern Approaches (2nd edition)* Oxford: Blackwell Scientific, 1985.
49. Rutter, M., Yule, W. and Graham, P.: Enuresis and behavioural deviance: Some epidemiological considerations. In Kolvin, I., MacKeith, R. and Meadow, S. R. (Eds) *Bladder Control and Enuresis* Clinics in Developmental Medicine Nos. 48/49. London: Heinemann/Spastics International Medical Publications, 1973.
50. Epstein, S.: The stability of behavior. I. On predicting most of the people much of the time. *Journal of Personality and Social Psychology, 37*:1097-1136, 1979.
51. Boudreault, M., Maziade, M., Thivierge, J., Caperaa, P., Cote, R., Boutin, P., Julien, Y. and Bergeron, S.: Cognitive functioning and reading achievement in pervasive ADD and situational ADD. Paper presented at the Joint Meeting of the American and Canadian Academies of Child Psychiatry, Toronto, October 11, 1984.
52. McGee, R., Silva, P. A. and Williams, S.: Behaviour problems in a population of 7-year-old children: Prevalence, stability and types of disorder—a research report. *Journal of Child Psychology and Psychiatry, 25*:251-260, 1984.
53. Rutter, M., Graham, P. and Chadwick, O.: Adolescent turmoil: fact or fiction? *Journal of Child Psychology and Psychiatry, 17*:35-56, 1976.
54. Macmillan, A., Kolvin, I., Garside, R. F., Nicol, A. R. and Leitch, I. M.: A multiple criterion screen for identifying secondary school children with psychiatric disorder: characteristics and efficiency of screen. *Psychological Medicine, 10*:265-276, 1980.
55. Kovacs, M.: The clinical interview: a developmental perspective. In Rutter, M., Izard, C. and Read, P. (Eds) *Depression in Young People: Developmental and Clinical Perspective* New York: Guilford Press, (in press), 1985.
56. Costello, A. J., Edelbrock, C. S., Dulcan, M. H., Kales, R. and Klavic, S. H.: *Report on the NIMH Diagnostic Interview Schedule for Children (DISC).* Report to the National Institute of Mental Health, Bethesda, MD., 1984.
57. Rutter, M. and Gould, M.: Classification. In Rutter, M. and Hersov, L. (Eds), *Child and Adolescent Psychiatry: Modern Approaches (2nd edition)* Oxford: Blackwell Scientific, 1985.
58. American Psychiatric Association: *Diagnostic and Statistical Manual of Mental Disorders—DSM-III (3rd ed).* American Psychiatric Association, Washington, DC., 1980.
59. Sandberg, S., Rutter, M. and Taylor, E.: Hyperkinetic disorder in psychiatric clinic attenders. *Developmental Medicine and Child Neurology, 20*:279-299, 1978.
60. Sandberg, S., Wieselberg, M. and Shaffer, D.: Hyperkinetic and conduct problem children in a primary school population: Some epidemiological considerations. *Journal*

of Child Psychology and Psychiatry, 21:293-322, 1980.

61. Taylor, E. and Sandberg, S.: Hyperactive behaviour in English schoolchildren: a questionnaire survey. *Journal of Abnormal Child Psychology, 12*:143-156, 1984.

62. Sandberg, S.: Patterns of stability and change in hyperactive behaviour during primary school years. (Submitted for publication), 1985.

63. Schachar, R., Rutter, M. and Smith, A.: The characteristics of situationally and pervasively hyperactive children: implications for syndrome definition. *Journal of Child Psychology and Psychiatry, 22*:375-392, 1981.

64. Sandberg, S.: On the overinclusiveness of the diagnosis of hyperkinetic syndrome. In Gittelman, M. (Ed), *Intervention Strategies and Hyperactive Children*. New York: M. E. Sharpe, 1981.

65. Sandberg, S.: Overactivity: Behaviour or syndrome? In Taylor, E. A. (Ed), *The Overactive Child* Heinemann/Spastics International Medical Publications (in press), 1985.

66. Taylor, E., Everitt, B., Thorley, G., Schachar, R., Rutter, M. and Wieselberg, M.: Conduct disorder and hyperactivity: A cluster analytic approach to the identification of a behavioural syndrome. (Submitted for publication), 1985.

67. Rutter, M., Graham, P. and Yule, W.: *A Neuropsychiatric Study in Childhood*. Clinics in Developmental Medicine Nos. 35/36. London: Heinemann/Spastics International Medical Publications, 1970.

68. Rutter, M., Chadwick, O. and Schachar, R.: Hyperactivity in minimal brain dysfunction: Epidemiological perspectives on questions of cause and classification. In Tartar, R. (Ed), *The Child at Psychiatric Risk* New York and Oxford: Oxford University Press, 1983.

69. Seidel, U. P., Chadwick, O. and Rutter, M.: Psychological disorders in crippled children: A comparative study of children with and without brain damage. *Developmental Medicine and Child Neurology, 17*:563-573, 1975.

70. Rutter, M., Chadwick, O. and Shaffer, D.: Head injury. In Rutter, M. (Ed), *Developmental Neuropsychiatry* New York: Guilford Press, 1983.

71. Prugh, D. G., Wagonfeld, S., Metcalf, D. and Jordan, K.: A clinical study of delirum in children and adolescents. *Psychosomatic Medicine, 42*:177-195, 1980.

72. Rutter, M.: Syndromes attributed to "minimal brain dysfunction" in childhood. *American Journal of Psychiatry, 139*:21-33, 1982.

73. Shaffer, D., O'Connor, P. A., Shafer, S. Q. and Prupis, S.: Neurological "soft signs": Their origins and significance for behavior. In Rutter, M. (Ed), *Developmental Neuropsychiatry* New York: Guilford Press, 1983.

74. Shaffer, D., Schonfeld, I. S., O'Connor, P. A., Stokman, C., Trautman, P., Shafer, S. and Ng, S.: Neurological soft signs and their relationship to psychiatric disorder and intelligence in childhood and adolescence. (Submitted for publication), 1985.

75. Shafer, S. Q., Shaffer, D., O'Connor, P. A. and Stokman, C. J.: Hard thoughts on neurological "soft signs". In Rutter, M. (Ed) *Developmental Neuropsychiatry* New York: Guilford Press, 1983.

76. Nichols, P. L. and Chen, T-C.: *Minimal Brain Dysfunction: A Prospective Study*. Hillsdale, New Jersey: Lawrence Erlbaum, 1981.

77. Schmidt, M. H., Esser, G., Allehaff, W., Eisert, H. D., Deisel, B., Laucht, M., Poustka, F. and Voll, R.: Prevalence and meaning of cerebral dysfunction in eight-year-old children in Mannheim. In Schmidt, M. H. and Remschmidt, H. (Eds) *Epidemiological Approaches in Child Psychiatry II* Stuttgart: Thieme Verlag, New York: Thieme-Stratton, 1983.

78. Gillberg, C.: Perceptual, motor and attentional deficits in Swedish primary school children. Some child psychiatric aspects. *Journal of Child Psychology and Psychiatry,* 24:377-404, 1983.
79. Shen, Y. and Wang, Y.: Study on MBD Children: Epidemiology, clinical investigation and biochemical study of MHPG-SO₄ in urine. Paper presented at UNICEF Workshop, Beijing, May 1984.
80. Shen, Y., Wang, Y. and Yang, X.: An epidemiological investigation of MBD children in six elementary schools in Beijing. (Submitted for publication), 1985.
81. Porter, R. and Collins, G. M. (Eds): *Temperamental Differences in Infants and Young Children.* Ciba Foundation Symposium 89. London: Pitman Medical, 1982.
82. Rutter, M.: Family, area and school influences in the genesis of conduct disorders. In Hersov, L. A. and Berger, M. with Shaffer, D. (Eds) *Aggression and Antisocial Behaviour in Childhood and Adolescence Journal of Child Psychology and Psychiatry Book Supplement No. 1.* Oxford: Pergamon Press, 1978.
83. Scarr, S. and McCartney, K.: How people make their own environment: A theory of genotype—> Environmental effects. *Child Development, 54*:424-435, 1983.
84. Maziade, M., Cote, R., Boudreault, M., Thivierge, J., and Caperaa, P.: The New York Longitudinal Study's model of temperament: Gender differences and demographic correlates in a French-speaking population. *Journal of the American Academy of Child Psychiatry, 23*:582-587, 1984.
85. Maziade, M., Caperaa, P., Laplante, B., Boudreault, M., Thivierge, J., Cote, R., and Boutin, P.: The predictive value of difficult temperament from ages 7 to 12 in a general population. *American Journal of Psychiatry* 1985.
86. Rutter, M.: *Children of Sick Parents: An Environmental and Psychiatric Study.* Institute of Psychiatry Maudsley Monographs No. 16. London: Oxford University Press, 1966.
87. Buck, C. and Laughton, K.: Family patterns of illness: the effect of psychoneurosis in the parent upon illness in the child. *Acta Psychiatrica Neurologica Scandinavica, 34*:165-175, 1959.
88. Pound, A., Cox, A., Puckering, C. and Mills, M.: The impact of maternal depression on young children. In Stevenson, J. (Ed), *Recent Research in Developmental Psychopathology* Monograph Supplement No. 4 to the Journal of Child Psychology and Psychiatry. Oxford: Pergamon Press, 1985.
89. Weissman, M. M., Prusoff, B. A., Gammon, G. D., Merikangas, K. R., Leckman, J. F. and Kidd, K. F: Psychopathology in the children (ages 6-18) of depressed and normal women. *Journal of the American Academy of Child Psychiatry, 23*:78-84, 1984.
90. Emery, R., Weintraub, S. and Neale, J. M.: Effects of marital discord on the school behavior of children of schizophrenic, affectively disordered and normal parents. *Journal of Abnormal Child Psychology, 10*:215-228, 1982.
91. Douglas, J. W. B.: Early hospital admissions and later disturbances of behaviour and learning. *Developmental Medicine and Child Neurology, 17*:456-480, 1975.
92. Quinton, D. and Rutter, M.: Early hospital admissions and later disturbances of behaviour: An attempted replication of Douglas' findings. *Developmental Medicine and Child Neurology, 18*:447-459, 1976.
93. Rutter, M.: Stress, coping and development: some issues and some questions. *Journal of Child Psychology and Psychiatry, 22*:323-356, 1981.
94. Dunn, J. and Kendrick, C.: *Siblings: Love, Envy and Understanding* Cambridge, Mass: Harvard University Press, 1982.
95. Wolkind, S. and Rutter, M.: Separation, loss and family relationships. In Rutter, M.

and Hersov, L. (Eds) *Child and Adolescent Psychiatry: Modern Approaches (2nd edition).* Oxford: Blackwell Scientific 1985.

96. Shannon, F. T., Fergusson, D. M. and Dimond, M. E.: Early hospital admissions and subsequent behavior problems in 6 year olds. *Archives of Disease in Childhood, 59*:815-819, 1984.

31

Obstetric Drugs and Infant Behavior: A Reevaluation

Helena C. Kraemer, Anneliese Korner, Thomas Anders, Carol Nagy Jacklin, and Sue Dimiceli

Stanford University

Poorly designed and analyzed studies ascribing effects of obstetric drugs on infant behavior may not only have misrepresented facts but may also have rendered well-designed and analyzed studies difficult to execute.

Strong claims have been made about adverse effects of obstetric drugs on the behavioral development of children (Brackbill, 1979). In some cases these claims have received wide coverage in the media. Yet there is growing skepticism about these claims (Kolata, 1979). The present paper focuses on two issues underlying skepticism: (a) problems of the confounding of obstetric drugs and various factors and (b) faulty statistical analysis.

Reprinted with permission from the *Journal of Pediatric Psychology*, 1985, Vol. 10, 345–353. Copyright 1985 by Plenum Publishing Corporation.

The studies reported were supported by the William T. Grant Foundation, the Distribution Fund, the National Institute of Child Health and Development (HD 09814-08), the Ford Foundation, the Spencer Foundation, and Grant RR-81 from the General Clinical Research Center's Program of the Division of Human Resources, and the National Institutes of Health. The authors thank E. Maccoby for her careful reading of the paper.

THE PROBLEM OF CONFOUNDING

Obstetric drug decisions are determined by the difficulty of individual labors. Therefore, drug use should be associated with any factor causative of, associated with, or resultant from, difficult labors: the health status or age of mother, parity, length of labor, level of anxiety, pain or tolerance for pain, and possibly socioeconomic status, home environments, etc. Any such factor related to infant behavior function and to use of obstetric drugs induces a correlation between obstetric drug use and infant behavior function. To interpret such a correlation as indicating a causal relationship is an error (Kenny, 1979). In short, infants found to be behaviorally disadvantaged in the group exposed to higher levels of obstetric drugs might have been so disadvantaged whether or not drugs had been used.

In rejoinder to such criticisms (Brackbill, 1979) points out that parity and length of labor have not been found to be significantly related to behavioral development. Thus, it is argued, obstetric drug decisions behave like random decisions with respect to behavioral parameters. Clearly if such decisions were indeed random, no correlations between parity, length of labor, and behavioral outcome would be found. However there are a remarkable number of ways that correlations may be found to be low when decisions are far from random, e.g., (a) The quality of measurement is poor (e.g., length of labor determined from hospital records). (b) Statistical tests are invalid (e.g., the product-moment correlation coefficient used for nonlinear relationships). (c) Important interactive effects are ignored (such as that between parity and length of labor). (d) Important cohort effects are ignored. (e) Sample sizes are too small to have sufficient power to detect associations.

Any or all of these may account for nonsignificant correlations even if the association between obstetric drug decisions and parity or length of labor were quite strong. Therefore, it is only as assumption, and a meager one at that, that obstetric drug decisions behave like random decisions.

In demonstration of this point, Table I presents the results of a study (Jacklin & Maccoby, 1982) conducted in two hospitals. There are significant differences in use of analgesics between hospitals. In each hospital, a first-born is more likely to be exposed to analgesia than one later born. Within each hospital and within each parity group, those with longer labor (over 8 hr) are more likely to be exposed to analgesia. This same relationship seems to hold with anesthesia at Stanford but not at El Camino. Similar results have been reported previously (Kraemer,

Table I. Parity,[a] Length of Labor, Hospital, and Their Effect on Use of Analgesia, Anesthesia

	% Use of analgesia							% Use of spinal/caudal anesthesia					
	Stanford (n = 82)			El Camino (n = 205)			Stanford (n = 82)			El Camino (n = 205)		
Labor (hr)	F %	L %	Total %	F %	L %	Total %	Labor (hr)	F %	L %	Total %	F %	L %	Total %
0–4	–	11	23	60	43	46	0–4	–	44	38	60	61	61
4+–8	55	18	38	91	50	68	4–8	50	59	54	65	61	62
8+–12	62	50	58	89	80	86	8–12	69	100	79	48	80	57
12+	88	–	64	75	–	75	12+	75	–	64	58	–	58
Total	62	20	44	83	49	63		57	60	58	58	62	60

[a] *F*, firstborn; *L*, later born.

Korner, & Thoman, 1972). The indications are clear that the results of any study that does not control (at least) for parity, length of labor, and locale should not be considered valid evidence for or against adverse effects of obstetric drug use.

Controlled Versus Noncontrolled Studies

The optimal method of control for such confounding factors in a drug evaluation is a randomized double-blind, controlled clinical trial. Only one such experimental study has been reported (Kron, Stein, & Goodard, 1966) and that study evaluated a drug (a standard dosage of 200 mg of secobarbital sodium 30 min before delivery) used in a way it is seldom used in obstetric drug practice (Kraemer et al., 1972). Currently, the proliferation of poorly controlled studies purporting to demonstrate adverse effects of obstetrical medication have made it nearly impossible to execute further such trials. Those who have reported the results of uncontrolled studies argue in their defense, that, at the very least, their results should motivate execution of more definitive studies. Yet they simultaneously argue (Brackbill, 1979) that "cumulative indications found in their studies make it ethically impossible to conduct randomized trials." Thus the use of results of studies utilizing poor scientific methodology perpetuate what may be invalid scientific conclusions.

An alternative acceptable method of control for such factors is a process of creating subgroups matched post hoc on these factors and assessing the effect of drugs within matched subgroups.

This paper reports the results of attempting such an analysis. The procedure was followed in three independent infant studies, one on strength and tactile sensitivity (Jacklin, Snow, & Maccoby, 1981), one on activity and irritability (Korner, Hutchinson, Koperski, Kraemer, & Schneider, 1981), and one on sleep (Anders, Keener, Bowe, & Shoaff, 1982).

In the reanalysis of each study, the following technique was used: An infant subject was randomly selected. If the infant was exposed to any analgesia, all infants included in the same study of the same sex, born in the same hospital, during the same year, and with lengths of labor within 1.5 hr of that of the target infant but who were *not* exposed to analgesia were identified. From this group, one infant was randomly selected as the match to the analgesia infant. Both target and match were withdrawn from the group. If no match was found, the target was dropped from the comparison. The process was repeated until all infants were either matched or dropped. A matched-pairs *t* test was used to compare various behaviors observed in that study between analgesia-exposed infants and their matches. (The analogous process was used to effect the Anesthesia Contrast.)

Using this procedure, it was found that 50–70% of subjects could not be matched. In the case of the Anders et al. (1981) study, when the subjects for whom length of labor could not be determined from the hospital record and the subjects for whom the matches could not be found were discarded, there were not enough matched subjects for a valid statistical test. The results of the other two studies appear in Table II.

Two results are noteworthy. First, there is no evidence of any drug effect. Second, matching procedures are extremely difficult to implement under retrospective circumstances, since any subgroup that does not contain a reasonable number of patients both for whom drugs were used and for whom drugs were not used tends to be excluded. Since the impact of the noncontrolled studies has been to decrease drug use and to limit use predominantly to patients with long labors, patients with very short labors tend to be excluded (since few are exposed to drugs) and patients with long labors, particularly nulligravida, tend to be excluded, since few are drug-free. One is left with a limited and unrepresentative sample. Once again, the impact of uncontrolled studies reported widely by the media, as some here have been, is to hamper the conduct of better designed studies.

Finally, yet another method to control the confounding factors is by mathematical analytic procedures, e.g., Multiple Regression or Analysis of Covariance (Cohen & Cohen, 1975). The problems noted above in connection with matching procedures, however, cause multicollinearity problems that compromise the statistical validity of these procedures as

Table II. Uncontrolled and Controlled Contrasts Relating to the Effect of Analgesia, Anesthesia on Newborn Behavior

	Analgesia contrast					Anesthesia contrast				
	Uncontrolled		Post hoc sample matched[a] loss %			Uncontrolled		Post hoc sample matched[b] loss%		
	n	t^c	n	t^c		n	t^c	n	t^c	
Jacklin et al. (1981)										
Tactile										
Insensitivity	196	−0.50	68	0.14	65	163	0.95	48	1.87	71
Prone head raise	202	1.02	68	−0.07	66	167	−0.12	52	0.28	69
Grip strength	188	0.16	62	−0.54	67	155	1.17	42	0.21	73
Korner (1981)										
Cry rate	61	0.83	28	−0.55	54	71	0.14	32	1.12	55
Noncry activity	69	0.10	34	−0.25	51	79	−0.72	42	0.44	47
Noncry style	65	1.16	32	−0.40	51	76	0.28	38	0.52	50
Anders (1982)										
Longest sustained sleep	30	1.09	−	−	−	30	0.28	−	−	−
Percentage quiet sleep	30	0.19	−	−	−	30	1.23	−	−	−
Out-of-crib frequency	30	2.02[a]	−	−	−	30	1.22	−	−	−
Longest quiet sleep	30	0.39	−	−	−	30	0.63	−	−	−

[a] $p \sim .053$.
[b] Matched by locale, sex, length of labor.
[c] A positive sign indicates a higher mean score for the Analgesia (Anesthesia) group than for the contrast group.

well. One cannot "correct" for the effects of length or difficulty of labors if those exposed to drugs are primarily those with long or difficult labors and those not so exposed, primarily those with short, uncomplicated labors. Thus, although these procedures might have once been acceptable, they are becoming less feasible as the impact of uncontrolled studies is increasingly evident.

Two such studies were done in the past and the conclusions of both indicate that the impact of drug use is either not significant or is trivial in comparison to the effects of parity and length of labor (Kraemer et al., 1972; Woodson & da Costa-Woodson, 1980). In short, the results of these studies are consistent with the present results in Table II.

FAULTY STATISTICAL ANALYSIS

The second area of criticism of these studies has been the statistical validity of the conclusions. If statistical significance had not been found in these studies, the issues discussed above would have been moot, since nonsignificant findings are generally not published in scientific journals. (One wonders: How many studies have found no adverse effect of obstetric drugs and have not been reported?) One must further be concerned with the question of whether the significant results reported have been mostly those that have used inadequate statistical methods and have reported false positive findings.

For example, Table II reports the two-sample t test used, as it frequently is, in uncontrolled studies. Here there appears to be a significant difference in out-of-crib frequency ($t_{28} = 2.02$, $p \sim .05$). This t test is based on the assumption of equal variances. In the analgesia-free group ($n = 23$), the mean frequency was 2.7 ± 1.4; in the analgesia-exposed group ($n = 7$), 4.4 ± 3.3. When, as here, a much larger variance appears in the much smaller group, it is known (Scheffé, 1959) that the usual t-test calculations tend to exaggerate the significance of the result. When a more appropriate test is used (a Mann-Whitney test), not only is the test result not statistically significant but it does not even approach significance ($p \sim .3$).

Arguments defending use of such statistical tests as t tests or tests of the product-moment correlation coefficients in circumstances when the assumptions on which the tests are based are violated are based on claims of a certain robustness, i.e., on the belief that the underlying assumption of normality does not matter too much. In fact this claim is correct but avoids the issues, since it is not the normality assumption that causes problems but such assumptions as those of linearity and equal variances (Scheffé, 1959; Kraemer, 1980).

Added to such concerns regarding the accuracy of calculations of significance levels is one related to the fact that each individual study tests not one but a number of behavioral parameters and, in some cases, assesses the same behavioral response separately in different subsamples. With so many tests, 5% or more might be significant by chance alone. Even if the claims of statistical significance on any *one* parameter were valid, many of the reported statistically significant results may be false positive findings (Miller, 1966).

But then, does not the fact that all reported effects are adverse indicate an overall adverse effect, even if not all were "really" significant (Brackbill, 1979)? The difficulty is that what is or is not termed adverse is frequently arbitrary. If drug-exposed infants cry more frequently, this may be interpreted as increased irritability; if less frequently, as increased lethargy. Any difference can be viewed as adverse. Unless there are standards, independent of the study, defining good and bad behavioral outcomes, the word "adverse" has no specific meaning.

CONCLUSION

Restricting unnecessary drug use is clearly desirable. If it were certain that the impact of uncontrolled study results were to restrict only the use of *unnecessary* drugs, whether or not the conclusions were valid substantively or statistically would be of scientific interest only. One would not question the value of their impact on medical practice or policy decisions. Unfortunately, the impact of such studies may have been to restrict *appropriate* drug use and thus to prolong unnecessary pain and discomfort for mothers; to cause distress or guilt in mothers of behaviorally disadvantaged children who elected or allowed drug use; to compromise optimal clinical decision making for labor management by obstetricians and anesthesiologists.

What is therefore of great concern is that the results of poorly designed ana analyzed studies not be allowed to preclude or compromise the conduct of carefully controlled studies necessary to establish the limits of safe use of obstetric drugs with respect to infant development.

What then is known of the effects of obstetric drugs from past studies that should form the basis of future studies?

1. From animal studies and a single, randomized clinical trial (Kron et al., 1966), potent drugs administered near the time of birth do have the potential of affecting infant behavior. It is not known which drugs, in which amounts, administered within which time limits, or to which patients, affect which aspects of infant behavior, or for how long. It is important that the possibility of adverse drug effects not be discounted just because the studies to-date documenting the possibility are not convincing.

2. Uncontrolled studies suggest a correlation between factors associated with use of obstetric drugs and behavioral development. To what extent it is the associated factors and not obstetric drug use itself that are implicated is not known. It should be remembered that such associated factors include potent influences such as birth order, maternal age and health, socioeconomic status, length and difficulty of labor, condition and position of the infant *in utero*, etc.

3. The few existing controlled nonexperimental studies have not demonstrated any statistically or clinically significant association between drug use and infant behavior. They include earlier (Kraemer, 1972; Woodson & da Costa-Woodson, 1980) and the three new studies reported here. Since there have been few of these studies, these must not be interpreted as demonstrating the safety of obstetric drug use.

In summary, we suggest that despite the large number of studies relating obstetric drugs to adverse effects on infant behavior, we yet know very little. What little information we have from the few controlled studies tends not to support the contention of adverse effects. Furthermore, very little will ever be known unless the poorly designed, controlled, or analyzed studies of the past are not used to preclude the conduct of better studies in the future.

Members of Use of Human Subjects Committees need be apprised of the situation, for, under the circumstances, randomized controlled trials are not unethical. Editors and reviewers dealing with submitted papers in this area must be very critical of studies at this stage and more willing to give positive consideration to well-designed and executed studies demonstrating no association between obstetric drugs and behavioral outcome. Researchers in this area should be encouraged to pursue this question by executing well-designed and well-controlled studies to resolve the important issues involved.

REFERENCES

Anders, T., Keener, M., Bowe, T., & Shoaff, B. (1982). A longitudinal study of nighttime sleep-wake patterns in infants from birth through one year. In J. Call & E. Galensen (Eds.), *Frontiers in infant psychiatry* (pp. 152-170). New York: Basic Books.

Brackbill, Y. (1979). Obstetrical medication and infant behavior. In J. D. Osofsky (Ed.), *Handbook in infant development* (pp. 76-125). New York: Wiley.

Cohen, J., & Cohen, P. (1975). *Applied multiple regression/correlation analysis for the behavioral sciences.* Hillsdale, NJ: Lawrence Erlbaum.

Jacklin, C. N., & Maccoby, E. E. (1982). Length of labor and sex of offspring. *Journal of Pediatric Psychology, 7,* 4, 355-360.

Jacklin, C. N., Snow, M. E., & Maccoby, E. E. (1981). Tactile sensitivity and muscle strength in newborn boys and girls. *Infant Behavior and Development, 4,* 261-268.

Kenny, D. A. (1979). *Correlation and causality.* New York: Wiley.

Kolata, J. B. (1979). Scientists attack report that obstetrical medications endanger children. *Science, 204,* 391-392.

Korner, A. F., Hutchinson, C. A., Koperski, J. A., Kraemer, H. C., & Schneider, P. A. (1981). Stability of individual differences of neonatal motor and crying patterns. *Child Development, 52,* 83-90.

Kraemer, H. C. (1980). Robustness of the distribution theory of the product moment correlation coefficient. *Journal of Educational Statistics, 2*(5), 115-128.

Kraemer, H. C., Korner, A. F., & Thoman, E. B. (1972). Methodological considerations in evaluating the influence of drugs used during labor and delivery on the behavior of the newborn. *Developmental Psychology, 6*(1), 128-134.

Kron, R. E., Stein, M., & Goodard, K. E. (1966). Newborn sucking behavior affected by obstetric sedation. *Pediatrics, 37,* 1012-1016.

Miller, R. B., Jr. (1966). Simultaneous statistical inference. New York: McGraw-Hill.

Scheffé, H. (1959). *The analysis of variance* (Chap. 10). New York: Wiley.

Woodson, R. H., & da Costa-Woodson, E. M. (1980). Covariates of analgesia in a clinical sample and their effect on the relations between analgesia and infant behavior. *Infant Behavior and Development, 3,* 205-213.

32

Assessment and Therapeutic Intervention of Black Children

Jeanne Spurlock
American Psychiatric Association

The need for a balance in addressing cultural differences and simi-larities in the diagnostic assessment and treatment of black children is the major focus of this article. Selected illustrations from the lit-erature and from the author's professional experiences point out some of the pitfalls, as well as steps to take that will promote accuracy in diagnosis and effective treatment. Several identified reference points are viewed to be of considerable significance in our multicultural society, and are advocated as warranting attention in the psychiatric care of any child.

Within any ethnic, racial, or religious group, there is a diversity among children and their families. Afro-American families are no different in this regard. This diversity underscores the necessity for diagnosticians to evaluate each primary patient and his or her family as an individual and unit. At the same time, it is essential for the diagnostician to be alert to the possibility of counter-transference reactions that are tied to various stereotypes of Afro-Americans. The diagnostician (or therapist) who views a black child only in terms of that child being a victim of racism and who dismissed any effort to evaluate intrapsychic factors mars the diagnostic process. Equally faulty is the clinician who is blinded to the

---

Reprinted with permission from the *Journal of the American Academy of Child Psychiatry,* 1985, Vol. 24, 168–174. Copyright 1985 by the American Academy of Child Psychiatry.

differences of race or of class. These premises underlie that which follows.

In those child psychiatry training and service programs with which I am familiar, a proper diagnostic assessment includes: 1) data collecting (from parents and/or other pertinent sources), 2) interviews with the identified patient and significant others, and 3) referral for selected, specific evaluation procedures (psychometric, projective, neurological, etc.). In evaluating Afro-American children the diagnostician, mindful of diversity within this racial group, should be especially alert to cultural characteristics, which could possibly affect the behavior ("normal" or "disordered") of the child being evaluated. The following clinical vignettes illustrate some features that have been viewed as characteristic of large segments of the Afro-American population.

THE ONE-PARENT/ABSENT FATHER FAMILY

During the course of a review of records (selected at random) in an East Coast, university based, child psychiatry clinic, the following information was culled from one of the records:

> Ellis (a fictitious name) is an 8-year-old black boy referred because of academic slowness and withdrawn behavior. The family was described as single parent although reference was made (in the social worker's history) to the mother's report that the father was a frequent visitor and regularly made financial contributions for the support of Ellis and his sister, 2 years his senior. Other background history included: 1) mother had been married to the father of the older children; this union terminated a decade prior to patient's birth; 2) following separation from the alcoholic husband, the family was supported by public assistance; and 3) 5 years prior to clinic contact, mother matriculated in a civil service training program, in which she did well; she was employed outside the home since Ellis began public school.
>
> The diagnostician noted that Ellis came from a fatherless home; that he apparently lacked a stable male figure with whom to identify. Also noted was that mother was less available to the child because of her outside employment.

My reaction to the recorded history was much less negative. I saw several significant and positive features: 1) the father, a frequent visitor and responsible for the financial support of his children, was very much in the life of the child (and may well have been available to participate in the diagnostic evaluation and treatment planning); and 2) the mother manifested apparent and significant strengths that might have been identified and effectively utilized in the treatment program. Missing from the protocol was any reference to the child's strengths. Could it have been that the child was devoid of any assets? Or, was it more likely that the diagnostician had failed to explore for, or record, those characteristics of health and strength?

In another case, paralleling that of Ellis and his family, there was no effort to elicit information about the child's early "mothering" by a maternal aunt, who continued to reside in the same building in which the mother and children lived. I speculated that the diagnostician might not have recognized the importance of examining the child's total support system, and/or of the significance of the extended family within the Afro-American culture. Even if the aunt/mother surrogate had been seen, it would have been essential for the diagnostician to explore carefully assets, as well as liabilities in this dual mothering experience in view of the reported negative impact of multiple mothering on a child's development.

According to Yarrow and Harmon (1980), even though ". . . there is some evidence of the harmful effects of multiple mothering in institutions, having more than one caretaker is not always associated with severe deprivations or traumatic discontinuities in care . . . It seems clear that the effects of multiple mothering depend on the specific patterns of interaction between the child and the mother figures and on the larger social context."

It has also been observed that having multiple parents has been a safeguard for many children: "Ghetto children also suffer from discontinuities in their mothering experience. Nevertheless, despite such problems, the majority of ghetto children survive as adults without developing flagrant and chronic psychiatric disorders. To a great extent, this can be explained by the presence of extended family arrangements which provide a safeguarding net through which children are not allowed to fall into a mire of neglect" (Wadeson (1975), p. 181).

"RICHES AND POVERTY" IN "CULTURAL DEPRIVATION"

Incompleteness or errors of diagnostic assessments of black children are often rooted in the concept of cultural deprivation or disadvantage. Chess (1969) noted that labeling has become a stereotype, which "no matter how benevolently intended, ignores the rich diversity of individuals within the group." Various positive role models are among the riches, even though the models may not meet the criteria established by white, middle-class professionals (Taylor, 1976).

During the course of a workshop discussion on the self-concept of black children, a male partcipant sharply challenged the global impression of the absence of positive role models in black communities across the country. In recalling his childhood experiences in a segregated southern town, he identified several such models; the most meaningful one was a railroad porter who was jet black in color. This man's childhood experiences parallel those of throngs of other Afro-American children I have known. For them, there was never a question about their worth. Their beginnings were rooted in the kind of environment that Powell (1973) determined to spawn positive self-esteem in its inhabitants—"a strong cohesive black community which has some power base in terms not only of numbers but also of achievements." Yet, even in the midst of powerlessness, large numbers of black youngsters grow up with a positive sense of self. Documentation has been provided by Ladner (1972), who conducted an in-depth study of female children and adolescents living in an inner-city public housing project:

> There is a wide range of views on what it means to be poor and black in the city today . . . The overwhelming majority of them seemed proud of their race and accepted it as a factor of life which, although problematic at times, was still real and did not need to be changed. Thus, there was no evidence of low self-esteem and severely damaged psyches . . . They did not seem to experience feelings of inadequacy . . . because of their racial status. As a whole, they are widely accepted by their peers . . . In other areas of their lives they saw themselves as desirable love objects, mothers, job holders, valued friends and individuals with much resourcefulness.

On the other hand, there are Afro-American children who do have a negative sense of self. In my experience, the chronicles of the development of many youngsters who have a demeaned self-concept are studded with encounters of rejection and/or belittlement by their parents or parent surrogates. As with any child, this kind of response from the parent(s) may be rooted in intrapsychic phenomena, which could be (or not) accentuated by family or extrafamilial stresses. A sharp rebuff from a harassed mother who has just returned from her "day work" employment, may well reinforce the sense of rejection that a 6-year-old experienced as a toddler, or even earlier, when his mother was too depressed or too fatigued to respond adequately to her child's emotional needs. A prediction, "you're gonna be no count, just like your father" (or mother) of a parent or grandparent, can be equally damaging.

PSYCHOPATHOLOGY—SOME ILLUSTRATIONS

Many black infants are born at risk because of limited, or nonexistent, prenatal care, especially among the adolescent mothers to be. Prematurity and its negative sequelae are not uncommonly found in many black infants born into families within the lower socioeconomic ranks (Pasamanick, 1959). The risks are compounded when the mother has been addicted to drugs and/or alcohol. Obviously the organic problems experienced early in life do not provide a sound foundation for healthy psychological development. The poor start in life is not infrequently accentuated by negative features of the external environment (such as overcrowded housing and excessive lead exposure) which may provoke or reinforce psychiatric symptomatology in the caretaker and then unfavorably affect the child. Any one of the aforementioned factors may serve as fertile soil for the development of psychopathology.

Developmental lags are not uncommon, and are often manifested by signs of intellectual retardation or minimal brain dysfunction (Lawrence, 1975). The appearance of pica and lead poisoning, a common side effect in these youngsters, is well known. Behavioral or academic problems account for a sizeable percentage of psychiatric referral of black children of elementary school age (Leal, 1981; Pizer, 1981; Simmons, 1981; Spurlock and Lawrence, 1979). Often, both behaviors are related to an attention deficit disorder. The diagnostician would do well to remain alert to the possibility of the learning problem being a "symptom choice" (Meers, 1970), as well as to assess for a specific developmental disorder (such as developmental reading disorder), or a neurotic disorder. It has been noted that the disordered behavior patterns in some youngsters reflect signs of depression (Spurlock and Lawrence, 1979). Of equal importance is the evaluation of the behavior disorder as a feature of a conduct disorder.

Behaviors that prompt psychiatric referral of preadolescents and adolescents are varied and range from antisocial behavior to vegetative, depressive features to substance abuse. Any one of the personality disorders may be an accurate diagnosis for any number of youths.

As previously noted, a range of psychiatric disorders are in evidence among the black child and adolescent populations. The signs and symptoms that lend to a *diagnosis* of separation anxiety disorder or schizophrenic disorder should not differ among blacks and whites, even though there may be some "cultural coloring" to the symptom picture.

TREATMENT MODALITIES AND TECHNIQUES

Sketches from the Literature

Findings derived from a number of studies reveal a common practice of basing treatment plans on racial and socioeconomic identification (Harrison et al., 1965; Hunt, 1962; Jackson et al., 1974). Families of lower socioeconomic status were found to have been offered short-term psychiatric intervention; they were not candidates for individual therapy. Biases of mental health professionals have been identified as partial explanations for these differences (Adams, 1970; Jackson et al., 1974). That is, black children and their parents have been viewed as not being psychologically aware and being poorly motivated for psychiatric intervention. The value of crisis intervention and brief, time-limited therapy, which have often been identified as methods of choice for chronically disturbed children of crisis-ridden inner city black families, has been challenged by some clinicians. Others have advocated a range of specific kinds of services ranging from the concrete to insight to advocacy (Lavietes, 1974; Lawrence, 1975; Leal, 1976; Malone, 1967). Reports of the successes in the use of psychoanalysis and psychoanalytically oriented psychotherapy have not been wanting, although limited in numbers (Meers, 1970; Spurlock and Cohen, 1969). In a number of clinical settings, major attention has been directed to services for preschool children. This particular focus is based on the need for early detection and intervention. The value of a multidisciplinary approach (including educational, pediatric, psychiatric and social services) has been stressed (Lawrence, 1975; Leal, 1976; Malone, 1967). This approach is particularly important in day care and residential treatment programs (Lawrence, 1975; Lockett, 1972; Westman, 1979).

Specific techniques for handling various patterns of resistance are the focal points of other references. Heacock (1976) addresses the significance of the child's aggression, the problems generated, and the need for firm limit-setting in the psychotherapeutic process. Pinderhughes and Rolland (1971) identified resistance in two major categories: 1) indirect expressions of hostile aggression (including lateness, missed appointments, etc.) and 2) reflection of a sense of·victimization (including denial of problems and transient paranoid feelings of persecution). Early identification and interpretation of resistance was emphasized.

Recognition of Racial Identity

As in many areas of our work, there is a difference of opinion about the value of introducing the subject of the child's (adolescent's) Afro-American identification at the initial appointment. I have found it to be advantageous to ask any patient, "How do you feel about seeing me, a black woman?" This question has appeared to put both black and white youngsters (as well as adults) at ease about the subject, even though pertinent associations may be reported at later times. In my experiences as a supervisor, I have observed that some trainees, both black and white, tend to deny any possibility of significance to the respective sameness or difference of their racial identity in the treatment of black patients. A mother's concern that we might meet in social situations and that this would cause her some embarrassment turned out to be a thin disguise for her conviction that the child's pediatrician (who was white) had depreciated the family by making a referral to me—a black child psychiatrist. Here, early on, important material surfaced. This mother showed evidence of having incorporated a negative stereotype of Afro-Americans as factual. This attitude was reflected in her intra- and extrafamilial relationships, and accounted for, in part, her daughter's self-effacing behavior. Obviously, racial identification was an issue that warranted being addressed in the therapeutic work with this child (referred because of poor academic performance) and her parents.

Vignettes from the Author's Experiences

The following illustrations are examples of effective psychotherapeutic encounters. They should not be viewed as the only techniques that can be successfully utilized in work with black children.

CONSULTATION SERVICES

Since so many poor, black children come to be identified on the caseloads of child care agencies (i.e., welfare, juvenile courts, placement, public health), valuable mental health services can be provided through psychiatric consultation to the agency or through the individual case worker, probation officers, or other service providers.

Often, a consultant's initial task is to point out the need for the service providers to become familiar with the culture and the community from which his or her charges come. Too frequently the consultant's knowledge is limited. It is essential that the providers know that some of the modes of behavior that they may identify as disordered may, indeed, be a nonpathological means of coping in a child's home environment. (Of course, this pattern is not confined to black children only; the possibility of such differences should be considered by providers who are responsible for children and adolescents from a background dissimilar to their own.)

Serving as a consultant to a family service agency, I have often found it necessary to point out that many black parents view physical discipline as commensurate with good child rearing, and not as abuse ("spare the rod and spoil the child"). The frequent tendency for the provider to identify primarily with the child can lead to the development of blind spots, which prevent the observation of any evidence of strengths. A treatment plan focused on the reinforcement of strengths in the family is often preferable to foster home placement of the child. On the other hand, it has often been necessary to help providers see that in their efforts to avoid cultural bias, they identify pathology as a cultural trait. This pattern was well illustrated by a 20-year-old college student, who had contacted me (at the suggestion of an instructor) for some information sources for a term paper. This young woman, the oldest of 10 children in a single parent family, volunteered the following information during the course of discussing her career goals. She identified her interest in human services, and allowed that the interest stemmed from her own personal (and her family's) experience. She emphasized that she would have "been stuck in despair" without some of the positive experiences with those providers who tended to "minimize the liabilities that were about to overpower any strengths that we might have had at the time, if we had any."

Service providers, not unlike many parents of their young clients, are frustrated and overwhelmed with their assigned responsibilities, and have benefited from efforts directed toward reducing their feelings of failure. As a consultant, I have found it helpful to encourage the service providers to recognize their own limitations and to be more open to alternative approaches for service delivery. Often, information about alternative services come from the families themselves. I have learned of numbers of serviceable support systems in the course of seeking information from parents about their religious affiliation and church programs. Teachers have reported their beneficial experiences in attending seminars which focused on culture's impact on psychosexual development. For example, a white, middle-class, third grade teacher, assigned to a black, inner city school, viewed all of her students to be culturally and intellectually limited. She reported a marked shift in her perception after attending several seminars with the aforementioned focus. The favorable experience of this one teacher has not been a universal reaction: the need for various kinds of reinforcement should not be underestimated. Consultation services provided as a part of liaison psychiatry should have the same goals regardless of the racial or ethnic identity of the patient and his or her family.

Crisis Intervention and Brief/Focused Psychotherapy

Many families subsisting in poverty tend to cope, although at great psychological costs, with daily occurrences of crises. At some point, however, a "strawlike" incident may provoke their travel to a hospital emergency room, or another service facility, along with pleas (if not demands) for immediate help in alleviating a longstanding painful problem. Here, again, it is essential that service providers not impose their value systems in determining the immediacy of need. (Ellis et al., 1979). Of course, there are other situations which any examiner will label as a crisis without hesitation. No matter who identifies the crises, the service provider has an obligation to meet the patient where he or she is, and must attend to determining which ways and means will provide symptom relief.

Medication may be the therapeutic agent of choice for immediate relief. On the other hand, a sensitive listener may find clues that can be used to help the patient reestablish ties with support systems within the immediate environment. Obviously, the service provider must have some familiarity with the nature of networking, a system that has permitted survival in many black communities. Here, reference is made not only to major and store-front religious groups, but also to aid societies, fraternal organizations, and social clubs.

Brief and focused psychotherapy is often indicated as a secondary step in crisis intervention, as in the case of 8-year-old Sarah. She had first been seen in the emergency room where she had been brought by her grandmother and several other relatives. The crisis occurred because Sarah had been sexually assaulted by a young adult uncle, who had returned home "high on some kind of dope." In a brief encounter with the family, the psychiatry resident noted the grandmother to be a reservoir of support. It was the grandmother who had been able to bring some order to the chaotic situation that confronted her when she returned home from her "day work" job, and arranged for the trip to the hospital. It was grandmother who was able to provide some comfort to Sarah, and persuade her to allow the nurse to examine her and to talk to the doctor. Providing support for the grandmother and guidance for handling of concrete problems (the child's anxiety, immediate child care and protection, and referral for help for the uncle) served as a focal point for the crisis intervention and the several subsequent sessions. The resident served as a connecting link with a member of the child abuse team, who was to follow the case. All involved agreed that on-going assessment would be an integral part of continued care.

Would the techniques of crisis intervention be any different for a family of another cultural background, or for a black middle-class family? The psychological pain triggered by an act of child abuse is experienced as "hurt" for any child, and the described repercussions might well be similar for many families. The first step in crisis intervention for any family is to assure treatment for any physical illness or injury and stop the psychological bleeding; then, to utilize those tools that are most useful in activating a reparative process. In outlining effective short-range psychiatric treatment of abused children referred to the Harlem Hospital Medical Center, Leal (1976) underscores the importance of determining the most therapeutic placement of the children returned to their families or foster home placement:

> In making the decision, the therapist should take into consideration the parents' abilities to be tolerant of the child's temperamental style as he or she negotiates the many developmental phases. Do they have the ability to recognize and accept their role in the child's trauma—whether it was direct or indirect: What potential do they have to develop more rational expectations for the child's behavior? What possibility is there that the parents will be able to meet their own affective, objective and socioeconomic needs appropriately through the supportive and insight-oriented psychiatric intervention that is available to them? If a foster home is being considered, what abilities do the guardians have to support and reinforce the child as he develops? (p. 224).

INDIVIDUAL PSYCHOTHERAPY

As noted in a previous section, there are numbers of documentations of the effectiveness of individual, psychodynamically oriented psychotherapy with black youngsters and their parents. There are no differences in the indications nor the goals. However, there may be a need for the introduction of parameters in the application of the techniques. Also, the therapist must remain alert to specific transferences and countertransferences. (It should be emphasized that these special considerations are not necessarily limited to work with black patients.)

It has been said that black patients tend to present as passive-aggressive and/or dependent; they tend to adopt defensive and adaptive behavior patterns that detract from the efficacy of psychotherapy. All of the above may well be valid for some black patients when there has been little or no attention to: 1) "educating" the patient about the process, 2) the identification of transference/counter-transference phenomena that can quickly convert into insurmountable barriers, 3) consideration of the use of parameters, and 4) weeding out of racial stereotyping that may have colored the assessment.

A first-year child psychiatry fellow, who had trained in general psychiatry in the same setting—a university based hospital on the fringes of an inner city black community—was well aware of the diversity of the families which had been assigned to him for diagnostic assessment and treatment. Many youngsters, like their parents, eyed authority with suspicion and held firm to a passive-aggressive stance. From his experience, he had come to know that many youngsters from this particular community were action oriented, and not readily accepting of an experience wherein one sat and talked to an authority figure for an extended period of time. Following suggestions from his supervisor, he made use of various parameters in the process of establishing and maintaining a therapeutic alliance. So it was for 8-year-old Adam, who was referred from a pediatric clinic because of hyperactivity, recurring nightmares, and episodic outbursts of near hysterical laughter. He was seen as a bright and inquisitive youngster, who needed to know all that went on (obviously, the latter characteristic was an asset to the psychotherapeutic process). For a number of reasons, not the least important being the child's and his mother's suspiciousness about the referral and the nature of the work of the clinic, both mother and child were introduced to two respective groups. The same resident and his co-therapist were assisted by established members of the group in "educating" the new members about the process. There was more than a hint that this kind of interaction assisted in the beginnings of the development of a therapeutic alliance. In the children's group, a major task was to convert ego syntonic behavior to ego dystonic. (The therapist remained alert to the fact that some behavior patterns that might be viewed as maladaptive in one cultural setting were adaptive in another. However, he was aware that some of the behavior patterns of some of the youngsters stunted their development.) Again and again assistance was provided by one child or another.

Within a period of several months, Adam began to focus much of his discussion on the content of his nightmares and dreams. This elicited some annoyance from other members of the group, who made it clear that they wanted and needed to stay with more concrete issues. The therapist pointed out that help comes from different sources, that one has different needs at different times, and suggested the possibility that Adam might be interested in figuring out a puzzle of his dreams in individual treatment sessions. Reference was made to an actual experience, previously discussed in the group as an example. (One of the girls, with a severe reading disability, had recently terminated group therapy several weeks after initial contact with a remedial reading tutor.)

There was no need to introduce parameters in working with Adam in individual treatment. The child responded to confrontations with apparent interest and eagerness to examine a bit of behavior, and readily supplied associations in the effort to "find other pieces to the puzzles of my life" (this was a reflection of his long-standing exposure to the "soaps"). As in other therapeutic encounters, the therapist was supportive of the child's self-mastery, and his movement in the direction of reinforcing those behaviors which decreased the sense of his inability to control his impulses.

A 16-year-old black girl of an interracial union (black mother and white father) was seen in consultation following an attempted suicide (by ingesting an unknown amount of a prescribed medication). At the time of a third visit, the consulting psychiatrist, a child psychiatry trainee, recommended outpatient psychotherapy after determining that the patient was no longer a suicidal risk. In addition to the overt depressive picture, a prominent feature of this adolescent's turmoil was her conflict about her racial identity. This identity conflict and her parents' handling of the matters of race (i.e., her father's tendency to ridicule black television characters and her mother's silence about race) prompted the therapist to focus on this early in the treatment. The therapist, a black woman, elected to be quite direct (in contrast to the patient's mother) about the issue. At the same time, the therapist remained alert to the possibility that the conflict about racial identity might have served to conceal or mask other roots of the patient's sense of low self-esteem. In this particular case, the patient's feelings about a physical handicap (which developed from an automobile accident 3 years prior to the suicidal gesture) were explored. In addition, strengths were identified and reinforced. (It was felt that treatment would have progressed more rapidly if the parents would have agreed to take part in family sessions or make a commitment for therapeutic intervention to resolve long-standing marital conflicts.)

A similar initial stance was taken in the treatment of an early adolescent black girl who had been adopted by white parents. I suggest that this approach be considered as an initial move in the therapeutic intervention with troubled black children (biological or adopted) of an interracial union or adopted by non-black parents. With the increase in the latter family structure, a growing number of white adoptive parents have sought guidelines to help them reinforce the racial identity of their black adopted children. Guidelines outlined by Comer and Poussaint (1975) are excellent reference points. They suggest that parents "discuss racial difference and adoption in a calm and natural way from time to time." They caution adoptive parents not to overprotect their black children about racial differences, and advise exposing them to the culture and history of various groups of black people. It should be noted that the efforts of white parents directed toward meeting their black child's need for black role models and peer companionship can alter the family's previous lifestyle in varying degrees. However, altered patterns of lifestyle are not limited to this type of family structure.

SUMMARY

In the diagnostic assessment and treatment planning for Afro-American children, a competent clinician will be alert to cultural differences and similarities, to the diversities within the racial group, and to the transferences and counter-transferences that may stem from class, cultural, and racial biases. These reference points are particularly significant in our multicultural society, and should be considered in the psychiatric care of any child. Stereotypes that have played a role in misdiagnosis and poor treatment planning for black youngsters should be avoided.

The reader has probably reflected on the numbers of children and parents seen in treatment who could not be reached, for whatever reason, by various techniques used. It should not be concluded that all black children are amenable to psychiatric intervention. Often, they are referred for our services "too late." In other instances, the noxious environment of their homes or communities serve to prevent or retard any therapeutic gains. The current curtailment of funding for the support of psychiatric care in various settings compound the difficulties and call for the combining efforts in child advocacy.

Unfortunately, for some black children, their lives are illustrated in a Langston Hughes (1974) poem:

> There are
> No clocks on the wall,
> And no time.
> No shadows that move
> From dawn to dusk
> Across the floor.
>
> There is neither light
> Nor dark
> Outside the door.
>
> There is no door!

However, for others there is a door, and these youngsters, aided by psychiatric intervention, can develop the strength to open it and move on.

REFERENCES

Adams, P. L. (1970), Dealing with racism in biracial psychiatry. *This Journal*, 9:33-43.

Chess, S. (1969), Disadvantages of "the disadvantaged child." *Amer. J. Orthopsychiat.*, 39:4-5.

Comer, J. P., & Pouissant, A. F. (1975), *Black Child Care.* New York: Simon & Schuster.

Ellis, W. A., Comer, J. P. & Rubenstein, S. (1979), Socioeconomic and racial considerations. In: *Basic Handbook of Child Psychiatry*, Vol. 3, ed. S. I. Harrison, New York: Basic Books, pp. 444-457.

Harrison, S. I., McDermott, J. F., Wilson, P. I. & Schrager, J. (1965), Social class and mental illness in children: choice of treatment. *Arch. Gen. Psychiat.*, 13:411-417.

Heacock, D. R. (1976), The black slum child and the problem of aggression. *Amer. J. Psychoanal.*, 36:219-226.

Hughes, L. (1974), *Selected Poems of Langston Hughes.* New York: Vintage Books.

Hunt, R. G. (1962), Occupational status in the disposition of cases in a child guidance clinic. *Int. J. Soc. Psychiat.*, 8:199-210.

Jackson, A. M., Berkowitz, H. & Farley, G. K. (1974), Race as a variable affecting the treatment involvement of children. *This Journal*, 13:20-31.

Ladner, J. A. (1972), *Tomorrow's Tomorrow: The Black Women.* New York: Doubleday.

Lavietes, R. L. (1974), Crisis intervention for ghetto children: contradictions and alternative considerations. *Amer. J. Orthopsychiat.*, 44:720-727.

Lawrence, M. M. (1975), *Young Inner-City Families: Development of Ego Strength Under Stress.* New York: Behavior Publications.

Leal, C. A. (1976), Treatment of abused and neglected preschool children in a city hospital. *Psychiat. Ann.*, 5:216-226.

——— (1981), Personal communication.

Lockett, H. J. (1972), The day treatment center. *J. Nat. Med. Assn.*, 64:527-532.

Malone, C. A. (1967), Child psychiatric services for low socioeconomic families. *This Journal*, 6:332-345.

Meers, D. R. (1970), Contributions of a ghetto culture to symptom formation. *The Psychoanalytic Study of the Child*, pp. 209-230.

Pasamanick, B. (1959), Influence of sociocultural factors in mental retardation. *Amer. J. Ment. Defic.*, 64:316-329.

Pinderhughes, C. A. & Rolland, R. (1971), Psychotherapy with black patients. Read at the Annual Meeting of the National Medical Association.

Pizer, E. (1981), Personal communication.

Powell, G. J. (1973), Self-concept in white and black children. In: *Racism and Mental Health*, ed. C. V. Willie, B. M. Kramer, & B. S. Brown. Pittsburgh: University of Pittsburgh Press.

Simmons, I. (1981), Personal communication.

Spurlock, J. & Cohen, R. L. (1969), Should the poor get none. *This Journal*, 8:16-35.

——— & Lawrence, L. E. (1979), The black child. In: *Basic Handbook of Child Psychiatry*, Vol. 3, ed. J. D. Noshpitz, New York: Basic Books, pp. 248-257.

Taylor, R. L. (1976), Psychosocial development among black children and youth: A reexamination. *Amer. J. Orthopsychiat.*, 46:4-19.

Wadeson, R. W. (1975), Psychoanalysis in community psychiatry: reflection on some theoretical implications. *J. Amer. Psychoanal. Assn.*, 23:177-189.

Westman, J. C. (1979), Psychiatric day treatment. In: *Basic Handbook of Child Psychiatry*, Vol. 3, New York: Basic Books, pp. 288-299.

Yarrow, L. J. & Harmon, R. J. (1980), Maternal deprivation. In: *Comprehensive Textbook of Psychiatry, III.* Baltimore: Williams & Wilkins, pp. 2727-2734.

33

Neuropharmacology of Methylphenidate and a Neural Substrate for Childhood Hyperactivity

C. T. Gaultieri
University of North Carolina, Chapel Hill

R. E. Hicks
University of Alabama, Birmingham

In 1977, a research group was assembled at the University of North Carolina with a multidisciplinary orientation around the problem of childhood hyperactivity and the pharmacology of stimulant drugs. The disciplines involved, in addition to psychiatry, were neuropharmacology (Breese), behavioral and experimental psychology (Schroeder and Hicks), analytic and medicinal chemistry (Patrick), and neuropsychology (Evans). The initial focus of the research program was the pharmacology of the frequently prescribed stimulant, methylphenidate (MPH), but the interest of the group eventually shifted to the broader question of a neural substrate for the syndrome of childhood hyperactivity. This is a summary of research developments from the North Carolina project and an incidental history of a shift from the solution of a traditional problem in psychopharmacology to a broader neuropsychological approach to developmental neuropsychiatry.

Reprinted with permission from *Psychiatric Clinics of North America*, 1985, Vol. 8, 875–892. Copyright 1985 by W. B. Saunders and Co.

The work described herein was supported by Grants HD 07201-06 and MH 36294-03 to Dr. Gualtieri.

METHYLPHENIDATE: PHARMACOLOGIC AND PHARMACOKINETIC
INVESTIGATIONS

The first concern of the research group was with the pharmacology of MPH and the clinical salience of MPH serum level (SL) determinations. MPH is by far the most often prescribed medication for hyperactivity[11] and stimulant medication is said to be taken by up to 700,000 American children.[108] Because definitive pharmacokinetic studies of MPH had not been done, it was thought that a careful study was in order and could conceivably improve clinical care for many youngsters. For example, it was not known whether problems such as response failure or the development of side effects were attributable to low or high SL, respectively. Our research in this area has been definitive and included studies of MPH in hyperactive children (HAC), in normal adults, and in "hyperactive adults" (HAA).[53,54]

At the time this work began in 1977, there had been only a few published studies on the pharmacology and metabolism of MPH. It had been established that MPH is poorly bound to plasma proteins,[28] differing in this respect from the neuroleptics and tricyclic antidepressants (TCAs), which are bound to a considerable degree to plasma proteins. Studies in man had been limited to the measurement of plasma levels and urinary output of ^{14}C-MPH and its inactive metabolite ritalinic acid (RA). It was known that peak ^{14}C-MPH levels occurred at about 2 hours after an oral dose. The estimated half-life (T½) ranged from 2 to 7 hours. Gastrointestinal absorption of ^{14}C-MPH was essentially complete.[40] However, the problems in measurement were severe, compromised by lack of internal standards, low sensitivity, thermal decomposition of drug, and large blood volume requirements for analysis.[29,42,61,99,124] No clinical correlation studies had been done, despite the wide prescription of MPH and the then-current psychiatric interest in blood-level correlations.

The first requirement was to develop a reliable and sensitive assay for MPH in blood. A gas chromatography-mass spectrometry method was developed that incorporated deuterated internal stands to quantify MPH and its active metabolite parahydroxy methylphenidate (p-OH-MPH). This method was subject to a rate of error no higher than 0.052 at one nanogram MPH per mm of solution. The lower level of quantifiable detection was 0.5 mg per ml. Test-retest accuracy in split samples analyzed separately by two laboratories yielded a correlation coefficient of 0.99.[120]

The development of an extremely sensitive and accurate analytic method was accompanied by chemical developments in the synthesis of assay standards and by basic pharmacologic studies of MPH in laboratory animals and normal volunteers.[84,120] Important information was obtained from these studies, for example, about the metabolism of MPH to RA, which is not active, and to parahydroxy MPH, which is active but which probably does not cross the blood-brain barrier.[84]

The pharmacokinetics of MPH were studied in hyperactive children (N = 26) and adults (N = 10) and in normal adults (N = 15). The early studies were intended to define the pharmacokinetic time profile of MPH in different groups. The profile was found to be similar for normal adults, HAA and HAC. Following an oral dose, concentration time profiles peak at 60 to 120 minutes and elimination half-lives range from 2.3 to 4.2 hours, with a mean of 3.4 hours. The pharmacokinetic time profile of MPH parallels the clinical activity of the drug over about 4 hours after an oral dose.[114] This is in contrast to d-amphetamine, which appears to peak at 3 to 4 hours, in spite of a duration of clinical activity that closely resembles that of MPH.[13]

In the pharmacokinetic studies, it was found that there was fourfold variation between individuals in peak SL, and substantial interindividual variation was also observed in 1 hour MPH SL in clinical studies of MPH effects in HAC and HAA. Interindividual variability in MPH SL was determined *not* to be a function of the 1-hour sampling time; variability in MPH blood levels at 2 to 3 hours was no smaller than at 1 hour,[54] nor were serum levels found to be affected by the subjects' fasting or eating state. Our original report in normal adults[55] was subsequently confirmed by Chan and associates[20] in HAC. This incidental finding is of considerable importance in the clinical management of HAC, as taking the drug on an empty stomach can cause anorexia and stomach aches in HAC. In fact, MPH can be administered before, during, or immediately after meals with no detectable loss of clinical activity. A further complicating factor in these studies was the discovery of substantial *intraindividual* variability in MPH blood levels.[54] In a given patient, serum levels were observed to vary by a factor of 20 on different days, even when controlling for oral dose, time after administration, the subject's eating-fasting state and activity level. This pattern of extreme variability, obviously not a function of the assay procedure, was a first hint of the relative inutility of MPH SL determinations.

Research having to do with the clinical utility of MPH blood level determinations included a double-blind crossover study of MPH in two doses (0.3 and 0.6 mg per kg) compared with placebo in 55 HAC, neuroendocrine and mood correlates of MPH blood levels along the pharmacokinetic curve in adults and children, and within-subject studies of the correlation between clinical response and variable blood levels. In the clinical study of 55 HAC (the "acute effects study"), MPH SLs drawn 1 hour after an oral dose were correlated with a number of response measures including clinical impressions, Conners rating scales (teachers and parents),[24] direct behavioral observations, and laboratory measures of attention and activity, neuroendocrine response (prolactin and growth hormone), and pulse and blood pressure change. Drug response was measured statistically in terms of absolute change from placebo and baseline levels, in terms of relative change in rating scale scores based on published norms,[48] in terms of the slope of the linear component of the dose-response function, and, borrowing a method from behavioral pharmacology, the logarithm of the drug score divided by the placebo score (log D/P). The results here were conclusive but negative. Correlation between response measures and MPH SL occurred at the level predicted by chance, regardless of the response measure or the statistical manipulation that was employed.

Prior to entry into the acute effects study, 26 of the HAC had undergone MPH pharmacokinetic time profile analysis. Following a 0.3 mg per kg oral dose, eight blood samples were drawn from 0 to 480 minutes. For each individual, a time profile was developed, and from this profile were derived the following measures: 1-hour MPH serum levels, peak MPH levels, time to peak, MPH half-life, and area under the pharmacokinetic curve (AUC). The dependent measures chosen for analysis were the various response measures to the 0.3 mg per kg dose in the acute effects study. No significant correlations were found between pharmacokinetic variables and any of the response measures.

The third phase of this research involved analysis of changes in secretion of the anterior pituitary hormones, growth hormone (GH) and prolactin (PRL), which are known to be under monoaminergic control and sensitive to MPH administration.[102] Again, there was no correlation between MPH SL levels and either GH level or PRL levels when a "detrended" analysis was employed. "Detrended" analysis is a method that controls for similar kinds of time profiles in the measures that are to be correlated. As levels of MPH, GH, and PRL will change after an oral dose of MPH, a spurious correlation might easily arise unless the analysis is "detrended."[82]

With respect to intraindividual variation in MPH SL, serial measurement of SL was done over several days in four HAC who were clear MPH responders in the Acute Effects Study. Serum levels were variable, indeed, but did not correlate within subjects with direct observations or ratings of behavior, laboratory measures of activity and attention, neuroendocrine or cardiovascular response.[51]

In at least some children on stimulant medications, the positive effects of treatment appear to wane over time. However, tolerance of MPH does not seem to be a pharmacologic phenomenon. In addition to acute studies of MPH, we conducted a follow-up study of 17 HAC who had been treated with MPH for 11 to 66 months (mean 22.5 months). MPH SLs relative to oral dose were not lower in these chronically treated children than in acutely treated children. When MPH effects were tested in a double-blind crossover design study similar in construction to the acute effects study, it was found that stimulant effects on behavior ratings, neuroendocrine, and cardiovascular measures and laboratory measures of attention and activity were undiminished even after months of treatment.[52] Tolerance to stimulant drugs in HAC may occur, but little is known about the frequency of the problem or its clinical significance. In this sample, however, evidence of neither clinical nor pharmacologic tolerance was found.

In summary, although MPH SLs are reliable from a procedural standpoint and a statistical standpoint as well, they are also (in a given individual) quite variable on a day-to-day basis, and this variability does not relate to the clinical variability that also occurs in HAC. The pharmacokinetic profile MPH is well-defined and similar across studies of HAC and adults, although clearance of the drug is more rapid in children. Along the pharmacokinetic time profile of the drug occasional associations can be demonstrated with certain measures, such as the neuroendocrine response and the euphoric response in adults. But neither 1-hour SLs nor any other pharmacokinetic parameter correlate with any of a host of measures employed to measure stimulant response. MPH SLs do not distinguish between drug "responders" and "nonresponders;" they are not correlated with the occurrence or severity of toxic effects; and they are not reflected, in between-subjects analyses, in correlated changes in any of the dependent measures.

Although there are reports in the literature that suggest that MPH blood levels are, in fact, correlated with clinical responses, these are preliminary reports based on limited kinds of response measures in relatively small samples of children.[71,102] In most such studies, no attempt is made to partial out the effects of dose on clinical response when the salience of SL is at issue. The clinically essential question, after all, is not whether blood levels correlate with response, but whether any additional variance in response is attributable to blood levels once the variance in response attributable to dose is partialled out. In other words, will blood levels predict any more about the patient's clinical response than dose will? In one study[131] this statistical manipulation was done, and no additional variance in response was explained by blood levels after the effects of dose were partialled out.

On the basis of this research, we concluded that MPH SLs are not statistically related to clinical response nor are they likely to prove clinically helpful. The reason for this dissociation may reside in the selective affinity of MPH for different tissues. For example, in preclinical studies conducted by colleagues in North Carolina, it was found that in rat brain, levels of MPH peak earlier and at much higher concentrations than SLs after intravenous or oral administration.[84]

A second explanation may be the lack of stereochemical stereospecificity of the present MPH assay, which does not differentiate between the d- and l-enantiomers of MPH (threo-dl-MPH). Present methods of MPH analysis cannot differentiate between the d- and l-enantiomers. Only 11 to 53 per cent of an oral dose of MPH is bioavailable;[20] most of an oral dose of MPH is metabolized by hydrolysis before reaching systemic circulation.[20,120] Enzymes that govern the hydrolysis of esters structurally similar to MPH exhibit extreme stereospecificity.[57] Thus, it is possible that the original 50:50 dl-mixture of MPH isomers present in the orally administered compound is selectively enriched in favor of one stereoisomer as a consequence of selective enzymatic degradation.[130] The relative potency of d- and l-enantiomers of MPH has not been examined.

The d-isomer of cocaine, a stimulant similar to MPH, possesses considerably more activity than the l-isomer.[92] Further, the erythro-dl- and three-dl isomers of MPH exhibit comparable toxicity.[116] It is possible that the d- and l-threo MPH isomers may likewise show differential pharmacologic profiles. A relevant example is amphetamine, in which the d-isomer is known to possess a more favorable therapeutic index than the racemic mixture, the isomers are metabolized differentially, and they are not equally retained in brain.[46]

A third explanation may be pharmacodynamic, rather than pharmacologic. That is, MPH response may be a function of neural sensitivity to the drug, rather than to drug level per se. This may be a function of interindividual differences of subgroups of HAC.

STIMULANTS AND NEUROLEPTICS

There is a singular aspect to the pharmacologic treatment of hyperactive children that has elicited comparatively little interest: that is, the fact that neuroleptic drugs—polar opposites to the psychostimulants, in neuropharmacologic terms—are also highly effective. The clinical disorder may be successfully managed by recourse to psychostimulants, which are indirect acting dopamine agonists,[70] or by neuroleptics, whose major therapeutic action is presumably a function of postsynaptic dopamine receptor blockade.[18]

In light of the extensive clinical, preclinical, and theoretical literature on childhood hyperactivity, it is surprising that this seeming paradox has elicited so little in the way of critical attention. The phenomen is difficult to reconcile with theories of childhood hyperactivity, for example, which posit as central to the disorder a unitary kind of neurotransmitter dysfunction (for example, Shaywitz and associates[101]). Several alternatives come to mind by way of explanation for the paradox. For example, it is possible that stimulant-responders and neuroleptic-responders represent different *subgroups* of hyperactive children. This alternative could not be tested, however, in the between-groups designs that have largely characterized the relevant literature. It is also possible that the neurochemical profiles of stimulants and neuroleptics are more complex than the preceding paragraph suggests. For example, neuroleptics in low doses are known to behave as dopamine agonists by virtue of their action on the presynaptic autoreceptor;[2] similarly, stimulant effects on the autoreceptor may actually inhibit dopamine release.[64] Alternatively, the therapeutic effects of neuroleptics and stimulants in HAC may be mediated through alternative pathways. Monoamine systems are highly interconnected, anatomically and functionally, and it is probably naive to reduce the action of any psychoactive drug to its effect on a single neurotransmitter system.[4] However, discussions on this order of pharmacologic ambiguity have not, as a rule, characterized the hyperactivity literature. The paradox stands: It is difficult to conceive of two classes of psychiatric medication so dissimilar as stimulants and neuroleptics. Nevertheless, a drug from either class may be, and frequently is, selected to treat the hyperactive child.

Recent therapeutic studies of drug treatment in HAC have not been oriented toward the neuroleptics, a consequence of the mounting concern over the long-term side effects of neuroleptics in children, especially tardive dyskinesia.[51] However, from the early 1960s to the mid-1970s, neuroleptic treatment played a prominent role in the pharmacologic literature on childhood hyperactivity. Unfortunately, the research literature in this area is fragmentary. There are only a handful of comparison studies. In many instances, the sample sizes are small (Alexandris and Lundel,[3] N = 21; Campbell and colleagues,[17] N = 15) or the subjects are diagnostically[17,21,58,96] or intellectually heterogeneous.[3,21,58] Many of the studies arrived at doses of neuroleptics or of stimulants that were "clinically titrated" to "therapeutically optimal levels,"[48,58,96,129] whereas fixed-dose studies based on weight or body surface formulae are currently preferred in pediatric pharmacologic research.[109,126] The doses employed as a consequence of the "optimal" titration method are probably excessively high by today's standards; neuroleptic doses, for example, ranged as high as 400 to 800 mg per day (chlorpromazine equivalents, Davis[27]).[17,45,58,112] Although the studies cited were all double-blind, between groups comparisons tended to be preferred[3,17,21,45,49,96,123,129] to cross-over designs.[58,110,127]

Despite these methodologic shortcomings, there is agreement across studies that the behavioral symptoms that characterize HAC (locomotor hyperactivity, impulsiveness, excitability, aggression) improve to a satisfactory extent with either neuroleptic or psychostimulant treatment. There is disagreement on whether symptoms of inattention and distractibility respond as well to neuroleptics as to stimulants. Weiss and coworkers[112] found that stimulants exerted positive effects on behavioral symptoms with no discernible effect on distractibility or inattention. In contrast, Gittelman-Klein and associates[45] reported that, on the basis of observers' ratings, attentional symptoms improved with both the stimulant MPH and the neuroleptic, thioridazine (THD). With respect to other cognitive tasks, the literature suggests that stimulants may lead to improvement or, at worst, no change,[123] whereas neuroleptics may cause deterioration in function or, at best, no change.[17,49,58,129] The favorable effects of psychostimulants on cognitive tasks and the detrimental effects of neuroleptics are, of course, well-supported in studies of normal adults.[56,72,121]

In summary, when psychostimulants and neuroleptic drugs are administered to hyperactive children, it appears that certain drug effects, especially cognitive and possibly attentional effects, are dissociable, whereas behavioral effects on troublesome symptoms like hyperactivity are exercised in common.

An opportunity to re-evaluate the comparative effects of stimulants and neuroleptics in HAC was afforded the authors by Werry at the University of Auckland (New Zealand), who generously permitted a reanalysis of raw data from a neuroleptic-stimulant comparison study that was elegant in conception and sophisticated in execution.[127,128] The study was a double-blind, placebo-controlled, cross-over design in 24 hyperactive or conduct-disordered boys and girls who had been referred to a child psychiatrist at a university hospital clinic. Each subject participated in a 12-week treatment study with four randomized, 3-week conditions: placebo, MPH (0.3 mg per kg) and two doses of haloperidol (HDL) (0.025 mg per kg and 0.050 mg per kg). Cognitive testing was done at the end of each treatment condition. Dependent measures included a short-term recognition memory task and the continuous performance task, seat movements on a stabilometric cushion, teachers' behavior ratings, and observed activity in a laboratory playroom. The cognitive measures were reported in the 1975 paper and the behavioral ratings in the 1976 paper.

The authors' analysis revealed favorable behavioral effects on symptoms of hyperactivity, aggression, and attention with MPH and both doses of HDL; however, the higher HDL dose did not lead to any further increment in behavioral ratings, whereas side effects, especially dystonia, were markedly increased.[128] On cognitive measures, MPH was found to improve performance on the memory task, at a high task difficulty level, whereas HDL, high dose, exercised a depressant effect at moderate task difficulty. Vigilance attention on the continuous performance task was improved by MPH and by low-dose HDL, compared with placebo and high-dose HDL.

Our reanalysis of these data revealed highly significant within-subjects correlations on behavioral response and cognitive improvement between MPH and low-dose HDL but not between MPH and high-dose HDL or between low- and high-dose HDL. In other words, the effects of stimulants and low-dose neuroleptics in HAC were exercised in common. Both classes of drug exerted positive effects on symptoms of locomotion or hyperactivity, impulsiveness, and inattention. More important, however, is that the behavioral effects were *correlated*; it is not simply that some HAC respond well to stimulants and others to neuroleptics. In essence, the same patients respond in the same direction and to the same degree with either medication. Thus, the paradox may not be resolved on the basis of clinical subgroups who respond differentially to stimulants and neuroleptics.

Low-dose neuroleptics may exert a stimulant-like effect by virtue of autoreceptor blockade.[2] In the Werry study, low-dose HDL did indeed exert a stimulant-like effect on the continuous performance task; this effect was lost at the higher dose and was not correlated with that of MPH. Yet both neuroleptic doses were effective in improving behavioral symptoms.

PREDICTION OF STIMULANT RESPONSE

Returning to the "pure" stimulant studies: If MPH SLs are not predictive of clinical response, it was natural to ask whether other clinical elements in the HAC might be predictive. In the acute effects study, an array of such factors were considered relative to clinical response: age, sex, race, social class, baseline behavior rating scales and observations, neurologic soft signs, minor physical anomalies, associated diagnoses, WISC-R and subtest scores, achievement testing, evidence of learning disability, perceptual motor testing, as well as measures of the child's adaptive function, social competence, and family environment. None of these measures were found to be correlated with or predictive of clinical response to medication.[59] This negative result is quite in keeping with other contributions to the stimulant literature.[8,132] Despite years of clinical research and attempts to predict clinical response on the basis of some aspect of the child's clinical picture, it is simply not possible to predict the clinical response to stimulant drugs. It is generally estimated that about 70 to 80 percent of HAC respond favorably to stimulants,[7] but neither clinical nor pharmacokinetic data, seemingly, are helpful in predicting who these children will be.

NONINTERCORRELATED DRUG EFFECTS

Although these two negative results from an exhaustive and meticulous series of clinical experiments were discouraging, we felt compelled to examine more closely the notion of drug "response." The idea of doing so would perhaps appear trivial to the practitioner who has grown confident in his or her own clinical judgment and those of trusted aides. It was believed, however, that a closer look at the concept of stimulant response was in order.

The traditional model represents a disorder or syndrome as a unitary entity, characterized by a constellation of symptoms that may vary in different individuals, but that respond in concert to a given intervention. We were surprised to learn that such is hardly the case for childhood hyperactivity. Stimulant response on different response measures were simply nonintercorrelated. Drug-induced improvement, for example, on the hyperactivity items of the Conners Teacher Rating Scale did not predict improvement on the distractibility items or in the Parent Rating Scale. Performance on the distractibility items of the Conners was not predictive of changes on laboratory measures of vigilant attention. Drug effects on attention were not predictive of changes in activity levels measured by a wristwatch actometer or in the Routh Activity Room.[95] When all of the dependent measures applied in the acute effects study were examined, it was startling to discover that the intercorrelation of response measures following MPH occurred at a level no greater than chance. Response to MPH in HAC is simply not a unitary phenomenon.[59]

RATE DEPENDENCY

Stimulant response, therefore, was a function of the dependent measure employed to gauge response. It was neither an integrated nor a unitary phenomenon. Although similar findings had been reported in HAC in the nondrug state, this was the first and most dramatic demonstration of nonintercorrelation of stimulant effects, for example, on the basis of single-minded attentional or arousal mechanisms.

If stimulant response cannot be predicted in terms of pharmacokinetic or clinical elements nor understood in terms of some unifying psychological constructs such as attention or arousal, it seemed as if some other conceptual base was called for. An appealing hypothesis in this regard was the idea of *rate dependency*. In preclinical studies, and in research with normal adult volunteers, it was known that the effects of stimulant medication on locomotor activity vary inversely with the state of the organism in the drug-free condition. Stimulants tend to decrease high rates of activity, whereas low rates are increased or remain unchanged. It has been hypothesized that this principle would also characterize the broader clinical response of HAC. Rate dependency,[33] the general term for this phenomenon, is well established in the behavioral pharmacology literature and occasionally is applied in the theoretical literature on childhood hyperactivity.[81,140] The idea of rate dependency is that the effects of stimulant drugs on any given measure will be largely a function of the *predrug* state of the organism on that measure. The state of the organism influences response to drug.[34]

The rate dependency hypothesis was primarily developed from single-subject operant paradigms in rats, pigeons, and other laboratory animals. It has been proposed as a clinically salient and useful idea; it is also consistent with our finding of nonintercorrelated response measures and the lack of predictive value for presumably relevant clinical factors. However, we were aware of substantial weaknesses in the rate dependency hypothesis. Operationally, the phenomenon may also be explicable in terms of drug effects on memory[59,83] or temporal judgment.[59,136] Rate dependency has been criticized on statistical grounds (regression to the mean) but the most telling argument against the wider relevance of rate-dependency is mathematical rather than statistical.[47]

When a traditional rate dependency analysis was actually applied to clinical data from the acute effects study, it was found that almost all of the dependent measures were rate-dependent. Dependent measures that were relatively unresponsive to MPH were among the most rate-dependent, whereas measures that were typically responsive to MPH were sometimes the least responsive when a rate-dependency analysis was applied. In fact, when we performed a traditional rate-dependency analysis to sets of computer-generated random numbers, they, too, were found to be rate-dependent. Our conclusion was that no direct information concerning the magnitude or direction of the effect of MPH could be gleaned from the statistical techniques of rate dependency.

Nevertheless, there are known to be instances in which the effect of a stimulant drug on a given response measure is related to the predrug response level of the subject.[1,67,90] This is well established, for example, in electrophysiologic studies of humans as well as in animals studies.[90,118] Although the mathematics of traditional rate dependency is questionable, the principle may have at least some validity.

A NEURAL HYPOTHESIS OF CHILDHOOD HYPERACTIVITY

It finally appeared that a unifying hypothesis of stimulant drug effects could be constructed. From our own clinical research and that of others cited, it seems as if stimulant drug effects on different dimensions are variable, unpredictable, and nonintercorrelated. The equivocal nature of stimulant effects[66] may be described as follows: "Neither performance nor arousal or vigilance should be viewed as steady-state phenomena . . . amphetamine probably acts by decreasing the amplitude of spontaneously occurring troughs in these hypothetical parameters."[107]

If the primary action of stimulant drugs is thus to *canalize* various parameters of arousal and reactivity, then their therapeutic benefit in HAC may be explicable on the basis of their trait of excessive variability. Inconsistent levels of arousal and reactivity do seem to characterize HAC[8,12,16,23,29,37,65,80,105,115] (see Hicks and Gualtieri[59] for review). Excessive variability in arousal and response would militate against efficient performance either on a psychological test or in the classroom or in a taxing social situation. The action of stimulants may be simply to reduce response variability, a homeostatic effect.[52,79,107]

The hypothesis of childhood hyperactivity as a dysregulatory or a heterostatic disorder has the advantage of suggesting a likely neural substrate for the disorder in anterior brain structures, especially the frontal cortex and caudate nucleus. The excessive intrasubject variability of autonomic, electrocortical, and behavioral response in HAC is also found in patients afflicted with frontal lobe lesions,[6,87] as is the evidence for relative uncoupling of CNS-ANS-behavioral processes.[50,60,98,103] It is not surprising that the orbital surface of the frontal lobe is essential to the coordination of various somatomotor and visceromotor activities. This area is unique in that (1) inputs from virtually all bilateral sensory systems converge;[98] (2) it constitutes the major neocortical representation of limbic output;[138] and (3) it constitutes the rostral end of a powerful descending, inhibitory, and synchronizing system.[22,98,134] Afferent information from all parts of the body and "affective marking" would be a prerequisite for the coordinating role of a cortical center that regulates many levels of the neuraxis (for review, see Hicks and Gualtieri[59]).

The neural model is derived from clinical observations of the striking similarity between HAC and patients with damage to the frontal lobes;[78,85,111] problems with excessive variability and dysregulation (heterostasis), distractibility and lack of impulse control, locomotion hyperactivity, attentional difficulties that take the form of diminished persistence of attending (orienting), distractibility from extraneous stimuli, and perseverative attending under certain conditions.[35,77,91,125,138] College students selected for poor performance on a vigilance attention task have been found to do especially poorly on neuropsychological tests of frontal lobe dysfunction.[15] In both the frontal lobe syndrome and in childhood hyperactivity, the apparent paradox of concurrent symptoms of perseveration and distractibility is explicable in terms of a diminished capacity for self-regulation: both classes of patients may persist in inappropriate behaviors that feedback indicates is inappropriate (and which they can describe as such), but they appear just as likely to discontinue behaviors that feedback indicates is correct.[37,139] Both groups are also liable to various "minor" motor abnormalities in addition to excess motor activity such as clumsiness and associated movements.[25,31,69,77] Both demonstrate striking deficiencies in various dimensions of impulse control, including low tolerance for frustration, low ability to delay gratification, antisocial behavior and delinquency, and impaired sphincter control.[75,125,138] Defective impulse control may also be partially responsible for the notorious lack of planning and poor judgment attributed to each group.[35,37,44,77,88,125,137] Antisocial or, at least, socially disapproved behavior characterizes both classes of patients: impulsiveness, undependability, destructiveness, and aggressiveness. Both exhibit profound deficits in interpersonal relations, in part a consequence of these impulsive behavioral patterns. Interpersonal relationships are probably influenced as well by another shared characteristic: disordered emotionality. Their apparent lack of modulation of emotional response is indicated by their mercurial lability, varying in extremes from anhedonic depression to uncontrolled excitement.[75,112,113,125,138]

Additional evidence to support the hypothesis is adduced by (1) animal models of HKS employing frontal and striatal lesions,[68,81,119,135] and (2) neurochemical studies of dopaminergic projections to frontal cortex.[9,10,14,19,43,63,74,89,100,101,104,117]

The frequent subsidence of the symptoms of hyperactivity in adolescence is consistent with frontal maturation in the second decade of life[133] and suggests a dysmaturational underpinning to the disorder.[69] Finally, direct support for the hypothesis was presented by Lou and colleagues[76] in a regional cerebral blood flow study of 11 HAC, all of whom evidenced cerebral hypoperfusion in the frontal lobes and caudate nucleus, which was correlated by administration of stimulant medication (MPH).

SUMMARY

What began as a simple chemical question about the clinical utility of MPH SL measurement has led our group across a broad expanse of research endeavors, from the problem of nonintercorrelated stimulant effects to a theory of hyperactivity as a dysregulatory disorder based on frontal-striatal dysfunction or dysmaturation. The transition has been from a traditional and fairly circumscribed question in psychopharmacology to a new interest in the neuropsychological approach to hyperactivity and its treatment. Biologic psychiatry and neuropsychology have developed as distinct disciplines well insulated from one another, but a degree of cross-fertilization is beginning to occur. Rather than thinking of childhood hyperactivity in terms of vague metapsychological concepts such as "attention" or "arousal," it will be perhaps more constructive to base a model for the disorder on the foundation of known elements of brain function.

Perhaps the most interesting research areas to pursue will be neuropsychological and neurodiagnostic (for example, PET). The specific locus of disorders, such as the HKS and the specific mechanisms of drug action, may not be so elusive after all.

REFERENCES

1. Abel, E. L.: Drugs and Behavior: A Primer in Neuropsychopharmacology. New York, John Wiley and Sons, 1974.
2. Ahlenius, S., and Engel, J.: Effects of small doses of haloperidol on timing behavior. J. Pharm. Pharmacol., 23:301-302, 1971.
3. Alexandris, A., and Lundell, F. W.: Effect of thioridazine, amphetamine, and placebo on the hyperkinetic syndrome and cognitive area in mentally deficient children. Can. Med. Assoc. J., 98:92-96, 1968.
4. Antelman, S. M., and Caggiula, A. R.: Norepinephrine-dopamine interactions and behavior. Science, 195:646-653, 1977.
5. Arnold, L. E., Huestis, R., Smeltzer, D., et al.: Levoamphetamine versus dextroamphetamine in minimal brain dysfunction: Replication, time response, and differential effect by diagnostic group and family rating. Arch. Gen. Psychiatry, 33:292-301, 1976.
6. Baranovskaya, O. P., and Homskaya, E. D.: Changes in the electroencephalogram frequency spectrum during the presentation of neutral and meaningful stimuli to patients with lesions of the frontal lobes. *In* Pribham, K. H., and Luria, A. R. (eds.): Psychophysiology of the Frontal Lobes. New York, Academic Press, 1973.
7. Barkley, R. A.: A review of stimulant drug research with hyperactive children. J. Child Psychol. Psychiatry, 18:137-165, 1977.
8. Barkley, R. A., and Jackson, T. L., Jr.: Hyperkinesis, autonomic nervous system activity, and stimulant drug effects. J. Child Psychol. Psychiatry, 18:347-357, 1977.
9. Berger, B.: Histochemical identification and localization of dopaminergic axons in rat and human cerebral cortex. Adv. Biochem. Psychopharmacol., 16:13-20, 1977.
10. Bjorklund, A., Divac, I., and Lindvall, O.: Regional distribution of catecholamines in monkey cerebral cortex: Evidence for a dopaminergic innervation of the primate prefrontal cortex. Neurosci. Lett., 7:115-119, 1978.
11. Bosco, J. J., and Robin, S. S.: Hyperkinesis: Prevalence and treatment. *In* Whalen, C. K., and Henke, B. (eds.): Hyperactive Children: The Social Ecology of Identification and Treatment. New York, Academic Press, 1980, pages 173-187.
12. Boyle, R. H., Dykman, R. A., and Ackerman, P. T.: Relationships of resting autonomic activity, motor impulsivity, and EEG tracings in children. Arch. Gen. Psychiatry, 12:314-323, 1965.
13. Brown, G. L., Hunt, R. D., Ebert, M. H., et al.: Plasma levels of d-amphetamine in hyperactive children. Psychopharmacology (Berlin), 62:133-140, 1979.
14. Brozoski, T. J., Brown, R. M., Ptak, J., et al.: Dopamine in prefrontal cortex of rhesus monkeys: Evidence for a role in cognitive function. *In* Usdin, E., Kopin, I. J., and Barchas, J. (eds.): Catecholamines: Basic and Clinical Frontiers. Vol. 2. New York, Pergamon Press, 1979.
15. Buchsbaum, M., and Wender, P.: Average evoked responses in normal and minimally brain dysfunctioned children treated with amphetamine. Arch. Gen. Psychiatry, 29:764-770, 1973.
16. Busby, K., Firestone, P., and Pivik, R. T.: Sleep patterns in hyperkinetic and normal children. Sleep, 4:366-383, 1981.
17. Campbell, M., Cohen, I. L., and Small, A. M.: Drugs in aggressive behavior. Am. Acad. Child Psychiatry, 21(2):107-117, 1982.
18. Carlsson, A.: Mechanism of action of neuroleptic drugs. *In* Lipton, M. A., DiMascio,

A., and Killam, K. F. (eds.): Psychopharmacology: A Generation of Progress. New York, Raven Press, 1978.

19. Carter, C. J., and Pycock, C. J.: Behavioural and biochemical effects of dopamine and noradrenaline depletion within the medial prefrontal cortex of the rat. Brain Res., 192:163-176, 1980.

20. Chan, Y. P., Swanson, J. M., Soldin, S. S., et al.: Methylphenidate hydrochloride given with or before breakfast: II. Effects on plasma concentration of methylphenidate and ritalinic acid. Pediatrics, 72:56-59, 1983.

21. Claghorn, J. L.: A double-blind comparison of haloperidol (Haldol) and thioridazine (Mellaril) in outpatient children. Curr. Ther. Res., 14(12):785-789, 1972.

22. Clemente, C. D., Chase, M. H., Knauss, T. K., et al.: Inhibition of a monosynaptic reflex by electrical stimulation of the basal forebrain or the orbital gyrus in the cat. Experientia, 22:844-845, 1966.

23. Cohen, N. J., and Douglas, V. I.: Characteristics of the orienting response in hyperactive and normal children. Psychophysiology, 9:238-245, 1972.

24. Conners, C. K.: Rating scales for use in drug studies with children. *In* Guy, W. (ed.): ECDEU Assessment Manual for Psychopharmacology. Rockville, Maryland, National Institute of Mental Health, 1976; DHEW Publication No. (ADM) 76-338, pages 303-312.

25. Damasio, A. R.: Frontal lobe dysfunction. *In* Heilman, K., and Valenstein, E. (eds.): Clinical Neuropsychology. Oxford, England, Oxford University Press, 1979.

26. Davis, G. D.: Effects of central excitant and depressant drugs on locomotor activity in the monkey. Am. J. Physiol., 188:619-623, 1957.

27. Davis, J. M.: Comparative doses and costs of antipsychotic medication. Arch. Gen. Psychiatry, 33:858-861, 1976.

28. Dayton, P. G., Perel, J. M., Israili, Z. H., et al.: Studies with methylphenidate: Drug interactions and metabolism. *In* Sellers, E. M. (ed.): Clinical Pharmacology of Psychoactive Drugs. Toronto, Alcoholism and Drug Addiction Foundation, 1975, pages 183-202.

29. Delbeke, F. T., and Debackere, M.: Isolation and detection of methylphenidate, phacetoperane, and some other sympathomimetic central nervous stimulants with special reference to doping: I. Gas chromatic detection procedure with electron capture detection for some secondary amines. J. Chromatogr., 106:412-417, 1975.

30. Delgado, J. M. R.: Inhibitory functions in the neostriatum. *In* Divac, I., and Oberg, R. G. E. (eds.): The Neostriatum. Oxford, England, Pergamon Press, 1979.

31. Denkla, M. B.: Childhood learning disabilities. *In* Heilman, K. M., and Valenstein, E. (eds.): Clinical Neuropsychology. New York, Oxford University Press, 1979.

32. Dews, P. B.: Studies on behavior: II. The effects of pentobarbital, methamphetamine and scopolamine on performances in pigeons involving discriminations. J. Pharmacol. Exp. Ther., 115:380-389, 1955.

33. Dews, P. B.: Studies on behavior: IV. Stimulant actions of methamphetamine. J. Pharmacol. Exp. Ther., 122:137-147, 1958.

34. Dews, P. B., and Wenger, G. R.: Rate dependency of the behavioral effects of amphetamine. *In* Thompson, T., and Dews, P. B. (eds.): Advances in Behavioral Pharmacology. Vol. 1. New York, Academic Press, 1977, page 167.

35. Douglas, V. I.: Higher mental processes in hyperactive children: Implications for training. *In* Knights, R. M., and Bakker, D. J. (eds.): Rehabilitation, Treatment, and Management of Learning Disorders. Baltimore, University Park Press, 1980.

36. Douglas, V. I.: Treatment approaches: Establishing inner or outer control? *In*

Whalen, C. K., and Henker, B. (eds.): Hyperactive Children: The Social Ecology of Identification and Treatment. New York, Academic Press, 1980.

37. Dykman, R. A., Ackerman, P. T., and Olgesby, D. M.: Selective and sustained attention in hyperactive, learning-disabled, and normal boys. J. Nerv. Ment. Dis., 167:288-297, 1979.

38. Dykman, R. A., Walls, R. C., Suzuki, T., et a.: Children with learning disabilities: Conditioning, differentiation, and the effect of distraction. Am. J. Orthopsychiatry, 40:766-782, 1970.

39. Everett, G. M.: Dopamine and the hyperkinetic child. Adv. Biochem. Psychopharmacol., 16:681-2, 1977.

40. Faraj, B. A., Israili, Z. H., Perel, J. M., et al.: Metabolism and disposition of methylphenidate-¹⁴C: Studies in man and animals. J. Pharmacol. Exp. Ther., 191:535-547, 1974.

41. Gaito, J.: Equal and unequal n and equal and unequal intervals in trend analyses. Educ. Psychol. Meas., 37:283-289, 1973.

42. Gal, J., Hodshon, B. J., Pintauro, C., et al.: Pharmacokinetics of methylphenidate in the rat using single-ion monitoring GLC-mass spectrometry. J. Pharm. Sci., 66:866-869, 1977.

43. Galey, D., Simon, H., and LeMoal, M.: Behavioral effects of lesions in the AIO dopaminergic area of the rat. Brain Res., 124:83-97, 1977.

44. Gerbner, M.: Study on the functional mechanisms of the dorsolateral frontal lobe cortex. *In* Pribham, K. H., and Luria, A. R. (eds.): Psychophysiology of the Frontal Lobe. New York, Academic Press, 1973.

45. Gittelman-Klein, R., Klein, D. F., Katz, S., et al.: Comparative effects of methylphenidate and thioridazine in hyperkinetic children: I. Clinical results. Arch. Gen. Psychiatry, 33:1217-1231, 1976.

46. Goldstein, M., and Anagnoste, B.: The conversion in vivo of D-amphetamine to (+)-p-hydroxynorephedrine. Acta Biochim. Biophys. Acad. Sci. Hung. 107:166-168, 1965.

47. Gonzalez, F. A., and Byrd, L. D.: Mathematics underlying the rate-dependency hypothesis. Science, 195:546-550, 1977.

48. Goyette, C. H., Conner, C. K., and Ulrich, R. F.: Normative data on revised Conners parent and teacher rating scales. J. Abnorm. Child Psychol., 6:221-236, 1978.

49. Greenberg, L. M., Deem, M. A., and McMahon, S.: Effects of dextroamphetamine, chlorpromazine, and hydroxyzine on behavior and performance in hyperactive children. Am. J. Psychiatry, 129:532-539, 1972.

50. Grueninger, W. F., and Grueninger, J.: The primate frontal cortex and allassostasis. *In* Pribham, K. H., and Luria, A. R. (eds.): Psychophysiology of the Frontal Lobes. New York, Academic Press, 1973.

51. Gualtieri, C. T., Quade, D., Hicks, R. E., et al.: Tardive dyskinesia and other clinical consequences of neuroleptic treatment in children and adolescents. Am. J. Psychiatry, 141:20-23, 1984.

52. Gualtieri, C. T., Hicks, R. E., Mayo, J. P., et al.: The persistence of stimulant effects in chronically treated children: Further evidence of an inverse relationship between drug effects and placebo levels of response. Psychopharmacology, 83:44-47, 1983.

53. Gualtieri, C. T., Hicks, R. E., Patrick, K., et al.: Clinical correlates of methylphenidate blood levels. Ther. Drug Monit., in press, 1985.

54. Gualtieri, C. T., Wargin, W., Kanoy, R., et al.: Clinical studies of methylphenidate

serum levels in children and adults. J. Am. Acad. Child Psychiatry, 21:19-26, 1982.
55. Gualtieri, C. T., Wargin, W., Kanoy, R., et al.: The effects of eating and fasting on the absorption of methylphenidate. Res. Commun. Psychol. Psychiatry Behav., 7:381-384, 1982.
56. Hartlage, L. C.: Effects of chlorpromazine on learning. Psychol. Bull., 64:235-245, 1965.
57. Hein, G. E., and Niemann, C.: Steric course and specificity of alpha-chymotrypsin-catalyzed reactions: I. J. Am. Chem. Soc., 84:4487-4494, 1962.
58. Helper, M. M., Wilcott, R. C., and Garfield, S. L.: Effects of chlorpromazine on learning and related processing in emotionally disturbed children. J. Consult. Clin. Psychol., 27:1-9, 1963.
59. Hicks, R. E., and Gualtieri, C. T.: Differential psychopharmacology of methylphenidate and the neuropsychology of childhood hyperactivity. *In* Bloomingdale, L. (ed.): Attention Deficit Disorders: Child Behavior Development Series. Vol. 6. Jamaica, New York, SP Medical and Science Books, in press, 1985.
60. Homskaya, E. D.: Verbal regulation of the vegetative components of the orienting reflex in focal brain lesions. Cortex, 1:63-76, 1964.
61. Hungund, B. L., Hanna, M., and Winsberg, B. G.: A sensitive gas chromatographic method for the determination of methylphenidate (Ritalin) and its major metabolite alpha-phenyl-2-piperidine acetic acid (ritalinic acid) in human plasma using nitrogen-phosphorous detector. Commun. Psychopharmacol., 2:203-208, 1978.
62. Hungund, B. L., Perel, J. M., and Hurwic, M. J.: Pharmacokinetics of methylphenidate in hyperkinetic children. Br. J. Pharmacol., 8:571-576, 1979.
63. Iversen, S. D.: Behavior after neostriatal lesions in animals. *In* Divac, I., and Oberg, R. G. E. (eds.): The Neostriatum. Oxford, Pergamon Press, 1979.
64. Iversen, S. D., Howells, R. B., and Hughes, R. P.: Behavioral consequences of long-term treatment. *In* Cattabeni, F., Racagni, G., Spano, P. F., et al. (eds.): Long-Term Effects of Neuroleptics. New York, Raven Press, 1980.
65. Juliano, D. B.: Conceptual tempo, activity, and concept learning in hyperactive and normal children. J. Abnorm. Psychol., 83:629-634, 1974.
66. Jungkunz, G.: Stimulants. *In* Hippius, H., and Winokur, G. (eds.): Psychopharmacology 1, Part 2: Clinical Psychopharmacology. Amsterdam, Excerpta Medica, 1983.
67. Kalat, J. W.: Animal models of childhood hyperkinesis. *In* Obiols, J., Ballus, C., Gonzalez-Monclus, E., et al. (eds.): Biological Psychiatry Today: Volume A. Amsterdam, Elsevier/North-Holland Biomedical Press, 1979.
68. Kennard, M. A., Spencer, S., and Fountain, G., Jr.: Hyperactivity in monkeys following lesions of the frontal lobes. J. Neurophysiol., 4:512-524, 1941.
69. Kinsbourne, M.: Minimal brain dysfunction as a neurodevelopmental lag. Ann. N.Y. Acad. Sci., 205:268-273, 1973.
70. Kuczenski, R.: Biochemical actions of amphetamine and other stimulants. *In* Creese, I. (ed.): Stimulants: Neurochemical, Behavioral, and Clinical Perspectives. New York, Raven Press, 1983.
71. Kupietz, S. S., Winsberg, B. G., and Sverd, J.: Learning ability and methylphenidate (Ritalin) plasma concentration in hyperkinetic children. J. Am. Acad. Child Psychiatry, 21:27-30, 1982.
72. Laties, V. G., and Weiss, G.: Performance enhancement by the amphetamines: A new appraisal. *In* Brill, H. (ed.): Neuropsychopharmacology. Amsterdam, Excerpta Medica, 1967.

73. Le Moal, M., Cardo, B., and Stinus, L.: Influence of ventral mesencephalic lesions on various spontaneous and conditioned behaviors in the rat. Physiol. Behav., 4:567-573, 1969.
74. Lindvall, O., Bjorklund, A., Moore, R. Y., et al.: Mesencephalic dopamine neurons projecting to neocortex. Brain Res., 81:325-331, 1974.
75. Lishman, W. A.: Brain damage in relation to psychiatric disability after head injury. Br. J. Psychiatry, 114:373-410, 1968.
76. Lou, H. C., Henriksen, L., and Bruhn, P.: Focal cerebral hypoperfusion in children with dysphasia and/or attention deficit disorder. Arch. Neurol., 41:825-829, 1984.
77. Luria, A. R.: The frontal lobes and the regulation of behaviors. *In* Pribham, K. H., and Luria, A. R. (eds.): Psychophysiology of the Frontal Lobes. New York, Academic Press, 1973.
78. Mattes, J. A.: The role of frontal lobe dysfunction in childhood hyperkinesis. Compr. Psychiatry, 21:358-369, 1980.
79. Matejeck, M., and Devos, J. E.: Assessment of spontaneous and drug-induced changes in vigilance by means of a new modification of the short-time spectral analysis of the EEG. Electroencephalogr. Clin. Neurophysiol., 43:476, 1977.
80. Mercier, L., and Pivik, R. T.: Spinal motoneuronal excitability during wakefulness and non-REM sleep in hyperkinesis. J. Clin. Neuropsychol., 5:321-336, 1983.
81. Millichap, J. G.: Neuropharmacology of hyperkinetic behavior: Response to methylphenidate correlated with degree of activity and brain damage. *In* Vernadakis, A., and Weiner, N. (eds.): Drugs and the Developing Brain. New York, Plenum Press, 1974.
82. Ostrom, C. W.: Time Series Analysis: Regression Techniques. Beverly Hills, Sage Publications, 1978.
83. Overton, D. A.: Discriminative control of behavior by drug states. *In* Thompson, T., and Pickens, R. (eds.): Stimulus Properties of Drugs. New York, Appleton-Century-Crofts, 1971.
84. Patrick, K. S., Ellington, K. R., and Breese, G. R.: Distribution of methylphenidate and p-hydroxymethylphenidate in rats. J. Pharmacol. Exp. Ther., 231:61-65, 1984.
85. Pontius, A. A.: Dysfunction patterns analogous to frontal lobe system and caudate nucleus syndromes in some groups of minimal brain dysfunction. J. Am. Med. Wom. Assoc., 28:285-292, 1973.
86. Porges, S. W., Walter, G. F., Korb, R. J., et al.: The influences of methylphenidate on heart rate and behavioral measures of attention in hyperaction children. Child Dev., 46:725-733, 1975.
87. Pribham, K. H., Ahumada, A., Hartog, J., et al.: A progress report on the neurological process disturbed by frontal lesions in primates. *In* Warren, J. M., and Abert, K. (eds.): The Frontal Granular Cortex and Behavior. New York, McGraw-Hill Book Co., 1964.
88. Pribham, K. H., and McGuinness, D.: Arousal, activation and effort in the control of attention. Psychol. Rev., 82:116-149, 1975.
89. Pycock, C. J., Carter, C. J., and Kerwin, R. W.: Effect of 6-hydroxydopamine lesions of the medial prefrontal cortex on neurotransmitter systems in subcortical sites in the rat. J. Neurochem., 34:91-99, 1980.
90. Reiter, L. W., Anderson, G. E., Laskey, J. W., et al.: Developmental and behavioral changes in the rat during chronic exposure to lead. Environ. Health Perspect., 12:119-123, 1975.

91. Ross, A. O.: Psychological Aspects of Learning Disabilities and Reading Disorders. New York, McGraw-Hill Book Co., 1976.

92. Ross, S. B.: On the mode of action of central stimulatory agents. Acta Pharmacol. Toxicol. (Kbh), 41:392-396, 1977.

93. Rosvold, H. E., Mishkin, M., and Szwarcbart, M. K.: Effects of subcortical lesions in monkeys on visual-discrimination and single-alternation performance. J. Comp. Physiol. Psychol., 51:437-444, 1958.

94. Rosvold, H. E., and Szwarcbart, M. K.: Neural structures involved in delayed response performance. In Warren, J. M., and Abert, K. (eds.): The Frontal Granular Cortex and Behavior. New York, McGraw-Hill Book Co., 1964.

95. Routh, D. K., Schroeder, C. S., and O'Tuama, L.: Development of activity level in children. Dev. Psychol., 10:163-168, 1974.

96. Saletu, B., Saletu, M., Simeon, J., et al.: Comparative symptomatological and evoked potential studies with d-amphetamine, thioridazine, and placebo in hyperkinetic children. Biol. Psychiatry, 10:253-275, 1975.

97. Sauerland, E. K., and Clemente, C. D.: The role of the brain stem in orbital cortex induced inhibition of somatic reflexes. In Pribham, K. H., and Luria, A. R. (eds.): Psychophysiology of the Frontal Lobes. New York, Academic Press, 1973.

98. Sauerland, E. K., Knauss, T., Nakamura, Y., et al.: Inhibition of monosynaptic and polysynaptic reflexes and muscle tone by electrical stimulation of the cerebral cortex. Exp. Neurol., 17:159-171, 1967.

99. Schubert, B.: Detection and identification of methylphenidate in human urine and blood samples. Acta Chem. Scand., 24:433-438, 1970.

100. Shaywitz, B. A., Yager, R. D., and Klopper, I. H.: Selective brain dopamine depletion in developing rats: An experimental model of minimal brain dysfunction. Science, 191:305-308, 1976.

101. Shaywitz, B. A., Klopper, J. H., Yager, R. D., and Gondon, G. W.: Paradoxical response to amphetamine in developing rats treated with 6-hydroxydopamine. Nature, 261:153-155, 1976.

102. Shaywitz, S. E., Hunt, R. D., Jatlow, P., et al.: Psychopharmacology of attention deficit disorder: Pharmacokinetic, neuroendocrine, and behavioral measures following acute and chronic treatment with methylphenidate. Pediatrics, 69:688-694, 1982.

103. Simernitskaya, E. G.: Application of the method evoked potentials to the analysis of activation processes in patients with lesions of the frontal lobes. In Pribham, K. H., and Luria, A. R. (eds.): Psychophysiology of the Frontal Lobes. New York, Academic Press, 1973.

104. Simon, H., Scatton, B., and Le Moal, M.: Dopaminergic A10 neurons are involved in cognitive functions. Nature, 286:150-151, 1980.

105. Small, A., Hibi, S., and Feinberg, I.: Effects of dextroamphetamine sulfate on EEG sleep patterns of hyperactive children. Arch. Gen. Psychiatry, 25:369-380, 1971.

106. Snyder, S. H., and Meyerhoff, J. L.: How amphetamine acts in minimal brain dysfunction. Ann. N.Y. Acad. Sci., 205:310-320, 1973.

107. Spiegel, R.: Effects of amphetamine on performance and on polygraphic sleep parameters in man. In Passouant, P., and Oswald, I. (eds): Pharmacology of the States of Alertness. Oxford, Pergamon Press, 1979.

108. Sprague, R. L., and Gadow, K. D.: The role of the teacher in drug treatment. School Rev., 85:109-140, 1976.

109. Sprague, R. L., and Sleator, E. K.: Methylphenidate in hyperkinetic children: Dif-

ferences in dose effects on learning and social behavior. Science, 198:1274-1276, 1977.

110. Sprague, R. L., Barnes, K. R., and Werry, J. S.: Methylphenidate and thioridazine: Learning, reaction time, activity, and classroom behavior in disturbed children. Am. J. Orthopsychiatry, 40:615-628, 1970.

111. Stamm, J. S., and Kreder, S. V.: Minimal brain dysfunction: Psychological and neurophysiological disorders in hyperkinetic children. *In* Gazzaniga, M. S. (ed.): Handbook of Behavioral Neurobiology: Vol. 2: Neuropsychology, New York, Plenum Press, 1979.

112. Starr, M. A.: Cortical lesions of the brain: A collection and analysis of the American cases of localized cerebral disease. Am. J. Med. Sci. (New Series), 87:366-391, 1984.

113. Still, G. F.: The Goulstonian Lectures on some abnormal psychical conditions in children. Lancet, 161(1):1008-1012, 1077-1082, 1163-1168, 1902.

114. Swanson, J., Kinsbourne, M., Roberts, W., et al.: Time response analysis of the effect of stimulant medication on the learning ability of children referred for hyperactivity. Pediatrics, 61:21-29, 1978.

115. Sykes, D. H., Douglas, V. I., and Morgenstern, G.: The effect of methylphenidate (Ritalin) on sustained attention in hyperactive children. Psychopharmacologia, 25:262-274, 1972.

116. Szporny, L., and Gorog, P.: Investigations into the correlations between monoamine oxidase inhibition and other effects due to methylphenidate and its stereoisomers. Biochem. Pharmacol., 8:263-268, 1961.

117. Tassin, J. P., Stinus, L., Simon, H., et al.: Relationship between the locomotor hyperactivity induced by A10 lesions and the destruction of the frontocortical dopaminergic innervation in the rat. Brain Res., 141:267-281, 1978.

118. Tecce, J. I., and Cole, J. O.: Amphetamine effects in man: Paradoxical drowsiness and lowered electrical brain activity (CNV). Science, 185:451-453, 1974.

119. Villablanca, J. R., and Olmstead, C. E.: The striatum: A fine tuner of the brain. Acta Neurobiol. Exp., 42:227-299, 1982.

120. Wargin, W., Patrick, K., Kilts, C., et al.: Pharmacokinetics of methylphenidate in man, rat, and monkey. J. Pharmacol. Exp. Ther., 226:382-386, 1983.

121. Weiss, B., and Laties, V. G.: Enhancement of human performance by caffeine and the amphetamines. Pharmacol. Rev., 14:1-36, 1962.

122. Weiss, G., Minde, K., Douglas, V., et al.: Comparison of the effects of chlorpromazine, dextroamphetamine, and methylphenidate on the behaviour and intellectual functioning of hyperactive children. Can. Med. Assoc. J., 104:20-25, 1971.

123. Weiss, G., Werry, J., Minde, K., et al.: Studies on the hyperactive child: V. The effects of dextroamphetamine and chlorpromazine on behaviour and intellectual functioning. J. Child Psychol. Psychiatry, 9:145-156, 1968.

124. Wells, R., Hammond, K. B., and Rodgerson, D. O.: Gas-liquid chromatographic procedure for measurement of methylphenidate hydrochloride and its metabolite, ritalinic acid, in urine. Clin. Chem., 20:440-443, 1974.

125. Wender, P. H.: Minimal Brain Dysfunction in Children. New York, Wiley-Interscience, 1971.

126. Werry, J. S., and Sprague, R. L.: Methylphenidate in children: Effect of dosage. Aust. N.Z. J. Psychiatry, 8:9-19, 1974.

127. Werry, J. S., and Aman, M. G.: Methylphenidate and haloperidol in children: Effects on attention, memory, and activity. Arch. Gen. Psychiatry, 32:790-795, 1975.

128. Werry, J. S., Aman, M. G., and Lampen, E.: Haloperidol and methylphenidate in hyperactive children. Acta Paedopsychiatr. (Basel), 42:26-40, 1976.

129. Werry, J. S., Weiss, G., Douglas, V., et al.: Studies on the hyperactive child: 3. The effect of chlorpromazine upon behavior and learning ability. J. Am. Acad. Child Psychiatry, 5:292-311, 1966.

130. Winitz, M., Block-Frankenthal, L., Izumiya, N., et al.: Studies on diastercoisomeric alpha-amino acids and corresponding alpha-hydroxy acids: VII. Influence of beta-configuration on enzymatic susceptibility. J. Am. Chem. Soc., 78:2423-2430, 1956.

131. Winsberg, B. G., Hungund, B. L., and Perel, J. M.: Pharmacological factors of methylphenidate metabolism in behaviorally disordered children. Psychopharmacol. Bull., 16:69-71, 1980.

132. Winsberg, B. G., Kaipietz, S. S., Sverd, J., et al.: Methylphenidate oral dose plasma concentrations and behavioral response in children. Psychopharmacology, 70:329-332, 1982.

133. Yakolev, P. I., and Lecours, A. R.: The myelogenetic cycles of regional maturation of the brain. *In* Minkowski, A. (ed.): Regional Development of the Brain in Early Life. Oxford, England, Blackwell, 1967.

134. Clemente, C. D., and Sterman, M. B.: Basal forebrain mechanisms for internal inhibition and sleep. Res. Publ. Assoc. Res. Nerv. Ment. Dis., 45:127-147, 1967.

135. Davis, G. D.: Effects of control excitant and depressant drugs on locomotor activity in monkey. Am. J. Physiol., 188:619-623, 1958.

136. Hicks, R. E., Perez-Reyes, M., Mayo, J. P., et al.: Cannibis, atropine, and temporal information processing. Neuropsychobiology, 1985, in press.

137. Milner, B.: Some cognitive effects of frontal-lobe lesions in man. Philos. Trans. R. Soc. Lond., (Biol.), 298:211-226, 1982.

138. Nauta, W. J. H.: The problem of the frontal lobe: A reinterpretation. J. Psychiatr. Res., 8:167-187, 1971.

139. Pribham, K. H., Konrad, K., and Gainsburg, D.: Frontal lesions and behavioral instability. J. Comp. Physiol. Psychol., 62:123-124, 1966.

140. Robbins, T. W., and Sahakian, B. J.: "Paradoxical" effects of psychomotor stimulant drugs in hyperactive children from the standpoint of behavioral pharmacology. Neuropharmacology, 18:931-950, 1979.

34

The Traumatic Impact of Child Sexual Abuse: A Conceptualization

David Finkelhor and Angela Browne
University of New Hampshire, Durham

A framework is proposed for a more systematic understanding of the effects of child sexual abuse. Four traumagenic dynamics—traumatic sexualization, betrayal, stigmatization, and powerlessness—are identified as the core of the psychological injury inflicted by abuse. These dynamics can be used to make assessments of victimized children and to anticipate problems to which these children may be vulnerable subsequently. Implications for research are also considered.

The literature on child sexual abuse is full of clinical observations about problems that are thought to be associated with a history of abuse, such as sexual dysfunction, depression, and low self-esteem. However, such observations have not yet been organized into a clear model that specifies how and why sexual abuse results in this kind of trauma. This paper is an attempt to provide such a model. Based on a review of the literature on the effects of sexual abuse,[6] the paper suggests a conceptualization of the impact of sexual abuse that can be used in both research and treatment.

Reprinted with permission from the *American Journal of Orthopsychiatry*, 1985, Vol. 55, 530–541. Copyright 1985 by the American Orthopsychiatric Association, Inc.

Preparation of this work was supported by grants from the National Center on Child Abuse and Neglect (90CA 0936/01) and the National Institute of Mental Health (MH15161).

The model proposed here postulates that the experience of sexual abuse can be analyzed in terms of four trauma-causing factors, or what we will call *traumagenic dynamics*—traumatic sexualization, betrayal, powerlessness, and stigmatization. These traumagenic dynamics are generalized dynamics, not necessarily unique to sexual abuse; they occur in other kinds of trauma. But the conjunction of these four dynamics in one set of circumstances is what makes the trauma of sexual abuse unique, different from such childhood traumas as the divorce of a child's parents or even being the victim of physical child abuse.

These dynamics alter children's cognitive and emotional orientation to the world, and create trauma by distorting children's self-concept, world view, and affective capacities. For example, the dynamic of stigmatization distorts children's sense of their own value and worth. The dynamic of powerlessness distorts children's sense of their ability to control their lives. Children's attempts to cope with the world through these distortions may result in some of the behavioral problems that are commonly noted in victims of child sexual abuse. This paper will describe the model and suggest some of its ramifications and uses. We will first describe each of the four dynamics and then show how each dynamic is associated with some of the commonly observed effects of sexual abuse. We will conclude by illustrating how the model can be used in clinical work and in research.

FOUR TRAUMAGENIC DYNAMICS

Traumatic sexualization refers to a process in which a child's sexuality (including both sexual feelings and sexual attitudes) is shaped in a developmentally inappropriate and interpersonally dysfunctional fashion as a result of sexual abuse. This can happen in a variety of ways in the course of the abuse. Traumatic sexualization can occur when a child is repeatedly rewarded by an offender for sexual behavior that is inappropriate to his or her level of development. It occurs through the exchange of affection, attention, privileges, and gifts for sexual behavior, so that a child learns to use sexual behavior as a strategy for manipulating others to satisfy a variety of developmentally appropriate needs. It occurs when certain parts of a child's anatomy are fetishized and given distorted importance and meaning. It occurs through the misconceptions and confusions about sexual behavior and sexual morality that are transmitted to the child from the offender. And it occurs when very frightening memories and events become associated in the child's mind with sexual activity.

Sexual abuse experiences can vary dramatically in terms of the amount and kind of traumatic sexualization they provoke. Experiences in which the offender makes an effort to evoke the child's sexual response, for example, are probably more sexualizing than those in which an offender simply uses a passive child to masturbate with. Experiences in which the child is enticed to participate are also likely to be more sexualizing than those in which brute force is used. However, even with the use of force, a form of traumatic sexualization may occur as a result of the fear that becomes associated with sex in the wake of such an experience. The degree of a child's understanding may also affect the degree of sexualization. Experiences in which the child, because of early age or developmental level, understands few of the sexual implications of the activities may be less sexualizing than those involving a child with greater awareness. Children who have been traumatically sexualized emerge from their experiences with inappropriate repertoires of sexual behavior, with confusions and misconceptions about their sexual self-concepts, and with unusual emotional associations to sexual activities.

Betrayal refers to the dynamic by which children discover that someone on whom they were vitally dependent has caused them harm. This may occur in a variety of ways in a molestation experience. For example, in the course of abuse or its aftermath, children may come to the realization that a trusted person has manipulated them through lies or misrepresentations about moral standards. They may also come to realize that someone whom they loved or whose affection was important to them treated them with callous disregard. Children can experience betrayal not only at the hands of offenders, but also on the part of family members who were not abusing them. A family member whom they trusted but who was unable or unwilling to protect or believe them—or who has a changed attitude toward them after disclosure of the abuse—may also contribute to the dynamics of betrayal.

Sexual abuse experiences that are perpetrated by family members or other trusted persons obviously involve more potential for betrayal than those involving strangers. However, the degree of betrayal may also be affected by how taken in the child feels by the offender, whomever the offender. A child who was suspicious of a father's activities from the beginning may feel less betrayed than one who initially experienced the contact as nurturing and loving and then is suddenly shocked to realize what is really happening. Obviously, the degree of betrayal is also related to a family's response to disclosure. Children who are disbelieved, blamed, or ostracized undoubtedly experience a greater sense of betrayal than those who are supported.

Powerlessness—or what might also be called disempowerment, the dynamic of rendering the victim powerless—refers to the process in which the child's will, desires, and sense of efficacy are continually contravened. Many aspects of the sexual abuse experience contribute to this dynamic. We theorize that a basic kind of powerlessness occurs in sexual abuse when a child's territory and body space are repeatedly invaded against the child's will. This is exacerbated by whatever coercion and manipulation the offender may impose as part of the abuse process. Powerlessness is then reinforced when children see their attempts to halt the abuse frustrated. It is increased when children feel fear, are unable to make adults understand or believe what is happening, or realize how conditions of dependency have trapped them in the situation.

An authoritarian abuser who continually commands the child's participation by threatening serious harm will probably instill more of a sense of powerlessness. But force and threat are not necessary: any kind of situation in which a child feels trapped, if only by the realization of the consequences of disclosure, can create a sense of powerlessness. Obviously, a situation in which a child tells and is not believed will also create a greater degree of powerlessness. However when children are able to bring the abuse to an end effectively, or at least exert some control over its occurrence, they may feel less disempowered.

Stigmatization, the final dynamic, refers to the negative connotations—e.g., badness, shame, and guilt—that are communicated to the child around the experiences and that then become incorporated into the child's self-image. These negative meanings are communicated in many ways. They can come directly from the abuser, who may blame the victim for the activity, demean the victim, or furtively convey a sense of shame about the behavior. Pressure for secrecy from the offender can also convey powerful messages of shame and guilt. But stigmatization is also reinforced by attitudes that the victim infers or hears from other persons in the family or community. Stigmatization may thus grow out of the child's prior knowledge or sense that the activity is considered deviant and taboo, and it is certainly reinforced if, after disclosure, people react with shock or hysteria, or blame the child for what has transpired. Children may be additionally stigmatized by people in their environment who now impute other negative characteristics to the victim (loose morals, "spoiled goods") as a result of the molestation.

Stigmatization occurs in various degrees in different abusive situations. Some children are treated as bad and blameworthy by offenders and some are not. Some children, in the wake of a sexual abuse experience, are told clearly that they are not at fault, whereas others are heavily shamed. Some children may be too young to have much awareness of social attitudes and thus experience little stigmatization, whereas others have to deal with powerful religious and cultural taboos in addition to the usual stigma. Keeping the secret of having been a victim of sexual abuse may increase the sense of stigma, since it reinforces the sense of being different. By contrast, those who find out that such experiences occur to many other children may have some of their stigma assuaged.

These four traumagenic dynamics, then, account in our view for the main sources of trauma in child sexual abuse. They are not in any way pure or narrowly defined. Each dynamic can be seen, rather, as a clustering of injurious influences with a common theme. They are best thought of as broad categories useful for organizing and categorizing our understanding of the effect of sexual abuse.

TRAUMAGENIC DYNAMICS IN THE IMPACT OF SEXUAL ABUSE

With the four traumagenic dynamics as an organizing framework, it is useful to reconsider the literature on the effects of sexual abuse. Although a great many behavioral and emotional problems have been related to a history of sexual abuse,[6] unfortunately the sum total of literature adds up to little more than a list of possible outcomes. This is conceptually frustrating and does not encourage deeper understanding of the phenomenon.

The notion of traumagenic dynamics, however, offers a way both to organize and theorize about many of the observed outcomes. Most of the outcomes, it will be noted, can be conveniently categorized according to one or two of these dynamics. It would seem as though certain traumagenic dynamics are more readily associated with certain effects. Obviously, there is no simple one-to-one correspondence. Some effects seem logically associated with several dynamics. But there are clear general affinities. In this section, we will briefly describe the effects that seem to be associated with the four dynamics (see Table 1).

Table 1
Traumagenic Dynamics in the Impact of Child Sexual Abuse

I. TRAUMATIC SEXUALIZATION

Dynamics
>   Child rewarded for sexual behavior inappropriate to developmental level
>   Offender exchanges attention and affection for sex
>   Sexual parts of child fetishized

Offender transmits misconceptions about sexual behavior and sexual morality

Conditioning of sexual activity with negative emotions and memories

Psychological Impact
Increased salience of sexual issues
Confusion about sexual identity
Confusion about sexual norms
Confusion of sex with love and care-getting/care-giving
Negative associations to sexual activities and arousal sensations
Aversion to sex-intimacy

Behavioral Manifestations
Sexual preoccupations and compulsive sexual behaviors
Precocious sexual activity
Aggressive sexual behaviors
Promiscuity
Prostitution
Sexual dysfunctions; flashbacks, difficulty in arousal, orgasm
Avoidance of or phobic reactions to sexual intimacy
Inappropriate sexualization of parenting

II. STIGMATIZATION

Dynamics
Offender blames, denigrates victim
Offender and others pressure child for secrecy
Child infers attitudes of shame about activities
Others have shocked reaction to disclosure
Others blame child for events
Victim is stereotyped as damaged goods

Psychological Impact
Guilt, shame
Lowered self-esteem
Sense of differentness from others

Behavioral Manifestations
Isolation
Drug or alcohol abuse
Criminal involvement
Self-mutilation
Suicide

III. BETRAYAL

Dynamics
Trust and vulnerability manipulated
Violation of expectation that others will provide care and protection

Child's well-being disregarded
Lack of support and protection from parent(s)

Psychological Impact
Grief, depression
Extreme dependency
Impaired ability to judge trustworthiness of others
Mistrust; particularly of men
Anger, hostility

Behavioral Manifestations
Clinging
Vulnerability to subsequent abuse and exploitation
Allowing own children to be victimized
Isolation
Discomfort in intimate relationships
Marital problems
Aggressive behavior
Delinquency

IV. POWERLESSNESS

Dynamics
Body territory invaded against the child's wishes
Vulnerability to invasion continues over time
Offender uses force or trickery to involve child
Child feels unable to protect self and halt abuse
Repeated experience of fear
Child is unable to make others believe

Psychological Impact
Anxiety, fear
Lowered sense of efficacy
Perception of self as victim
Need to control
Identification with the aggressor

Behavioral Manifestations
Nightmares
Phobias
Somatic complaints; eating and sleeping disorders
Depression
Disassociation
Running away
School problems, truancy
Employment problems
Vulnerability to subsequent victimization
Aggressive behavior, bullying
Delinquency
Becoming an abuser

Traumatic Sexualization

There are many observed effects of sexual abuse that seem readily connected to the dynamic of traumatic sexualization. Among young child victims, clinicians have often noted sexual preoccupations and repetitive sexual behavior such as masturbation or compulsive sex play. Some children display knowledge and interests that are inappropriate to their age, such as wanting to engage school age playmates in sexual intercourse or oral-genital contact.[1,3,12,21,22] Some children who have been victimized, especially adolescent boys, but sometimes even younger children, become sexually aggressive and victimize their peers or younger children. Clinicians have remarked about promiscuous and compulsive sexual behavior that sometimes characterizes victims when they become adolescents or young adults, although this has not been confirmed empirically.[7,22,40] There are also several studies suggesting that victims of sexual abuse have a high risk for entering into prostitution.[5,19,32]

The sexual problems of adult victims of sexual abuse have been among the most researched and best established effects. Clinicians have reported that victimized clients often have an aversion to sex, flashbacks to the molestation experience, difficulty with arousal and orgasm, and vaginismus, as well as negative attitudes toward their sexuality and their bodies.[8,12,29,34,38] The frequently demonstrated higher risk of sexual abuse victims to later sexual assault may also be related to traumatic sexualization,[11,13,17,30] and some victims apparently find themselves inappropriately sexualizing their children in ways that lead to sexual or physical abuse.[14,18,21,34,36] All these observations seem connected to the traumagenic dynamic of sexualization.

Such problems and behavior, as well as victims' self-reports, suggest the various psychological effects produced by traumatic sexualization. At its most basic level, sexual abuse heightens awareness of sexual issues, which may be particularly true among young children who might not otherwise be concerned with sexual matters at their stage of development. Part of the preoccupation is associated simply with the sexual stimulation of the abuse and the conditioning of behavior that may go along with it, but it is also very much a function of the questions and conflicts provoked by the abuse about the self and interpersonal relations. Confusion often arises especially about sexual identity. Victimized boys, for example, may wonder whether they are homosexuals. Victimized girls wonder whether their sexual desirability has been impaired, and whether later sexual partners will be able to "tell."

Traumatic sexualization is also associated with confusion about sexual norms and standards. Sexually victimized children typically have misconceptions about sex and sexual relations as a result of things offenders may have said and done. One common confusion concerns the role of sex in affectionate relationships. If child victims have traded sex for affection from the abuser over a period of time, this may become their view of the normal way to give and obtain affection.[17,20,24] Some of the apparent sexualization in the behavior of victimized children may stem from this confusion.

Another impact that traumatic sexualization may have is in the negative connotations that come to be associated with sex. Sexual contact associated in a child's memory with revulsion, fear, anger, a sense of powerlessness, or other negative emotions can contaminate later sexual experiences. These feelings may become generalized as an aversion to all sex and intimacy, and very probably also account for the sexual dysfunctions reported by victims.

Stigmatization

Other effects of sexual abuse seem naturally grouped in relation to the dynamic of stigmatization. Child victims often feel isolated, and may gravitate to various stigmatized levels of society. Thus they may get involved in drug or alcohol abuse, in criminal activity, or in prostitution.[3,4,17] The effects of stigmatization may also reach extremes in forms of self-destructive behavior and suicide attempts.[4,11,17,21,34,35]

The psychological impact of these problems has a number of related components. Many sexual abuse victims experience considerable guilt and shame as a result of their abuse.[2,10,11] The guilt and shame seem logically associated with the dynamic of stigmatization, since they are a response to being blamed and encountering negative reactions from others regarding the abuse. Low self-esteem is another part of the pattern, as the victim concludes from the negative attitudes toward abuse victims that they are "spoiled merchandise"[3,9,18,21,34,38] Stigmatization also results in a sense of being different based on the (incorrect) belief that no one else has had such an experience and that others would reject a person who had.

Betrayal

A number of the effects noted in victims seem reasonably to be connected with the experience of betrayal that they have suffered, in the form of grief reactions and depression over the loss of a trusted figure.[1,3,7,20,21] Sexual abuse victims suffer from grave disenchantment and disillusionment. In combination with this there may be an intense need to regain trust and security, manifested in the extreme dependency and clinging seen in especially young victims.[20,23] This same need in adults may show up in impaired judgment about the trustworthiness of other people[4,9,21,34,36,38] or in a desperate search for a redeeming relationship.[34, 35] As mentioned before, several studies of female incest victims have remarked on the vulnerability of these women to relationships in which they are physically, psychologically, and sexually abused.[4,11,13,17,25,30] Some victims even fail to recognize when their partners become sexually abusive toward their children. This seems plausibly related to both an overdependency and impaired judgment.

An opposite reaction to betrayal—characterized by hostility and anger—has also been observed among sexually abused girls.[4,9,26] Distrust may manifest itself in isolation and an aversion to intimate relationships. Sometimes this distrust is directed especially at men and is a barrier to successful heterosexual relationships or marriages. Studies have noted marital problems among sexual abuse victims that also may represent the surfacing of mistrust and suspicion.

The anger stemming from betrayal is part of what may lie behind the aggressive and hostile posture of some sexual abuse victims, particularly adolescents,[1,8,10,21,27,39,41] Such anger may be a primitive way of trying to protect the self against future betrayals. Antisocial behavior and delinquency sometimes associated with a history of victimization are also an expression of this anger and may represent a desire for retaliation. Thus, betrayal seems a common dynamic behind a number of the observed reactions to sexual abuse.

Powerlessness

There is also a configuration of effects of sexual abuse that seem plausibly related to the dynamic of powerlessness. One reaction to powerlessness is obviously fear and anxiety, which reflect the inability to control noxious events. Many of the initial responses to sexual abuse among children are connected to fear and anxiety. Nightmares, phobias, hypervigilance, clinging behavior, and somatic complaints related to anxiety have been repeatedly documented among sexually abused children.[1, 2,7,8,10,14,15,21,22,26,33,35,39] These fears and anxieties may extend into adulthood as well.

A second major effect of powerlessness is to impair a person's sense of efficacy and coping skills. Having been a victim on repeated occasions may make it difficult to act without the expectation of being revictimized.

This sense of impotence may be associated with the despair, depression, and even suicidal behavior often noted among adolescent and adult victims. It may also be reflected in learning problems, running away, and employment difficulties, which researchers have noted in victims who feel unable to cope with their environments.[1,2,7,17,22,24,26] Finally, it seems readily related to the high risk of subsequent victimization (noted in previous sections) from which sexual abuse victims appear to suffer: these victims may feel powerless to thwart others who are trying to manipulate them or do them harm.

Attempts to compensate for the experience of powerlessness may account for a third cluster of effects. In reaction to powerlessness, some sexual abuse victims may have unusual and dysfunctional needs to control or dominate. This would seem particularly to be the case for male victims, for whom issues of power and control are made very salient by male sex role socialization.[16,28] Some aggressive and delinquent behavior would seem to stem from this desire to be tough, powerful, and fearsome, if even in desperate ways, to compensate for the pain of powerlessness. When victims become bullies and offenders, reenacting their own abuse, it may be in large measure to regain the sense of power and domination that these victims attribute to their own abuser. All these effects seem related to the traumatic dynamic of powerlessness that is integral to the sexual abuse experience.

The preceding should give a sense of how the four traumagenic dynamics are connected to the common patterns of reactions seen among victims. It should be clear, however, that the reactions are overdetermined. Some effects seem plausibly connected to two or even three traumagenic dynamics; for example, depression can be seen as growing out of stigmatization, betrayal, or powerlessness. There is no one-to-one correspondence between dynamics and effects. It may be that stigma-related depression has different manifestations and therefore calls for a different therapeutic approach than depression related to powerlessness. Such hypotheses suggested by the model are worthy of further clinical and empirical investigation.

CLINICAL ASSESSMENT USING THE MODEL OF TRAUMAGENIC DYNAMICS

Of the many possible uses for the conceptual model described here, an obvious one is in making clinical assessments of the possible effects of abuse. Up to the present, clinicians have evaluated abuse experiences on the basis of unsystematic and untested assumptions about what causes trauma. There have been some attempts to classify abuse experiences to aid in assessment, but these classifications have various shortcomings.

One common classification scheme looks at the characteristics of the offender: for example, whether the abuse was at the hands of a "regressed" or "fixated" abuser.[16] However, this conceptualization provides little insight into the nature of the trauma experienced by the child. More often, experiences have been classified according to simple dichotomies which reflect collective clinical judgment about what kinds of abuse are "more traumatic." Thus, abuse is commonly distinguished by whether it occurred inside or outside the family, on the belief that abuse inside the family has more serious effects on the child. Abuse is also commonly categorized according to whether or not penetration occurred and whether force was used.

This approach to assessing the potential for trauma has real limitations. Beyond the fact that its assumptions are largely untested, the approach results in an overly simplistic classification of experiences as either more or less serious. Nothing about the *character* of the effect is inferred, and nothing about how the trauma is likely to manifest itself is suggested.

The model of traumagenic dynamics proposed here allows for a more complex assessment of the potential for trauma. With the assistance of these concepts, the clinician can evaluate an abuse experience on four separate dimensions. The question is not whether it was more or less serious, but rather what specific injurious dynamics were present. The characteristics of the experience itself can be examined for their contribution to each of the traumagenic processes. On the basis of the configuration of traumagenic dynamics most present in an experience, the clinician can anticipate what would be the most likely types of effects.

Thus, a clinician might proceed through the model dynamic by dynamic, asking first: How traumatically sexualizing was this experience? Facts about the experience, such as whether intercourse occurred, how long it went on, and the degree to which the child participated, all might contribute to an assessment of the degree of sexualization. Next a clinician would ask: How stigmatizing was the experience? Factors such as how long it went on, the age of the child, the number of people who knew about it, and the degree to which others blamed the child subsequent to the disclosure would all add to the assessment of this dynamic. Similarly, with regard to betrayal, facts about the relationship between the victim and the offender, the way in which the offender involved the victim, and the attempts—successful and unsuccessful—of the victim to get assistance and support from other family members would all be taken into account. Finally, the facts about the presence of force, the degree to which coercion was brought to bear, the duration of the abuse, and the circumstances under which the abuse was terminated would be particularly relevant to a determination of the degree to which powerlessness was a major dynamic.

Once an assessment is made about the experience according to the four traumagenic dynamics, a clinician should be able to draw inferences about some of the predominant concerns of the victim and about some of the subsequent difficulties to be expected. An assessment based on the traumagenic dynamics would also be useful for formulating intervention strategies. If, for example, assessment suggested greatest trauma in the area of stigmatization, interventions might be aimed specifically at reducing this sense of stigma. Such interventions might include involvement with a survivors group, where the victim could get support from other victims, or other activities to repair the sense of a stigmatized and devalued self.

TRAUMAGENESIS BEFORE AND AFTER ABUSE

Although the sexual abuse itself is assumed to be the main traumatic agent in victims, it is important to emphasize that any assessment approach to understanding trauma must take into account the child's experiences both prior to *and* subsequent to the abuse. Abuse will have different effects on children depending on their prior adjustment and on how others respond to it. The conceptual framework being proposed here is easily adapted to this need.

The four traumagenic dynamics do not apply solely to the abuse event. They are ongoing processes that have a history prior to and a future subsequent to the abuse. They can be assessed in each phase. In the pre-abuse phase, the traumagenic dynamics need to be understood particularly in relation to a child's family life and personality characteristics prior to the abuse. For example, a child who was a previous victim of physical or emotional abuse may have already been suffering from a disempowering dynamic before the abuse occurred. However, an eldest child with important responsibilities, living in a fairly healthy family environment, may have acquired a well developed sense of personal efficacy and powerfulness. In such a context, the disempowering aspects of a sexual abuse experience may have only a minor or transient effect. If the child had experienced an unstable family configuration, in which the loyalty of significant others was in doubt, then the dynamic of betrayal may have already been strongly potentiated. However, the betrayal dynamic from the sexual abuse experience might be substantially less for a child who had a sense of trust firmly established.

The operation of the traumagenic dynamics can also be assessed in the events subsequent to the sexual abuse. Two main categories of subsequent events have particular importance: *1)* the family reaction to disclosure, if and when it occurs, and *2)* the social and institutional response to the disclosure. For example, much of the stigmatization accompanying abuse may occur *after* the experience itself, as a child encounters family and societal reactions. A child who was relatively unstigmatized by the molestation itself may undergo serious stigmatization if later rejected by friends or blamed by family and if having been abused remains a focus for a long time. The dynamic of powerlessness is also greatly affected by a child's experiences subsequent to sexual abuse. If, for instance, a great many authorities become involved in the experience and the child is forced to testify, forced to leave home, forced to tell the story on repeated occasions, and subjected to a great deal of unwanted attention, this can also greatly increase the child's sense of powerlessness. But, if the child has a sense of having been able to end the abuse and obtain support and protection, this may greatly mitigate any sense of powerlessness that resulted from the experience itself. Thus, in assessing the experience, the contributions of the pre- and post-abuse situation must be included in relation to the four traumagenic dynamics.

IMPLICATIONS FOR RESEARCH

The four traumagenic dynamics described in this paper have implications for both research and intervention. Perhaps most importantly, they can be used as a conceptual guide in the development of assessment instruments. Up until now, research on child sexual abuse has been conducted using either broad psychological inventories like the MMPI[37] or the California Psychological Inventory[31] or else ad hoc, investigator-invented measures. The broad inventories have subscales like neuroticism or self-acceptance that can assess a variety of pathological conditions, but these are not necessarily the pathologies related most closely to sexual abuse. The ad hoc measures, by contrast, are more sensitive to the specific pathology that may result from sexual abuse, but they are not based on any theory, and often suffer from lack of methodological rigor.

This model of traumagenic dynamics can be the basis for developing instruments specifically designed to assess the impact of sexual abuse.

Sections of the instruments would be geared to tap each of the four dynamics. Two separate instruments might be developed, one for direct administration to the children and another for completion by parents or professionals. Forms of the instruments might be tailored for different age groups. Such instruments are badly needed to further research on sexual abuse.

CONCLUSION

This paper has tried to suggest a framework for a more systematic understanding of the effects of sexual abuse. It has introduced four traumagenic dynamics, which are seen as the four links between the experience of sexual abuse and the sequelae that have been widely noted. Developing a conceptualization of these links may serve as a step in the direction of advancing our understanding of sexual abuse and mitigating the effects of these experiences on its victims.

REFERENCES

1. Adams-Tucker, C. 1981. A sociological overview of 28 abused children. Child Abuse Neg. 5:361-367.
2. Anderson, S., Bach, C., and Griffith, S. 1981. Psychosocial sequelae in intrafamilial victims of sexual assault and abuse. Presented at the Third International Conference on Child Abuse and Neglect, Amsterdam.
3. Benward, J. and Densen-Gerber, J. 1975. Incest as a causative factor in anti-social behavior: an exploratory study. Presented to the American Academy of Forensic Science, Chicago.
4. Briere, J. 1984. The effects of childhood sexual abuse on later psychological functioning: defining a "post-sexual-abuse syndrome." Presented to the Third National Conference on Sexual Victimization of Children, Washington, DC.
5. Brown, M. 1979. Teenage prostitution. Adolescence 14:665-675.
6. Browne, A. and Finkelhor, D. 1984. The impact of child sexual abuse: a review of the research. Presented at the Second National Conference of Family Violence Researchers, Durham, NH.
7. Browning, D. and Boatman, B. 1977. Incest: children at risk. Amer. J. Psychiat. 134:69-72.
8. Burgess, A. and Holmstrom, L. 1978. Accessory to sex: pressure, sex, and secrecy. *In* Sexual assault of children and adolescents. A. Burgess et al. Lexington Books, Lexington, Mass.
9. Cortois, C. 1979. The incest experience and its aftermath. Victimology 4:337-347.
10. De Francis, V. 1969. Protecting the Child Victim of Sex Crimes Committed by Adults. American Humane Association, Denver.
11. De Young, M. 1982. The Sexual Victimization of Children. McFarland & Company, Jefferson, N.C.

12. Finch, S. 1967. Sexual activity of children with other children and adults. Clin. Pediat. 3:1-2.
13. Fromuth, M. 1983. The long term psychological impact of childhood sexual abuse. Unpublished doctoral dissertation, Auburn University, Auburn, Ala.
14. Gelinas, D. 1983. The persisting negative effects of incest. Psychiatry 46:312-332.
15. Goodwin, J. 1982. Sexual Abuse: Incest Victims and Their Families. John Wright—PSG, Inc., Boston.
16. Groth, N. 1979. Men Who Rape. Plenum, New York.
17. Herman, J. 1981. Father-Daughter Incest. Harvard University Press, Cambridge, Mass.
18. Herman, J. and Hirschman, L. 1977. Father-daughter incest. Signs 2:735-756.
19. James, J. and Meyerding, J. 1977. Early sexual experiences and prostitution. Amer. J. Psychiat., 134:1381-1385.
20. Jones, C. and Bentovim, A. Sexual Abuse of Children: Fleeting Trauma or Lasting Disaster. Unpublished manuscript. The Hospital for Sick Children, London.
21. Justice, B. and Justice, R. 1979. The Broken Taboo. Human Sciences Press, New York.
22. Kaufman, I., Peck, A. and Tagiuri, C. 1954. The family constellation and overt incestuous relations between father and daughter. Amer. J. Orthopsychiat. 24:266-279.
23. Lustig, N. et al. 1966. Incest: a family group survival pattern. Arch. Gen. Psychiat. 14:31-40.
24. Meiselman, K. 1978. Incest. Jossey-Bass, San Francisco.
25. Miller, J. et al. 1978. Recidivism among sexual assault victims. Amer. J. Psychiat. 135:1103-1104.
26. Peters, J. 1976. Children who are victims of sexual assault and the psychology of offenders. Amer. J. Psychother. 30:398-421.
27. Reich, J. and Gutierres, S. 1979. Escape/aggression incidence in sexually abused juvenile delinquents. Crim. Just. Behav. 6:239-243.
28. Rogers, C. and Terry, T. 1984. Clinical intervention with boy victims of sexual abuse. *In* Victims of Sexual Aggression, I. Stewart and J. Greer, eds. VanNostrand Reinhold, New York.
29. Rosenfeld, A. et al. 1979. Incest and sexual abuse of children. J. Amer. Acad. Child Psychiat. 16:327-339.
30. Russell, D. 1983. Intrafamily child sexual abuse: a San Francisco survey. Final Report to the National Center on Child Abuse and Neglect.
31. Seider, A. and Calhoun, K. 1984. Childhood sexual abuse: factors related to differential adult adjustment. Presented at the Second National Conference for Family Violence Researchers, Durham, N.H.
32. Silbert, M. and Pines, A. 1981. Sexual child abuse as an antecedent to prostitution. Child Abuse Neg. 5:407-411.
33. Sloane, P. and Karpinski, E. 1942. Effects of incest on the participants. Amer. J. Orthopsychiat. 12:666-673.
34. Steele, B. and Alexander, H. 1981. Long-term effects of sexual abuse in childhood. *In* Sexually Abused Children and their Families, P. Mrazek and C. Kempe, eds. Pergamon Press, Oxford.
35. Summit, R. 1983. The child sexual abuse accommodation syndrome. Child Abuse Neg. 7:177-193.
36. Summit, R. and Kryso, J. 1978. Sexual abuse of children: a clinical spectrum. Amer. J. Orthopsychiat. 48:237-251.

37. Tsai, M., Feldman-Summers, S. and Edgar, M. 1979. Childhood molestation: variables related to differential impact of psychosexual functioning in adult women. J. Abnorm. Psychol. 88:407-417.
38. Tsai, M. and Wagner, N. 1978. Therapy groups for women sexually molested as children. Arch. Sex. Behav. 7:417-429.
39. Tuft's New England Medical Center (Division of Child Psychiatry). 1984. Sexually Exploited Children: Service and Research Project. Final report for the Office of Juvenile Justice and Delinquency Prevention, U.S. Department of Justice, Washington, DC.
40. Weiss, M. et al. 1955. A study of girl sex victims. Psychol. Quart. 29:1-27.
41. Wisconsin Female Juvenile Offender Study. 1982. Sex Abuse among Juvenile Offenders and Runaways. Summary report, Madison, Wisc.

35

Psychological Adaptation of Siblings of Chronically Ill Children: Research and Practice Implications

Dennis Drotar

Case Western Reserve University School of Medicine

Peggy Crawford

Frances Payne Bolton School of Nursing, University Hospitals of Cleveland

Studies of the psychological adjustment of physically healthy siblings to their sibling's chronic illness indicate that there is no one-to-one correspondence between the presence of a chronic illness and risk for psychological disturbance in nonafflicted children. Although the presence of a chronic illness may increase siblings' subjective distress, effects of a chronic illness on the psychological adjustment of siblings are selective and vary with age, sex, and type of illness. Chronic illness is a stressor which, in interaction with other variables, may contribute to increased risk of psychological disturbance for some siblings. Although the variables which mediate the effects of a chronic illness on siblings are as yet poorly understood, the quality of family functioning and relationships has both direct and indirect effects on siblings and deserves primary consideration in the comprehensive care of chronically ill children. Future research might profitably focus on individual differences in sibling adaptation, especially on factors which contribute to positive adjustment, the role of the family context as a mediating influence, and evaluation of preventive interventions designed to enhance sibling adaptation.

Reprinted with permission from *Developmental and Behavioral Pediatrics*, 1985, Vol. 6, 355–362. Copyright 1985 by Williams & Wilkins Co.

Understanding of the adaptational difficulties and/or psychological sequelae experienced by siblings of chronically ill children is necessary for delivery of pediatric comprehensive care to this population.[1] Clinical observations have suggested that healthy siblings' adjustment may be disrupted by the experience of their ill siblings' chronic condition[2-8] and that parents struggle with the demands of conjoint allocation of time and energies to chronically ill children and their siblings.[9-11] Systematic studies of sibling psychological adaptation are relatively new and represent a welcome trend toward a family-centered perspective in chronic illness research. This report considers research concerning psychological adaptation of healthy siblings and the implications for research and comprehensive care concerning chronically ill children and their families.

DESCRIPTIVE AND CONTROLLED STUDIES

Reports based on interviews and/or projective test data, which dominated the early literature, have called attention to sibling adaptational problems. A number of studies have dealt with sibling adaptation to childhood cancer, a condition which is well recognized as placing extraordinary demands on families. Binger et al[11] noted that half of the well siblings of childhood leukemics had difficulty coping. Problems described by parents included enuresis, headaches, poor school performance, school phobia, depression, severe separation anxiety, and persistent abdominal pain. Some siblings complained about the parents' preoccupation with the sick child as rejection of themselves and expressed guilt and fear.

Subsequent studies based on psychological tests also underscored the psychological plight of siblings. Spinetta and Deasy-Spinetta[12,13] found that children with cancer fared worse than controls, and that siblings fared the same, or worse, than children with cancer on a number of psychological measures. Families were rated as meeting siblings' emotional needs less adequately than those of patients. Four- to six-year-old siblings had a lower self-concept than that of patients and viewed their parents as more distant psychologically from them than did patients. Siblings also were described as having negative responses to experiences concerning disease stage, visibility of illness, and patients' level of pain and discomfort. These findings strongly suggested that sibling emotional adjustment needed to be addressed by professional care givers.

Somewhat similar findings were reported by Cairns et al,[14] who noted that siblings showed even more distress than patients in areas such as perceived social isolation and fear of confronting family members with negative feelings. On the other hand, less severe problems have been found among siblings of survivors of childhood cancer.[15,16] Koocher and O'Malley[15] found that almost one-fourth of siblings said they felt jealous of the patient during the course of treatment, and one-fifth admitted residual feelings of jealousy. One-third worried about getting cancer themselves. Siblings' scores on a death anxiety questionnaire were within the normal range but higher than those of long-term survivors. In contrast, some siblings reported feelings of enhanced closeness to other family members. Most appeared to have resolved anger toward the patient once treatment ended.

Although these descriptive studies focused attention on siblings as a risk population, they did not provide precise estimates of the frequency of sibling adaptational problems or inferences about factors which influence adaptation. However, a number of controlled studies using objective measures have delineated patterns of psychological adaptation among siblings of chronically ill children. Tew's and Lawrence's[17] finding (based on teacher reports) that the frequency of maladjustment among siblings of children with spina bifida was four times that of siblings of normal control children is one of the most striking differences thus far reported. An interesting additional finding was that the mothers of children with spina bifida had higher stress scores than mothers of children with psychiatric problems or brain disorder. In addition, highly stressed mothers of spina bifida patients were more likely to have children with adjustment problems

Other controlled studies have reported less dramatic rates of sibling maladjustment and more complex findings. Lavigne and Ryan[18] found that siblings of pediatric hematology, cardiology, and plastic surgery patients were more likely to show symptoms of irritability and social withdrawal based on parental reports than members of a comparison group. Among younger children, the siblings of patients undergoing plastic survery showed the highest level of general psychopathology among the illness groups studied. Among children ages 7 to 13, male siblings of patients with blood disorders were more likely to show signs of emotional disturbance than female siblings. No group differences were found in aggression or learning problems or as a function of illness severity.

In a very well controlled study, Vance et al[19] studied siblings of children with nephrotic syndrome and healthy children from closely matched families in a comprehensive psychosocial assessment. The frequency of serious problems experienced by the siblings of children with nephrotic syndrome was much less than anticipated. However, nearly twice as many siblings of children with nephrosis were described as not having enough friends, as compared with siblings in the control families. Parents and teachers agreed that the school performance of siblings of nephrotic children was significantly worse than that reported by parents of control children. Siblings in the intermediate and adolescent age groups had lower security and social confidence than their peers. The authors suggested that the effects of a chronic illness on siblings may vary with family coping style.

Using a psychiatric screening inventory, Breslau et al[20] found that the proportion of siblings (ages 6 to 18) of children with cystic fibrosis, cerebral palsy, myelodysplasia and multiple handicaps with serious mental disorders was not different from that of the normative sample. However, siblings scored higher on Mentation Problems, Fighting, and Delinquency subscales. Type and severity of disability bore no relationship to sibling psychological functioning, nor did sex, age, or birth order. However, among siblings younger than the disabled children, males had greater impairments than females, whereas among siblings older than the disabled group, females were worse off. Little direct support was found for the hypothesis that siblings of chronically ill children suffer from lack of parental attention. Sibling adjustment was not related to level of disability. On the other hand, the fact that the siblings of disabled children demonstrated more aggressive behavior suggests that attention-seeking aggressive acts may be one pattern of sibling maladaptation.

Although they are not directly relevant to chronic illness, Gath's programmatic studies[21-24] have also documented individual differences in sibling adaptation to a chronic condition, Down's syndrome. Gath[24] found little evidence that the advent of an infant with Down's syndrome had major effects upon the behavior of other children in the family, based on teacher or parental reports. Although there was little evidence of significant health/emotional or behavioral disturbance among siblings of Down's syndrome infants, as compared to those of controls, individual differences in levels of risk were reported: female siblings were much more likely to have emotional or behavioral problems. These difficulties were usually of an antisocial nature and were most evident at school. Gath felt that such differences may be explained by a difference in the roles of boys and girls with respect to the child and may be mediated via overburdening of the mother.[22] The salient factor may be exposure to greater domestic responsibility than is usual for girls of their age. In another study, children most at risk were those whose mother was over

40 at the birth of the baby, those from large families, and those from social classes IV and V.[23]

The absence of severe adjustment problems among siblings of chronically ill children, as compared to those of controls, has now been replicated in various populations (e.g., juvenile diabetes, cystic fibrosis) and with a number of measures.[25-27] Moreover, variation in findings has necessitated attention to the question of individual differences in levels of risk among siblings. For example, Hoare[28] assessed degree of psychiatric disturbance, based on parent and teacher scales, among school age siblings of epileptic children. Although the siblings of newly diagnosed children with epilepsy were not excessively disturbed, compared with siblings from population norms, school age siblings of chronic epileptic children were more disturbed than those of newly diagnosed children with epilepsy and children in the general population. Ferrari[29] compared the siblings of male children with those of children having pervasive developmental disability, juvenile onset diabetes, and children with no identifiable chronic illness. The few group differences again indicated that siblings of chronically ill children were not uniformly at greater risk for psychosocial impairment. However, the degree of intragroup variability suggested that analysis of adjustment within the sample might be a productive approach. Siblings' behavior problem scores were predicted by self-concept, sibling time postdiagnosis, and maternal social support. One significant conclusion was that sibling adjustment depends not only upon child variables but upon the family environment. Certain illness-related adaptational patterns were suggested by the findings. For example, siblings of diabetic children were much more likely to complain of somatic symptoms and request insulin injections than siblings in the other groups. On the other hand, the siblings of developmentally disabled children were more likely to demonstrate internalizing or externalizing behavior problems relative to other groups. Finally, findings that siblings of diabetic children displayed the most prosocial behavior toward peers based on teacher reports and the high social competence of siblings of pervasively disabled children were suggestive of positive effects of living with a chronically ill sibling.

The results of controlled studies of sibling adaptation parallel those of psychological adjustment of children with chronic illness[30] in the following ways: (1) absence of a one-to-one correspondence between the pressures of a chronically ill sibling and psychological disturbance in well siblings; (2) sibling maladjustment is selective and varies with age, sex, and the outcome measure employed; and (3) chronic illness is a stressor which, in interaction with other variables, may contribute to increased risk of psychological disturbance for some siblings.

The findings concerning sibling adaptation indicate that the effects of a chronic illness on siblings are much more complex than initially thought and require more comprehensive explanatory models, especially those which consider family systems influences. Although the manner in which the relationships and perceptions of family members affect sibling adjustment is as yet poorly understood, a number of investigators have pursued this line of inquiry. Klein and Simmons[31] studied chronically ill children ages 8 to 20 with acute and serious renal problems, normal siblings, and mothers, providing separate perspectives on the meaning of the disease to the child and his family. One of the more interesting findings was the relationship between severity of disease as estimated by the mother and sibling adjustment. Greater perceived severity was related to lower self-esteem in siblings, a tendency to conceal feelings, and higher anxiety. Moreover, there was an intriguing contrast between the way in which ill children described the personal costs of their disease versus descriptions given by healthy siblings. Most often, the sibling reported that the illness caused considerable sacrifices for the ill child, whereas the sick child minimized these problems.

Bush[32] also found support for an interrelationship between family concept and sibling adjustment in families of diabetic children, children with chronic emotional disorders, and healthy children. Although perceived family satisfaction, family effectiveness, parent adjustment, and sibling adjustment did not differentiate the three groups, perceived family satisfaction and perceived family effectiveness were significantly related to adjustment of family members, including siblings. These findings suggest that family communication and functioning may mediate individual adjustment, which has been documented in chronically ill children by Pless and others[33-35] and proposed for siblings.[36]

The influence of family structure on sibling adjustment has generally received little systematic attention. However, Breslau[37] hypothesized a difference between older siblings of children with congenital disability who have lived their earliest years in a "normal" family environment versus younger siblings, especially those in a close age-spacing relationship who were born into families marked by the presence of a disabled child (cystic fibrosis, cerebral palsy, myelodysplasia, and multiple handicaps). The findings partially confirmed expected relationships. Younger male siblings, specifically those in close age-spacing relationship to the disabled child, scored higher on psychological impairment than other male siblings. Female siblings were more psychologically adjusted than older siblings, and age spacing did not relate to adjustment in this group.

CONCEPT AND METHOD IN STUDIES OF SIBLING ADAPTATION

Studies of the psychological adaptation of siblings have increased in methodological sophistication over time. The import of early descriptive research on sibling adaptation was limited by small sample sizes, subjective methods, and single group designs. Subsequent research has utilized better controls and outcome measures, but has not yielded clear-cut findings. It should be recognized that research on sibling psychological adaptation is an extremely difficult endeavor which requires researchers to grapple with a number of problems, such as control of variables expected to influence adaptation,[19] choice of outcome measures, and development of explanatory models to guide hypotheses. The absence of theory to guide predictions of sibling adaptation remains a significant stumbling block to research progress. Much of existing research has been implicitly guided by a deficit-centered perspective in which a chronic disease has been hypothesized to exert negative effects on siblings in a global fashion. The possibility of either positive effects and/or more subtle effects on personality and cognition generally has not been considered, with certain exceptions.[38]

Investigations of psychological outcome among siblings of chronically ill children must address inevitably difficult state of the art methodological problems in the assessment of child psychopathology,[39,40] as well as dilemmas raised by the relative utility of interview versus objective measures[19] and parental report versus direct measures of child functioning.[40] Such problems require investigators to carefully consider the choice of specific outcome measures in light of investigatory aims and psychometric properties of measures. Inconsistencies in findings in studies of sibling adaptation may relate to differences in populations and in measures employed. For example, measures of psychopathology may yield very different findings than assessments of developmental competencies such as self-esteem.

The problem of research design concerning sibling psychological adaptation transcends the formidable problem of ruling out extraneous (nonillness-related) influences. The construction of a complex, multidimensional subject variable such as a chronic illness as an experimental variable is inherently misleading for a number of reasons: The effects of living with a chronically ill sibling are inevitably mediated by a complex array of variables including siblings' direct experience with their ill sibling and indirect influences, especially the effects of the illness on maternal physical or mental health.[20] The quality of family functioning may have a significant effect on all family members, including the siblings of chronically ill children. On the other hand, potential influences on psychological adaptation, such as parental treatment or birth order, may not be shared by well and chronically ill siblings.[37,42]

The complexity of factors which mediate sibling adjustment has a number of implications for research design. When differences between a sibling population and a comparison group are obtained, it is usually difficult to determine the processes which gave rise to these differences unless the study is designed to explicitly test hypotheses about factors which contribute to intrasample variation. For this reason, hypothesis testing studies designed to differentiate among sets of factors expected to influence sibling adaptation may be a productive research strategy. Studies should also clearly differentiate among illness versus nonillness-related stressors. Recent evidence, which questions the role of single stressors in the development of psychological disturbance in children,[43] suggests that a chronic illness may be productively construed as one set of stressors among many[44,45] that can contribute to psychological outcomes among well siblings.

TOWARD A FAMILY-CENTERED PERSPECTIVE OF SIBLING ADAPTATION

Although a strong disease-centered orientation has generally contributed to the neglect of a family-oriented conceptual framework in research and comprehensive care concerning well siblings, recent advances in understanding of family system influences on childhood psychological outcome have an important application to studies of sibling adaptation to chronic disease.[46-54] For example, the quality of marital and/or sibling relationships is as yet an unexplained variable which might be expected to influence sibling adaptation. The marital relationship may be expected to have an influence on sibling adaptation by affecting maternal adaptation[46] and/or availability to siblings and by influencing family communication and cohesion.[48-50] The nature and quality of the sibling relationship may have a unique influence on the coping of well siblings.[55-57] For example, to the extent that their relationship with their ill sibling is negative, one might expect the perceived resentment of well siblings to be heightened. On the other hand, to the extent that the sibling and/or family relationships are close and collaborative, the experience of a sibling's illness could conceivably enhance psychological resilience. The nature of sibling adaptation may depend less upon illness-related stress per se than upon how the family manages communication, problem solving, and the relationships among physically healthy and ill siblings.

Studies of the relationships among well and chronically ill siblings should be a fruitful area of future investigation. Until recently, the sibling relationship has been a neglected area of study in child developmental research.[55] However, in keeping with a general shift from an individual to family-centered paradigm, a growing number of developmental researchers have documented patterns of sibling interaction throughout the life span and their relevance to psychological development.[57-64] Some of these findings are potentially applicable to studies of sibling adaptation to chronic illness: for example, siblings may contribute to one another's social development: (1) by reinforcing certain patterns of behavior while discouraging others; (2) by serving as models who furnish information about the appropriateness or inappropriateness of response; (3) by helping to provide a forum in which children participate in the formation of rules that govern their conduct; and (4) through mutual identification. Sibling relationships provide a context in which siblings can experiment with new behavior and roles, master aggressive feelings, and perform valuable tangible services for one another, such as balancing the power of parents and translating reality.[55-64] Specific roles may vary with developmental level and birth order. For example, salient roles for elder siblings include teaching and caretaking of their younger siblings.[59,63-64] Empirical evidence suggests that the quality of sibling relationships may affect social development. For example, Bryant[60] found that in small families, the more older brothers engaged them in interctions that were supportive and challenging, the more accepting younger siblings were of differences in their peers. In addition, the more their older siblings showed them concern and control, the more younger female siblings accepted individual differences in peers. Finally, there is emerging evidence of the importance of relationships among siblings throughout the life span.[62]

Although sibling relationships among families of chronically ill children have not been studied, Bush,[65] following the work of others,[55,56,66] has developed the intriguing hypothesis (now being tested in her research) that well siblings' perceptions of similarity or identification with their ill sibling relate to their psychological adjustment. Adjustment is expected to be poorer among siblings who perceive themselves as either extremely similar or extremely dissimilar to their ill sibs than among siblings who demonstrate more balanced perceptions of both similarities and differences. The rationale for this hypothesis is that siblings who perceive themselves as very similar to their ill brother or sister are more likely to be overidentified with them. On the other hand, siblings who perceive themselves as very much unlike their ill sib may be defending against underlying fears of identification which may reflect a maladaptive level of anxiety.

CLINICAL IMPLICATIONS

Because research on well siblings' psychological adaptation has not directly focused on pediatric comprehensive care to chronically ill children, this work has only partial relevance to clinical practice. However, consistent research findings that a chronic illness does not necessarily result in heightened psychologic risk for well siblings certainly provide important information for practitioners and a point of potential reassurance to parents. On the other hand, research concerning sibling adaptation has not resulted in specific recommendations concerning what practitioners should do to help the siblings of chronically ill children cope with illness-related stresses. In the context of comprehensive care, unique clinical dilemmas arise from such questions as what to tell the siblings and how to deal with siblings' sense of responsibility, feelings of vulnerability, concerns that they are not being cared for, and parental feelings that they are not doing enough for well siblings.[1-9] Practitioners who work with the families of chronically ill children face a number of troubling questions in their day-to-day work with these families, such as: (1) Does it help or hurt to involve siblings in clinic visits and in the care of their sibling? (2) If so, what should their role be? (3) What anticipatory guidance should be given to parents to best help them ameliorate stresses on siblings? Practitioners are called upon to work with families in the absence of information concerning basic questions which could well form a research agenda for the future, such as: How do parents manage time and energy with respect to chronically ill children and their siblings? How are healthy siblings involved in their chronically ill siblings' disease management? What patterns of sibling coping are most productive? What strategies of pediatric comprehensive care best facilitate sibling coping?

It is useful for practitioners to consider the special coping tasks that are faced by families[67,68] and well siblings of chronically ill children.[69] Such tasks vary with parameters of a chronic illness such as illness duration, demands of illness management, and disease course (including hospitalizations and physical deterioration). Factors such as increased isolation from parents, lack of information about their sibling's condition, readjustment of family routines, and witnessing sibling's pain appear to be potential stressors for physically healthy siblings. Sourkes[69] has noted that healthy siblings must develop a reasonable account of the causation of their sibling's illness, cope with their sibling's physical changes, and maintain a relationship with their sibling and an independent adjustment at the same time. Such tasks can be considered either as stress-inducing burdens or as opportunities for healthy siblings to learn greater maturity and competencies with which to cope with demanding life experiences of all sorts.

It may be useful for practitioners to consider ways in which children's adjustment can be enhanced by the experience of their sibling's chronic illness. Our clinical experience suggests that the goals and structure of pediatric comprehensive care may have a bearing on the nature of the well sibling's understanding of medical treatment and potentially on their psychological adjustment.[1] To the extent that the healthy siblings are involved in illness-related management in accord with age expectations and given accurate information about their ill sib's condition, their sense of involvement in the family and mastery of illness-related stresses may be enhanced. On the other hand, to the extent that well siblings are uninvolved, misinformed, and do not have a role in their brother or sister's illness experience, they may feel anxious, resentful, and isolated.[7] Pediatric practitioners are in a primary position to inform and involve well siblings concerning their sibling's illness, foster adaptive sibling relationships, and recognize counterproductive patterns of psychological adaptation.

Practitioners may find a number of strategies to be helpful in improving sibling psychological adaptation. One basic principle is a concerted effort to involve family members, including siblings, starting at the point of diagnosis and continuing throughout the course of the illness or handicap.[1–10,70–75] Involvement of healthy siblings provides practitioners with direct access to the quality of their psychological functioning, which is not only a potential antidote for the neglect of sibling concerns, but also can be instructive in its own right. Siblings are often keen observers of family life and can bring a unique perspective about family functioning that is relevant to the clinical management of the ill child. For example, well siblings sometimes voice specific concerns or observations about the chronically ill child's adjustment that are not fully appreciated by other family members. Involvement of physically healthy siblings in pediatric visits can increase their sense of participation in their sibling's illness experience in ways that enhance their self-esteem.[1] Involvement of siblings in pediatric visits also is a primary means of identifying those who demonstrate coping difficulties before these problems seriously disrupt their functioning.

In addition to involving siblings in pediatric visits, clinical observations suggest that well siblings may be productively involved in interventions designed to lessen family dysfunction.[1] For example, in families with chronically ill children where well siblings have taken over parent-like functions to their detriment, it may be helpful to support more adaptive roles between siblings and parents by reinforcing parental power and control.[76,77] On the other hand, in emotionally isolated families, it may be useful to strengthen sibling relationships by helping them to communicate more effectively with one another. Laviguer et al[78,79] noted that having both siblings and parents assume therapeutic roles was advantageous in modifying children's disruptive behavior at home. The intervention was most successful when both parents and siblings reduced attention to the disturbed sibling's disruptive behavior and produced benefits over and beyond those contributed by changing the parenting behaviors alone.[78-80]

Despite general agreement that the psychological needs of siblings may be underemphasized in comprehensive care of chronically ill children,[1-9] there have been few descriptions of formal or informal intervention strategies for siblings.[74,75] Given the demanding nature of comprehensive care of childhood chronic illness, it may be difficult for practitioners to determine how best to address the needs of well siblings. Parent groups may provide an effective way to address sibling concerns. In our experience, many parents have difficulty reconciling the demands of healthy versus ill siblings, feel guilty about their taking time away from well siblings and, hence, may very much appreciate an opportunity to discuss the well siblings' problems.

Cunningham et al[81] have described an innovative sibling group experience, offered as part of a comprehensive care program in pediatric oncology, to provide emotional support for siblings and information concerning treatment regimens and accompanying stresses. Recurrent themes in these discussions included concern with the special attention given to the ill patient by the parents, the lack of control over parents' caretaking arrangements, loneliness, embarrassment or shame with the discussion of the illness with peers and with the ill sibling, and variation in information about the illness. A 1-year follow-up underscored the value of this group in helping to define and discuss common problems, minimizing guilt and resentment, and relieving anxiety and emotional concerns into more satisfactory channels. Parent groups also have been utilized with the siblings of children with Down's syndrome.[82] To our knowledge, such interventions have not yet been systematically evaluated but hold promise as a potential modality of preventive intervention with well siblings.

SUMMARY AND RECOMMENDATIONS FOR FUTURE RESEARCH

The disparate aims and methods employed in studies of sibling adaptation preclude an easy summary of their effects. In general, studies demonstrate that chronic illness is a stressor which may increase the subjective sense of stress on the part of many well siblings and, in some instances, decrease psychological competencies and increase psychopathology. However, the effect of a chronic illness per se on healthy siblings' psychological adjustment may not be as dominant as initially thought and is selective, depending on populations studied and individual characteristics of siblings, especially sex and age. Research on the psychological adjustment of chronically ill children generally has been guided by a disease or deficit-centered perspective, which has neglected the possibility that a chronic illness presents opportunities for positive self-extension among siblings, just as it does for chronically ill individuals. Research on sibling adaptation also has tended to underemphasize the role of family functioning and relationships, including sibling relationships, as a potential mediator of illness-related effects on siblings' psychological adaptation.

The question of the effects of a chronic illness on the adjustment of physically healthy siblings may be framed as: Under what circumstances, and by what processes, does the experience of living with a chronically ill sibling affect various psychological outcomes? To this end, the following recommendations for future research can be considered.

(1) Studies should focus on individual differences in psychological outcomes as a complement to research designs that emphasize group differences. The strategy of identifying factors that differentiate siblings with positive mental health outcomes and/or coping skills from those with poorer outcomes, which has now been used productively in studies of stress and competence in a number of populations, has special advantages.[42,44]

(2) Increasing evidence for psychological strengths among well siblings suggests that future research could effectively focus on the study of competencies among this population.[82,83] Objective documentation of factors which predict competence in siblings of chronically ill children might eventually facilitate development of preventive interventions to enhance their psychological competence and quality of life.

(3) Research concerning sibling adaptation can be effectively categorized from a family-centered framework and designed to test alternative models of family influence on sibling adjustment. Family influences that are potentially relevant to sibling adjustment include family support, cohesion, and flexibility.[83-88]

(4) It would be productive to expand the focus of investigation from questions concerning whether the siblings of chronically ill children are more disturbed than those of comparison groups to more pragmatic, process-related topics, such as the strategies used by well siblings of chronically ill children to cope with various illness-related demands. Greater specificity in research-based definitions of sibling coping tasks might also result in a greater yield of useful recommendations for practitioners.

(5) Studies should begin to consider the role of illness-related variables (e.g., treatment regimens, duration of disease) in sibling adjustment. For example, one important but as yet unanswered question concerns the changes in physically healthy siblings' adjustment which occur as a function of change in their ill sibling's disease, especially physical deterioration.

(6) A final area of needed research concerns evaluation of psychosocial interventions with siblings of chronically ill children. As a first step, descriptive reports of psychosocial interventions currently being used with siblings in various settings would be instructive. Dissemination of such information might eventually facilitate the development and evaluation of interventions with a preventive, life enhancement focus such as family-centered comprehensive care, sibling, or parent groups. One would hope that such research could eventually involve cross-center collaboration which, despite the enormous logistical problems involved, holds maximum promise of generalizability. Applied preventive intervention research has the potential of uniting research and practice in ways that are likely to be of maximum benefit to chronically ill children and their families.

REFERENCES

1. Drotar, D., Crawford, P., Bush, M.: The family context of childhood chronic illness: Implications for psychosocial intervention, in Eisenberg, M., Sutkin, L. C., Jansen, M. (eds): Chronic Illness and Disability through the Life Span. New York, Springer, 1984.
2. Sourkes, B.: Facilitating family coping with childhood cancer. J Pediatr Psychol 2:65-68, 1977.
3. Power, P. W., Dell Orto, A. E. (eds): Role of the Family in the Rehabilitation of the Physically Disabled. Baltimore, University Park Press, 1980.

4. Kramer, R. F: Living with childhood cancer: Impact on the healthy siblings. Oncol Nurs Forum 11:44-51, 1984.
5. Sourkes, B. M.: Siblings of the pediatric cancer patient, in Kellerman, J. (ed): Psychological Aspects of Childhood Cancer. Springfield, IL, Charles C. Thomas, 1980, pp 47-69.
6. Friedrich, W. N.: Ameliorating the psychological impact of chronic physical disease on the child and family. J Pediatr Psychol 2:26-31, 1977.
7. Townes, R., Wold, D.: Childhood leukemia, in Pattison, E. (ed): The Experience of Dying. Englewood Cliffs, NJ, Prentice-Hall, 1977.
8. Binger, C. M.: Childhood leukemia: Emotional impact on the siblings, in Anthony, E. J., Koupernick, E. (eds): The Child and His Family: Impact of Disease and Death. New York, Wiley, 1973, vol 2.
9. McCollum, A. T.: The Chronically Ill Child: A Guide for Parents and Professionals. New Haven, CT, Yale University Press, 1981.
10. Phillips, S., Bohannon, W. E., Gayton, W. F., Friedman, S. B.: Parent interview findings regarding the impact of cystic fibrosis on families. Dev Behav Pediatr 6:122-127, 1985.
11. Binger, C. M., Ablin, A. R., Feuerstein, M. D., Kushner, J. H., Zoger, S., Mikkelsen, C.: Childhood leukemia: Emotional impact on patient and family. N Engl J Med 280:414-418, 1969.
12. Spinetta, J. J.: The sibling of the child with cancer, in Spinetta, J. J., Deasy-Spinetta, P. (eds): Living with Childhood Cancer, St. Louis, CV Mosby, 1981.
13. Spinetta, J. J., Deasy-Spinetta, P. (eds): Living with Childhood Cancer. St. Louis, CV Mosby, 1981.
14. Cairns, N., Clark, G. M., Smith, S. D., Lansky, S. B.: Adaptation of siblings to childhood malignancy. J Pediatr 95:484-487, 1979.
15. Koocher, G. P., O'Malley, J. E.: The Damocles Syndrome. Psychological Consequences of Surviving Childhood Cancer. New York, McGraw-Hill, 1981.
16. Gogan, J. C., O'Malley, T. E., Foster, D. J.: Treating the pediatric cancer patient: A review. J Pediatr Psychol 2:42-48, 1977.
17. Tew, B. J., Lawrence, K. M.: Mothers, brothers and sisters of patients with spina bifida. Dev Med Child Neurol (Suppl 29) 15:69-76, 1973.
18. Lavigne, J. V., Ryan, M.: Psychological adjustment of siblings of children with chronic illness. Pediatrics 63:616-627, 1979.
19. Vance, J. C., Fazan, L. E., Satterwhite, B., Pless, I. B.: Effects of nephrotic syndrome on the family: A controlled study. Pediatrics 65:948-955.
20. Breslau, N., Weitzman, M., Messenger, K.: Psychologic functioning of siblings of disabled children. Pediatrics 67:344-353, 1981.
21. Gath, A.: The mental health of siblings of a congenitally abnormal child. J Child Psychol Psychiat 13:211-218, 1972.
22. Gath, A.: The school age siblings of Mongol children. Br J Psychiatr 123:161-167, 1973.
23. Gath, A.: Sibling reactions to mental handicap: A comparison of the brothers and sisters of mongol children. J Child Psychol Psychiatr 15:187-198, 1974.
24. Gath, A.: Down's Syndrome and the Family. New York, Academic Press, 1978.
25. Gayton, W. F., Friedman, S. B., Tavormina, J. F., Tucker, F.: Children with cystic fibrosis. 1. Psychological test findings of patients, siblings and parents. Pediatrics 59:888-894, 1977.
26. Drotar, D., Doershuk, C. F., Stern, R. C., Boat, T. F., Boyer, W., Matthews L.: Psychosocial functioning of children with cystic fibrosis. Pediatrics 67:338-343, 1981.

27. Lavigne, J. V., Irassman, H. S., Marr, T. J., Chasnoff, I. J.: Parental perceptions of the psychological adjustment of children with diabetics and their siblings. Diabetes Care 5:420-426, 1982.

28. Hoare, P.: Psychiatric disturbance in the families of epileptic children. Dev Med Child Neurol 26:14-19, 1984.

29. Ferrari, M.: Chronic illness: Psychosocial effects on siblings. I. Chronically ill boys. J Child Psychol Psychiatry 25:459-476, 1984.

30. Drotar, D.: Psychological perspectives in childhood chronic illness. J Pediatr Psychol 6:211-228, 1981.

31. Klein, S. D., Simmons, R. G.: Chronic disease and childhood development: Kidney disease and transplantation, in Simmons, R. G. (ed): Research in Community Mental Health. Greenwich, CT. Jai Press, 1979, vol 1.

32. Bush, M.: Family concept and adjustment of siblings and parents on children with chronic illness and emotional disorder. Unpublished Master's Thesis, Case Western Reserve University, Cleveland, Ohio, 1981.

33. Pless, I. B., Roghmann, K. J., Haggerty, R. J.: Chronic illness: Family functioning and psychological adjustment: A model for the allocation of preventive mental health services. Int J Epidemiol 1:271-278, 1977.

34. Pless, I. B., Pinkerton, P.: Chronic Childhood Disorder-Promoting Patterns of Adjustment. Chicago, Year Book Medical Publishers, 1975.

35. Spinetta, J., Maloney, L. J.: The child with cancer: Patterns of communication and denial. J Consult Clin Psychol 46:1540-1541, 1978.

36. Caldwell, S. M., Pickert, J. W.: Systems theory applied to families with a diabetic child. Fam Syst Med 3:34-44, 1985.

37. Breslau, N.: Siblings of disabled children: Birth order and age spacing effects. J Abnorm Child Psychol 10:85-96, 1982.

38. Carandang, M. L. U., Folkins, C. H., Hines, P. A., Steward, M. S.: The role of cognitive level and sibling illness in children's conceptualization of illness. Am J Orthopsychiatry 49:474-481, 1979.

39. Achenbach, T.: DSM III in light of empirical research on the classification of child psychopathology. J Am Acad Child Psychiatry 9:395-420, 1982.

40. Achenbach, T., Edelbrock, C. S.: Taxonomic issues in child psychopathology, in Ollendick, T. H., Hersen, M. (eds): Handbook of Child Psychology, New York, Plenum, 1983.

41. Breslau, N.: The psychological study of chronically ill and disabled children: Are healthy siblings appropriate controls? J Abnorm Child Psychol 11:379-391, 1983.

42. Rowe, O. C., Plomin, R.: The importance of nonshared environmental influences in behavioral development. Dev Psychol 17:517-531, 1981.

43. Rutter, M.: Invulnerability, or why some children are not damaged by stress, in Shamsie, S. J. (ed): New Directions in Children's Mental Health, New York, Spectrum, 1979.

44. Kalnin, I. V., Churchill, M. D., Terry, G. E.: Concurrent stresses in families with a leukemic child. J Pediatr Psychol 5:81-92, 1980.

45. Garmezy, N., Masten, A. S., Tellegen, S.: The study of stress and competence in children: A building block for developmental psychopathology. Child Dev 55:97-111, 1984.

46. Parke, R. D.: Perspectives on father-infant interaction, in Osofsky, J. (ed): Handbook of Infant Development. New York, Wiley, 1979.

47. Belsky, J.: Early human experience: A family perspective. Dev Psychol 17:3-23, 1981.

48. Moos, R., Moos, B.: A typology of family social environments. Fam Process 15:357-371, 1976.
49. Olson, D. H., Sprenkle, D., Russell, C. S.: A circumplex model of marital and family systems. I. Cohesion and adaptability dimensions, family types and clinical applications. Fam Process 14:1-35, 1979.
50. Olson, D. H., Russell, C. S., Sprenkle, D. H.: Model of marital and family systems. Fam Process 22:69-83, 1983.
51. Olson, D. H., McCubbin, H. I.: Families: What makes them work? Beverly Hills, CA, Sage, 1983.
52. Beavers, W. C., Voeller, M. N.: Family models comparing the Olson circumplex model with the Beavers systems model. Fam Proc 22:85-98, 1983.
53. Kucia, C., Drotar, D., Doershuk, C., Stern, R. C., Boat, T. F., Matthews, L.: Home observation of family interaction and childhood adjustment to cystic fibrosis. J Pediatr Psychol 4:479-489, 1979.
54. Moise, J. R.: Psychosocial adjustment of children and adolescents with sickle cell anemia. Unpublished Master's Thesis, Case Western Reserve University, 1979.
55. Bank, S. P., Kahn, M. D.: The sibling bond. New York, Basic Books, 1982.
56. Bank, S. P., Kahn, M. D.: Sisterhood-brotherhood is powerful: Sibling subsystems and family therapy. Fam Proc 14:311-337, 1975.
57. Lamb, M., Sutton-Smith, B. (eds): Sibling Relationships: Their Nature and Significance Across the Life Span, Hillsdale, NJ, Erlbaum, 1982.
58. Brody, G. H., Stoneman, Z.: Children with atypical siblings: Socialization outcomes and clinical participation, in Lahey, B. B., Kazdin, A. E. (eds): Advances in Clinical Child Psychology, New York, Plenum, 1983.
59. Circerrelli, V. G.: Sibling influence throughout the life span, in Lamb, M. & Sutton-Smith, B. (eds): Sibling Relationships: Their Nature and Significance Across the Life Span. Hillsdale, NJ, Erlbaum, 1982.
60. Bryant, B. K.: Sibling relationships in middle childhood, in Lamb, M., Sutton-Smith, B. (eds): Sibling Relationships: Their Nature and Significance Across the Life Span. Hillsdale, NJ, Erlbaum, 1982.
61. Sutton-Smith, B.: Birth order and sibling status effects, in Lamb, M., Sutton-Smith, B. (eds): Sibling Relationships: Their Nature and Significance Across the Life Span. Hillsdale, NJ, Erlbaum, 1982.
62. Antonucci, J.: Attachment: A life span concept. Hum Dev 19:135-152, 1976.
63. Weisner, T. W., Gallimore, R.: My brother's keeper: Child and sibling care taking. Curr Anthropol 18:169-191, 1977.
64. Weisner, T. S.: Sibling interdependence and child caretaking: A cross-cultural view, in Lamb, M., Sutton-Smith, B. (eds): Sibling Relationship: Their Nature and Significance Across the Life Span. Hillsdale, NJ, Erlbaum, 1982.
65. Bush, M.: The Sibling relationship and adaptation to childhood cancer. Unpublished Ph.D. prospectus. Case Western Reserve University, Cleveland, Ohio, 1985.
66. Schacter, F. F., Shore, E., Feldman-Rotman, S., Marquis, R., Campbell, S.: Sibling deidentification. Dev Psychol 12:412-427, 1976.
67. Parsons, T., Fox, R.: Illness, therapy and the modern urban American family. J Soc Issues 8:31-44, 1982.
68. Anthony, E. J.: The impact of mental and physical illness on family life. Am J Psychiatry 127:138-145, 1970.
69. Sourkes, B.: Siblings of the pediatric cancer patient, in Kellerman, J. (ed): Psychological Aspects of Childhood Cancer. Springfield, IL, Charles C. Thomas, 1980.

70. Lascari, A., Stehbens, J.: The reactions of families to childhood leukemia and evaluation of a program of emotional management. Clin Pediatr 12:210-214, 1973.
71. Kagen-Goodheart, L.: Re-entry: Living with childhood cancer. Am J Orthopsychiatry 47:651-658, 1977.
72. Jaffee, D. T.: The role of family therapy in treating physical illness. Hosp Community Psychiatry 29:169-174, 1979.
73. Koch, C., Herman, T., Donaldson, M.: Supportive care of the child with cancer and his family. Semin Oncol 1:81-86, 1974.
74. Crocker, A. C.: The involvement of siblings of children. In Milwsky, A. (ed): Coping with Crisis and Handicap, New York, Plenum, 1981.
75. Crocker, A. C.: Brothers and sisters, in Mulick, J. A., Pueschel S. M. (eds): Parent-Professional Partnerships in Developmental Disability Services. Cambridge, MA, Academic Guild, 1983.
76. Minuchin, S.: Families and Family Therapy. Cambridge, MA, Harvard University Press, 1974.
77. Minuchin, S., Rosman, B., Baker, L.: Psychosomatic Families. Cambridge, MA, Harvard University Press, 1978.
78. Laviguer, H., Peterson, R. F., Sheese, J. G., Peterson, L. W.: Behavior treatment in the home: Effects on the untreated sibling and long-term follow-up. Behav Ther 4:431-441, 1973.
79. Laviguer, H.: The use of siblings as an adjunct to the behavioral treatment of children in the home with parents as therapists. Behav Ther 7:602-613, 1976.
80. Humphreys, L., Forehald, R., McMahon, R., Roberts, M.: Parent behavioral training to modify child noncompliance: Effects on untreated siblings. J Behav Ther Psychiatry 10:58-62, 1978.
81. Cunningham, C., Betsa, N., Gross, S.: Sibling groups: Interaction with siblings of oncology patients. Am J Pediatr Hematol Oncol 3:135-139, 1981.
82. Murphy, A., Pueschel, S., Duffy, T., Brady, E.: Meeting with the brothers and sisters of children with Down's syndrome. Children Today, 5:20-23, 1976.
83. Harter, S.: The Perceived Competence Scale for Children. Child Dev 53:87-97, 1982.
84. Kohn, M., Rossman, B. C.: A social competence scale symptom checklist for the preschool child. Dev Psychol 6:430-444, 1972.
85. Litman, T. J., Venters, M.: Research on health care and the family: A methodological overview. Soc Sci Med 13:379-385, 1979.
86. McCubbin, H. I., Patterson, J. A.: Systematic Assessment of Family Stress, Resources and Coping in the Universe: Tools for Research, Education and Clinical Intervention. Minneapolis, MN, University of Minnesota Press, 1981.
87. VanderVeen, F., Novak, A. L.: Family concept of the disturbed child: A replication study. Am J Orthopsychiatry 44:763-772, 1974.
88. Moos, R. H., Moos, B. S.: Family Environment Scale Manual. Palo Alto, CA, Consulting Psychologist's Press, 1981.
89. Drotar, D., Ganofsky, M. A., Makker, S. P., DeMaio, D.: A family-oriented supportive approach to renal transplantation in children, in Levy, N. (ed): Psychological Factors in Hemodialysis and Transplantation. New York, Plenum, 1981.

Part X

INTERVENTION PROGRAMS

The Head Start program, which was started in the 1960s with great expectations of what it could accomplish for impoverished disadvantaged preschool children, has been subject to criticism by a number of mental health professionals for its limitations and "failures." Edward Zigler, who was a member of the original planning committee in 1965 and has been actively involved with the program over the years in his professional and governmental positions, presents an assessment of Head Start over the 20 years of its existence.

No one is in a better position than Zigler to give such a broad overview of the accomplishments of the program as well as its limitations and problems. He reminds us of facts in the history of Head Start that need reiteration. For example, he reminds us that the great variation in policy and quality in different Head Start programs stems from the original decision to structure Head Start as a decentralized set of community projects, conducted equally by parents and professionals, rather than a centralized, uniform, and professionally run program. He still believes that this was a wise decision, because it led to the active involvement of parents in the program. He spells out the positive effects of parental involvement and how this model has helped to spawn a myriad of medical and social service programs, which emphasize the role of the parents, for the improvement of the lives of disadvantaged families. Zigler is frank in pointing out the price paid for setting up Head Start as a network of decentralized community projects, but feels the price was well worth paying. He is critical of the romantic unrealistic expectations that many workers had at the inception of Head Start, but also emphasizes its many accomplishments. He feels that Head Start's future seems secure, but does express concern about maintaining the quality of the program, especially in these days of ruthless federal budget cuts in social service programs. But he dreams about what Head Start could do given adequate resources—a dream we all share and need to fight for.

The paper by Provence evaluates the efficacy of early intervention

667

programs, using Head Start, the Perry Preschool Program, and the Yale Child Welfare Program as illustrations. She details not only the short-term but also the long-term positive effects of such programs. Like Zigler, she emphasizes the importance of parent involvement. Provence also points up the trend away from programs that focus primarily on cognitive approaches and toward those that provide more comprehensive services to children and families. She endorses this trend, as well as the use of broad measures of adaptation and social competence for measuring the effectiveness of a program rather than relying on changes in IQ. She is realistic about the limitations, in our knowledge of the effectiveness of different types of programs, but is optimistic about our ability to deal with the problem of careful evaluation of early intervention programs.

Shore's paper deals with a different type of intervention, namely the clinician in the role of child advocate in the courtroom. This highly important issue has been given very little attention, either in the literature or in professional meetings. Shore provides us with vivid concrete examples of this issue, and underlines the opportunities, responsibilities, and hazards that the clinician faces in the courtroom, especially when what may be important for legal purposes may be psychologically detrimental to the child. But these issues must be faced because, as Shore points out, there are currently too many procedures in the legal system that are damaging to the child in the name of protecting her or his interests. There are, however, many young lawyers who are extremely sensitive to these issues, with whom the clinician can work to protect the children and their families. But this is only a beginning, and Shore emphasizes the need to take action to bring about changes in the present legal system so that children are adequately protected.

36

Assessing Head Start at 20: An Invited Commentary

Edward Zigler

Yale University

In a critique of the articles by Valora Washington and Ura Jean Oyemade, one of the originators of Head Start points up the accomplishments of the program over the past two decades, takes note of some of its limitations, and assesses the prospects for Head Start in the current era of conservative fiscal policy.

I was asked to comment on these two excellent papers in light of my long involvement with Head Start. A member of the original planning committee in 1965, I was also responsible for Head Start as first Director of the Office of Child Development, 1970-1972, and I acted as chairperson of the Presidential committee that evaluated the project on its 15th anniversary. Given my background, I read Washington and Oyemade's papers from an historical perspective, and I welcome the chance to review Head Start at 20.

As will be apparent, I agree with some of Washington and Oyemade's criticisms and disagree with others. Of course, I would rather praise Head Start for its accomplishments than condemn it for its faults. But it does not follow that I am deaf to constructive criticism. As I have said before,[11] Head Start is less a static program than an evolving concept, constantly in need of evaluation.

Reprinted with permission from the *American Journal of Orthopsychiatry*, 1985, Vol. 55, 603–609. Copyright 1985 by the American Orthopsychiatric Association, Inc.

Ignoring Head Start's "evolutionary" nature, neither Washington nor Oyemade give sufficient credit to the part Head Start plays as a national laboratory for early childhood intervention.[8,15] In this role Head Start has spawned a myriad of medical and social service programs intended to improve the lives of economically disadvantaged families. Examples include Parent and Child Centers (for children younger than Head Start age), Project Follow Through (for school-age children), Health Start, Home Start, Education for Parenthood, and the Child Development Associate Credentialing and Training Program (a promising source of affordable, trained day care workers) and the Child and Family Resource Program.

Another point needs clarification. Both authors refer to "the Head Start program." While there is a single Head Start policy, there are over 2000 locally administered Head Start programs of varying quality. This problem of variability led Head Start in the early 1970s to issue performance standards mandating that certain services be offered nationally (*e.g.*, health benefits). Still, Head Start remains essentially a collection of locally run, autonomous programs. Washington and Oyemade praise this aspect of Head Start but ignore its price in terms of quality control. Neither a blizzard of memos from Washington, D.C., nor regional monitoring to the limit of Head Start's scarce resources could guarantee homogeneity. Thus, I am not surprised by Washington's charge that there are instances of Head Start workers being paternalistic to parents, or occasions when the Home Start Program was conducted by noncommunity people. I can state unequivocally, however, that such practices are totally antithetical to the national policy of Head Start.

Still, the problems Washington raises do reveal an inherent, structural tension within Head Start between a centralized, uniform, professionally run program on the one hand, and a decentralized set of community projects, conducted equally by parents and professionals, on the other. For 20 years, Head Start has chosen the second course; wisely, in my opinion. Given this history of long-term, deep parental involvement in Head Start, the charge that Head Start disparages either the culture or the abilities of its participants seems absurd. In fact, in the early '70s it was decided that Head Start parents ought to have primary authority in determining the nature of local programs.

This decision was not a facile one. We knew that parents would make mistakes and learn from them, just as we at the national office made mistakes and learned from them. We thought from the beginning that parents are their children's best advocates and that parental control would most effectively guarantee Head Start's quality. Today, 20 years later, I can say with certainty that our faith in Head Start parents was not misplaced. We did not and should not, however, go to the opposite extreme and romanticize the poor.

The poverty fighters of the sixties made two errors. The "deficit model," which equated lower-class existence with "cultural deprivation" was one widely shared misconception.[4,12] The opposite mistake was the glorification of the poor, reminiscent of earlier "noble savage" views. For example, it is one thing to assert the legitimacy of black dialect; it is quite another to insist, as some did, on its superiority. The Head Start planners tried to traverse a road midway between these two extremes. We knew economically disadvantaged parents, like more affluent ones, come in all varieties. Some are gifted parents, some are not. Head Start planners felt, however, that all parents could gain by learning about the nature of the developing child. While our first effort at parent education probably contained too much on child development in too many lectures, parents soon corrected our excesses. They did want some information about children, but redirected our educational efforts to matters of more immediate interest, such as home economics. In any case, it is wrong to assert that Head Start officials displayed disdain toward parents. Every formal action of Head Start over the past 20 years negates this criticism.

It is an analogous error to assert that Head Start displayed hostility toward the cultures of participating children. Improving children's confidence was always a primary goal of Head Start; clearly, any disparagement of their culture could be detrimental to a healthy sense of self. One caveat is in order, however. Many of today's workers champion a "non-evaluative" cultural relativism. While in sympathy with the wish to accept rather than demean cultural differences, I am concerned that this view tends to overemphasize dissimilarities between children, and ignore basic, universal needs for healthy growth.[13] From its inception, Head Start committed itself to the view that there are certain environmental nutrients that are universally beneficial to development. For example, all children require good health care and nutrition. By the same token, regardless of culture, programs should instill curiosity and engagement in children and acquaint them with the norms and even icons of the mainstream school culture they will have to join (*e.g.*, high test scores are "better" than low). Interestingly, and somewhat ironically in view of Oyemade's criticism, Head Start parents of all backgrounds tend to champion training in cognitive skills (*e.g.*, reading, writing and arithmetic) more vigorously than do the early childhood authorities who often implement the programs.

Discussions of racism in Head Start and comments about a program devised by "whites" strike me as simultaneously irrelevant and incorrect. Two distinguished black scholars, Perry Crump and Mamie Clark, were members of the original Head Start planning committee. I vividly recall Mrs. Clark's reproofs at any hint that Head Start might disparage the black culture or attenuate its strength; it was no accident many early Head Start programs convened in local black churches. It should be remembered, too, that Edmund Gordon, a leading black scholar, assumed leadership of the vital research component of the project. In any case, 20 years after the beginning of Head Start we should be well beyond the time that programs are assessed according to the skin color of those who mounted them. Blacks, like whites, possess no monolithic approach either to early childhood intervention or to curing the ills of society. It is regressive to assert that whites can only help whites and that blacks can only help blacks. Head Start must remain open to the insights and skills of everyone who can contribute to it. To do otherwise would make Head Start an instrument of the discrimination it has always opposed.

Evidence that further negates the charge of racism is the magnitude of minority involvement in Head Start, which is greater than that in any other national American program. Again, there is no need to idealize Head Start. There have been power struggles between blacks and whites, and even among different minority groups, each group hoping to lay claim to what it regards as its legitimate degree of control. Nevertheless, over the years, Head Start has been a place where members of different ethnic and socioeconomic groups learned to cooperate to achieve common goals. While still imperfect with regard to racial mix, Head Start continues to represent the best our nation has ever been able to do.

Oyemade is correct in noting the initial grandiose and unrealistic expectations for the Head Start program. The error of thinking that we could solve the problem of poverty in America with an eight-week intervention for preschoolers, or even with total educational reform, is now obvious.[5,6,10,16] Yet, she ignores recent findings of long-term positive effects of participation in Head Start. These effects have been found on variables closely associated with poverty, *e.g.*, teenage pregnancy, welfare dependence, unemployment, and delinquency.[1,3,9] In view of Moynihan's[6] caution that we not exaggerate these findings, I hasten to add that even though relatively better off in early adulthood than nongraduates, graduates of early intervention programs achieve poorer socioeconomic status than their middle-class age-mates. The lesson we can learn from this research is not that Head Start is a failure because one year of preschool intervention does not result in complete economic parity at adulthood, however. On the contrary, the moral is the surprising amount such a relatively minimal intervention can accomplish. The task for future research is to discover the processes that lead from a one-year intervention to the considerable long-term effects now documented. Yet Washington and Oyemade seem to be setting the same trap for themselves today that we fell into 20 years ago. Both suggest we could make major inroads on poverty if we would only expand Head Start. Such a view is unrealistic, and I continue to counsel that we respect Head Start for its accomplishments without unduly raising hopes for fundamental social changes.

Washington and Oyemade raise a second point related to Head Start's proposed role in solving the problem of poverty; its community involvement component. Few recall that at the inception of the War on Poverty, Head Start was not an independent program in the Office of Economic Opportunity (OEO) but was part of OEO's Community Action Program. The Community Action people viewed themselves as poverty warriors, and Head Start was considered only one of many weapons in their arsenal. The late '60s and early '70s were a period of politics by confrontation; marches and sit-ins were common forms of persuasion in attempts to increase society's responsiveness to the poor. It is hardly surprising that when the *status quo* was attacked, established members of society retaliated. Mayors and governors lost little time informing their Congressmen that Community Action funds, including Head Start's, were financing militants. This reactionary wave reached its peak when Head Start was most vulnerable: by 1970 the Nixon administration had a three-year plan to phase out Head Start. Clearly, Head Start's problem in the early '70s was not changing the system, but survival.

Head Start officials were in a dilemma. Ahead of their time in adopting an ecological approach to human development, Head Start planners had recognized that a better future for children and their families required major social changes.[2] Yet, Head Start's venue was limited by pragmatic political and financial considerations to early childhood intervention programs. Furthermore, by the '70s Head Start had learned that community involvement was a mixed blessing. Friction had developed between some of the Community Action programs and Head Start. For example, Head Start workers in New Orleans complained the program was being used as make-work for Community Action loyalists, rendering it impossible for them to mount an optimal intervention program. In fairness, though, it should be noted that in most places Community Action efforts and Head Start programs were and are truly synergistic. From the early '70s on, Head Start money has continued to flow through Community Action programs, and confrontation has dissipated. However, at no time did the thrust for control attenuate parental involvement in Head Start. It is a tribute to parents that while many continued in their efforts to affect other community institutions on behalf of their children, they learned to do so in a way that did not endanger their Head Start base. Certainly part of this change is the result of a changing *Zeitgeist,* in which the militancy and "non-negotiable demands" of the '60s and early '70s have been replaced by subtler and, one hopes, more effective efforts to make social institutions more responsive.

Both Washington and Oyemade correctly point out that the fears in the Head Start community over the Reagan administration's attitudes toward the program were well founded. Washington makes some mention of a three-year planning document which could dismantle the community involvement aspect of Head Start. As an ex-Washington bureaucrat, I've come to the conclusion that, like Goldwyn's famous verbal agreements, three-year planning documents are rarely worth the paper they are written on. Given the "Perils of Pauline" nature of the history of Head Start, it is understandable that there is constant fear for its future. Nevertheless, we must be clear on the facts: It is a fact that even before Reagan took office, Casper Weinberger, acquainted with Head Start through an earlier incarnation as Secretary of Health, Education and Welfare, announced the Reagan administration's support for Head Start on national television. It is a fact Head Start was placed in the Reagan administration's "safety net," and that the program now has its largest yearly budget ever. It is a fact that Reagan made no major structural changes in the Head Start program, which continues to operate within the conceptual framework developed 20 years ago.

My own reading of the situation is that over the Reagan years, decision makers have increased their commitment to Head Start. The fate of the Child Development Associate (CDA) program, which grew out of Head Start, offers some support on this point. A year or two ago this effort seemed doomed, but under Assistant Secretary for Human Development Services Dorcas Hardy's leadership, the Reagan Administration has made a strong commitment to the program. Though gratified by this support, I and other CDA proponents are concerned that the fees required to obtain the certificate will be prohibitive for the economically disadvantaged. There is hope of relief, however: a recent bill by Congressman George Miller would ensure that no one would be denied CDA training because they could not afford it. The Reagan Administration thus deserves considerable credit for its recent support of Head Start.

At this point, Head Start's future seems secure. The question we must answer is not why Head Start has done so poorly during the Reagan years, but why it has done so well. The forces that have kept Head Start alive in the '80s include: *a*) effective support by parents, staff and advocacy groups, such as the Children's Defense Fund; *b*) a positive image in the media; *c*) strong bipartisan congressional support; *d*) robust, reliable research demonstrating the long-term, cost-effective benefits of Head Start, and *e*) powerful converts to the program within the Reagan Administration who, after working with Head Start, have become advocates—a common sequence of events in my experience. However, the points made by Washington and Oyemade concerning recent reductions in Head Start are valid, and tend to dampen my enthusiasm.

My main concern about Head Start is one of quality maintenance. I refer the reader to *Head Start in the 1980's,*[7] which listed a myriad of concerns centered on the observed diminution of the Head Start program. More recently, I also noted my concern about the falling quality of the Head Start program.[14] I share Washington's concern about the recent "numbers" approach to Head Start, which involves an attempt to serve ever larger numbers of children with relatively constant resources. Some sympathy must be displayed toward those public servants responsible, however. With less than 20% of the eligible families being served, there is constant pressure to include more children in the program. Even liberal Head Start advocates have often asked for inclusion of more children. My own fear is that if we submit to the numbers pressure, Head Start will become little more than a token effort. I would rather serve fewer children and do so well, than admit more children and serve them badly.[14] The original planners had a vision of what every Head Start family should receive. Twenty years later this vision remains largely unfulfilled, and including more children will only further delay its realization. The error of trying to do more with fewer resources makes me hesitate to embrace many of the changes in Head Start that Washington and Oyemade propose. Does Head Start really have the resources to provide day care for all the economically disadvantaged families that need it? Can Head Start finance large-scale, expensive interventions for children under three? Given the current political realities, this cannot be an expansive period for Head Start. It is rather a time to guard and, one hopes, reconstruct the quality features of the Head Start model program.

This does not mean we cannot dream. Head Start will continue to evolve; Washington and Oyemade give us some fine leads as to what the next stage of its evolution might be. Its most natural transformation would be into a "cafeteria" of programs from which families could select services to fit their needs. Head Start should offer programs for both preschool and school-age children. It should begin dealing with such virulent problems as teenage pregnancy and child abuse. To reiterate, Head Start should evolve in the direction of a general family support program,[12] such as the one we mounted several years ago. This project, the Child and Family Resource Program (CFRP), was pronounced the wave of the future by the usually unenthusiastic Government Accounting Office. As happens too often in the federal government, however, this exceptional intervention was terminated before it could receive the attention and acclamation necessary to assure its survival. Nevertheless, despite the pragmatic political and financial problems Head Start faces, I am gratified by what seems to be a growing, research-based consensus that individualized, multi-resource, family-oriented interventions such as Head Start's CFRP are optimal. I am encouraged still more by the similarity between many of Washington and Oyemade's proposed reforms and my own, as represented by CFRP. In the final analysis, then, I feel that the authors of these two fine papers and I agree on much more than we disagree.

REFERENCES

1. Berruta-Clemant, J. et al. 1984. Changed Lives. High/Scope Press, Ypsilanti, Mich.
2. Bronfenbrenner, U. 1979. The Ecology of Human Development. Harvard University Press, Cambridge, Mass.
3. Consortium for Longitudinal Studies. 1983. As the twig is bent . . . Earlbaum, Hillsdale, N.J.
4. Horowitz, F. and Padden, L. 1973. The effectiveness of environmental intervention programs. *In* Review of Child Development Research (Vol. 3), B. Caldwell and H. Ricciuti, eds. University of Chicago Press, Chicago.
5. Lazerson, M. 1970. Social reform and early childhood education: some historical perspectives. Urban Ed. 5:84-102.
6. Moynihan, D. 1984. On the present discontent. Presented to the convocation for the 104th Anniversary of the School of Education, State University of New York, Albany.
7. Office of Human Development Services. 1980. Head Start in the 1980's, Review and Recommendations. A Report Requested by the President of the United States. Head Start Bureau, Administration of Children, Youth and Families, USDHHS, Washington, D.C.
8. Richmond, J., Stipek, D. and Zigler, E. 1979. A decade of Head Start. *In* Project Head Start: A Legacy of the War on Poverty, E. Zigler and J. Valentine, eds. Free Press, New York.
9. Seitz, V., Rosenbaum, L. and Apfel, N. 1985. Effects of family support intervention: a ten year follow-up. Child Devlpm. 56:376-391.
10. Zigler, E. Formal schooling for four year olds?—No. Amer. Psychol. (in press)
11. Zigler, E. 1979. Head Start: not a program but an evolving concept. *In* Project Head Start: A Legacy of the War on Poverty, E. Zigler and J. Valentine, eds. Free Press, New York.

12. Zigler, E. and Berman, W. 1983. Discerning the future of early childhood intervention. Amer. Psychol. 38:894-906.

13. Zigler, E. and Kegan, S. 1982. Child development knowledge and educational practice: using what we know. *In* Policy Making in Education, A. Lieberman and M. McLaughlin, eds. University of Chicago Press, Chicago.

14. Zigler, E. and Lang, M. Should parents be encouraged to teach infants to read? a developmental view. Pediat. Nurs. (in press)

15. Zigler, E. and Seitz, V. 1980. Early childhood intervention programs: a reanalysis. Schl. Psychol. Rev. 9:354-368.

16. Zigler, E. and Valentine, J., eds. 1979. Project Head Start: A Legacy of the War on Poverty. Free Press, New York.

37

On the Efficacy of Early Intervention Programs

Sally Provence

Yale University Child Study Center

This article summarizes some of the recent literature on early intervention programs and their short and long-term results. The trend away from programs that focus primarily on cognitive approaches toward more comprehensive services to children and families is considered a step forward. Similarly, the use of broad measures of adaptation and social competence for measuring program effectiveness rather than cross-sectional IQ outcomes appears to be a sound approach. Evaluations of Headstart, The Perry Preschool Program, and the Yale Child Welfare Program are cited as illustrations.

In a recent publication, Greenspan and White[1] have examined concerns about the efficacy of early intervention programs, pointing out that questions about their success have increased along with their proliferation. These authors report previous efforts to discover whether or not types of preventive intervention currently being offered to children and families in the early years of life have been successful, draw conclusions about the current state of the art, and suggest research approaches to investigate the complex and challenging questions the field now faces. They note that preventive interventions for infants and young children involve an enormous range of activities, among them infant

Reprinted with permission from *Developmental and Behavioral Pediatrics*, 1985, Vol. 6, 363–366. Copyright 1985 by Williams & Wilkins Co.

stimulation programs, curricula in day care centers, home-based counseling ranging from attention to nutritional states to cognitive development, preschool programs for 2 to 4 year olds, and, more recently, comprehensive "clinical" approaches. These comprehensive clinical approaches have tried to include the ingredients of many approaches listed above with simultaneous focus on the child and family in the context of the child's physical, cognitive, and emotional functioning and the child's and family's individual differences.

Preventive interventions also are being used increasingly with children at risk of or with established physical and mental handicaps. Here, too, a variety of programs are encompassed under the definition of "early intervention." They include, for example, vestibular stimulation for children with cerebral palsy, language therapy for hearing-impaired children, auditory and kinesthetic stimulation for low birthweight infants, and other interventions. The intensity of such programs varies from a few seconds of vestibular stimulation once per day to 40 hours/week of intensive educational programming beginning in the earliest months. Objectives range widely from prevention to complete resolution of problems.

Greenspan and White[1] point out that such a variety of programs, with different goals and strategies, did not emerge accidentally. The diversity evolved from the experience, clinical intuition, and perceptions of thousands of professionals in medicine, psychology, education, social work, nutrition, and other disciplines. It is difficult to estimate how many children might be involved in such programs, but it seems safe to say that while many who need preventive or early intervention services are not served, there are indeed millions of children who are served each year. Headstart, for example, includes more than 100,000 children each year; the U.S. Department of Education's Handicapped Children Early Education Program has funded more than 300 demonstration projects in the last 15 years, 22 of which have been approved for national dissemination, resulting in more than 2000 replications in other states. Twenty-four states now mandate services for preschool handicapped children, and similar legislation is pending in several more states.

The question as to whether the types of interventions currently being offered are likely to be successful, given the challenges these programs are facing, is not an easy one to answer. Greenspan and White[1] point out that one must ask what types of programs are most effective with what types of children. For example, is a program which focuses only on teaching cognitive skills likely to succeed when there are multiple problems in the family, including severe social and emotional difficulties?

Similarly, is a program that can offer outreach only once every 2 weeks likely to be helpful for a family that is in constant crisis? Is it effective to work with the child's emotional functioning and disregard motor or cognitive lags? How long must a program last, or how early must it start to produce clinically important results?

White and Casto[2] performed a comprehensive meta analysis of more than 150 preventive intervention studies of children from birth to 5 years which revealed that early interventions generally have an immediate positive effect of considerable magnitude across many different types of interventions, various subgroups of children, and a number of outcome measures. Yet, the lack of comprehensive approaches to both intervention and evaluation in most of the studies they analyzed limited the conclusions they could draw about the duration of the effect, and about which types of programs are most effective with which types of children and families. Their analysis included studies in which children participating in an intervention were compared with children who received no intervention, and in which one type of intervention was compared with another. The studies also included different types of problems and populations ranging from high risk populations (socially, emotionally, or economically disadvantaged) to infants and children with developmental delays and handicaps.

Greenspan and White[1] note that, "There is compelling evidence that preventive intervention results in a positive immediate effect across a range of outcome variables and for many different types of children and intervention programs" (p. 3). Furthermore, they believe that effects reported may well be lower than those actually achieved; this is because most investigators focused primarily on outcomes of cognitive functioning and largely ignored outcomes such as social competence, family functioning, and adaptability, which are more closely related to the goals of most intervention programs. They caution, however, that evidence for longer term impact is less compelling. For handicapped children, long-term effects of intervention are far from clear because the issue remains largely uninvestigated; Greenspan and White urge that this gap in the research literature be addressed. For disadvantaged children, studies of the effects 3 years or more after the early intervention report differing outcomes. However, three programs—Headstart, The Perry Preschool Project, and the Yale Child Welfare Research Project—are examples of efforts that do demonstrate long-term benefits of participation.

Zigler[3] makes the following comments in his valuable discussion of Headstart: "It is important to note at the outset that whether Headstart is thought to be a success or failure is determined by the factors one chooses to consider in making such an assessment. Thus if Headstart is appraised by its success in universally raising the IQs of poor children and maintaining these IQs over time, one is tempted to write it off as an abject failure. On the other hand if one assesses Headstart by the improved health of the tens of thousands of poor children who have been screened, diagnosed and treated, it is clearly a resounding success. The problem appears to be that as a nation we are not clear about the exact nature of the Headstart program or about its goals. It is my belief that a realistic and proper assessment of Headstart proves that it has been a success" (p. 496). Zigler emphasizes that the creators of Headstart hoped to bring about greater social competence in disadvantaged children, defining social competence as an individual's every day effectiveness in dealing with his environment. He notes, "A child's social competence may be described as ability to master appropriate formal concepts, to perform well in school, to stay out of trouble with the law, and to relate well to adults and other children. We have sought to achieve this broad goal by working with the child directly—providing services to improve his health, intellectual ability and social-emotional development all of which are components of social competence. We also work with a child's family in the community in which he lives since programs that ignore these parts of a child's life cannot produce maximum benefits" (p. 496). Zigler speaks of the influence of the environmental mystique on attitudes toward Headstart, commenting that the position held by many persons at the time it began was that young children are so malleable that rather minimal intervention in the early years would have major and lasting impact. The theorists whose work gave rise to this mystique were themselves rebelling against an earlier view of child development that emphasized hereditary factors, a maturationally determined sequence of development, a relatively nonmalleable child, and a fixed IQ. He notes further that because the environmental mystique represented the dominant position in the theoretical literature, permeated the popular press, and became established in the minds of parents, it is easy to see why the preschool programs of the 1960s had such strong cognitive orientation. The "whole child" approach, with its commitment to the view that a child's emotional and motivational development is just as important as his cognitive development, has continued to be somewhat suspect. Zigler says, "What we have learned from the evidence is what we could have predicted at the outset—mainly that intellectual gains discovered at the end of the summer or a one year compensatory program often dissipate if nothing more is done for the child after he leaves the program. However, excellent or even some moderately good programs have reported more durable IQ and achievement score gains, of which the magnitude was determined in large part by two factors: (1) whether the parents extended the remedial program to the home through their own efforts; and (2) whether the preschool program was followed by further special educational effort once the child reached elementary school. Headstart's comprehensive design in encompassing day care, education, nutrition, parent involvement, and career development is clearly its unique quality. Headstart's contribution to children's performance in school may turn out to be less important than incidental, with unanticipated effects as illustrated by the results of parent involvement in local Headstart programs. Parents who participated in Headstart were able to exercise control over their own lives by influencing decisions about the care of their children. According to the parents' own testimony their improved self-esteem changed their relation to their children and their communities" (p. 506). Zigler makes a strong plea that Headstart be expanded to encompass a broader range of American families, with full subsidies remaining for the poor and a sliding fee instituted for the middle class. Headstart's benefits should not be denied children because they already seem to have a fair start in life. It has become an effective, flexible, and comprehensive program for children and families. As a national laboratory for serving the nation's children, Headstart has introduced new ways to combine educational, health, and social welfare services that can benefit all children. Zigler's position is increasingly shared by other early childhood specialists.

The Perry Preschool Project was a longitudinal experiment designed to reveal the effects of early intervention on disadvantaged children. Begun in Ypsilanti, Michigan, in 1962, the study compared an experimental group that received a daily preschool program (with weekly home visits) and a control group that received no intervention program. Follow-up reports of the study were conducted when the children were 15 and 19 years of age. The study carried out by Weikart and Schweinhart[4] was originally designed to test the hypothesis that early intervention has positive effects on children. The findings are presented in terms of a set of interconnected pathways defining the effects of early intervention over time: Two basic conditions of the study were (1) an experimental design with experimental and control groups assigned on an essentially random basis, and (2) an early intervention program of daily preschool education and weekly home visits lasting at least one school year.

The study examined the lives of 124 children who were born with the odds against them—poor, apparently destined for school failure, and black in a country which discriminates against blacks. Each year, from 1962 to 1965, children were assigned to an experimental group or a control group so as to ensure group equivalence in initial cognitive ability, sex ratio, and socioeconomic status. Children in the experimental group attended a group preschool program 12½ hours/week and were visited at home with their mothers 1½ hours/week (for one school year for the first cohort of children, for two school years for the remaining cohorts). The goal of the program was to contribute to the intellectual development and education of each child. Between ages 3 and 15 years, children were assessed by a total of 48 measures, including IQ tests, school achievement tests, child rating scales, parent and youth interviews, and school records. Improvement in cognitive ability at school entry of children who attended preschool was indicated by their increased IQs during kindergarten and first grade. Greater school achievement for these children was shown by higher achievement test scores during elementary school and substantially higher scores at 8th grade when compared to those of control group children. Greater commitment to schooling was shown, in particular, by higher value placed on schooling by teenagers.

The Perry Preschool Project is considered one of the best designed of the studies available on long-term effects of intervention programs for disadvantaged children. The group of children served had better school attendance, needed fewer special education services, had a higher proportion of graduates, and had lower rates of school dropout, delinquency, and teen-age pregnancy.[5] The findings support current views that broad measures of adaptation and social competence may be more valuable than cross-sectional IQ tests for studying program effectiveness.

The Yale Child Welfare Program[6] was one of a number of comprehensive research and demonstration projects undertaken in the 1960s to help disadvantaged families. It was planned with the expectation that services could be designed to reduce the risk factors associated with poverty for both parents and children. A coordinated set of pediatric, educational, and social services, including developmental day care, were provided from the birth of firstborn children to age 30 months. Each of the families was assigned a pediatrician, a social worker who made home visits, and a developmental examiner. The responsibility of this family team was to deliver individualized services according to the perceived needs of each family. Child care staff and teachers also became important for the children who attended day care or toddler school. Supporting the parents in their parental roles and in their own development was a centrally important effort. The short-term effect of this program was revealed in the superior performance of the intervention group on developmental and adaptive functioning measures over the matched controls at age 30 months. Five years later, at follow-up, project families showed general upward mobility; more mothers were employed, had obtained additional education, and had smaller families than was the case in the comparison group. The project children had higher IQ scores, better school achievement, and markedly better school attendance than a group of randomly chosen children from the same neighborhoods. In the 10-year follow-up study of these families, Seitz and her colleagues[7] found that the beneficial effects of participation in the program were still in evidence. They concluded that "The results of the present study suggest that early, intensive family support intervention has significant potential for improving long-range family functioning in at least certain kinds of impoverished families" (p. 386). They further commented, "We tentatively postulate that the causal link between the intervention program and the children's better social and school adjustment is to be found in the greater parental nurturance brought about by the program . . . There is no question that current mother-child relationships are better in intervention than in control families" (p. 386).

Provence and Naylor,[6] in a retrospective evaluation of the Yale program, argue for the long-range benefits to families of programs in which parents' capacity to nurture their children is addressed, in addition to the provision of coordinated clinical, social, and educational services. Long-term benefits of early intervention programs appear to be closely linked to the inclusion of parents as active participants in efforts to bring about change and facilitate development.

In conclusion, the state of the art regarding the influence of early intervention programs can be thought of, as Greenspan and White[1] suggest, as a glass half empty because of the gaps in our knowledge or as a glass half full because of what has been learned about the benefits of many of the early childhood programs. Those of us committed to the importance of early intervention much prefer the optimistic attitude, while supporting continuing efforts at careful evaluation of its effectiveness.

REFERENCES

1. Greenspan, S. I., White, K. R.: The efficacy of preventive intervention: A glass half full?, in Provence, S. (ed): Zero to Three. Bull Natl Center Clin Infant Prog 5(4):1-5, 1985.
2. White, K. R., Casto, G.: An integrative view of early intervention efficacy studies with at-risk children: Implications for the handicapped, in Analysis and Intervention in Developmental Disabilities, in press, 1985.

3. Zigler, E.: Project Head start: Success or failure?, in Zigler, E., Valentine, J. (eds): Project Head Start: A Legacy of the War on Poverty. New York, The Free Press, 1979, pp 495-507.

4. Schweinhart, L. J., Weikart, D. P.: Young children grow up: The effects of the Perry Preschool Program on youths through age 15. Ypsilanti, MI, The High/Scope Press, 1980.

5. Berrento-Clement, J. R., Schweinhart, L. J., Barnett, W. S., Epstein, A. S., Weikart, D. P.: Changed lives: The effects of the Perry Preschool Program on youths through age 19. Ypsilanti, MI, The High/Scope Press, 1984.

6. Provence, S., Naylor, A. K.: Working with disadvantaged parents and their children: Scientific and practice issues. New Haven, CT, Yale University Press, 1982.

7. Seitz, V., Rosenbaum, L. K., Apfel, N. H.: Effects of family support intervention: A ten-year follow-up. Child Dev 56:376-391, 1985.

38

The Clinician as Advocate—Interventions in Court Settings: Opportunities, Responsibilities, and Hazards

Milton F. Shore

Silver Spring, Maryland

Clinicians in the role of child advocate in the courtroom may find themselves in conflict because what may be important for legal purposes may be psychologically detrimental to the child. One recent example is where children who were well prepared for courtroom testimony performed so well in court that the jury (and another psychologist) believed they could not have been adversely affected by an experience of long periods of isolation in storage rooms in public school. The result was a hung jury. Some recent attempts to integrate both clinical and legal dimensions in the courtroom are noted.

A California teenager is arrested and jailed because she would not testify against her stepfather who is accused of sexual abuse against her. Two teenage girls were removed from their home and placed in an adequate foster home because one of them revealed to a psychotherapist that her father had molested her, a fact that by law had to be reported to protective services, which took the action. A child was asked to recall in vivid detail in a courtroom the pain and suffering of physical

---

Reprinted with permission from the *Journal of Clinical Child Psychology*, 1985, Vol. 14, 236–238. Copyright 1985 by Lawrence Erlbaum Associates, Inc.

abuse—an event that precipitated a whole series of nightmares for many nights before it was brought out in court. A 7-year-old boy sits alone for hours in a hallway of a courtroom while parents and lawyers are arguing about the custody arrangements and what would be in his best interest. These are all examples of legal actions that, in the name of protecting the child have, in fact, further punished the victim and clearly impaired the child's mental health.

The usual role of the clinician with regard to courts has been as an expert witness. For example, a child is seen for diagnostic and/or treatment services, and a report is presented to the court orally or in writing. The clinician describes any damage done and the child's functioning, from which several recommendations are then made. The traditional role of the clinician, thus, is as an outsider who has knowledge and expertise that can aid the court in making a decision. The clinician does not deal with issues related to the handling of the case, nor with the courtroom procedures themselves, and rarely with the effects of the various other legal procedures on the child's mental health.

As clinicians become more ecologically oriented and as they become more involved in advocacy, they, of necessity, become aware of the broader aspects of the mental health of the child with regard to the legal system. Indeed, many lawyers have become more sensitive to these broader mental health issues. Thus, more nontraditional ways of using mental health services in courtroom settings have taken place. This is particularly true in such areas as civil rights cases and class action suits where the issues are much broader than the individual child. Sometimes, in the name of much broader legal issues, an individual child may be neglected or subjected to experiences that are painful and destructive.

Such issues were brought home to the author when he was involved in a case where a group of black elementary school children had, in the name of "assertive discipline," been placed in windowless storage rooms in a local public elementary school for 3 to 5 days for minor misbehaviors in the classroom. The school was 50% black. Although some 26 (25 black) children, ages 7 to 12, were involved, only 5 black families decided to bring suit against the school system, the principal, and vice-principal, on the grounds of deprivation of civil rights and of cruel and unusual punishment. The children's lawyers, an extremely dedicated and caring group, were very sensitive to the impact of the suit on the children's education (would the school system retaliate?) and of the court procedures and the trial on the psychological functioning of the children. Questions asked were: Should the children remain in the school where the events occurred, or would they be damaged further by remaining in that setting? Would the adversarial procedure in cross-examination of these young children hurt them further? What should be done to ease the fears of the parents that somehow the educational system would retaliate? Would the court procedures be intimidating and overwhelming to these lower class families whose only experience with courts had been negative ones? The author served both as expert witness and consultant to the parents and the lawyers.

One of the major issues and ironies became clear very early on—what might be of value to the court and especially to the jury (i.e., clear evidence in court of the psychological damage done to the children by being placed in the storage room) may not be of help to the child but might, indeed, further hurt the child. For example, if the children remained in the school, given the newspaper publicity and the focus on the racial issues in the community and the school, there seemed little doubt that exacerbation of the children's problems was very likely. Anonymous telephone threats of potential physical harm to the children by unidentified people in the community did occur. The staff of the school split along racial, social class, humanitarian, and personal lines with one group strongly supporting the principal's claim that he was "returning discipline" to the school and the other stating that racial discrimination was evident and had been documented by a federal report. Being caught in the crossfire, the children could only be damaged further. Yet the court needed evidence and the jury had to be convinced of the damage done. In the imprecise and subtle areas of psychological harm, the author's responsibilities as a clinician were to see that the situation not be traumatic so that the children's mental health would be further jeopardized. But how does one balance the role? How does one deal with the multiple, and sometimes conflicting, roles of diagnostician, consultant, and advocate?

A recommendation to the lawyers (which was implemented immediately) was that the children be removed from the particular school that had punished them severely and placed in schools that were more benign and understanding. (Contact with the new schools indicated that these other schools did not see the children as problem children or in need of other than routine discipline to control them.) The families were also referred to resources in the community to help work out the psychological sequelae resulting from the experience (e.g., nightmares, fears of separation, resistance to school, panic attacks). Advice and support were also given to the families.

Because the lawyers were concerned that the courtroom experiences might negatively affect the children, it was recommended that the children be taken to a courtroom in one of the local law schools where the courtroom procedure would be acted out. The children would go through the complete experience of presenting their case and being cross-examined.

These various techniques for alleviating the stress of the courtroom procedures and supporting the families were carried out, and the children presented their case remarkably well in the courtroom, indeed, with pride, confidence, and extraordinary calm. (It was remarkable how these children who had been labeled "uncontrolled" by the principal and vice-principal manifested excellent control during the 2-week trial.) Many people were extraordinarily surprised at how well these children had been prepared. Furthermore, although they were only 9 to 14 years of age, they were able to handle certain harassments and provocations in the courtroom when the defense lawyers tried to confuse them, then tried to point out contradictions in their testimony.

But the fact that these children were able to function in a new school and were able to perform so well in the courtroom was also, in some ways, their undoing. The psychologist for the insurance company and for the school used this coping behavior as evidence that the children were not distressed or upset by the experience and, in fact, concluded that on the basis of observations in the courtroom (no testing or interviewing of the children or the families had been done and he had criticized the use of the Rorschach), they did not need any psychological help. In fact, the psychologist stated that, from his behavioral observations, it was clear that these children had not been damaged in any way. The jury, it appears, concluded that these children had not experienced trauma, although the clinical material was very vivid in showing the effect of the isolation (one child had panicked when, 1 year later, he had seen "The Elephant Man" on television and the Elephant Man was being placed in a closed room). Thus, those features that would have made a stronger case legally and probably influenced the jury would not have been in the best interest of the child from a mental health point of view. The final verdict was a hung jury.

Clearly, mental health professionals cannot isolate themselves, or limit themselves, to being only expert witnesses. But the hazards of hurting the child in the interests of the case become great. Two systems—the adversarial system of the courtroom and the helping system of the mental health professions—come into conflict. It is hoped that changes will occur within the legal system that will be more consonant with assisting, not damaging, the child, yet also be used to obtain adequate evidence. Steps have already been taken by some courts, which have instituted informal hearings with the child represented by counsel. They have also selected adults who can take testimony from the young children in their home, in writing, or on videotape, which can be presented in the court-room, rather than having the child appear in the courtroom, and more use of the judge's chambers rather than courtroom settings as a way of gathering information. But there are currently too many procedures in the legal system that are damaging to the child in the name of protecting his or her interests. It is necessary that clinicians take an active role in altering these procedures through helping lawyers and judges become aware of the iatrogenic factors in court procedures and court settings. This does not mean abrogating due process procedures in these cases. Luckily, there are many young lawyers who are extremely sensitive to these issues and are able to integrate the legal and psychological dimen-sions. However, the problems become greater when there are jury trials; for juries tend to respond differently than judges, the latter having options and often less subject to social fashions. If we do not adequately protect the children and their families, the dangers are that they will not have the courage to oppose or take action against injustice to bring about the types of changes necessary to move us toward a more just and eq-uitable society.

T - #0254 - 101024 - C0 - 212/152/38 [40] - CB - 9780876304372 - Gloss Lamination